Essentials of Communication Sciences & Disorders

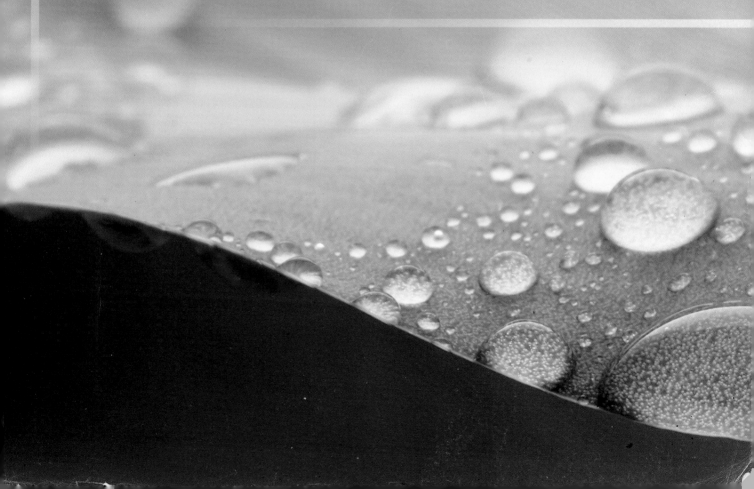

Essentials of Communication Sciences & Disorders

Paul T. Fogle, Ph.D., CCC-SLP

Private Practice
Sacramento/Elk Grove, California

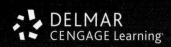

DELMAR
CENGAGE Learning

Australia • Brazil • Japan • Korea • Mexico • Singapore • Spain • United Kingdom • United States

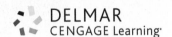
DELMAR
CENGAGE Learning

Essentials of Communication Sciences & Disorders, 1st Edition
Paul T. Fogle, Ph.D., CCC-SLP

Vice President, Careers and Computing:
Dave Garza

Director of Learning Solutions:
Matthew Kane

Associate Acquisitions Editor: Tom Stover

Managing Editor: Marah Bellegarde

Senior Product Manager: Laura J. Wood

Editorial Assistant: Anthony Souza

Vice President, Marketing: Jennifer Baker

Marketing Director: Wendy E. Mapstone

Marketing Manager: Matthew Williams

Senior Director, Education Production:
Wendy A. Troeger

Production Manager: Andrew Crouth

Senior Content Project Manager:
Kara A. DiCaterino

Senior Art Director: David Arsenault

Library of Congress Control Number: 2011942788

ISBN-13: 978-0-8400-2254-7

ISBN-10: 0-8400-2254-9

Delmar
5 Maxwell Drive
Clifton Park, NY 12065-2919
USA

Cengage Learning is a leading provider of customized learning solutions with office locations around the globe, including Singapore, the United Kingdom, Australia, Mexico, Brazil, and Japan. Locate your local office at:
international.cengage.com/region

Cengage Learning products are represented in Canada by
Nelson Education, Ltd.

To learn more about Delmar, visit **www.cengage.com/delmar**

Purchase any of our products at your local college store or at our preferred online store **www.cengagebrain.com**

Notice to the Reader

Publisher does not warrant or guarantee any of the products described herein or perform any independent analysis in connection with any of the product information contained herein. Publisher does not assume, and expressly disclaims, any obligation to obtain and include information other than that provided to it by the manufacturer. The reader is expressly warned to consider and adopt all safety precautions that might be indicated by the activities described herein and to avoid all potential hazards. By following the instructions contained herein, the reader willingly assumes all risks in connection with such instructions. The publisher makes no representations or warranties of any kind, including but not limited to, the warranties of fitness for particular purpose or merchantability, nor are any such representations implied with respect to the material set forth herein, and the publisher takes no responsibility with respect to such material. The publisher shall not be liable for any special, consequential, or exemplary damages resulting, in whole or part, from the readers' use of, or reliance upon, this material.

Printed in the United States of America
1 2 3 4 5 6 7 16 15 14 13 12

Contents

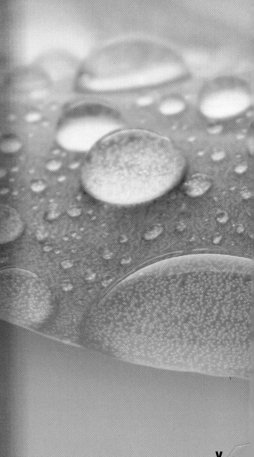

CHAPTER 6

Language Disorders in Children — 140

CHAPTER 7

Literacy Disorders in Children — 178

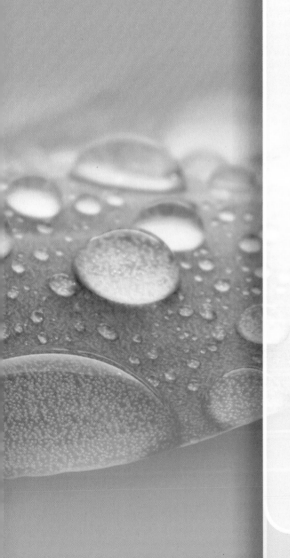

CHAPTER 8

Fluency Disorders 200

CHAPTER 9

CHAPTER 10

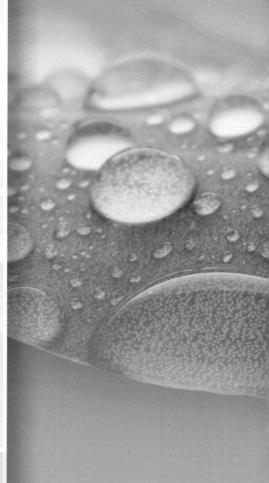

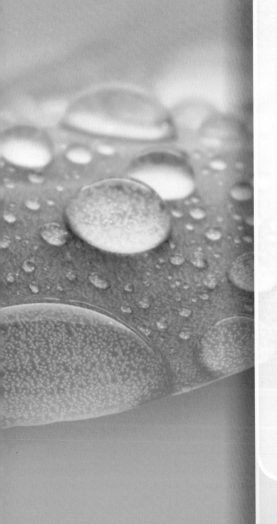

INTRODUCTION

Essentials of Communication Sciences & Disorders is a shorter version of the extensive 920-page *Foundations of Communication Sciences & Disorders* text (Fogle, 2008). Both texts were written for students just beginning their education in speech-language pathology and audiology (communicative disorders). The *Essentials* text focuses on what is considered the vital information beginning students need, whereas the *Foundations* text goes well beyond that level of information. Both texts are based on the skills and knowledge specified in the American Speech-Language-Hearing Association's (ASHA's) 2005 Standards for the Certificate of Clinical Competence (CCC) that address the Knowledge and Skills Acquisition Summary (KASA). Both texts are written in a student-friendly manner so they are both understandable and interesting.

Other Groups of Students

There are other groups of students for whom the *Essentials* text is written—students who take an introductory course in speech-language pathology and audiology who have no intention of going into the major. During the years I have taught the introductory course, students from a wide range of majors have taken the course because someone recommended it, it sounded interesting, or it just worked well into their schedules. Some of these students find the information very interesting and change their majors. For them, the course is serendipitous. These students often bring into their new major valuable perspectives from their past majors, such as premedicine, predentistry, prepharmacy, education, psychology, business, and many others. The professions of speech-language pathology and audiology are all the richer for having students enter who come from other majors. However, for the students who take the introduction to speech-language pathology and audiology course who do not change their major, they and their future professions often benefit from having an understanding of how this course and this book can relate to their work. In addition, students later realize that much of what they learn may help them in their personal lives as parents and possible caregivers to their own parents. As instructors of the introductory course, we know that the information we present relates to life in general and not just to the disciplines of speech-language pathology and audiology.

DESIGN OF THE TEXT

This text was designed for students to enjoy. One of the first things students notice is that all of the illustrations, photos, and figures

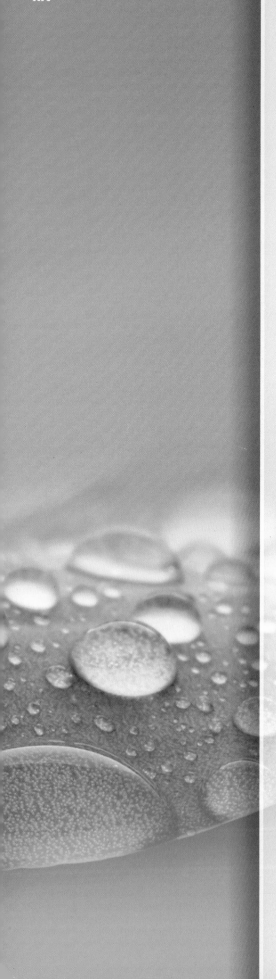

are in full color. Students also find the writing clear and understandable, with many colorful stories and examples of real-life cases. In other words, we have created an inviting place for students to learn.

The text presents much of the most recent literature in each chapter. This text also cites literature that is not often cited in introductory texts. There are many references from professional journals outside of speech-language pathology and audiology that are relevant to our professions. These were included to help students understand that there is important information from other professions that relates directly and indirectly to our work.

Essentials of Communication Sciences & Disorders includes literature from numerous foreign journals that are not normally cited by an American author. This was done for several reasons. First, there is a vast amount of literature published in journals around the world that adds important information to our understanding of the many disorders we work with, as well as providing directions for assessment and treatment. Second, this text was written for an international market because speech-language pathology and audiology are practiced in countries around the world. Third, it is important for students to realize that in many countries where they may choose to travel or live and work, they are in a fraternity of speech-language pathologists (SLPs) and audiologists (Auds) with whom they can immediately relate.

CONCEPTUAL APPROACH TO THE TEXT

The conceptual approach to this text is based on several considerations, which may be seen as themes throughout the book. First and foremost, solid, up-to-date information is the foundation of this text. Second, our work is always a team approach, and the most important person on the team is the person with the communication disorder. Third, all of our therapy involves working with the central and peripheral nervous systems. Fourth, people of all ages with communication impairments have emotional and social reactions to their problems. As clinicians, we must work with our clients and patients holistically; we must work with the whole person and not just the disorders that we diagnose and treat. Likewise, the family members of our clients and patients often experience their own emotional and social effects from their loved one's problems. Fifth, there is a joy in being a therapist—a person in a helping profession. As clinicians, we receive much satisfaction from our work. People recognize that we are excited about our work even after doing therapy for many years.

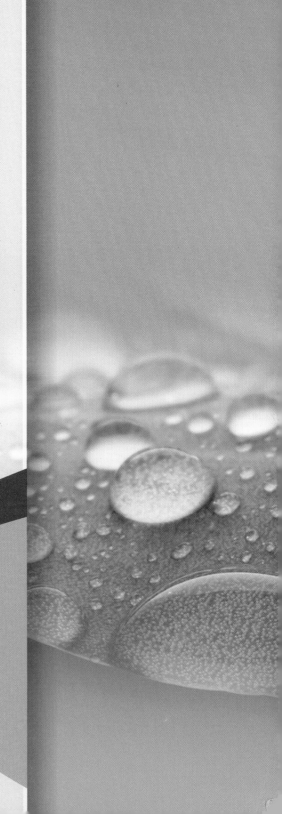

ORGANIZATION AND FEATURES OF THE TEXT

Essentials of Communication Sciences & Disorders was carefully organized for the benefit of students and for ease in teaching. Each chapter begins with learning objectives, a list of key terms, a chapter outline, and an introduction. When an important term is first introduced in the text, it is placed in bold type to highlight it. The term is defined in the margin of the text, and all definitions are compiled in a comprehensive glossary at the back of the book.

Throughout each chapter there are various application questions designed to help students consider how they might use the information they are learning in their personal lives. Most chapters also have case studies and personal clinical stories that are relevant to the material. These features are intended to help paint a vivid picture of the profession, long before students have the opportunity to participate in a clinical practicum.

 Multicultural considerations are discussed in nearly all chapters as the text material relates specifically to this important area. The multicultural considerations are indicated with a special margin icon, so while the content is part of the main narrative, it can still be easily identified.

Each chapter ends with a Summary that highlights some of the basic concepts discussed. Numerous study questions are provided that are based on Bloom's (1956) taxonomy of educational objectives. That is, three general levels of question difficulty are presented for each chapter: (1) knowledge/comprehension, (2) application, and (3) analysis/synthesis. By answering these questions, students can demonstrate several levels of learning. Each chapter ends with an extensive list of references that students may use to further research the information and concepts presented.

A Word About Words

Many of the terms we use in our profession have Greek or Latin origins, some of which date back 1,000 to 2,000 years. When possible, the end-of-the-book glossary definitions include etymologies of words. Having an understanding of the etymology of words may be helpful in learning the words. Words evolve and meanings change, and the etymology may provide a sense of the history of a word and how it relates to its current use. Also, as with English, the ancient Greek and Latin languages had synonyms for words, and students may find some variability in the terms we use and their etymologies (e.g., in Latin, *aqua* and *lympha* both mean water). Several sources were consulted for definitions of terms and their etymologies, including the *Cambridge International Dictionary of English* (1999), *Mosby's Nursing and Allied Health Dictionary* (2009), Nicolosi, Harryman, and Kresheck's *Terminology of Communication Disorders: Speech-Language-Hearing* (5th ed.) (2004), the *Oxford Dictionary of English Etymology* (1994), *Webster's New Universal Unabridged Dictionary* (2003), and the glossaries of many of the texts that are cited in the various chapters.

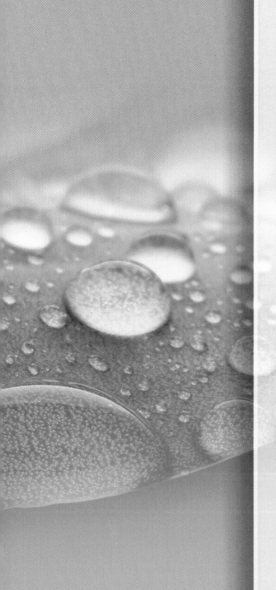

CHAPTERS

Chapter 1: Essentials of Communication and Its Disorders

Chapter 1 introduces the study of human communication and disorders of communication, including communication modalities and classification of communication disorders. It also discusses the concept that there are always emotional and social effects of a communication disorder on the person and the family, and these are discussed further in each chapter on the various disorders.

Chapter 2: Speech-Language Pathologists and Audiologists

A discussion of the professions and the professionals is placed early in the text because students want to know whether these are professions they want to work in and are these the kinds of professionals they want to work with. Some of the topics include the professional organizations, professional ethics, personal qualities (attributes) of effective professionals, the team approach, work settings of SLPs and Auds, and the employment outlook.

Chapter 3: Anatomy and Physiology of Speech and Language

This chapter discusses each of the speech systems (respiratory, phonatory, resonatory, and articulatory) and the essential information about the nervous system that is needed by students in an introductory course on communicative disorders. The numerous illustrations are helpful in understanding both the anatomy and physiology of the structures.

Chapter 4: Speech and Language Development

This chapter begins with theories (perspectives) of speech and language development. The material on speech and language development attempts to provide a sequential but "blended" (i.e., the stages overlap) explanation of how children learn speech and language through early adolescence.

Chapter 5: Articulation and Phonological Disorders in Children

This is one of the longest chapters in the book but it also includes information beyond articulation and phonological disorders.

The material on General American English and Etiologies of Communication Disorders provides foundations from which all other information about children's speech and language disorders can build. Beyond articulation and phonological disorders, there also are discussions about childhood apraxia of speech and dysarthria in children. The ending material in this chapter, as well as in all succeeding chapters, deals with the emotional and social effects of the disorders discussed in the chapter.

Chapter 6: Language Disorders in Children

This chapter begins with essential background information on definitions of language disorders, language disorder vs. language delay, language disorder vs. language difference, prevalence vs. incidence, and severity levels. The discussions of language disorders in this chapter generally follow a chronological sequence, from young children through adolescence. The essential components of a language evaluation are presented and a discussion of operationally defined goals and an outline of a therapy session are included.

Chapter 7: Literacy Disorders in Children

A solid case for literacy disorders being within the scope of practice of SLPs is presented, as well as ASHA guidelines for the roles and responsibilities of SLPs in literacy for children and adolescents. Common problems of children with literacy disorders are discussed and the essentials of assessment and intervention for reading and writing problems are presented.

Chapter 8: Fluency Disorders

This chapter begins with a discussion of normal fluency and defining stuttering, with emphasis on overt and covert behaviors. The essential information about stuttering and theories of its etiology are presented. The rest of the chapter focuses on working with children who stutter and working with adolescents and adults who stutter. The emotional and social effects of stuttering are discussed.

Chapter 9: Voice Disorders in Children and Adults

The various voice disorders are discussed in groupings or classifications relating to functional etiologies and faulty usage, organic etiologies, and neurological etiologies. Both the otolaryngologist's and

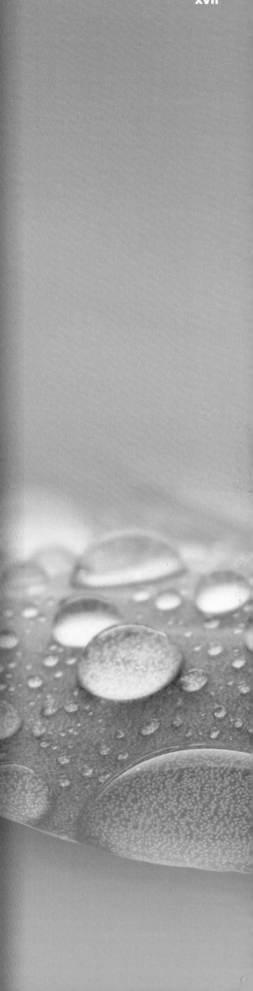

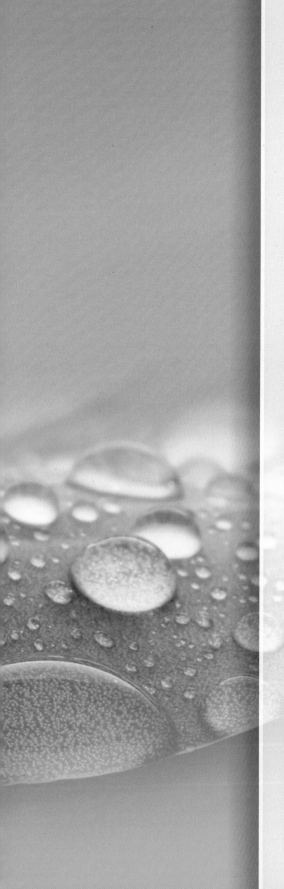

the speech pathologist's assessments are discussed. Three foundational voice therapy approaches are presented: physiologic voice therapy, hygienic voice therapy, and symptomatic voice therapy. Laryngectomy and alaryngeal speech are discussed.

Chapter 10: Cleft Lip and Palate

This chapter presents the primary etiologies of clefts of the lip and palate associated problems with clefts and craniofacial anomalies, including articulation disorders. Surgical management of cleft lip and palate and speech assessment and therapy are discussed. The numerous photographs of real people with clefts enhance the student's understanding of the complexity of these problems.

Chapter 11: Neurological Disorders in Adults

This is a relatively long chapter because the area of neurological disorders in adults is extensive and complex. The essentials of the etiologies of neurological disorders are presented, from strokes to traumatic brain injuries to dementia. The aphasias and cognitive disorders are discussed, and assessment and general principles of therapy for the disorders are included.

Chapter 12: Motor Speech Disorders and Dysphagia/Swallowing Disorders

Apraxia and dysarthria in children were discussed earlier in Chapter 5: Articulation and Phonological Disorders. These disorders, however, are more commonly seen in adults and are discussed in more detail in this chapter. General principles of assessment and therapy for apraxia and dysarthria are presented. SLPs are considered the medical experts in the area of dysphagia/swallowing disorders and this section of the chapter emphasizes the phases of the normal swallow followed by discussions of the various swallowing disorders and their diagnosis and treatment.

Chapter 13: Special Populations with Communication Disorders

This chapter introduces several diverse topics, including intellectual disabilities, autism and pervasive developmental disorders, attention deficit disorders, auditory processing disorders, traumatic brain injury in children, cerebral palsy, and augmentative and alternative communication. There are numerous references that students can use for further information on each of these special populations and their communication disorders.

Chapter 14: Hearing Disorders in Children and Adults

The chapter on hearing disorders is traditionally the last chapter in introductory textbooks; however, its placement does not diminish its importance. This chapter is relatively long but numerous figures that add visual information are included. The chapter begins with discussions of the anatomy and physiology of the ear and central auditory nervous system. These are followed by information on the types and causes of hearing impairments, communication disorders associated with hearing impairments, hearing assessment, and amplification for individuals with hearing impairments. Discussions about aural rehabilitation and the emotional and social effects of hearing impairments end the chapter.

Epilogue

The Epilogue is intended to help students understand that what they have in the book and the introductory course is more than just information about communication disorders, but about the kinds of interesting work speech-language pathologists and audiologists do on a daily basis. The textbook they have and the information they have learned in the course can help them not only in their professional lives but also in their personal lives.

ALSO AVAILABLE

CourseMate to accompany Essentials of Communication Sciences and Disorders

INSTANT ACCESS CODE ISBN-13: 978-1-111-64251-8
PRINTED ACCESS CARD ISBN-13: 978-1-111-64252-5
CourseMate includes:
- an interactive eBook, with highlighting, note taking and search capabilities
- interactive learning tools including:
  - Quizzes
  - Flashcards
  - Animations
  - Games and activities
  - Internet Search Terms
  - and more!
- Engagement Tracker, a first-of-its-kind tool that monitors student engagement in the course.

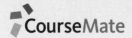 Go to **www.cengagebrain.com** to access these resources, and look for this icon to find resources related to your text.

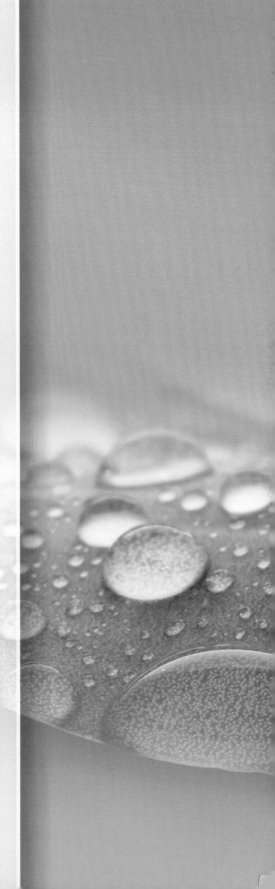

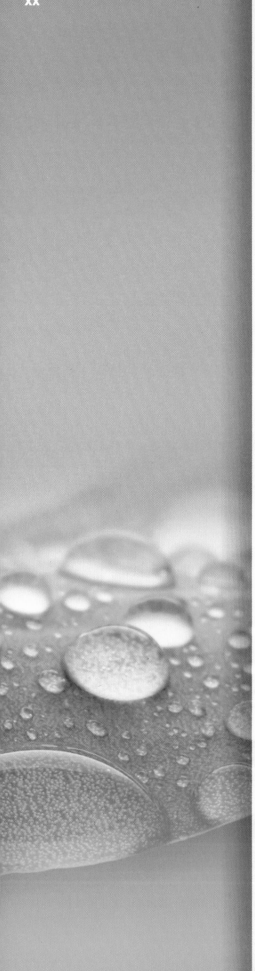

Instructor Companion Website to Accompany Essentials of Communication Sciences and Disorders

ISBN-13: 978-0-840-02255-4

Spend Less Time Planning and More Time Teaching!

With Delmar, Cengage Learning's Instructor Companion Website to Accompany *Essentials of Communication Sciences and Disorders,* preparing for class and evaluating students has never been easier! As an instructor, you will find this tool offers invaluable assistance by giving you access to all of your resources – anywhere and at any time. Features:

- The **Instructor's Manual** contains a course syllabus, teaching tips, and answers to the end of chapter study questions; it is available in Adobe Acrobat PDF® format.

- The **Computerized Testbank** in **ExamView®** makes generating tests and quizzes a snap. With hundreds of questions and different styles to choose from, including multiple choice, true/false, completion, matching, and short answer, you can create customized assessments for your students with the click of a button. Add your own unique questions and print answers for easy class preparation.

- Customizable instructor support slide presentations in **PowerPoint®** format focus on key points for each chapter. Use for in-class lectures or as hand outs for note taking.

- Use the **Image Library** to enhance your instructor support slide presentations, insert art into test questions, or add visuals wherever you need them. These valuable images, which include all artwork form the textbook, are organized by chapter and are easily searchable.

- **Animations** offer enhanced visual aids to help students comprehend important concepts. Animations include The Process of Respiration, The Process of Hearing, The Process of Phonation, and more!

ExamView® is a registered trademark of eInstruction Corp.

PowerPoint® is a registered trademark of the Microsoft Corporation.

To access these resources, contact your sales representative or go to http://login.cengage.com.

ACKNOWLEDGMENTS

This text emphasizes the team approach when working with clients and patients. Likewise, the writing of this book was a team approach with so many people contributing their time, energy,

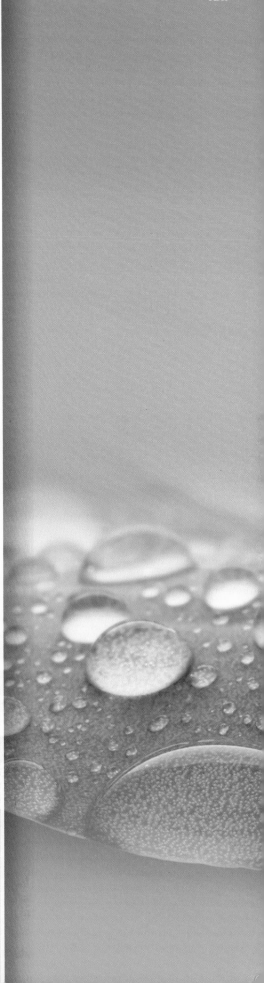

and talents to my education, professional development, and ultimately this writing.

Mr. Rex Fisher, my high school biology and anatomy and physiology teacher, and eventually my friend, introduced me to the fascinating study of life and the human body. These became the foundations of my life's work.

Dr. Joseph and Mrs. Vivian Sheehan inspired my interest in stuttering, trained me well at the Psychology Adult Stuttering Clinic at the University of California, Los Angeles (UCLA), and encouraged me to pursue my doctorate in speech-language pathology.

Dr. Dean Williams, professor and expert in stuttering at the Wendell Johnson Speech and Hearing Center, the University of Iowa, was my mentor and dissertation advisor. His statement to the students in one of his classes remains an inspiration to me: "I hope all of you find someone who helps you become more than what you ever thought you could be." Dr. Williams was that person for me.

Sherry Dickinson, Senior Acquisitions Editor, Delmar Cengage Learning, had the foresight to suggest the need for this text, and Tom Stover, Associate Acquisitions Editor, supported this project.

Laura Wood, Senior Product Manager, Delmar Cengage Learning, provided her expertise and diligence in all steps during the writing, editing, and production of this book. Her insightful comments and dedicated work were essential from the inception to the completion.

Marlene Salas-Provance, Ph.D., MHA, CCC-SLP, contributed significantly to the Multicultural Considerations material throughout this text. Dr. Salas-Provance is the Director of the Graduate Program in Communication Disorders at New Mexico State University; President and CEO of Bilingual Advantage, Inc.; past Coordinator of ASHA Division 14, Communication Disorders and Sciences in Culturally and Linguistically Diverse Populations; past President of the Hispanic Caucus, an ASHA-related professional organization; and is a founding steering committee member and coordinator (2012–2014) of ASHA's Special Interest Group 17, Global Issues in Communication Sciences and Related Disorders. She serves as New Mexico's representative on ASHA's Speech-Language Pathology Advisory Council (2011–2013). She is an ASHA Fellow and a recipient of ASHA's Certificate of Recognition for Special Contributions in Multicultural Affairs.

Barbara Hutchinson, M.A., CCC-SLP, carefully reviewed and edited Chapters 1–7 of this text. Her suggestions were very helpful in strengthening and making clearer each of those chapters.

Rotary International and Rotaplast International Cleft Palate Team provided opportunities for me to travel to Venezuela, Egypt, and India to work with infants, children, and adults with cleft lips

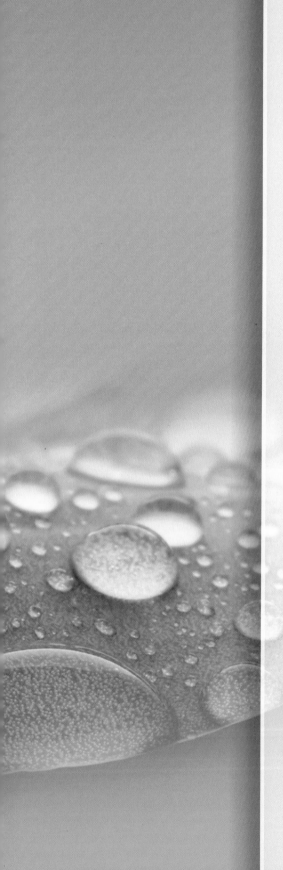

and palates, and from those "missions" photographs have been included in this text.

The libraries of Macquarie University, Sydney, Australia; Canterbury University, Christchurch, New Zealand; and the University of Reading, Reading, England, provided excellent facilities for research for the international emphasis of this text.

Tom Stock of Stock Photography provided many of the beautiful photographs of children and adults with communication disorders.

Tiana Pendleton, M.S., CCC-SLP arranged for her patients and colleagues to participate in a photo shoot at St. Peter's Hospital in Albany, New York, and helped ensure the accuracy of each photograph.

Carol Fogle, R.N., my wife of over 40 years, whose love, support, and encouragement for all of my projects has allowed me to contribute to the profession I love. My daughters Heather Brooke Morrison and Heather Lea Fogle are appreciated and loved for being such joys in my life.

Reviewers

Tausha Beardsley, M.A., CCC-SLP
   Clinical Instructor
   Wayne State University
   Detroit, MI

Dana J. Boyd, MS, CCC-SLP
   Clinic Director
   University of Montevallo
   Montevallo, Alabama

Chris Gaskill, PhD, CCC-SLP
   Assistant Professor
   The University of Alabama
   Tuscaloosa, AL

John K. Gould, PhD, CCC-SLP
   Assistant Professor
   Elms College, Division of Communication Sciences
      and Disorders
   Chicopee, Massachusetts

Chip Hahn, MS, AuD, CCC-A/SLP
   Visiting Assistant Professor
   Miami University (OH)
   Oxford, Ohio

Nancy L. Martino, PhD, CCC-SLP
    Xavier University of Louisiana
    New Orleans, LA

Kate Battles Skinker, M.A., CCC-SLP
    Instructor, Director of Undergraduate Program
    University of Maryland
    College Park, Maryland

Suzanne Swift, Ed.D., CCC-SLP
    Chair, Health and Human Services, Associate Professor of CDIS
    Eastern New Mexico University
    Portales, New Mexico

ABOUT THE AUTHOR

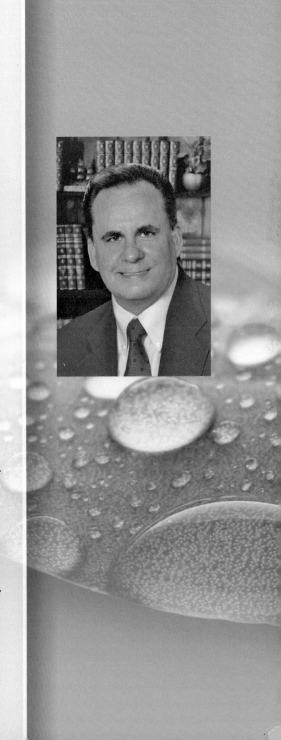

Paul T. Fogle, Ph.D., CCC-SLP, (Fogle is pronounced with a long o, as in FO-GULL) has been studying, training, and working in speech-language pathology for over 40 years. Although he earned all of his degrees in speech-language pathology, he minored in psychology throughout each degree. He earned his Bachelor of Arts in 1970 and his Masters of Arts in 1971, both at California State University, Long Beach. After receiving his M.A., he worked for two years as an Aphasia Classroom Teacher for the Los Angeles County Office of Education and started the first high school aphasia class in California, teaching and working with adolescents who had sustained traumatic brain injuries, strokes, and other neurological impairments. Between 1970 and 1973, Dr. Fogle worked as a therapist at the University of California, Los Angeles (UCLA) Psychology Adult Stuttering Clinic, training under Dr. Joseph Sheehan and Mrs. Vivian Sheehan. Concurrently, he trained on human brain autopsy procedures at Rancho Los Amigos Medical Center in Southern California.

Dr. Fogle earned his doctorate in 1976 from the University of Iowa. He specialized in neurological disorders in adults and children, and stuttering. His dissertation was directed by Dr. Dean Williams and he was awarded membership in Sigma Xi, the Scientific Research Society of North America, for his research. Since receiving his Ph.D. he has taught undergraduate courses on Introduction to Speech-Language Pathology and Audiology, Anatomy and Physiology of Speech and language, Speech Science, and Organic Disorders. At the graduate level he has taught Neurological Disorders in Adults, Motor Speech Disorders, Dysphagia/Swallowing Disorders, Gerontology, Voice Disorders, Cleft Palate and Oral-Facial Anomalies, and

Counseling Skills for Speech-Language Pathologists. Since the early 1990s, he has been training in counseling psychology and family therapy. Most recently he has been receiving education and training in the area of neuropsychology.

Dr. Fogle has worked extensively in hospitals, including Veteran Administration Hospitals, university hospitals, and acute, subacute, and convalescent hospitals. He has maintained a year-round private practice for over 30 years. He has presented numerous seminars, workshops, and short courses on a variety of topics at state, ASHA, international (IALP), and Asia-Pacific Society for the Study of Speech-Language Pathology and Audiology conventions and conferences. Dr. Fogle has presented all-day workshops and seminars in cities around the United States and in countries around the world on counseling skills for speech-language pathologists and audiologists, and on auditory processing disorders and attention deficit disorders. He has been involved with forensic speech-language pathology (court testifying as an expert witness) for over 25 years and has published and presented on this topic. Most recently he has been the speech-language pathologist on Rotaplast (Rotary) International Cleft Palate teams in Venezuela, Egypt, and India.

Dr. Fogle's primary publishing has been textbooks and clinical materials. He is the author of *Foundations of Communication Sciences and Disorders* (Delmar Cengage Learning, 2008) and coauthor of *Counseling Skills for Speech-Language Pathologists and Audiologists* (1st ed. 2004, 2nd ed. 2012, Delmar Cengage Learning), *Ross Information Processing Assessment-Geriatric* (1st ed. 1996, 2nd ed. 2012, Pro-Ed), *The Source for Safety: Cognitive Retraining for Independent Living* (LinguiSystems, 2008), and the *Classic Aphasia Therapy Stimuli* (CATS) (Plural Publishing, 2006). His website is: www.PaulFoglePhD.com and his e-mail address is paulfoglephd@gmail.com.

LETTER TO STUDENTS

Dear Students,

Welcome! Thank you for purchasing this textbook for the beginning of your study about the professions of speech-language pathology and audiology. I hope that you find not only interest in the information but a genuine joy in its learning. If you do, there is a good chance you will find that joy will remain with you throughout your life as you continue to learn about and work in these remarkable professions.

You will find several themes throughout this book that will help you in your learning and work as either a speech-language pathologist or audiologist.

First, our work is always a team approach, and the most important person on the team is the person with the communication disorder because without that person no other team members are needed.

Second, all of our therapy is "brain therapy;" that is, whether we are working with a child or adult with an articulation disorder, language disorder, stuttering problem, neurological disorder, or other disorder, we are working with neurons, axons, dendrites, and synapses within the person's brain to change the muscles that relax and contract for specific behaviors to occur. More subtly, when we are helping people change their attitudes, beliefs, feelings, and reactions toward their communication problems (e.g., stuttering), we are working with the brain.

Third, people of all ages with communication impairments have emotional and social reactions to their problems. A problem may be physical, for example a cleft palate or a hearing loss, but there are always emotional and social effects of the problem. This tells us that, as clinicians we must work with our clients and patients holistically—the whole person and not just the disorders that we diagnose and treat. Likewise, the family members of our clients and patients commonly have their own emotional reactions to their loved one's problems. The therapy we provide one person often has subtle to profound effects on the lives of a constellation of people. If you are going to be a speech-language pathologist or audiologist, you are going to touch countless lives.

Fourth, there is a joy to being a therapist, a person in a helping profession. We give our time, energy, and talents to others, but we receive back more than we give. Yes, you can make a living and support yourself with your profession, but we go into our profession and stay in it not so much because of the financial rewards, but because of the satisfaction we receive knowing that we have helped others have better lives. Ultimately, that becomes our greatest reward.

I hope that you enjoy reading and studying this book as much as I enjoyed writing it for you.

Best Wishes,

Paul T. Fogle, Ph.D., CCC-SLP
www.PaulFoglePhD.com

How to Use *Essentials of Communication Sciences & Disorders*

LEARNING OBJECTIVES

After studying this chapter, you will:
- Be able to discuss vowels and consonants and how they are produced.
- Be able to discuss the etiologies of articulation and phonological disorders.
- Understand the essentials of articulation disorders.
- Understand the essentials of phonological disorders.
- Understand the essentials of childhood motor speech disorders.
- Be able to discuss the assessment of articulation and phonology.
- Be able to discuss the general principles of therapy for articulation and phonological disorders.
- Be familiar with multicultural considerations of children with articulation and phonological disorders.
- Appreciate the emotional and social effects of articulation and phonological disorders on children.

KEY TERMS

addition	childhood apraxia of speech (CAS)	dysarthria
allophone	connate	failure to thrive

CHAPTER OUTLINE

Introduction
The Respiratory System
  Structures of Respiration
  Muscles of Respiration
  The Respiratory Process
The Phonatory System
  Framework of the Larynx
  The Vocal Folds
The Resonatory System
  Embryological Development of the Upper Lip and Palates
  Hard and Soft Palates
The Articulatory System
  The Skeletal Structures of Articulation
  Facial Muscles
  Tongue
  Dentition
The Nervous System

Application Question

What are your comfort foods? How would you feel if the foods you need or crave for comfort were the very foods you could not have, particularly when you needed them most—when you are sick, anxious, or depressed?

Parentese

Parentese (also called *motherese* and *baby talk*, but more professionally called *child-directed speech*) refers to how parents and other caregivers often talk to infants. Adults using parentese typically (1) use a high-pitched voice with greater pitch variation; (2) use one- and two-syllable words in short, simple sentences; and (3) speak at a slower rate with clearer articulation, sometimes emphasizing every syllable (Berko-Gleason, 2001).

Learning Objectives

Each chapter provides a list of the main concepts to be presented. Read these objectives before reading the chapter to focus your study and then review these objectives as a study tool.

Key Terms

This brief list provides the most important terms from each chapter. Each term is highlighted in the chapter and definitions are included in the margins. You will also find these terms listed in the glossary at the back of the book. These are an excellent tool for review and study.

Chapter Outline

To help you understand the organization of information, a chapter outline has been provided. This prepares you for the information to come and helps show the relationship and order of concepts.

Application Questions

Throughout every chapter application questions give you the chance to think about the material being discussed in terms of your own experiences. Consider these questions as you read the chapter to strengthen your comprehension of information and empathy for your clients and their families.

Sidebars

Throughout the chapters you will find boxes of additional information related to the core concepts under discussion. These boxes provide greater depth about the profession, disorder, or other information in the chapter. These interesting boxes enrich your reading and awareness of the field of communication sciences and disorders.

Personal Story

In these features, the author shares his personal experiences to paint a vivid picture of what it means to be a professional in this field. These stories highlight the clinician's experiences and the challenges and opportunities faced by professional speech-language pathologists and audiologists.

Multicultural Considerations

Rather than confine discussion of multicultural issues to a box or sidebar, these discussions occur as part of the main text to more accurately reflect the reality of professional practice. A special icon appears in the margin next to sections on multicultural issues, allowing you to quickly find this information when you need it.

Case Study

Where appropriate, case histories are included to highlight individual experiences with a particular disorder, as well as the clinician's approach to the case.

Study Questions

Each chapter concludes with study questions that offer three different levels of difficulty: knowledge/comprehension, application, and analysis/synthesis. These questions can be used for self-study or as part of course assignments.

References

A comprehensive listing of key resources used to write the chapter, these references are also ideal if you are looking for additional information on the topics covered in the chapter. Reliable and well respected, the chapter references are a good place to start when preparing for a term paper, report, or research project.

A $40,000 Phone Call
Personal Story

A private client of mine who was in his late 20s was already successful farming orchard crops. John had avoided the telephone all of his life; he even had his wife make the initial phone call to set up the first appointment with me. After several weeks of therapy, John was increasingly working on overcoming his feared situations, especially those involving the telephone. At the beginning of one appointment, he smiled, shook my hand, and thanked me for helping him make $40,000 that week. He told me that for the first time he made a phone call to talk directly to one of his buyers and from that conversation landed an additional $40,000 contract that he had never expected to obtain. Beyond all of the emotional and psychological "costs" of stuttering, for many people their fears and avoidances can be financially costly. ■

Multicultural Considerations

All cultures have their own food preferences and unique ways of preparing foods. In addition, cultures have rituals around food and meals. There may be religious and dietary preference and taboos related to the use of special spices and food preparation practices, when and where meals are served, and even who is present during meals (some cultures have rigid rules as to whether both males and females can be present) (Shoemaker, 1997). Patients in hospitals are presented "institutional food" that the kitchen staff tries to make as nutritious and enjoyable as possible. However, many patients would agree that the food is often rather bland and not always appetizing or appealing.

For patients who are accustomed to "ethnic" foods because of their ethnic and cultural backgrounds, the hospital food presented may be totally foreign to them. A patient with dysphagia may be a visitor to this country or a long-time resident, but has not adopted the food choices tion methods of this country. The hospital kitchen staff can-

---

CASE STUDY
Daddy Wanted to Hear "Daddy"

I was conducting a research study on the speech-sound development of 11-month-old babies with cleft palate. One of the babies produced many glottal stops. The parents were proud of their daughter because she produced this sound to communicate in an expressive manner. It sounded like "uh uh uh." She was a "daddy's girl," and Daddy was happy with the glottal stops but was hurt because the baby had only one recognizable word, "mamma." No matter how hard the father worked with her, she would never say "daddy." When I explained to him that it was physically impossible at this time for her to make a /d/ sound, he was so relieved he just squeezed his little girl and said, "You do love daddy, I knew you did!" In addition, I took the opportunity to tell the parents not to reinforce the glottal stop sounds and taught them how to help their other speech sounds with...

STUDY QUESTIONS
Knowledge and Comprehension

1. Define voice disorder.
2. Explain hoarseness.
3. What is an otolaryngologist?
4. Why might the interview of a client with a voice disorder be sensitive?
5. What is acute (traumatic) laryngitis, and what are some common causes?

REFERENCES

Alexander-Passe, N, (2010). *Dyslexia and depression: The hidden sorrow.* London South Bank University: London.

ASHA. (2001). *Roles and responsibilities of speech-language pathologists with respect to reading and writing for children and adolescents: Practice guidelines.* Rockville, MD: ASHA.

ASHA. (2009). *National Outcomes Measurement System Fact Sheet: Do SLP services have an impact on students' classroom performance? What teachers think.* Rockville, MD: ASHA.

Catts, H. W., Fey, M. E., Tomblin, J. B., & Zhang, X. (2002). A longitudinal investigation of reading outcomes in children with language

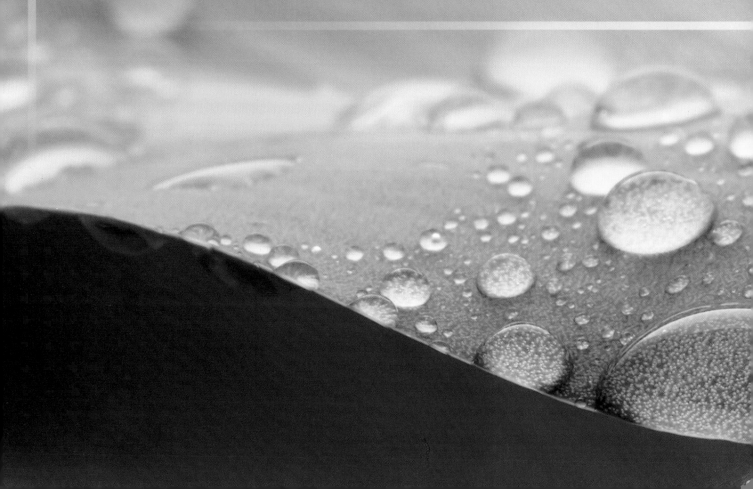

Essentials of
Communication
Sciences &
Disorders

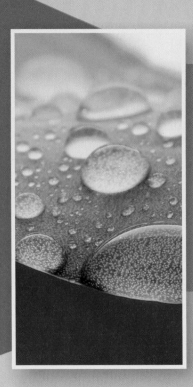

CHAPTER 1
Essentials of Communication and Its Disorders

LEARNING OBJECTIVES

After studying this chapter, you will:

- Know the modalities of communication.
- Be familiar with each of the speech systems.
- Be able to discuss the essentials of oral language: phonology, morphology, syntax, semantics, and pragmatics.
- Understand various classifications of communication disorders.
- Be able to define each of the communication disorders.
- Be aware of the emotional and social effects of communication disorders on the person and the family.

KEY TERMS

acquired disorder
aphasia (dysphasia)
aphonia
articulation disorder
articulator/articulation
audiologist
clinicians
cluttering
cognition
cognitive disorder
communicate
communication
  (communicative) disorder
conductive hearing loss
congenital disorder
consonant
context

dementia
disability
disorder/impairment
dysphonia
etiology
expressive language
functional disorder
General American English (GAE)
grammar
habilitate/habilitation
handicap
hearing impairment
hoarseness
hypernasal/hypernasality
hyponasal/hyponasality
  (denasal/denasality)
idiom

KEY TERMS continued

incidence
inner speech
intelligibility
language
language delay
language differences
language disorder
linguistics
modality
morpheme
morphology
motor speech disorder
organic disorder
perception
phoneme
phonological disorder
phonology
pragmatics
prevalence
quality of life
receptive language

rehabilitate/rehabilitation
resonance disorder
semantics
sensorineural hearing loss
sign
speech
speech disorder
speech-language pathologist/
     speech pathologist/speech
     therapist
stuttering (disfluency)
suprasegmentals/paralinguistics/
     prosody (prosodic) features
syllable
symptom
syndrome
syntax
traumatic brain injury (TBI)
voice disorder
vowel
World Health Organization (WHO)

CHAPTER OUTLINE

INTRODUCTION

Welcome! You are beginning the study of a basic human need: the need to **communicate**. When two people are interacting, a message is always being communicated, even when neither person is speaking. The old adage still holds true: *We cannot not communicate.* Our ability to communicate is often taken for granted until we have some difficulty communicating or see someone else having difficulty. This text is about the difficulties children and adults of all ages (newborns to end of life) have with **communication disorders**. As **clinicians**, we need to have a solid foundation in the understanding of the **modalities** of communication, that is, the various ways we communicate. Although **speech-language pathologists (SLPs)** and **audiologists (Auds)** focus on the *auditory-verbal* modalities (hearing and speaking), the *nonverbal modalities* (body language and facial expressions) are essential to our understanding what a person is saying and communicating our messages in return.

In a way, good communication is like a dance in which each person takes turns leading and following. The individuals try to stay "in step" with one another, "reading" every nuance of choice of words, tone of voice, *inflections* (variations of pitch during speech), pauses, hesitations, facial expressions, postures, and gestures (i.e., *total communication*) so that there is an easy and enjoyable flow during the conversation. When we meet someone new, it usually does not take long before we decide whether or not we can "dance" well together and whether we even want to try to dance again. We use communication to survive and thrive in our homes, communities, schools, and work places. With a communication disorder, surviving and thriving are much more difficult. Reed (2005) presents the modes we use in communicating (see Figure 1–1). As clinicians, we learn to be increasingly aware of the interactions of these modalities and the effects of subtle to complete breakdowns in these modalities.

THE STUDY OF HUMAN COMMUNICATION

Thirty-thousand-year-old cave paintings of geometric symbols and animals are the earliest forms of communication designed to preserve human experiences. Three-thousand-year-old Egyptian pictographic hieroglyphs were a formal writing system that used symbols for words and letters of the Egyptian alphabet that were carved into stone and later

---

communicate/ communication

Any means by which individuals relate their wants, needs, thoughts, knowledge, and feelings to another person.

communication (communicative) disorder

Speech, language, voice, resonance, cognitive, or hearing that noticeably deviates from that of other people, calls attention to itself, interferes with communication, or causes distress in both the speaker and the listener; any speech, language, voice, resonance, cognitive, or hearing impairment, disability, or handicap that interferes with a person conveying his wants, needs, thoughts, knowledge, and feelings to another person.

clinicians

Health care professionals, such as physicians, nurses, physical therapists, occupational therapists, speech-language pathologists, audiologists, psychiatrists, or psychologists involved in clinical practice who base their practice on direct observation and treatment of patients and clients.

modality

Any sensory avenue through which information may be received, i.e., auditory, visual, tactile, taste, and olfactory (smell).

speech-language pathologist/speech pathologist/speech therapist

A professional who is specifically educated and trained to identify, evaluate, treat, and prevent speech, language, cognitive, and swallowing disorders.

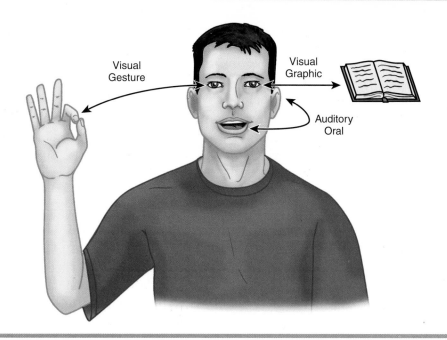

Visual
Gesture

Visual
Graphic

Auditory
Oral

Figure 1-1

Modes of communication.

Source: Adapted from Reed, 2005.

painted on papyrus. The evolution of communication from basic sounds and signs to more sophisticated systems is one of the most important developments in human history. More recently, Wolfgang von Kempelen (1734–1804), a Hungarian author and inventor, described, illustrated, and constructed mechanical devices that could produce speech sounds for words. His devices (see Figure 1-2) were composed of bellows for the lungs, a vibrating reed for the vocal folds, and a leather tube whose shape helped produce different vowel sounds, with constrictions controlled by fingers for generating consonants. To study the production of plosive sounds (e.g., p, b, t, d, k, g), he included movable "lips" and a hinged "tongue" in his device. The device could produce intelligible whole words and short sentences. Von Kempelen may be considered the first speech scientist (Gedeon, 2006).

audiologist

A professional who is specifically educated and trained to identify, evaluate, treat, and prevent hearing disorders, plus select and evaluate hearing aids, and **habilitate** or **rehabilitate** individuals with hearing impairments.

habilitate/habilitation

The process of developing a skill to be able to function within the environment; the initial learning and development of a new skill.

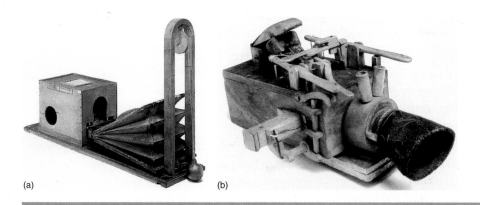

(a)   (b)

Figure 1-2

Von Kempelen's (1791) (a) "lungs" and "voice box" and (b) articulating mouth.

Source: *Science and technology in medicine: An illustrated account based on ninety-nine landmark publications for five centuries,* 2005, pages 138 and 141, "Wolfgang Von Kempelen," Andras Gedeon, Figure 25:4 and 25:8. With kind permission of Springer Science and Business Media.

COMMUNICATION MODALITIES

Communication means conveying messages through one or more modalities; that is, listening, speaking, reading, and writing. We normally think of communication as being between two or more people; however, much of what we "hear" every day is us talking to ourselves. We commonly have an internal monologue (**inner speech**) going on inside of our heads that we refer to as *thinking* (Luria, 1961; Vygotsky, 1962). We silently (and sometimes not so silently) talk to ourselves and even argue with ourselves, wrestling with decisions from the mundane (Where am I going to have lunch?) to the profound (What am I going to do with my life?). Our verbal communication is mostly a reflection of our wants, needs, thoughts, feelings, and knowledge (i.e., sharing information).

However, spoken words may communicate only a small portion of a person's total message. SLPs and Auds also need to become skilled in "reading" facial expressions and nonverbal communication as well (Fogle, 2009). Burgoon, Guerrero, & Floyd (2010) reviewed 100 studies on *verbal* (oral) and *nonverbal* (body postures, gestures, eye contact, and facial expressions) communication and, among other points, determined the following:

- Verbal content is more important for factual, abstract, and persuasive communication; nonverbal content is more important for judging emotions and attitudes.
- When verbal and nonverbal channels conflict, adults rely more on nonverbal cues (i.e., people believe what they see more than what they hear).

When we think of communication disorders, we usually think of talking and listening. Most of your education and training in speech-language pathology and audiology will focus on these modalities. However, because communication may involve three different input modalities (auditory, visual, and tactile) and three different output modalities (speaking, gesturing, and writing), SLPs and Auds work with more than just speech and hearing. Any or all of the input and output modalities may be involved in a communication disorder.

Hearing

Normal hearing is essential for the development of normal **speech** and **language**. The hearing mechanism includes the *outer, middle,* and *inner ear* (see Figure 1–3). The outer ear is made of cartilage and forms the *pinna* or *auricle* and the *ear canal* that leads to the eardrum (*tympanic membrane*). Sound waves are directed from the outer ear into the ear canal where they reach the eardrum and cause it to vibrate. The vibration of the eardrum causes three small bones (*ossicles*) in the enclosed middle ear to vibrate, which in turn sets into vibration the fluid in the next chamber—the inner ear or *cochlea*. The fluid in the cochlea stimulates minute structures (*hair cells*) that transmit nerve impulses

rehabilitate/ rehabilitation

Restoration to normal or to as satisfactory a status as possible of impaired functions and abilities.

inner speech (internal discourse, stream of consciousness)

The nearly constant internal monologue a person has with himself at a conscious or semi-conscious level that involves thinking in words; a conversation with oneself.

speech

The production of oral language using phonemes for communication through the process of respiration, phonation, resonation, and articulation.

language

According to Owens (2012), "a socially shared code or conventional system for representing concepts through the use of arbitrary symbols [sounds and letters] and rule-governed combinations of those symbols [grammar]."

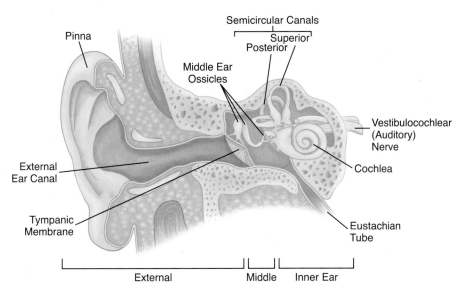

Figure 1–3

The human peripheral auditory system has three divisions: external, middle, and inner ear. The external ear consists of the pinna (or auricle) and the external ear canal (or external auditory meatus). The tympanic membrane (eardrum) closes off the medial end of the external ear canal. The middle ear is an air-filled cavity that contains the three middle-ear ossicles. The middle-ear cavity is connected to the nasopharynx by the Eustachian tube. The inner ear includes the cochlea, vestibule, and three semicircular canals. The cochlea contains the end organ for hearing. The vestibule and three semicircular canals contain the end organs for balance and motion detection, respectively.
© Cengage Learning 2013.

through a nerve to the brain that interprets the sound and its meaning. If speech sounds are not perceived normally by infants and young children, they will not be able to understand the speech of others or hear their own speech to make appropriate adjustments in voice and articulation and develop normal speech and language.

Speech Systems

Speech is the result of several physiological systems interacting and functioning in near perfect timing and harmony (the individual speech systems will be discussed in more detail in Chapter 3). To produce a single sound, the *respiratory system* (lungs, diaphragm, and chest muscles) must have adequate inhalation and controlled exhalation (see Figure 1–4). The *phonatory system* is composed of the *vocal folds* and other muscles inside and outside the *larynx*. The numerous muscles within the larynx that are necessary to close and open the vocal folds must have sufficient strength for the vocal folds to vibrate and create sound. The vocal folds must have the proper tension for subtle changes of loudness, pitch, and quality from instant to instant. But the voice does more than just produce sounds to speak words; it also gives a tone to the voice that can convey the true meaning of the message, which may in some cases be

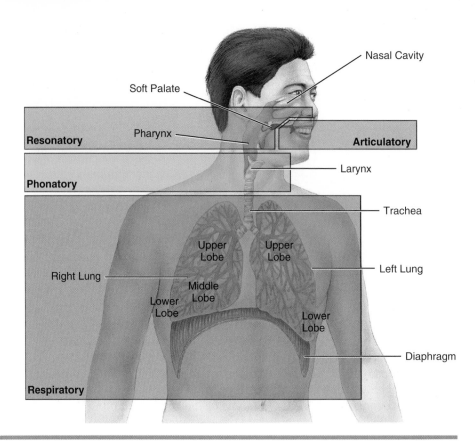

Figure 1-4

The speech systems: respiratory, phonatory, resonatory, and articulatory.

© Cengage Learning 2013.

articulator/articulation

In speech, the mandible, lips, tongue, and soft palate are the articulators; *articulation* refers to the movements of the articulators for speech sound production that involves accuracy in placement, timing, direction of movement, and pressure of the articulators on one another; the totality of motor processes involved in the planning and execution of speech.

intelligible

The degree to which a person's utterances are understood by the average listener; influenced by articulation, rate of speech, fluency, vocal quality, and intensity of voice.

syllable

Either a single **vowel** (V) or a vowel and one or more **consonants** (C); e.g., V+ consonant (VC), VCC, CV, CCV, CVC, etc.

the opposite of what the words mean (as in sarcasm). A simple sigh can convey numerous meanings just by its tone.

The *resonatory system* in the throat, nose, and mouth modifies the sounds produced by the larynx. For example, a tense throat (*pharyngeal region*) can significantly alter the sound produced by the vocal folds. The position of the *soft palate* (the back of the roof of the mouth) determines whether sounds will come through the mouth (soft palate up for *oral sounds* [e.g., p, t, s]) or the sound will come through the nasal passages (soft palate down for *nasal sounds* [e.g., m, n, ng]). The *articulatory system* (**articulators**) includes the *maxilla* (upper jaw), *mandible* (lower jaw), lips, teeth, and tongue. The articulators modify the sounds that enter the *oral cavity* (mouth) into words. Incredibly fast and precise movements of the articulators and their muscles allow us to produce **intelligible** speech.

Oral/Spoken Language

When sounds are organized into **syllables** and words are organized into grammatical sentences, spoken language is generated. As noted previously, language has been defined as "a socially shared code or conventional system for representing concepts through the use of arbitrary symbols [sounds and letters] and rule-governed combinations of those symbols [grammar]" (Owens, 2012). Spoken language is our primary and usually most efficient form of communication. There are approximately

7,000 "living languages" (languages widely used as a primary form of communication by specific groups of people) and an unknown number of dead or extinct languages (Lewis, 2009).

Spoken language gives the listener not only the *content* (the words in the message) but the **suprasegmentals** (also called **paralinguistics** or **prosody [prosodic] features**) that help the listener understand the true intent of the message by using voice inflections for emphasis or deemphasis (e.g., the difference between "I scream" and "ice cream"). Suprasegmentals include *prosody* (rate and rhythm), *intonation* (pitch change within an utterance), and *stress* (combination of pitch, loudness, and duration). Suprasegmentals are important in conveying the emotional aspects of messages, such as happiness, sadness, fear, and surprise. When we cannot see a person's face (e.g., while on the telephone), we usually can still discern the emotions behind the messages based on the suprasegmentals.

Linguistics

Linguistics is the scientific study of language, and *linguists* are individuals who specialize in the study of linguistics. Traditionally, linguists divide language into several components: *phonemes* (sounds), *morphemes* (groups of sounds that form words or parts of words), *syntax* (rules for combining words into sentences), *semantics* (meaning of the language or message), and *pragmatics* (the rules governing the use of language in social situations). *Linguistic competence* is a person's underlying knowledge about the system of rules of a language. Linguistic competence helps us recognize when a sentence is grammatically correct or incorrect.

Phonology

Phonology is the study of speech sounds (**phonemes**) and the rules for using them to make words in a language. The English language has a limited number of phonemes, but an almost limitless variety of sound combinations can be used in words and to make up new words. Each year, hundreds of words are added to our language that must follow phonological rules (see Chapter 4, Speech and Language Development). Consider all of the new words that were created when automobiles first arrived on the scene, or when televisions and computers were invented. Whenever there is a significant technological advancement such as computers, a large number of words are added to our language (e.g., *Google*—the search engine).

For new words to be accepted by the public, certain phonological rules for combining sounds must be followed. For example, a single letter is not used as a new word, nor is a combination of more than two consonants with no **vowels**. A combination of three or more vowels also is not considered to follow English phonological rules. Some foreign languages are difficult for English speakers to learn because their phonologies use consonant and vowel combinations not used in English. Many people

---

consonant

Speech sounds articulated by either stopping of the outgoing air stream or creating a narrow opening of resistance using the articulators.

suprasegmentals/ paralinguistics/prosody (prosodic) features

Voice inflections used in a language such as stress, intensity, changes in pitch, duration of a sound, and rhythm that help listeners understand the true intent of a message and that convey the emotional aspects of a message, such as happiness, sadness, fear, or surprise.

linguistics

The scientific study of the structure and function of language and the rules that govern language; includes the study of phonemes, morphemes, syntax, semantics, and pragmatics.

phonology

The study of speech sounds and the system of rules underlying sound production and sound combinations in the formation of words.

phoneme

The shortest arbitrary unit of sound in a language that can be recognized as being distinct from other sounds in the language.

vowel

Voiced speech sounds from the unrestricted passage of the air stream through the mouth without audible stoppage or friction.

trying to learn English as a second language find it difficult because the pronunciation of a word may vary considerably depending on the context, and the differences in the pronunciation can significantly change a word's meaning. For example, "He could lead if he got the lead out." "The girl had tears in her eyes because of the tears in her dress." "Since there is no time like the present, he decided to present the present."

Authors of fiction books sometimes create new words by following phonological rules of English; for example, J.R.R. Tolkien, in *The Lord of the Rings* trilogy, created a great number of new words, including *hobbit, glede,* and *Fallohides.* J. K. Rowling, the author of the *Harry Potter* books, also created *quidditch* and *muggle* (*muggle* is now in the *New Oxford English Dictionary*). These words "sound like they could be words," just as any new technical word must follow accepted English phonological rules to eventually become part of our vocabulary (e.g., *byte, megabyte,* and *telecommunication*).

Morphology

Morphology is the study of the way words are formed out of basic units of language—**morphemes**. Morphemes are one or more letters or sounds that may be used as prefixes, such as *un*comfortable; base (root) words, such as *comfort*; or suffixes such as *able.* When a morpheme is able to stand alone, that is, it does not need any other morphemes attached to it to make it a true word, it is called a *free morpheme* (e.g., *horse, culture,* and *accept*). Morphemes that cannot stand alone and must be attached to a free morpheme are referred to as *bound morphemes* (e.g., prefixes such as *pre-, dis-,* and *mis-*; suffixes such as the plural *-s,* the past tense *-d,* and the gerund *-ing*; and base words such as *-celerate-* and *audio-*). Table 1–1 shows how prefixes, base words, and suffixes (morphemes) combine to make whole words.

Syntax

Syntax and morphology are the two major categories of language structure (i.e., **grammar**). Syntax is the study of the rules for acceptable sequences (order) and word combinations in sentences. Various languages

Glossary (margin)

morphology

The study of the structure (form) of words.

morpheme

The smallest unit of language having a distinct meaning, for example, a prefix, root word, or suffix.

syntax

Rules that dictate the acceptable sequence and combination of words in a sentence to convey meaning; the study of sentence structure.

grammar

The rules of the use of morphology and syntax in a language.

TABLE 1–1 Examples of Whole Words, Prefixes, Base Words, and Suffixes

WHOLE WORD	PREFIX	BASE WORD	SUFFIX
miscommunication	mis	communicate	tion
indefensible	in	defense	ible
disorienting	dis	orient	ing

© Cengage Learning 2013.

have different word orders for sentences. In an English declarative sentence, the subject comes before the verb: "David is going to work." However, when the subject (*David*) and the auxiliary or helping verb (*is*) are reversed in order, the sentence becomes a question—"*Is David* going to work?" English syntax has the adjective preceding the noun (e.g., the green room); however, the syntax of Spanish and French has the adjective following the noun (e.g., the room green). Most English sentences flow from subject to verb to objects or complements. Most sentences conform to variations of the following patterns:

Subject/verb/direct object (*The woman took her purse.*)

Subject/verb/indirect object (*The horse ran to the barn.*)

Subject/verb/subject complement (*The man worked hard.*)

Native speakers of a language develop a grammatical intuition by which they can recognize when a sentence is not quite grammatically correct, but they may have some difficulty pinpointing or explaining what is not correct. When people who have learned English as a second language are speaking, they may use some incorrect word order or omit morphemes (e.g., the plural -*s*) that a native speaker of English recognizes and may be a little uncomfortable with, feeling a need to correct the nonnative speaker.

Semantics

Semantics is the study of meaning in language that is conveyed by the words, phrases, and sentences communicated. Semantics may be thought of as the *content expressed* by the speaker and the *content understood* by the listener. Miscommunication occurs when there is a discrepancy between the two.

Social and cultural factors play significant roles in the way we use and understand language. For example, a word's meaning in one region of the United States may be considerably different from its meaning in another region. In many western regions of the United States *dinner* is the evening meal but in many midwestern and southern regions *dinner* is the noon meal and *supper* is the evening meal. Among English-speaking countries, there can be significant differences in the use of words for the same thing. For example, in England a *restroom* is sometimes called a *water closet* and in Australia a *napkin* is a *diaper*. The differences in the semantic use of words and the meanings of words can certainly affect communication, even among people who do not have communication disorders.

Idioms (figures of speech) are a way of expressing a thought by referring to one thing in terms of another (see Figure 1–5). We use countless idioms in our language, most of which when analyzed word by word make little or no sense, although we assume that the listener will automatically know what we mean when we say "I'm all ears," "He has butterflies in his stomach," "She has a heart of gold," and "He put his foot in his mouth."

Application Question

How good is your grammatical intuition; that is, how easily do you automatically detect or recognize grammatical errors in other people's speech? In your own speech?

semantics

The study of meaning in language conveyed by words, phrases, and sentences.

idiom

An expression in the usage of a language that is peculiar to itself either grammatically (e.g., "Zip your lip.") or in having a meaning that cannot be derived from the normal combination of words (e.g., "Keep your eyes on the ball, your shoulder to the wheel, and your nose to the grindstone.").

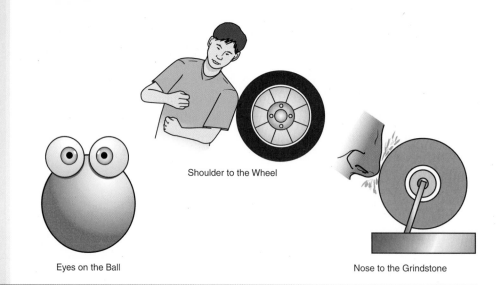

Figure 1–5

How an idiom might look. ("Keep your eyes on the ball, your shoulder to the wheel, and your nose to the grindstone.")

© Cengage Learning 2013.

Eyes on the Ball

Shoulder to the Wheel

Nose to the Grindstone

pragmatics

The rules governing the use of language in social situations; includes the speaker–listener relationship and intentions and all elements in the environment surrounding the interaction—the context.

context

The circumstances or events that form the environment within which something exists or takes place; also, the words, phrases, or narrative that come before and after a particular word or phrase in speech or a piece of writing that helps to explain its full meaning.

Pragmatics

Pragmatics are the rules governing the use of language in social situations. Some elements included in pragmatics are the *relationship* of the people talking, the **context** or environment they are in (e.g., social vs. business), and the *intentions* of the communication (e.g., friendliness or hidden agendas). The context in which a message is framed significantly affects its true meaning. Pragmatics places greater emphasis on the functions of language than on the structure of language.

Pragmatics are culturally based or influenced. For example, in some regions of the world, such as the Middle East, an initial business meeting may be devoted to sharing about family and friends, and the business may not be discussed until a later meeting. Also, the beginning of each new business meeting may be devoted to extended casual conversation rather than moving to the task at hand. When businesspeople do not know the cultural traditions of the people they are dealing with, disastrous consequences may result.

Reading and Writing

Many speech-language pathologists are involved in the area of literacy with children who have reading and writing disabilities, particularly in the public schools. Reading and writing may be more challenging for the brain to process and, therefore, more difficult to develop than auditory-verbal abilities. In a way, we have two languages: listening-speaking (*auditory-verbal* or *aural-oral*) and reading-writing (*visual-graphic*). The auditory-verbal language is developed in the early years of life; however, the reading-writing language does not normally start developing until the early years of schooling. Also, a person may become verbal and be considered a good communicator, but that does not mean he is an equally good reader or writer.

DISORDERS OF COMMUNICATION

When we listen to someone talk, we typically (consciously or subconsciously) pay attention or notice several features. We notice the person's articulation and how clearly and easily we can understand him. We pay attention to the person's voice and whether we think it is appropriate for the person's age and gender, and whether it is relatively smooth and clear. We hear whether a person has a resonance problem and sounds like he is either "talking through his nose" or sounds like he has a "stuffy nose." We listen for the person's language skills and whether good syntax is being used with a reasonably appropriate choice of words. We notice whether the person's speech is relatively fluent or whether he has unusual pauses and hesitations, repetitions of sounds and words, or prolongations of sounds. We also notice whether the person's hearing is adequate when we are talking to him or whether we have to speak louder than normal or repeat ourselves often. We also may notice whether the person seems embarrassed or frustrated with his own communication. In social conversations, when we notice problems in any of these areas we usually try not to let the speaker know that we are aware of them. However, in our professional work as speech-language pathologists and audiologists we need to recognize, analyze, diagnose, and treat a person's communication disorders.

Charles Van Riper's (1978) classic definition of communication disorder is commonly used by SLPs; that is, speech (or language) is disordered when it deviates from that of other people, calls attention to itself, interferes with communication, or causes distress in both the speaker and the listener. However, based on the earlier definition of *communication* (i.e., any means by which individuals relate their wants, needs, thoughts, knowledge, and feelings to another person), a communication disorder, therefore, may be defined as any voice, resonance, articulation, language, cognitive, or hearing impairment that interferes with people relating their wants, needs, thoughts, knowledge, and feelings to another person.

As professionals, SLPs and Auds try to provide objectivity in their definitions of terms and diagnoses of communication disorders. In reality, the subjective feelings of clients and patients and their listeners are what determine how much a communication disorder actually affects an individual. Some individuals have very negative reactions to even minor communication problems, whereas others appear (or try to appear) remarkably tolerant, unconcerned, or unaware of even fairly significant problems. In essence, a communication disorder can affect our **quality of life**, and the task of SLPs and Auds is to help improve the quality of life of our clients, patients, and their families. The term **handicap** is generally avoided because of its negative connotations, with the terms **disability** and **impairment** now more commonly used.

Prevalence refers to the number of individuals diagnosed with a particular disorder at a given time. **Incidence** is the rate at which a disorder appears in the normal population over a period, typically one year.

quality of life

A global concept that involves a person's standard of living, personal freedom, and the opportunity to pursue happiness; a measure of a person's ability to cope successfully with the full range of challenges encountered in daily living; the characterization of health concerns or disease effects on a person's lifestyle and daily functioning.

handicap

Loss or limitation of opportunities to take part in the life of the community on an equal level with others (**World Health Organization [WHO]**); a congenital or acquired physical or intellectual limitation that hinders a person from performing specific tasks.

World Health Organization (WHO)

An agency of the United Nations established in 1948 to further international cooperation in improving health conditions throughout the world.

disability

Any restriction or lack (resulting from an impairment) of ability to perform an activity in the manner or within the range considered normal for a human being (World Health Organization [WHO]); the impairment, loss, or absence of a physical or intellectual function; *physical disability* is any impairment that limits the physical functions of limbs or gross or fine motor abilities; *sensory disability* is impairment of one of the senses (e.g., hearing or vision); *intellectual disability* encompasses intellectual deficits that may appear at any age.

disorder/impairment

Any loss or abnormality of psychological, physiological, or anatomical structure or function that interferes with normal activities (World Health Organization [WHO]).

prevalence

The estimated total number of individuals diagnosed with a particular disorder at a given time in a population, or the percent of people in a population with the disorder.

incidence

The rate at which a disorder appears in the normal population over a period, typically one year.

speech disorder

Any deviation of speech outside the range of acceptable variation in a given environment.

language disorder

An impairment of receptive and/ or expressive linguistic symbols (morphemes, words, semantics, syntax, or pragmatics) that affects comprehending what is said or verbally expressing wants, needs, thoughts, information, and feelings.

cognitive disorder

An impairment of attention, perception, memory, reasoning, judgment, and/or problem solving (i.e., thinking).

congenital disorder

A disorder that is present at birth.

syndrome

A complex of **signs** and **symptoms** resulting from a common etiology or appearing together that presents a clinical picture of a disease or inherited anomaly.

sign

An objective finding of a disease or change in condition as perceived by an examiner, such as a physician.

The prevalence of disorders is more clinically relevant and, therefore, more commonly reported than is the incidence. It is nearly impossible to determine the precise prevalence of communication disorders in the United States or any country, and it is likely that overall estimates are underestimated because not all communication disorders are diagnosed or diagnosed with the same criteria, or systematically reported to calculate their totals. In the United States, approximately 25% of all children between 3–21 years of age receive services from a speech-language pathologist or audiologist at some time. More than 25% of all children with learning or physical disabilities also have one or more communication disorders (e.g., articulation and language, language and literacy, speech, language, and hearing). Males are more likely to have communication disorders at all ages than females (American Speech-Language-Hearing Association [ASHA], 2008a; Catts & Kamhi, 2005; National Dissemination Center for Children with Disabilities, 2010).

CLASSIFICATIONS OF COMMUNICATION DISORDERS

There are numerous approaches to classifications of **speech** and **language disorders**, but in general they are divided into *articulation* (articulation disorders, phonological disorders, and motor speech disorders), *language* (receptive language and expressive language), *fluency* (stuttering and cluttering), *voice* (aphonia and dysphonia), *resonance* (hypernasality and hyponasality), *cognition* (developmental and acquired disorders), *literacy* (reading disorders and writing disorders), and *hearing* (conductive, sensorineural, and mixed losses) (see Figure 1–6). A swallowing disorder is not a communication disorder but is a major area of concern for SLPs, particularly in medical settings. In addition to the term *disorder*, clinicians often use the terms *impairment*, *disability*, or *problem* as synonyms when discussing clients and patients of all ages.

SLPs and Auds often try to determine *dichotomies* (i.e., either this or that) when classifying disorders. For example, a disorder may be considered *congenital* or *acquired*, *organic* or *functional*, an *articulation disorder* or *phonological disorder*, a *receptive language disorder* or an *expressive language disorder*, a *child communication disorder* or an *adult communication disorder*, or a *stroke* or *traumatic brain injury (TBI)*. In many cases two or more disorders may occur concurrently (i.e., a *mixed*, *coexisting*, or *comorbid* disorder), such as a child who has articulation and language disorders or an adult who has both language and **cognitive disorders**.

Congenital disorders are those that are present at birth and are usually considered either hereditary (e.g., some **syndromes**), problems caused during the pregnancy (e.g., maternal drug or alcohol use), or a complication at birth (e.g., fetal *anoxia* [no oxygen] or *hypoxia*

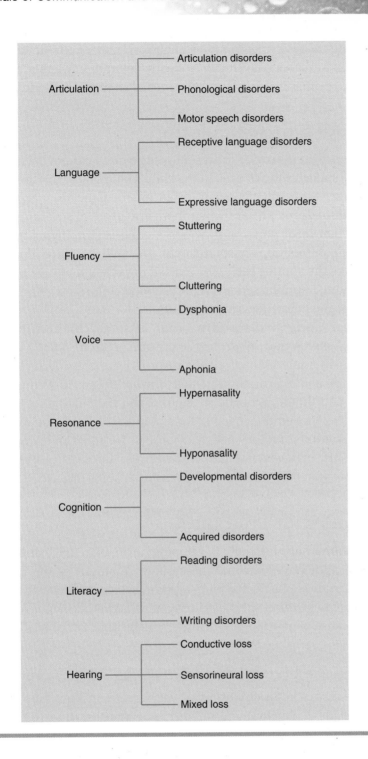

Figure 1-6

Major categories of communication disorders.

© Cengage Learning 2013.

[inadequate oxygen]). **Acquired disorders** are those that begin after an individual has developed normal communication abilities, such as a hearing loss from loud noise exposure, or a speech, language, or cognitive disorder caused by a **traumatic brain injury**.

When considering the **etiology** or cause of a disorder, some clinicians will use the terms **functional disorder** and **organic disorder**. A functional disorder is a problem or impairment that has some behavioral and/or emotional components but no known anatomical, physiological, or neurological basis. An organic disorder has an anatomical, physiological,

symptom

A subjective indication of a disease or change in condition as perceived by the patient or other nonmedical or rehabilitation specialist, such as a family member.

acquired disorder

A disorder that begins after an individual has developed normal communication abilities, such as a hearing loss from loud noise exposure or a speech, language, or cognitive disorder caused by a traumatic brain injury.

traumatic brain injury (TBI) (head trauma, acquired brain injury-ABI)

An acquired injury to the brain caused by an external force that results in partial or total functional disability, including physical, communication, cognitive, and psychosocial impairments.

etiology

The cause of an occurrence (e.g., a medical problem that results in a disorder or disability).

functional disorder

A problem or impairment with no known anatomical, physiological, or neurological basis that may have behavioral or emotional causes or components.

organic disorder

A problem or impairment with a known anatomical, physiological, or neurological basis.

articulation disorder

The incorrect production of speech sounds due to faulty placement, timing, direction, pressure, speed, or integration of the movements of the mandible, lips, tongue, or velum.

phonological disorder

Errors of phonemes that form patterns in which a child simplifies individual sounds or sound combinations.

or neurological basis and may have behavioral and/or emotional components. In many cases it is difficult to clearly determine whether a disorder is purely or primarily a functional disorder or an organic disorder.

Disorders of Articulation

An **articulation disorder** is present when a child cannot correctly *produce* (say) speech sounds used in the child's language. Most articulation disorders are the result of inaccurate placement of the tongue. A **phonological disorder** is present when there are errors of several *phonemes* (sounds) that form patterns in which a child is simplifying individual sounds or combinations of sounds (i.e., the child is unintentionally trying to make the sounds easier for himself to say). Ninety-two percent of SLPs working in public schools report serving children with articulation or phonological disorders (ASHA, 2010).

Motor speech disorders occur in some children (*childhood apraxia of speech* and *dysarthria* [e.g., with *cerebral palsy*]) but more commonly in adults. Motor speech disorders are considered the result of neurological impairments that affect the *motor* (i.e., movement) planning and coordination, or the strength of the articulators for the rapid and complex movements needed for smooth, effortless, and intelligible speech. In adults, motor speech disorders are most often caused by strokes, TBIs, or *neuromuscular diseases* (i.e., diseases of the nervous system that affect the muscles), such as Parkinson's disease.

Disorders of Language

Many children have difficulty developing normal language abilities and these difficulties may become increasingly apparent as the child gets older and more sophisticated language is expected. Adults who have had normal language all of their lives may have acquired language impairments because of neurological disorders such as strokes or head injuries.

Language Disorders in Children

Language disorders in children can vary greatly in how they manifest during language development in both **receptive language** (how well a child understands what he hears) and **expressive language** (how well a child can verbally communicate his messages), with age of a child being a significant factor. Children who have difficulty understanding language commonly have difficulty expressing themselves. Some children are slow to develop language and may be considered to have a **language delay**, but then develop normal language. Parents often refer to these children as "slow talkers" and "late bloomers." Language disorders are associated with more than 75% of children who have learning disabilities (Barnes, Fletcher, & Fuchs, 2007). Some causes of language disorders include hearing loss, traumatic brain injuries, autism, various genetic syndromes, and intellectual disabilities. Most of these children have articulation disorders in conjunction with their language disorders or language delays (ASHA, 2008a). Ninety percent of SLPs working in schools report that they work with children who have language impairments (ASHA, 2010).

Children's culturally and linguistically diverse backgrounds can significantly affect their expressive language. However, expressive language affected by cultural and linguistic diversity is not a disorder—it is a *difference*. **Language differences** are variations in speech and language production that are the result of a person's cultural, linguistic, and social environments. When determining whether a particular child's language is a disorder or a difference, we must consider two norms: **General American English (GAE) (Standard American English [SAE])** and the cultural norms of the child (Hegde, 2007; Paul, 2006). A 1983 American Speech-Language-Hearing Association position paper (p. 24) on social dialects stated "No dialect variety of English is a disorder or a pathological form of speech or language. Each social dialect is considered adequate as a functional and effective variety of English."

Language Disorders in Adults

Impaired language in adulthood may be a continuation of the language problems of a child or adolescent. However, generally we think of language disorders in adults as being acquired because of neurological impairments such as strokes and head injuries. These adults have lived their entire lives, often at very high functioning levels, and then because of medical problems or accidents have communication disorders that they could never have imagined. Damage to the brain's left hemisphere can cause both language impairments (**aphasia**) and motor speech disorders. It is estimated that between 5% to 10% of adults have neurological impairments that result in language disorders (ASHA, 2008c).

Disorders of Fluency

Stuttering (disfluency) is likely the most common problem people think of when they think of a speech disorder. (Note: Most current authorities on stuttering use *dis*fluency rather than *dys*fluency [Bloodstein & Bernstein Ratner, 2008; Guitar, 2006; Manning, 2010; Ramig & Dodge, 2010; Ward, 2006; Yairi & Ambrose, 2005]). Probably most adults have encountered someone who stutters, and the media (including cartoons) have parodied people who stutter countless times. Stuttering is usually heard as repetitions of sounds, syllables, or words; prolongations of sounds; and abnormal stoppages or "silent blocks" while a child or adult is talking. There can be visible tension and struggle behaviors, such as blinking their eyes, looking away just as they begin to stutter, and a variety of facial grimaces and unusual arm, hand, and other body part movements. Stuttering can be one of the most emotionally difficult of all the communication disorders (Bloodstein & Bernstein Ratner, 2008). About 5% of preschool-age children have episodes of disfluency, and in

---

motor speech disorder

Impaired speech intelligibility that is caused by a neurological impairment that affects the motor (movement) planning or the strength of the articulators needed for rapid, complex movements in smooth, effortless speech.

receptive language/ comprehension/ decoding

What a person understands of what is said.

expressive language/ production/encoding

The words, grammatical structures, and meanings that a person uses verbally.

language delay

An abnormal slowness in developing language skills that may result in incomplete language development.

language differences

Variations in speech and language production that are the result of a person's cultural, linguistic, and social environments.

General American English (GAE)/ Standard American English (SAE)

The speech of native speakers of American English that is typical of the United States and that excludes phonological forms easily recognized as regional dialects (e.g., Northeastern or Southeastern) or limited to particular ethnic or social groups, and that is not identified as a nonnative American accent; the norm of pronunciation by national radio and television broadcasters.

aphasia/dysphasia

An impairment in language processing that may affect any or all input modalities (auditory, visual, and tactile) and any or all output modalities (speaking, writing, and gesturing).

stuttering/disfluency (dysfluency)

A disturbance in the normal flow and time patterning of speech characterized by one of more of the following: repetitions of sounds, syllables, or words; prolongations of sounds; abnormal stoppages or "silent blocks" within or between words; interjections of unnecessary sounds or words; circumlocutions (talking around an intended word); or sounds and words produced with excessive tension.

cluttering

Speech that is abnormally fast with omission of sounds and syllables of words, abnormal patterns of pausing and phrasing, and often spoken in bursts that may be unintelligible; frequently includes abnormalities in syntax, semantics, and pragmatics.

voice disorder

Any deviation of loudness, pitch, or quality of voice that is outside the normal range of a person's age, gender, or geographic cultural background that interferes with communication, draws unfavorable attention to itself, or adversely affects the speaker or listener.

dysphonia

A general term that means a voice disorder, with the person's voice typically sounding rough, raspy, or hoarse.

the general population approximately 1% of school-age children and adults stutter (Yairi & Ambrose, 2005).

Cluttering is considered a fluency disorder that shares some characteristics of stuttering but differs in several important ways. Cluttered speech is abnormally fast with omissions of sounds and syllables so that words sound compressed or *truncated* (reduced in length). A person who clutters has abnormal patterns of pausing and phrasing, and has bursts of speech that may be unintelligible.

Disorders of Voice

A **voice disorder** occurs when the loudness, pitch, or quality (i.e., "smoothness") of a person's voice is outside the normal range for the person's age, gender, or the speaking environment, or the voice is unpleasant to hear. Children and adults can have severe voice disorders that leave them without a functional voice for communicating essential messages. Most voice disorders in children and adults are diagnosed as **dysphonias** in which the person's voice sounds rough, raspy, or **hoarse**. Dysphonia may be caused by laryngitis, masses on the vocal folds (e.g., vocal nodules [cheerleaders nodules]), neurological damage that causes weakness of the vocal folds, or psychological causes, such as tension in the vocal mechanism (*larynx*). **Aphonia** is a complete loss of voice, which is rare, and typically has psychological causes such as emotional stress. Following the complete loss of voice the person may use whispering or writing to communicate and often avoids communication. Voice disorders have been reported to occur in 6% to 23% of children and almost 30% of SLPs report that they serve children or adults with voice disorders (ASHA, 2008a).

Disorders of Resonance

Resonance disorders involve abnormal structures or functioning of the *hard* and *soft palates* (the roof of the mouth, front to back) that cause the voice to be directed into the nasal cavities on oral sounds or not directed into the nasal cavities on nasal sounds (i.e., /m/, /n/, and "ng"). Most resonance disorders in children are the result of cleft palates, with an overall prevalence of about 0.001% to 0.002% of the general population (i.e., 1 to 2 per 1,000 live births) (Peterson-Falzone, Hardin-Jones, & Karnell, 2009). **Hypernasality** is the result of clefts of the hard and soft palates or weakness of the soft palate. In hypernasality, oral consonants and vowels that should exit the mouth pass into the nasal passages where they are *resonated* (i.e., increased vibration and amplification of sounds) and listeners perceive the person's speech as though the person is "talking through his nose." **Hyponasality (denasality)** occurs because of partial or complete obstruction of the nasal passages (e.g., enlarged adenoids), causing the /m/, /n/ and "ng" sounds to not have their normal nasal resonance. Acquired resonance disorders in adults are usually the result of a weak soft palate that is caused by strokes and head injuries.

Disorders of Cognition

Cognition is the act or process of thinking or learning that involves perceiving, memory, reasoning, judgment, and problem solving. Cognitive disorders in children are usually associated with intellectual disabilities. The majority of children who have intellectual disabilities also have mild to profound language delays, with some children never developing functional language skills or the ability to live independently. Relatively intact cognitive abilities are important for development of both speech and language.

Adults may have acquired cognitive disorders, which are usually the result of damage to the right hemisphere or the frontal lobes of the brain. Cognitive disorders affect attention, **perception**, memory, reasoning, judgment, and problem solving (in a word, *thinking*). Mild to moderate TBIs can result in significant cognitive disorders in individuals of all ages, and severe neurological impairments can result in any combination of aphasia, motor speech disorders, and cognitive disorders. Approximately 1% to 2% of children and adults have TBIs that result in long-term disability (Zaloshnja, Miller, Langlois, et al., 2008). Many elderly people develop **dementia**, which is a neurological disorder that is a progressive deterioration of cognitive functioning and personality. Alzheimer's disease is just one form of dementia. It is estimated that approximately 8% to 15% of people between 65 and 70 years of age have some level of dementia; this percent increases significantly every 5 years (Plassman, Langa, Fisher, et al., 2007).

Hearing Impairments

Hearing is the foundation for development of speech and language. **Hearing impairments** can cause numerous speech and language delays and disorders in children that can affect them throughout their lives. Adults may acquire hearing impairments at any age from loud noises, medical problems that affect the ear, or the progressive hearing losses that often come with age. The two primary types of hearing impairments are conductive and sensorineural. A **conductive hearing loss** is a decrease in the loudness of a sound because of poor conduction of sound through the outer or middle ear. In severe conductive hearing losses, the fluid in the *cochlea* (hearing portion of the inner ear) may not be set into motion sufficiently to stimulate the nerves in the cochlea and, therefore, little or no auditory information is sent to the brain. Conductive hearing losses can have numerous causes, including malformations of the outer ear (*pinna*), occlusion of the ear canal from ear wax (*cerumen*), damage to the eardrum (*tympanic membrane*) or the three small bones in the middle ear (*ossicles*), or middle ear infections (*otitis media with effusion*).

---

hoarseness

A common symptom of dysphonia that is a combination of breathiness and harshness that affects how pleasant and smooth a voice sounds.

aphonia

A complete loss of voice followed by whispering for oral communication that typically has psychological causes such as emotional stress.

resonance disorder

Abnormal modification of the voice by passing through the nasal cavities during production of oral sounds (*hypernasality*) or not passing through the nasal cavities during production of nasal sounds (*hyponasality*).

hypernasal/hypernasality

A resonance disorder that occurs when oral consonants and vowels enter the nasal cavity because of clefts of the hard and soft palates or weakness of the soft palate, causing a person to sound like he is "talking through his nose."

hyponasal/hyponasality (denasal/denasality)

Lack of normal resonance for the three English phonemes, m, n, and ng, resulting from partial or complete obstruction in the nasal tract.

cognition/cognitive processing/cognitive functioning

The act or process of thinking or learning that involves perceiving, memory, abstraction, generalization, reasoning, judgment, and problem solving; closely related to intelligence.

perception/perceive

The process of detecting, discriminating, and recognition of a stimulus.

dementia

A neurological disease that causes intellectual, cognitive, and personality deterioration that is more severe than what would occur through normal aging.

hearing impairment/ hearing loss

Abnormal or reduced function in hearing resulting from an auditory disorder.

conductive hearing loss

A reduction in hearing sensitivity because of a disorder of the outer or middle ear.

sensorineural hearing loss

A reduction of hearing sensitivity produced by disorders of the cochlea and/or the auditory nerve fibers of the vestibulocochlear (VIII cranial) nerve.

In a **sensorineural hearing loss** there is a reduction of hearing sensitivity caused by disorders of the cochlea and/or the auditory nerve fibers of the vestibulocochlear (VIII cranial) nerve. This type of hearing loss typically results in difficulty discriminating speech sounds and, consequently, understanding speech. Infants may be born with sensorineural hearing losses or they may develop losses in childhood because of infections such as measles, mumps, and chicken pox. In older children, adolescents, and young adults, sensorineural hearing losses are often caused by listening to loud music for long periods of time (Thaker & Jongnarangsin, 2007). In older adults sensorineural hearing losses are common with advancing age.

Hearing loss is the most common of all physical impairments. In infants and children, approximately 1 in every 22 newborns in the United States has some kind of hearing problem, and 1 in every 1,000 infants has a severe to profound hearing loss. Of school-age children, 83 out of 1,000 have a significant hearing loss (ASHA, 2008b; National Dissemination Center for Children with Disabilities, 2010). Approximately 4.5% of adults 18 to 44 years of age, 14% of adults 45 to 64 years of age, and 54% of adults 65 years of age and older have some degree of hearing loss (Pleis & Lethbridge-Cejku, 2007).

EMOTIONAL AND SOCIAL EFFECTS OF COMMUNICATION DISORDERS

Communication disorders can have untold emotional and social effects on people of all ages. Many of these effects are likely undocumented and even unacknowledged by the individuals. However, beyond the individuals with the communication disorders are the parents, grandparents, siblings, husbands and wives, and other family members who are bewildered and anguished by their loved one's communication problems. A communication disorder affects a family, not just the person who has it, and it is essential to educate the family about the communication disorder their loved one has (Flasher & Fogle, 2012; Tye Murray, 2012). Each chapter in this text that deals with a disorder has a discussion of the emotional and social effects of that disorder on the person and the family.

As clinicians, we always need to keep in mind the entire person (and the family) with whom we are working, not just the disorder the person has. We need to place considerable importance on developing good, caring, working relationships with clients and their families in order to optimally carry out therapy and provide the necessary family education and training. Good people skills and counseling skills are essential when working with clients of all ages and their families (Flasher & Fogle, 2012).

CHAPTER SUMMARY

Speech-language pathologists and audiologists work with all areas of communication, including hearing, speaking, reading, writing, and nonverbal communication. For speech, we need to consider the various systems involved, including respiration, phonation, resonation, and articulation. We work with all areas of speech and language, including phonology, morphology, syntax, semantics, and pragmatics. Communication disorders may affect articulation, language, fluency, voice, resonance, cognition, and hearing. Communication disorders can have untold emotional and social effects on children, adolescents, and adults, and their families.

STUDY QUESTIONS

Knowledge and Comprehension

1. What are the four speech systems?

2. Explain morphology. In two three-syllable words, indicate each morpheme.

3. What are pragmatics? What are some elements included in pragmatics?

4. What is a communication disorder?

5. What are receptive language and expressive language?

Application

1. When talking with clients and their families, why is it helpful to understand that verbal content is usually more important for factual communication and nonverbal content is more important for judging emotions and attitudes?

2. How do suprasegmentals help us communicate?

3. Discuss the importance of good pragmatics when working with clients and their families.

4. Discuss how being familiar with the major categories of communication disorders could be helpful in your personal life.

5. Discuss the importance of appreciating and understanding the emotional and social effects of language disorders in children.

Analysis/Synthesis

1. What does the sentence, "We cannot not communicate." mean?

2. Explain the differences between speech and language.

3. How are *linguistic competence* and *grammatical intuition* similar and different?

4. Why might determining dichotomies be helpful in diagnosing a speech or language disorder?

5. How might cognitive disorders in children affect their language abilities?

REFERENCES

American Speech-Language-Hearing Association [ASHA]. (1983). Position paper: Social dialects and implications of the position on social dialects. *ASHA, 25*(9), 23–27.

ASHA. (2008a). *Communication facts.* Science and Research Department, Rockville, MD: ASHA.

ASHA. (2008b). *Incidence and prevalence of communication disorders and hearing loss in children in the United States: 2008 edition.* http://www.asha.org. Accessed August 27, 2010.

ASHA. (2008c). *Incidence and prevalence of speech, voice, and language disorders in adults in the United States: 2008 edition.* http://www.asha.org. Accessed August 27, 2010.

ASHA. (2010). *2010 School Survey report: Caseload characteristics.* Rockville, MD: ASHA.

Barnes, M. A., Fletcher, J., & Fuchs, Lynn. (2007). *Learning disabilities: From identification to intervention.* New York, NY: The Guilford Press.

Bloodstein, O., & Bernstein Ratner, N. (2008). *A handbook on stuttering* (6th ed.). Clifton Park, NY: Delmar Cengage Learning.

Burgoon, J. K., Guerrero, L., & Floyd, K. (2010). *Nonverbal communication.* New York, NY: Pearson.

Catts, H. W., & Kamhi, A. G. (2005). *Language and reading disabilities* (2nd ed.). Boston, MA: Allyn & Bacon.

Flasher, L. V., & Fogle, P. T. (2012). *Counseling skills for speech-language pathologists and audiologists* (2nd ed.). Clifton Park, NY: Delmar Cengage Learning.

Fogle, P. T. (2009). *Counseling skills: Recognizing and interpreting nonverbal communication (body language, gestures, and facial expressions),* Gaylord, MI: Northern Speech/National Rehabilitation Services.

Gedeon, A. (2006). *Science and technology in medicine: An illustrated account based on ninety-nine landmark publications from five centuries.* New York, NY: Springer Science.

Guitar, B. (2006). *Stuttering: An integrated approach to its nature and treatment.* Philadelphia, PA: Lippincott Williams & Wilkins.

Hegde, M. N. (2007). *Pocket guide to assessment in speech-language pathology* (3rd ed.). Clifton Park, NY: Delmar Cengage Learning.

Lewis, M. P. (Ed.). 2009. *Ethnologue: Languages of the world* (16th ed.). Dallas, TX: SIL International.

Luria, A. (1961). *The role of speech in the normal and abnormal processes in the child.* Baltimore, MD: Penguin.

Manning, W. H. (2010). *Clinical decision making in fluency disorders* (3rd ed.). Clifton Park, NY: Delmar Cengage Learning.

National Dissemination Center for Children with Disabilities. (2010). *Disability fact sheet.* Washington, DC: NDCCD.

Owens, R. E., Jr. (2012). *Language development: An introduction* (8th ed.) San Antonio, TX: Pearson/Allyn & Bacon.

Paul, R. (2006). *Language disorders from infancy through adolescence: Assessment and intervention* (3rd ed.). St. Louis, MO: Mosby.

Peterson-Falzone, S. J., Hardin-Jones, M. A., & Karnell, M. P. (2009). *Cleft palate speech* (4th ed.). St. Louis, MO: Mosby.

Plassman, B. L., Langa, K. M., Fisher, G. G., Heeringa, S. G., Weir, D. R., Ofstedal, M. B., & Burke, J. R. (2007). Prevalence of dementia in the United States: The aging, demographics, and memory study. *Neuroepidemiology, 29,* 125–132.

Pleis, J. R., & Lethbridge-Cejku, M. (2007). Summary health statistics for U.S. adults: National Health Interview Survey, 2006. National Center for Health Statistics. *Vital Health Statistics, 10*(235), table 11.

Ramig, P. R., & Dodge, D. M. (2010). *The child and adolescent stuttering treatment and activity resource guide* (2nd ed.). Clifton Park, NY: Delmar Cengage Learning.

Reed, V. A. (2005). *An introduction to children with language disorders* (3rd ed.). Boston, MA: Pearson Allyn and Bacon.

Thaker, J., & Jongnarangsin, K. (2007). iPods and pacemakers. *ASHA Leader,* June 19, 5.

Tye Murray, N. (2012). Counseling for adults and children who have hearing loss. In L. Flasher & P. Fogle, *Counseling Skills for Speech-Language Pathologists and Audiologists* (2nd ed.). Clifton Park, NY: Delmar Cengage Learning.

Van Riper, C. (1978). *Speech correction: Principles and methods* (6th ed.). Englewood Cliffs, NJ: Prentice-Hall.

Vygotsky, L. (1962). *Thought and language.* Cambridge, MA: MIT Press.

Ward, D. (2006). *Stuttering and cluttering: Framework for understanding and treatment.* East Sussex, England: Psychology Press.

Yairi, E., & Ambrose, N. G. (2005). *Early childhood stuttering.* Austin, TX: Pro-Ed.

Zaloshnja, E., Miller, T., Langlois, J. A. & Selassie, A. W. (2008). Prevalence of long-term disability from traumatic brain injury in the civilian population of the United States, 2005. *Journal of Head Trauma Rehabilitation, 23*(6), 394–400.

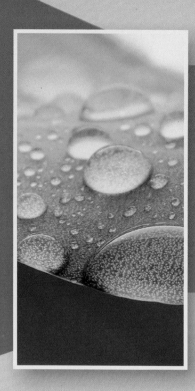

CHAPTER 2
Speech-Language Pathologists and Audiologists

LEARNING OBJECTIVES

After studying this chapter, you will:

- Appreciate that speech-language pathologists and audiologists help many people beyond the clients and patients directly receiving therapy.

- Be aware of numerous personal qualities of effective professionals.

- Recognize that as professionals we are always using a team approach.

- Know the basic educational and clinical experience requirements to become a nationally certified and state-licensed speech-language pathologist or audiologist.

- Be aware of the scope of practice of speech-language pathologists and audiologists.

- Know the variety of work settings in which speech-language pathologists and audiologists practice.

- Understand the employment outlook for speech-language pathologists and audiologists.

- Be aware of the professional organizations that oversee speech-language pathologists and audiologists.

- Be familiar with the National Student Speech-Language-Hearing Association (NSSLHA).

KEY TERMS

acute care hospital

American Speech-Language-
  Hearing Association (ASHA)

Clinical Fellowship

clinical intuition

continuing education units
  (CEUs)

convalescent hospital

diagnosis

evaluation/assessment

inpatient

National Student Speech-
  Language-Hearing
  Association (NSSLHA)

outpatient

scope of practice

speech-language pathology
  assistant (SLPA)

subacute hospital

telecommunication devices
  for the deaf (TDD)

therapy/treatment

CHAPTER OUTLINE

Introduction
Beginning Your Study of Speech-Language Pathology
  and Audiology
A Brief History of the Professions
Professional Organizations
  Student Organizations
  State Associations
Professional Ethics
Personal Qualities (Attributes) of Effective Professionals
The Team Approach
Communication Disorders Professionals
  Speech-Language Pathologists
  Audiologists
  Speech, Language, and Hearing Scientists
  Speech-Language Pathology Assistants
  Audiology Assistants
Chapter Summary
Study Questions
References

INTRODUCTION

Speech-language pathology and audiology are wonderful professions filled with caring and amiable professionals who serve interesting people with challenging disabilities. Speech-language pathology and audiology are professions that likely will be increasingly fascinating as you study them. It eventually becomes nearly impossible to separate the individual from the profession. The knowledge and skills you learn as a speech-language pathologist or audiologist become an important part of who you are as a person and how you interact and communicate with others.

BEGINNING YOUR STUDY OF SPEECH-LANGUAGE PATHOLOGY AND AUDIOLOGY

This textbook is designed to answer your questions about speech-language pathology and audiology, and it will likely give you a picture of the scope of these professions that is broader than what you imagined. Speech-language pathologists and audiologists learn about and are concerned about people from the moment of conception to their last breaths of life. Every age of infants, children, adolescents, young adults, middle-aged adults, and elderly adults have unique challenges that may affect their speech, language, cognitive, hearing, and swallowing functions. You will learn about many of these challenges through this course and this text. If you decide to major in communication disorders, you will learn about each of the areas introduced in this text in more depth. If, however, you choose to take only this course, you will still learn information that will be invaluable throughout your adult life.

Some clinicians feel that speech-language pathology and audiology are the best majors for preparation for adult life and parenthood. During their education and training students learn about normal and abnormal development of infants and children; how to work with children one-on-one and in small groups of two or three; how to talk with children about what is bothering them and how to talk with parents regarding their concerns about their children; how to motivate children to work hard to improve their communication and academic skills and how to work with children who are fearful of failure and who need special care to learn to trust you and themselves; how to work with adults and elderly people with a variety of neurological problems and the sensitive and sometimes emotional issues that accompany impairment or loss of communication abilities; about the problems of the hearing impaired at all ages and the effects not only on the child with a hearing loss but also the parents and family of the child; and how to be a patient, active listener—a trained listener—which is perhaps the most important interpersonal skill you can develop.

Communication disorders can affect people throughout their life span—for example, children born with hereditary disorders and syndromes, cleft lips and palates, hearing impairments, auditory processing disorders, and cerebral palsy. Adults with acquired communication disorders caused by strokes or traumatic brain injuries may never be able to communicate easily and effectively again, which can prevent returning to work or force them to work at a lower-level (and lower-paying) job.

The person with a communication disorder is, in a way, the tip of an iceberg. A child or adult with a communication disorder affects the family around him, as well as countless other people with whom the child or adult tries to communicate (see Figure 2–1). Therefore, when we help individuals improve their communication abilities we also are helping many other people, both directly and indirectly—most of whom we never meet.

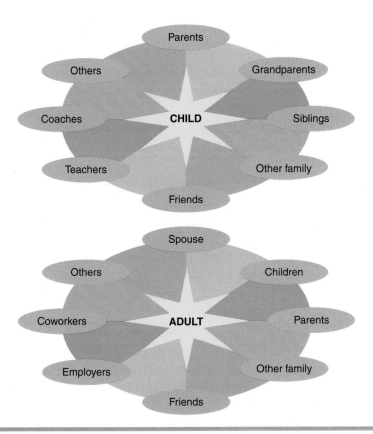

Figure 2–1

Who is really helped?

© Cengage Learning 2013.

Person-First Language

Students and professionals in speech-language pathology and audiology must keep in mind that the problems individuals experience do not define who they are. People are not their problems; problems are something people experience. Therefore, as clinicians and researchers we follow the "client/person first" convention as closely as possible; in other words, we refer to "a boy with an articulation disorder," "a girl with a hearing impairment," "a woman with a voice disorder," and so on. Professionally, we avoid phrases such as "He's an articulation client," "She's hearing impaired," "She's a voice case," and so on, because the wording implies that the person's problem is his or her identity. It is easy to slip into the habit of referring to the problem that the person has rather than to the person who has a problem. We need to learn early and maintain our vigilance to always use person-first language.

A BRIEF HISTORY OF THE PROFESSIONS

The professions of speech-language pathology and audiology are relatively new compared to medicine and education. The common origins of these professions can be traced back to Alexander Graham Bell, whose father and grandfather had been *elocutionists* (individuals who studied formal speaking in pronunciation, grammar, style, and tone) in Edinburgh, Scotland, in the 1860s. A. G. Bell and his father were interested in people who were deaf or hard of hearing (both A. G. Bell's mother and wife were deaf) and developed and applied a formal system of speech rehabilitation for the deaf. A. G. Bell recognized the need for the professions of speech-language pathology and audiology. In the early 1900s, groups with special interests in *speech correction* in the United States were formed within the National Association of Teachers of Speech (NATS), a professional society for individuals with interests in rhetoric, theater, and public speaking. In 1925, the American Academy of Speech Correction (AASC) was unofficially chartered by a group within NATS. The AASC members included physicians, psychologists, professors of English and speech, phonetician, and *speech correctionists*. The AASC eventually evolved to become the American Speech and Hearing Association (ASHA). In the 1970s when language disorders became an essential area of the profession, the organization became the **American Speech-Language-Hearing Association** but retained the abbreviation ASHA (Lubinski, Golper, & Frattali, 2007), Moeller (1975), in her *Speech Pathology & Audiology: Iowa Origins of a Discipline,* discussed the beginnings of our professions in psychology and psychiatry. In 1924, Lee Edward Travis, a doctoral student at the University of Iowa with training in psychology and medicine became "the first individual in the world to be trained by clearly conscious design at the doctoral level for

American Speech-Language-Hearing Association (ASHA)

The professional organization that represents speech-language pathologists and audiologists and sets standards for their education, training, and certification. The organization was formerly called the American Speech and Hearing Association, and retained the ASHA abbreviation.

a definite and specific professional objective of working experimentally and clinically with speech and hearing disorders."

Rehabilitation is a relatively new concept. Even after World War I, when thousands of injured soldiers were released from hospitals, little rehabilitation was provided (certainly, there was no speech therapy or hearing aids for hearing losses caused by acoustic traumas from explosions). If soldiers were medically able to be discharged, they were sent home; how they functioned when they arrived was not the concern of the medical personnel. After World War II, rehabilitation of injured individuals (including those with head injuries) became an important focus of their overall treatment.

Special education and special services for children struggling educationally were not federally mandated and widespread until the 1960s. During that decade and the following decades, important federal legislation was enacted to provide the necessary services to school-age and even preschool children:

- 1965—The *Elementary and Secondary Education Act (Public Law 89-10)* was enacted. This law required states to provide funds so that students with special needs, including the gifted, would be evaluated and appropriately educated.
- 1975—The passage of the *Education of All Handicapped Children Act (Public Law 94-142)* mandated that all school-age children with disabilities must be provided a free and appropriate education in the least restrictive environment. This included providing all related services, such as speech-language therapy, physical therapy, and occupational therapy, for children to maximally benefit from their education.
- 1986—The *Education of the Handicapped Amendments (Public Law 99-457)* provided federal funds to states to develop programs for children with disabilities from birth through 2 years of age, and provisions for Public Law 94-142 were extended to children with disabilities between 3 and 5 years of age.
- 1990—The *Individuals with Disabilities Act (IDEA)* came into being, and the *Americans with Disabilities Act (ADA) (Public Law 101-336)* mandated improved access for individuals with handicaps to buildings and facilities and provided effective communication for people with disabilities, including the use of interpreters, sign language, and **telecommunication devices for the deaf (TDD)**.

The professions of speech-language pathology and audiology have grown as the services they provide have been increasingly valued and funded. From the early years of emphasis on stuttering and articulation disorders grew a profession that touches every communication problem known to science. With the addition of swallowing disorders to our scope of practice, speech-language pathologists can work with disorders of anatomy and physiology that involve the oral, pharyngeal (*pharynx*), laryngeal (*larynx*), and respiratory systems, regardless of a person's communication abilities.

telecommunication devices for the deaf (TDD)

Telephone systems used by those with significant hearing impairments in which a typewritten message is transmitted over telephone lines and is received as a printed message.

PROFESSIONAL ORGANIZATIONS

ASHA is the primary scholarly and professional organization for individuals in the field of communication sciences and disorders in the United States. ASHA considers communication sciences and disorders to be a single discipline with two separate professions: speech-language pathology and audiology. ASHA also establishes the "Scope of Practice in Speech-Language Pathology" and "Scope of Practice in Audiology." These documents are available on the ASHA website at http://www.asha.org. ASHA's Certificates of Clinical Competence (CCC) in Speech-Language Pathology (CCC-SLP) and Audiology (CCC-A) are nationally recognized professional credentials that indicate individuals have met rigorous academic and professional standards, and that they have the knowledge, skills, and expertise to provide high-quality clinical services. SLPs and Auds must engage in ongoing professional development to keep their certification current. In addition to being members of ASHA, many audiologists are also members of the American Audiological Association (referred to as "Triple A"—AAA). AAA is separate from ASHA and has its own national conventions designed to meet the needs of audiologists.

As the need for speech-language pathology and audiology services has increased, membership in ASHA has steadily grown. As of 2010, ASHA had a membership of more than 140,000, including members from countries other than the United States. Speech and hearing associations around the world have their own memberships, for example:

- Speech Pathology Australia
- Royal College of Speech and Language Therapists (Great Britain)
- Canadian Association of Speech-Language Pathology and Audiology
- Israeli Speech, Hearing, and Language Association
- Japanese Association of Speech-Language-Hearing Therapists
- Russian Association of Phoniatricians and Speech Therapists
- Swedish Association of Phoniatrics and Logopedics

Children and adults worldwide experience communication disorders, and perhaps in countries where there is the greatest need (the "developing countries") there are the fewest professionals and resources to provide help.

National Student Speech-Language-Hearing Association (NSSLHA)

The preprofessional association for students interested in the study of communication sciences and disorders.

Student Organizations

Students can join the **National Student Speech-Language-Hearing Association (NSSLHA)** while undergraduates or graduate students (full or part time, national or international). NSSLHA provides students with a closer affiliation to professionals in the discipline, as well as monthly professional publications and other support designed specifically for them (see http://www.nsslha.org).

NSSLHA also has developed an excellent manual for students, titled *Communication Sciences Student Survival Guide* (NSSLHA, 2010), which provides, among other things, information on financing your education and advice (from students' perspectives) about enhancing your education and involvement in the profession throughout your education.

State Associations

Each state has its own state association for speech-language pathologists and audiologists, which provides professional support, public awareness, opportunities for professional growth, and advocates for the professions and the individuals they serve. Both states and ASHA have annual conventions and provide numerous opportunities for continuing education and professional development.

Individual state licensing boards also regulate the practice of speech-language pathology and audiology. State licensing requirements generally follow the requirements for ASHA certification. Most states also have continuing education requirements for licensure renewal. Medicare, Medicaid, and private health insurers generally require a practitioner to be licensed to qualify for reimbursement of clinical services.

PROFESSIONAL ETHICS

In order to be nationally certified professionals, the members must adhere to a code of ethics. Ethics is the process of deciding what is the right thing to do in a moral dilemma (Aiken, 2008). Ethics are standards of conduct that guide our professional behavior. They define acceptable versus unacceptable behaviors and promote high and consistent standards of practice.

The establishment of a code of ethics has been a major function of ASHA since its founding in 1925. For speech-language pathologists and audiologists, ethical practice transcends employment settings, levels of experience, and nature of clientele. Once a speech-language pathologist or audiologist signs the agreement to follow the ASHA Code of Ethics and holds a current Certificate of Clinical Competence, he or she must abide by the ASHA Code regardless of certification held or the location of services provided (Miller, 2007). Failure to abide by the Code of Ethics could result in loss of certification or licensure. Refer to ASHA's website (http://www.asha.org) for a copy of the Code of Ethics.

PERSONAL QUALITIES (ATTRIBUTES) OF EFFECTIVE PROFESSIONALS

Speech-language pathologists and audiologists are professionals. Several personal qualities (attributes) of effective professionals have been identified in the literature (Flasher & Fogle, 2012):

- *Encouraging*—The ability to encourage may be one of the most important qualities of clinicians. Encouragement helps people learn to believe in their potential for improvement.

Personal Story — Elizabeth Smith, M.Ed., CCC-SLP

On an unusual snowy day in Atlanta, Georgia, in March 1983, kindergartner Elizabeth Smith was walking to a friend's nearby house when she stepped on a downed power line that had been hidden under the snow. While she was unconscious, she was rushed to the hospital, and over the next 6 weeks she underwent a series of surgeries that included amputation of both arms at her shoulders and her left leg at the high thigh level. This was followed by physical and occupational rehabilitation for the young girl with triple amputations. She eventually returned to school, and over the next 5 years, with the help of the hospital rehabilitation staff and her schoolteachers, she learned to walk using a prosthetic leg. Although she was fitted with prosthetic arms, she abandoned them because they felt heavy and awkward. Instead, she learned to use her one foot to perform most functions her arms and hands would have done: she learned to eat, type, write, apply makeup, brush her hair, and most everything else people use two arms and hands to do (see Figure 2–2).

Elizabeth said that her hospital stay after the accident inspired her to go into rehabilitation as an adult—as a speech-language pathologist. She said that during her hospital stay as a child, "Rehabilitation was difficult, but I could always communicate." In college, Elizabeth decided that becoming a speech-language pathologist would put all of her interests and talents to good use: verbal skills, interest in science, teaching ability, and talent for interacting with people. In 1999, Elizabeth graduated magna cum laude with a B.A. in speech communication from Georgia State University in Atlanta, followed by a master's degree in communication disorders, which included an internship at a skilled nursing facility (nursing home). Here, she learned even more about overcoming her own clinical challenges on the job, such as working with patients who have feeding and swallowing problems. Her first professional work

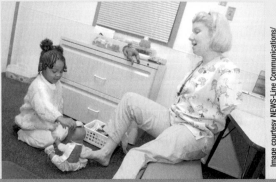

Image courtesy NEWS-Line Communications/
© Cengage Learning 2013

Figure 2–2
Elizabeth Smith on the job.

after completing her master's degree was as a public school speech-language pathologist, but she eventually decided that hospital work in a rehabilitation center for children was her passion. Only a few work-environment accommodations have been made for her, such as lowering the therapy table and having files and materials stored at a comfortable height to make it easier for her to use her foot. Even with its occasional challenges, Elizabeth says of her work, "It is my dream job." ◼

- *Emotionally stable*—Most speech-language pathologists and audiologists are at least fairly well-adjusted people.
- *Self-aware*—Self-awareness is related to self-acceptance, self-esteem, and self-realization. Self-awareness is important to maintain our emotional stability.
- *Patient*—One of the hallmark characteristics of speech-language pathologists and audiologists is patience; that is, the ability and willingness to persevere during the often long, slow road of speech and language development or rehabilitation of our clients and patients. It also means not becoming anxious or frustrated about a person's slow rate of improvement and realizing that most people are doing about as well as they can at the moment.
- *Sensitive to others*—Sensitivity requires awareness of others, particularly the sometimes almost unobservable emotional responses to what is being said or what is happening in the person's life.
- *Empathic*—Speech-language pathologists and audiologists attempt to understand the client from the client's point of view; that is, they try to understand what the person is thinking, feeling, and experiencing and communicate this understanding back to the client.

Application Question

Which of the personal qualities do you feel are some of your strongest? Your weakest? How could you strengthen your weakest qualities?

THE TEAM APPROACH

As professionals working with communication disorders, we are members of a team—in all of our work, we take the team approach. We are typically working with other professionals, as well as family members of clients. At minimum, the people on the team are the client and the clinician, with the client always being the most important team member because without the client there would be no need for any other team members. In most cases, the team includes several others, such as family members of the client, the clinician's supervisor or administrator, teachers, and reading specialists in a school setting. Depending on the setting and the needs of the client or patient, physicians, nurses, physical therapists, occupational therapists, respiratory therapists, and other professionals may all be involved directly with helping the person (see Figure 2–3).

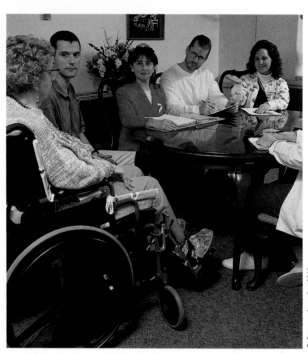

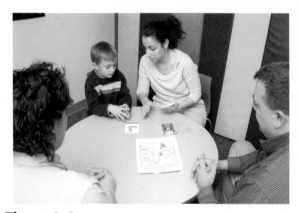

© Cengage Learning 2013

Figure 2-3

The team approach always includes the client/patient, family, and other professionals.

Typical treatment teams for different settings are as follows:

- University clinic: Client, family, student clinician, and supervisor
- School: Child, family, school speech-language pathologist, and classroom teacher
- Hospital: Patient, family, physician, nurse, dietitian, speech-language pathologist , physical therapist, and occupational therapist

Countless other people are indirectly involved with helping clients and patients, including secretarial and administrative staff, custodial and maintenance workers, and kitchen workers. The list of the "behind the scenes" people is long, and if any of these people are not doing their job well it can affect the person we are trying to help. After clinicians have been working for a while, they begin to realize that what makes the "machinery" of the work environment function are the people who are the least acknowledged for their contributions. We as communication specialists need to show our appreciation for all people who are part of the big picture of helping people with communication disorders.

COMMUNICATION DISORDERS PROFESSIONALS

The field of communication (communicative) disorders involves interrelated professionals who begin with earning a bachelor's degree (either a B.A. or a B.S., depending on the institution) in speech-language pathology, communication (communicative) disorders, or speech and hearing sciences (other terms may be used). Students also may earn an undergraduate degree in another major and then begin their education at the graduate level, although they must take a series of undergraduate speech-language pathology and audiology courses to prepare for the more advanced courses in the major. After earning a bachelor's degree, a student needs to attend graduate school and it is at this level that individuals begin to specialize in either speech-language pathology or audiology. The entry-level requirement for speech-language pathologists to work professionally is an M.A. (Master of Arts) or M.S. (Master of Science). The entry-level requirement for audiologists is a doctoral degree, either a Ph.D. (Doctor of Philosophy) or Au.D. (Doctor of Audiology). After receiving a master's degree in speech-language pathology or a doctorate in audiology, passing the national examination, and becoming nationally certified and state licensed (to be discussed later), individuals become independent practitioners. In some countries (e.g., Great Britain, Australia, and New Zealand), a bachelor's degree in speech-language pathology (therapy or logopedics) is a professional degree; however, students begin their education in speech-language pathology in their freshman year of college, and their senior year is roughly equivalent to a graduate year in the United States.

Some individuals in speech-language pathology choose to continue their graduate education after their master's degree by pursuing a Ph.D. or Ed.D. (Doctor of Education). During their doctoral studies, which usually take 3 to 5 years after earning an M.A. or M.S., the individuals continue to specialize in either speech-language pathology or audiology. A few individuals also choose to become *dual certified*, that is, they must meet all educational, training, examination, and professional experience to qualify to be both a certified speech-language pathologist and an audiologist. In all clinical settings for SLPs and Auds, those with Ph.D.s have wide opportunities as teachers and professors, clinicians, and researchers. The following is a brief explanation of the work of speech-language pathologists and audiologists.

The Need for New Ph.D.s

Most men and women who earned Ph.D.s in the 1960s and 1970s in either speech-language pathology or audiology and who became university professors are retiring or have retired. This leaves a significant number of faculty positions in universities around the country struggling to be filled. For individuals with doctoral degrees interested in teaching at a university and doing research, employment prospects are excellent. If students beginning their education and training in speech-language pathology and audiology can look beyond the master's degree and consider pursuing a doctorate, they may find the rewarding (and relatively flexible) career as a university professor to their liking.

Speech-Language Pathologists

The American Speech-Language-Hearing Association has designated our professional title as *speech-language pathologist*; however, many other English-speaking countries prefer to use the designation *speech-language therapist* (e.g., England, Ireland, and New Zealand). What we are called by other professionals, clients, patients, and their family members depends somewhat on the setting in which we are working. For example, in public schools we are more likely to be called speech therapists, speech-language therapists, speech teachers (mostly by children), or speech and hearing specialists. In medical settings, we are commonly referred to by physicians, nurses, and patients as speech therapists or speech pathologists. Rarely is the entire designation *speech-language pathologist* used, perhaps because of the number of sounds and syllables in the complete title. Also, the terms **therapy** and *therapist* are positive terms that suggest helping (e.g., physical therapy, occupational therapy, and respiratory therapy) and include us as regular members of the rehabilitation team. The term *pathology* in the medical field typically connotes diseased tissue, and *pathologist* refers to a physician specializing in the study of diseases.

Outside of university clinics, the term *clinician* is not commonly used. (Interestingly, in textbooks we typically refer to ourselves as *clinicians* rather than *therapists*.) Many universities that train students to become speech-language pathologists refer to their departments as the Department of Communication (or Communicative) Disorders, Department of Communication Sciences and Disorders, or other variations around the term *communication*. However, in many countries around the world students train in a Department of Phoniatrics and Logopedics and become *logopedists*.

The education, coursework, and clinical training of speech-language pathologists are specified by ASHA. The national professional organization specifies coursework and clinical training requirements and standards to help with consistency throughout the country in the quality of new professionals. Upon completion of an M.A. or M.S. in the major, individuals are eligible to take the national *Praxis Examination* administered by the Educational Testing Service (ETS). In addition, to earn ASHA certification, individuals must complete a 36-week **Clinical Fellowship** of full-time work (35 hours per week) or the equivalent part-time experience totaling a minimum of 1,260 hours. After successful completion of all of these requirements, the person becomes a nationally certified speech-language pathologist.

Most states have licensing boards that specify criteria that must be met to be eligible for a state license to work in hospitals and practice independently. States also have credentialing boards that specify education and training criteria to work in public schools. ASHA, as well as most states, requires SLPs to earn **continuing education units (CEUs)** throughout their professional careers to keep abreast of new developments in the field and to maintain their state license or credential. CEUs are essential to the continued professional development of clinicians

---

therapy/treatment

Treatment of any significant condition to prevent, alleviate, or cure it; note: *therapy* and *treatment* are interchangeable.

Clinical Fellowship

A 36-week full-time (35 hours per week) or the equivalent part-time mentored clinical experience totaling a minimum of 1,260 hours begun after all academic coursework and university clinic training are completed; required by ASHA to be eligible for the Certificate of Clinical Competence (CCC).

continuing education units (CEUs)

Additional education or training required by ASHA and most states throughout a professional's career to help the professional remain current in the field.

Application Question

How could attending state and national conferences be valuable to your professional development and career?

and researchers and to strengthening the profession. CEUs are provided in numerous settings, such as national and state conferences and conventions, one- or two-day seminars and workshops provided at the local level, ASHA professional publications, and online coursework in an array of areas. SLPs may continue their formal education at any time by entering one of the many fine doctoral programs throughout the United States. An earned doctorate (Ph.D., Ed.D., or Au.D.) is usually required to be a university professor.

Scope of Practice

The **scope of practice** or work of speech-language pathologists may be described in a few words: we identify, evaluate, diagnose, and help (treat) people with communication and swallowing disorders. The following is a brief description of the primary roles in which speech-language pathologists may be involved when working with clients and patients.

Evaluate Communication and Swallowing Delays and Disorders

When a speech-language pathologist suspects a communication, cognitive, or swallowing problem, a thorough **evaluation** is in order (note: the terms *evaluation* and *assessment* may be used interchangeably). The evaluation generally includes an interview and standardized or *clinician-devised* assessments (i.e., nonstandardized tests designed for specific patients). The purposes of the evaluation are to determine, if possible, the cause of the problem, the nature of the problem, whether it is progressive or static, the characteristics of the problem, what makes it better and what makes it worse, the severity of the problem, treatment goals, and the potential for habilitation or rehabilitation.

Diagnose Communication and Swallowing Delays and Disorders

Making a **diagnosis** means the SLP makes a professional decision and commitment as to the specific diagnostic terms that may be used to represent the client's or patient's communication, cognitive, or swallowing problems. Specific diagnostic terms, with their associated billing codes, are necessary for SLPs to be reimbursed by insurance companies, Medicare, or other third-party payers. A written description of a client's or patient's problems in a formal report is essential, as is *documentation* (reporting) of all therapy goals, rationales, and treatment procedures.

Treat Communication and Swallowing Delays and Disorders

Most speech-language pathologists love doing therapy and developing creative strategies for helping clients and patients. Our best therapy is always based on sound research and theoretical principles with *evidence-based practice* (EBP) as the goal. Evidence-based practice is the integration of (a) clinical expertise, (b) best current evidence, and (c) client/patient perspectives to provide high-quality services reflecting the interests, values, needs, and choices of the individuals we serve.

scope of practice

ASHA's delineation of the general and specific areas in which speech-language pathologists and audiologists may engage with the appropriate and necessary education, training, and experience.

evaluation/assessment

The overall clinical activities designed to understand an individual's communication abilities and disabilities before a treatment program is determined and established. Also called assessment.

diagnosis

The determination of the type and cause of a speech, language, cognitive, swallowing, or hearing disorder based on the signs and symptoms of the client or patient obtained through case history, observations, interviews, formal and informal evaluations, and other methods.

The *art of therapy* involves flexibility and thinking on our feet. It also includes the understanding of when and how to use particular therapy approaches and techniques. No two therapy sessions are the same. Each session has its own uniqueness in the client's responses to the approaches, techniques, materials, and stimuli we present. In addition, the personal interactions and dynamics between the client and the clinician can vary from session to session and sometimes from moment to moment. Our insightfulness into our clients and their problems, our **clinical intuition**, and our counseling skills help make a challenging therapy session into a productive therapy session (Flasher & Fogle, 2012).

Work Settings

Speech-language pathologists work in a variety of work settings, with considerable diversity among clients and patients. The work settings can roughly be divided into educational and medical settings. The largest employer of speech-language pathologists is the public schools, with the legal mandate in the United States to provide services to every child from birth to 21 years of age, and to students who are in adult transition programs who need and qualify for services. Many SLPs also work in infant and early childhood programs funded by local and state agencies. Speech-language pathologists are working with increasingly complex clinical cases, including children with multiple handicaps, most with unidentified etiologies and others that are related to premature birth, mothers who abused substances during pregnancy, and children with HIV or AIDS.

On the other end of the educational spectrum, increasing numbers of speech-language pathologists are being employed by community colleges to provide services to older students and to direct or be involved with programs for people of all ages who have sustained neurological damage. Some speech-language pathologists also provide clinical supervision in university training programs and may do some clinical teaching.

Many SLPs work in medical settings of all types, including **acute care hospitals**, **subacute hospitals**, **convalescent hospitals**, and **inpatient** and **outpatient** clinics. *Home health care* (i.e., therapy in the patient's home) is an increasingly popular employment opportunity for SLPs. Home health care is designed to provide rehabilitation services without the high cost of hospitalization. *Private practice* provides opportunities for SLPs to work with a variety of clients or to specialize in a specific age group or disorder. Private practice also allows speech-language pathologists to have considerable independence and flexibility in their work schedules and allows them to develop their entrepreneurial skills (Fogle, 2001).

Aging presents an increasing number of clinically complex cases with multiple impairments. For example, it is not uncommon to see a patient with a hearing loss, stroke, heart disease, cancer, and visual impairments, along with arthritis and diabetes mellitus. Because speech-language pathologists are good communicators with good to excellent interpersonal skills, they are often advanced into administrative positions

---

clinical intuition

A decision-making process that is used unconsciously by experienced clinicians that is rapid, subtle, and based on the entire context of the situation, but does not follow simple, cause-and-effect logic.

acute care hospital

A hospital where patients are treated for brief but severe episodes of illness, injury, trauma, or during recovery from surgery.

subacute hospital

A level of care needed by patients who do not require acute care but who are medically fragile and require special services, e.g., respiratory therapy, intravenous tube feeding, and complex wound management care.

convalescent hospital/ skilled nursing facility (SNF)/extended care facility/nursing home

A medical facility, such as a skilled nursing facility, extended care facility, or nursing home, that provides extended medical, nursing, or custodial care for individuals over a prolonged period, e.g., during the course of a chronic illness or the rehabilitation phase after an acute illness or injury.

inpatient

A patient who has been admitted to a hospital or other health care facility for at least an overnight stay.

outpatient

A patient who is not hospitalized but is being treated in an office, clinic, or medical facility.

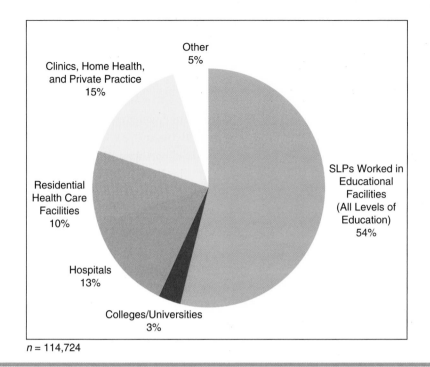

$n = 114{,}724$

Figure 2–4

ASHA-certified speech-language pathologists by primary employment setting.

Source: ASHA Summary Membership and Affiliation Counts, year ending 2010.

in various work settings, which increases their opportunities in a variety of ways (Lubinski, Golper, & Frattali, 2007).

Speech-language pathologists can devote their time to the age groups they most enjoy—for example, early childhood, school-age, adolescence, adult, or elderly. Many SLPs like working in more than one setting. For example, some clinicians work in public schools during the day as their primary job and work in hospitals or their own private practice for a few hours after leaving the school in the afternoon.

Job opportunities in foreign countries are plentiful; all industrialized countries have speech-language pathologists. In addition, military bases worldwide often provide speech-language pathologists for the dependents of service men and women who are being educated in schools on the base. Various military and VA hospitals have speech-language pathologists on staff. Figure 2–4 shows the primary employment settings of speech-language pathologists in 2010.

Employment Outlook

In articles on "The 50 Best Jobs in America" in the November 2009 and 2010 issues of *Money* magazine, speech-language pathology was rated as one of the best, with job satisfaction rated as very high. According to the U.S. Department of Labor's Bureau of Labor Statistics, in its *Occupational Outlook Handbook* (2010), the job outlook is very good for speech-language pathologists. The report projected that between 2010 and 2018 employment of speech-language pathologists is expected to grow by 19%, which is faster than the average for all other occupations. The outlook for a strong job market also exists in Canada, England, Australia, New Zealand, and other English-speaking countries

Application Question

Many people are surprised by our relatively broad scope of practice, the variety of clients and patients SLPs work with, and the array of work settings in which SLPs are employed. Are there any surprises for you?

with shortages of SLPs. If you are bilingual, your job market is even broader.

The number of jobs in all types of medical settings will continue to increase for SLPs, partly because of the growing elderly population's susceptibility to strokes. Also, because of the number of premature (i.e., under 5 pounds [2.7 kg]) and micropremature infants (i.e., under 2 pounds [.91 kg]) surviving, there will be increased needs for our services throughout much of their early development and education. As health care professionals and the public become more aware of the importance of identifying and diagnosing speech, language, and hearing problems, SLPs in clinics, home health care, and private practice are expected to see increasing needs for their services.

Anticipated growth in elementary, secondary, and special education enrollments, as well as other federally mandated services, has created more employment opportunities for speech-language pathologists in schools. There will continue to be a long-term shortage of speech-language pathologists in inner cities, rural, and less densely populated areas. Overall, speech-language pathologists will continue to be in great demand in many work settings and most communities in the United States and many other countries. Having a job you enjoy should never be a problem.

Audiologists

Audiologists are professionals who, "by virtue of academic degree, clinical training, and license to practice and/or professional credential, are uniquely qualified to provide a comprehensive array of professional services related to . . . the audiologic identification, assessment, diagnosis, and treatment of persons with impairments of auditory and vestibular function, and to the prevention of impairments associated with them" (American Academy of Audiology, 2004).

ASHA, in conjunction with the *American Academy of Audiology* (AAA), determines the education, coursework, and clinical training of audiologists. Audiologists must earn either a Ph.D. or Au.D., complete a clinical fellowship in audiology, and pass the national (ASHA) examination in audiology. Audiologists need to be licensed, credentialed, or both in their state of employment and must earn CEUs. In some states, in order for audiologists to work with and dispense hearing aids, they must also become licensed hearing instrument specialists.

Scope of Practice

Audiologists evaluate an individual's hearing loss to determine the type and extent of the loss. They further assess the benefits of amplification (e.g., hearing aids) and habilitation or rehabilitation to maximize the person's hearing ability. Many audiologists are able to sell and dispense hearing aids or other amplification devices as part of their practice. Most states have enacted legislation requiring universal screening of newborn infants, which has become an important new area of practice for audiologists. Another area of practice for some audiologists involves testing for balance disorders that may be associated with inner ear problems. As with speech-language pathologists, the scope of practice of audiologists is expanding.

Work Settings

Audiologists work in a variety of settings, including public schools, hospitals, clinics, private practices, and industry. Some audiologists also function as consultants to various agencies and help determine appropriate hearing conservation and protection requirements for state and local government employees, as well as industry standards. Some audiologists work in two or more settings in any one week—for example, private practice, industry, and consulting. Audiologists also teach and supervise in university programs. Even when a university does not offer an audiology program, an audiologist still must provide the basic coursework and training in audiology and aural rehabilitation for the speech-language pathology majors. Figure 2–5 shows the primary employment settings of audiologists in 2010.

Employment Outlook

The 2010 *Occupational Outlook Handbook* from the U.S. Department of Labor's Bureau of Labor Statistics reported that the job outlook is good for audiologists, projecting that between 2010 and 2018 there will be approximately a 25% increase in the need for audiologists. The number of jobs in all types of medical settings will continue to increase for audiologists, partly because of the growing elderly population susceptible to hearing losses. On the other end of the age spectrum, micropremature infants (weight less than 1 pound, 12 ounces [800 grams]) tend to have increased needs for audiological services throughout much of their early

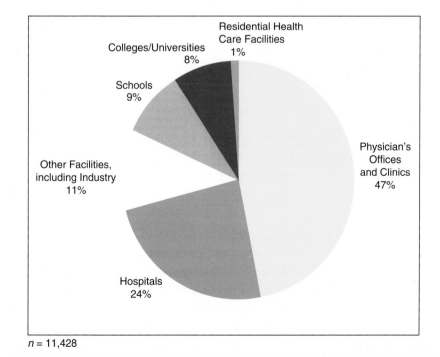

n = 11,428

Figure 2–5

ASHA-certified audiologists by primary employment setting.

Source: ASHA Summary Membership and Affiliation Counts, year ending 2010.

development and education. As health care professionals and the public become more aware of the importance of protecting hearing, identifying and diagnosing hearing problems, and wearing hearing aids as willingly as most people wear contact lenses or eyeglasses, audiologists are expected to see increasing needs for their services.

Audiologists also expect to see employment opportunities in schools grow if enrollment increases in elementary, secondary, and special education classes. The long-term shortage of audiologists in inner cities and less densely populated areas, including rural communities, is likely to continue. Overall, audiologists are and will be needed in many work settings and most communities worldwide.

Speech, Language, and Hearing Scientists

Speech, language, and hearing scientists are a relatively small portion of the professions (less than 5%). They have doctorates and mostly work in universities but also in government agencies, research centers, laboratories, or industry. Some also provide clinical services in either speech-language pathology or audiology. Depending on their specialty (speech, language, or hearing), these scientists usually are involved with *basic research*—that is, investigating the anatomy and physiology of the speech and hearing mechanisms, the physics and acoustics of speech-sound production, or the acquisition and structure of language. In many cases, they generate grants to carry on their research.

Speech, language, and hearing scientists are the skeletal framework of speech-language pathology and audiology because without them the normative data would not be available for clinicians to compare the normal with the abnormal or to understand the scientific rationales for many clinical procedures. The research data collected by scientists are essential to those who provide direct services to clients and patients of all ages. A firm grounding in normal communication processes through courses such as anatomy and physiology, speech science, and hearing science provides the foundation from which clinicians can better understand, diagnose, and treat communication disorders and delays.

Speech-Language Pathology Assistants

speech-language pathology assistant (SLPA)

A support person who performs tasks as prescribed, directed, and supervised by ASHA certified SLPs.

For individuals who do not want to or cannot pursue a B.A. and M.A. in speech-language pathology, ASHA established **speech-language pathology assistants (SLPAs)** as support personnel who, following academic and/or on-the-job training, perform tasks prescribed, directed, and supervised by ASHA certified speech-language pathologists. Individuals may earn an Associate of Arts degree (AA) in speech-language pathology assistant training programs. According to ASHA guidelines and state licensure laws, no speech-language pathologist can employ an SLPA without a certified speech-language pathologist as a supervisor. SLPAs are more commonly employed in school-based programs than in medical settings or clinics. ASHA is the credentialing body that offers a national registration process to ensure basic knowledge and competencies are developed for those wanting to become SLPAs. Many SLPAs eventually choose to pursue a B.A. and M.A. to become state licensed and ASHA certified speech-language pathologists (Moore & Pearson, 2003).

The following is a list of SLPA responsibilities taken from Background Information and Criteria for the Registration of Speech-Language Pathology Assistants (ASHA, October, 2000).

- Assist the SLP with speech-language and hearing screenings (without interpretation).
- Follow documented treatment plans or protocols developed by the supervising SLP.
- Document patient/client performance (e.g., tally data for the SLP to use; prepare charts, records, and graphs) and report this information to the supervising SLP.
- Assist the SLP during assessment of patients/clients.
- Assist with informal documentation as directed by the SLP.
- Assist with duties such as preparing materials and scheduling activities as directed by the SLP.
- Collect data for quality improvement.
- Perform checks and maintenance of equipment.
- Support the SLP in research projects, in-service trainings, and public relations programs.
- Assist with departmental operations (e.g., scheduling, record keeping).
- Exhibit compliance with regulations, reimbursement requirements, and other responsibilities associated with the assistant position.

Audiology Assistants

The American Academy of Audiology has defined the functions of audiology assistants (AAA, 2006).

> An audiology assistant is a person who, after appropriate training and demonstration of competence, performs delegated duties and responsibilities that are directed and supervised by an audiologist. The role of the assistant is to support the audiologist in performing routine tasks and duties so that the audiologist is available for the more complex evaluative, diagnostic, management and treatment services that require the education and training of a licensed audiologist (p. 5).

The duties of an audiology assistant may include equipment maintenance, hearing aid repair, neonatal screening, preparation of patients for electrophysiologic and balance testing, hearing conservation, air-conduction hearing evaluation, assisting the audiologist in testing, record keeping, clinical research, and other tasks after full and complete training and delineation by the supervising audiologist.

The minimal educational background for an audiology assistant is a high school diploma or equivalent, and competency-based training.

Some community colleges and online training programs offer an Associate Degree in Audiology for training of audiology assistants. However, the state licensed audiologist who employs and supervises an assistant must assure that the assistant can perform all duties and responsibilities that are delegated (AAA, 2010).

CHAPTER SUMMARY

You have begun learning about the professions and professionals of speech-language pathology and audiology, and you are in good company. Most countries with speech-language pathologists and audiologists have strong national organizations that help support and regulate the professions. There are excellent job opportunities throughout the United States and in many other countries for both professions. The people who study and work in these professions are interesting and caring people who enjoy helping others. These professionals are team players who interact regularly with colleagues, as well as many other professionals.

STUDY QUESTIONS

Knowledge and Comprehension

1. By helping a child with a communication delay or impairment, whom in the child's life are you also helping?

2. By helping an adult with a communication impairment, whom in the adult's life are you also helping?

3. Why is it important, as students and professionals, to use person-first language?

4. What is the "team approach" and why is it important in the work of speech-language pathologists and audiologists?

5. What is the American Speech-Language-Hearing Association (ASHA)?

6. What is the National Student Speech-Language-Hearing Association (NSSLHA)?

Application

1. Discuss how you might use some of the information you learn in this text and course in your personal life, even if you do not become a speech-language pathologist or audiologist.

2. What are three qualities of effective professionals? How could you apply these to your personal life?

3. How are public laws affecting the work of speech-language pathologists and audiologists?

4. What are some specific things you could do to keep yourself abreast of new developments in the profession?

Analysis/Synthesis

1. What are the similarities and differences between speech-language pathologists and audiologists?

2. Why is it important for a professional organization (e.g., ASHA) to specify the education, coursework, and training of individuals entering a profession?

3. Why might speech-language pathologists be referred to by different titles, depending on the setting in which they work?

REFERENCES

Aiken, T. D. (2008). *Legal and ethical issues in health occupations.* Philadelphia, PA: W. B. Saunders.

American Academy of Audiology. (2004). Audiology: Scope of practice. *Audiology Today, 16*(3), 44–45.

American Academy of Audiology. (2006). Position statement on audiologist's assistants. *Audiology Today, 18*(2), 27–28.

American Academy of Audiology. (2010). Audiology assistant task force report. *Audiology Today, 22*(3), 68–73.

ASHA. (2000). Background information and criteria for the registration of speech-language pathology assistants. Rockville, MD: ASHA.

Bureau of Labor Statistics. (2010). *Occupational outlook handbook, 2004–2005 edition.* Washington, DC: U.S. Department of Labor.

Flasher, L. V., & Fogle, P. T. (2012). *Counseling skills for speech-language pathologists and audiologists* (2nd ed.). Clifton Park, NY: Delmar Cengage Learning.

Fogle, P. T. (2001). Professors in private practice: Rediscovering the joy of therapy. *Advance for Speech-Language Pathologists & Audiologists,* 18–19.

Lubinski, R., Golper, L. A. C., & Frattali, C. (2007). *Professional issues in speech-language pathology and audiology* (3rd ed.). Clifton Park, NY: Delmar Cengage Learning.

Miller, T. D. (2007). Professional ethics. In R. Lubinski, L. Golper, & C. Frattali (Eds.). *Professional issues in speech-language pathology and audiology* (3rd ed.). Clifton Park, NY: Delmar Cengage Learning.

Moeller, D. (1975). *Speech pathology & audiology: Iowa origins of a discipline.* Iowa City, IA: The University of Iowa Press.

Moore, S. M., & Pearson, L. D. (2003). *Competencies and strategies for speech-language pathology assistants.* Clifton Park, NY: Delmar Cengage Learning.

NSSLHA. (2010). *Communication sciences: Student survival guide.* Clifton Park, NY: Delmar Cengage Learning.

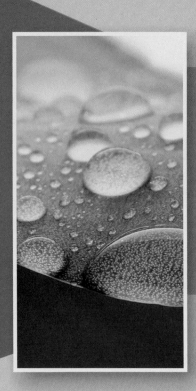

CHAPTER 3
Anatomy and Physiology of Speech and Language

LEARNING OBJECTIVES

After studying this chapter, you will:

- Understand the essentials of the anatomy and physiology of respiration.
- Be able to discuss the contributions of the respiratory system to the production of speech.
- Understand the essentials of the anatomy and physiology of phonation.
- Be able to discuss the contributions of the phonatory system to the production of speech.
- Understand the essentials of the anatomy and physiology of resonation.
- Be able to discuss the contributions of the resonatory system to the production of speech.
- Understand the essentials of the anatomy and physiology of articulation.
- Be able to discuss the contributions of the articulatory system to the production of speech.
- Understand the essentials of the anatomy and physiology of the nervous system.
- Be able to discuss the contributions of the nervous system to speech, language, and cognition.

KEY TERMS

abduct
adduct
alveolar ridge
alveolar sacs
anoxia

arytenoid cartilages
auditory comprehension
axon
Bernoulli's law

brainstem
Broca's area
cartilage
central nervous system

KEY TERMS continued

cerebellum
cerebral hemisphere
cortex
cricoid cartilage
decibels (dB)
deciduous teeth
deglutition
dendrite
dentition
diaphragm
epiglottis
executive functions
expiration
   (exhalation)
false vocal folds
   (ventricular folds)
formulate
frequency
hard palate
hertz (Hz)
incisors
inspiration

integrate
intensity
intonation
labia
larynx
malocclusion
mandible
mastication
maxilla
motor
myofunctional
   therapy
neuron
occlusion
open bite
orbicularis oris
peripheral nervous
   system
phonation
process
produce
protrude

range of motion
reflex
resonance
respiration
retract
sensory
soft palate
   (velum)
spinal cord
synapse
thoracic cavity
thyroid cartilage
tongue (lingua,
   glossus)
trachea
true vocal folds
uvula
velopharyngeal
   closure
voice quality

CHAPTER OUTLINE

INTRODUCTION

Therapy to improve speech usually focuses on helping children and adults do something different with their articulators (mandible, lips, and tongue) to be more intelligible to their listeners or to have smoother, more fluent speech. However, clinicians need to know and understand the anatomy and physiology of each of the speech systems (respiratory, phonatory, resonatory, and articulatory) and the nervous system to evaluate and treat clients with all types of communication disorders. The foundations of speech are the *anatomy* (structures) and *physiology* (functions and movements) of each of the speech systems. Before any muscle contracts or relaxes in order for each speech system to perform with near perfect timing, the brain must actively decide what will be communicated and how. Most of the processes involved with producing speech are never consciously thought about until we make a speech error or have a communication disorder. Clinicians need to be aware of each speech system (and sometimes specific muscle groups) when working with clients and patients in order to help them make subtle changes so they can better communicate their messages.

THE RESPIRATORY SYSTEM

Other than the beating of our heart, our respiratory system works harder than any other organ in our body. Every minute while sitting quietly, we breathe (one inhalation and one exhalation) about 15 times, or about once every 4 seconds. In 1 hour we breathe about 900 times and in 1 day we breathe more than 20,000 times. To **produce** voice (**phonation**) and speech, humans have learned to control **respiration** by taking quick, short **inspirations (inhalations)** and sustaining the **expirations (exhalations)**. An intricate and interdependent balance exists between respiration and phonation. The first demand of the respiratory system is to supply freshly oxygenated blood to every cell in our bodies and to rid our bodies of the carbon dioxide (CO_2) that is produced when we use up the oxygen (O_2). Producing voice is an *overlaid function* (i.e., not necessary to sustain life) of the respiratory system.

Structures of Respiration

The bones in the chest (*rib cage* and *sternum/breastbone*) provide protection and a framework for the respiratory system. The **thoracic cavity (thorax)** is the upper part of the trunk that contains the principle

---

produce/production

In speech, to create an utterance (sound, syllable, word, sentence, or longer) that is spontaneous or imitated.

phonation (voice)

The vibration of air passing between the two vocal folds that produces sound that is used for speech.

respiration (ventilation, pulmonary ventilation, breathing)

The movement of air into and out of the lungs that allows for the exchange of oxygen and carbon dioxide.

inspiration (inhalation)

The process of drawing air into the lungs.

expiration (exhalation)

The process of breathing air out of the lungs.

thoracic cavity (thorax, rib cage, chest)

The upper part of the trunk that contains the organs of respiration (lungs) and circulation (heart).

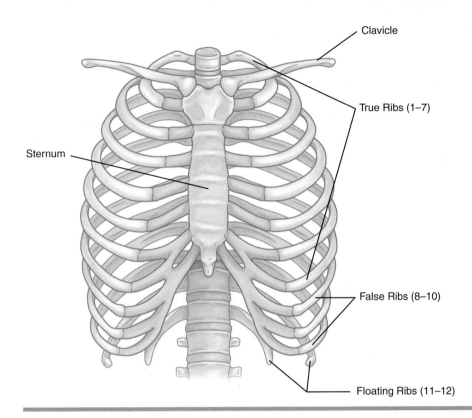

Clavicle

True Ribs (1–7)

Sternum

False Ribs (8–10)

Floating Ribs (11–12)

Figure 3–1

Anterior view of the skeletal framework for respiration.

© Cengage Learning 2013.

organs of respiration (lungs) and circulation (heart). The thorax extends from the *clavicle* (collarbone) and first rib down to the twelfth rib. The ribs attach to the sternum in the center of the chest and the *vertebral (spinal) column* is in the back. The bones of the thoracic cavity (plus the *pelvis*) provide attachments for the many muscles involved in respiration (see Figure 3–1).

During quiet breathing, inspired air enters through the nostrils and flows into the nose and *nasal cavities,* where it is warmed, moistened, and filtered. From the nasal cavities, the air passes through the *larynx* and flows past the open *vocal folds*. The **trachea**, or "windpipe," begins just below the larynx and continues down to where it divides into the lungs. The trachea is a tube about 4 to 5 inches (10 to 13 cm) long and 1 inch (2.5 cm) in diameter and is formed by about 20 rings made of **cartilage** (see Figure 3–2). The bottom of the trachea divides into the *mainstream (primary) bronchi,* which enter into the left and right lungs. The bronchi continue to divide into smaller diameter branches and extend out much like the branches of a tree.

Muscles of Respiration

Twenty-six pairs of muscles are involved in the processes of inspiration and expiration. Most are used during quiet breathing, and additional muscles are used during forced inspiration or expiration. We will only discuss some of the most important muscles involved in respiration.

trachea (windpipe)

The tube that begins just below the larynx and continues down to where it divides into the lungs; carries air down to and up from the lungs.

cartilage

Firm, fibrous, and strong connective tissue that does not contain blood vessels.

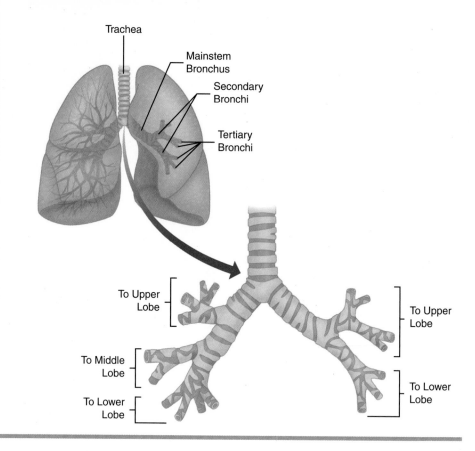

Figure 3–2

Trachea and bronchial tree.

© Cengage Learning 2013.

diaphragm

A large, dome-shaped muscle that separates the thoracic and abdominal cavities and is the main muscle of respiration; during inspiration it moves down to increase the volume in the thoracic cavity, and during expiration it moves up to decrease the volume.

The **diaphragm** is the primary muscle involved with respiration. It is a large, dome-shaped muscle that separates the thoracic and abdominal cavities. During inspiration, it moves down and increases the volume in the thoracic cavity; during expiration, it moves up and decreases the volume. In the thoracic cavity, the volume changes affect the air pressures, which allow air to passively or actively flow into or out of the lungs (see Figure 3–3). Between each rib are muscles that help raise and lower the ribcage during inspiration and expiration (the muscles you eat when eating pork spare ribs). The muscles over the stomach are important in *forced exhalation* when we pull in our stomachs to try to blow out air. When these muscles are well developed they are sometimes called "six-pack abs."

The Respiratory Process

During a single, quiet respiratory cycle, several neurological and physiological processes are occurring. The respiratory center in the brainstem sends messages to the muscles we use for inhalation. The diaphragm contracts and lowers, and the rib cage slightly raises and expands. The volume (space) inside the thoracic cavity increases, which decreases the air pressure inside the lungs. The difference in air pressure between the environmental air and the pressure in the lungs causes air from the outside to flow through the nose, down the trachea, and into the lungs to equalize the pressure (inhalation). The millions of **alveolar sacs** (similar to the holes in a sponge) that make up the lungs are expanded

alveolar sacs (alveoli, air sacs)

The spongy tissue of the lungs where gas exchange takes place; walls of alveoli are one cell thick and porous, allowing rapid transfer of fresh O_2 into the capillary bed surrounding the alveoli, and of CO_2 from the capillary bed into the alveoli to be exhaled.

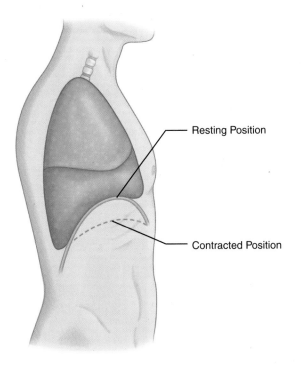

Resting Position

Contracted Position

LATERAL VIEW

Figure 3-3

Lateral-view schematic of the diaphragm showing relative positions during quiet (passive) inspiration and expiration.

© Cengage Learning 2013.

and stretched slightly (much like a balloon that is blown up part way). Because the alveolar sacs cannot remain in a stretched position for long, they begin to relax (deflate), which forces the air back out of the lungs and up the trachea. At the same time, the expanded chest relaxes down, creating more *intrathoracic air pressure* and contributing to the air being forced out of the lungs (exhalation) (Seikel, King, & Drumright, 2010).

THE PHONATORY SYSTEM

The voice is probably one of the speech systems that we most take for granted. The anatomy and physiology of the **larynx** (voice box) are both simple and complex. The simplicity of the anatomy is that the individual structures of the larynx are basically stacked on top of one another; the complexity is that each structure can move in various subtle ways that can alter the loudness, pitch, and quality of the voice. The simplicity of the physiology of the larynx is that the various muscles both inside and outside the larynx can only contract and relax; the complexity is that the precise combinations and amounts of muscle contraction and relaxation can provide the beautiful, pure sounds of opera singers or the grating, strident voices of some people.

Framework of the Larynx

The larynx is located between the top of the trachea and just below the horseshoe-shaped *hyoid bone* that helps support it. Several cartilages make up the larynx, including (1) the circular shaped **cricoid cartilage**

larynx (pl. larynges) (voice box)

Located just above the trachea, the structure that contains cartilages, muscles, and membranes that produce voice by air passing between the vocal folds.

cricoid cartilage

A solid circle of *cartilage* (nonvascular dense supporting connective tissue) shaped like a signet (class) ring located below and behind the thyroid cartilage and on top of the first tracheal ring.

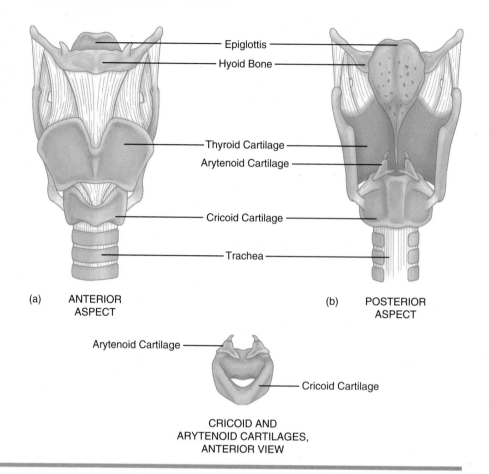

Figure 3–4

(a) Anterior and
(b) posterior views
of the larynx.

© Cengage Learning 2013.

thyroid cartilage

The largest of the *laryngeal cartilages* that is the main structure of the larynx and encloses and protects the vocal folds; its *anterior* (front) point is popularly referred to as the "Adam's apple."

arytenoid cartilages

A pair of pyramid-shaped cartilages that sit on top of the posterior edge of the cricoid cartilage and rotate to open and close the vocal folds and pivot back and forth to help change the pitch of the voice.

epiglottis

A large cartilage that is wide at the top and narrow at the bottom that is attached to the anterior edge of the cricoid cartilage and drops over the vocal folds like a lid to prevent food and liquid from entering the trachea and lungs when swallowing.

that sits on top of the first tracheal ring and is below and behind the thyroid cartilage; (2) the large **thyroid cartilage** that is the main structure of the larynx and encloses and protects the vocal folds (its *anterior* [front] point is popularly referred to as the "Adam's apple" [*laryngeal prominence*]); (3) the two pyramid shaped **arytenoid cartilages** that sit on top of the *posterior* (back) portion of the cricoid cartilage and rotate to open and close the vocal folds and pivot back and forth to help change the pitch of the voice; and (4) the **epiglottis**, a large cartilage that is wide at the top and narrow at the bottom (like a leaf or egg that comes to a sharp point) that has an important role protecting the airway during swallowing (see Figure 3–4).

The Vocal Folds

Two pairs of vocal folds, the **true vocal folds** and the **false vocal folds** (**ventricular folds**), stretch across the airway. When talking about the *vocal folds* we are referring to the true vocal folds unless we specifically say *false (ventricular) vocal folds.* (Note: SLPs prefer the term "vocal folds" over "vocal cords" because they are two folds of tissue with attachments on the sides of the thyroid cartilage rather than two "cords" [thick strings] with attachments at either end, although the term *cord* is acceptable in some medical literature.) The true vocal folds are muscles covered with mucous membranes that make them look pearly white (see Figure 3–5).

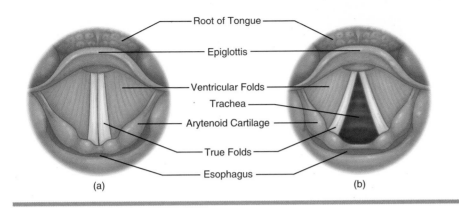

Root of Tongue

Epiglottis

Ventricular Folds

Trachea

Arytenoid Cartilage

True Folds

Esophagus

(a)   (b)

Figure 3–5

Superior view of the vocal folds (a) closed and (b) open.

© Cengage Learning 2013.

---

true vocal folds

Paired muscles (thyroarytenoid and vocalis) covered with mucous membranes with a pearly white appearance inside the thyroid cartilage at the level of the Adam's apple that open and close extremely rapidly to produce voice; closure during swallowing protects the trachea and lungs from penetration of food and liquid.

false vocal folds

Paired, thick folds of mucous membranes with few muscle fibers that lie just above the true vocal folds in the larynx at the level of the laryngeal prominence (*Adam's apple*); they do not vibrate during speech but close tightly during swallowing to prevent material from entering the trachea.

abduct/abduction

The opening of the vocal folds away from the midline.

adduct/adduction

The closing of the vocal folds toward the midline.

The biological function of the vocal folds is to prevent food and liquid from entering the trachea and lungs, and their overlaid function is to produce voice. Each vocal fold is composed of two joined muscles that are covered by a *mucous membrane* (membrane that protects a structure, secretes mucus, and absorbs water, salts, and other materials).

The vocal folds lie in the midline at the level of the laryngeal prominence. When looking down upon the true vocal folds, they have a V shape when open, with the upper point of the V facing anteriorly and the two lower points attaching to the two arytenoid cartilages posteriorly. The space between the open vocal folds is referred to as the *glottis*. Because the trachea below the vocal folds is circular, the shape and position of the vocal folds create a constriction for air passing into or out of the larynx. The false vocal folds lie slightly superior to the true vocal folds inside the thyroid cartilage and are composed of thick mucous membranes with few muscle fibers. They do not vibrate during speech but close tightly during swallowing to prevent material from entering the trachea.

Vocal Fold Vibration

During normal breathing the vocal folds are at rest and partially open (**abducted**), but when we want to phonate the vocal folds must close (**adduct**). (Note: *Abduct* is usually pronounced "A-B-duct," with the "A" and "B" pronounced as the first two letters of the alphabet to prevent confusion between the similar sounding *adduct* and *abduct*.) To produce voice, the vocal folds are told by the brain to close and simultaneously the respiratory system is sent a message to exhale air. As the air coming up the trachea reaches the closed vocal folds *subglottic air pressure* (air pressure below the vocal folds) builds up and blows the vocal folds open in the shape of a football or rugby ball with both the anterior and the posterior points closed. However, because the vocal folds have been told by the brain to stay closed, their elasticity, along with **Bernoulli's law** (a law of physics involving airflow and air pressure) causes them to instantaneously close again, which causes subglottic air pressure to build and then blow them open again. One complete open-close (abduct-adduct) sequence is referred to as a complete *vibratory cycle*. Every time the open phase occurs in the vibratory cycle, a small "puff" of air escapes and travels up to our mouths to be articulated.

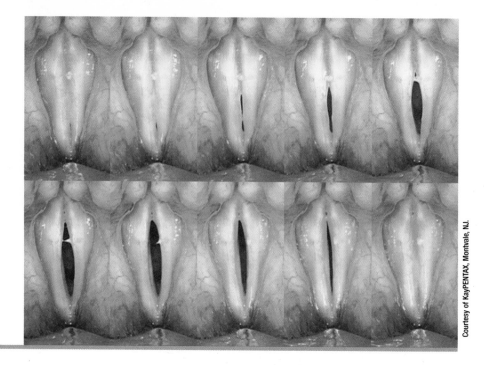

Courtesy of KayPENTAX, Montvale, NJ.

Figure 3-6

Stroboscopic film images of the vocal folds during one complete vibratory cycle.

Bernoulli's law (principle)

A law in physics that states when air flowing through a tube (e.g., trachea) reaches a constriction (e.g., vocal folds) there is an increase in speed of the flow of air that causes decreased pressure on the walls of the constriction that results in a slight negative pressure (i.e., slight vacuum) at the constriction; in voice, this slight negative pressure contributes to the vocal folds closing during vibration; (Daniel Bernoulli, Swiss scientist, 1700–1782).

frequency

In speech, the number of complete cycles (opening, closing) per second that the vocal folds vibrate; *pitch* is the psychological perception of frequency.

hertz (Hz)

The unit of vibration adopted internationally to replace cycles *per second* (CPS).

It is the extremely rapid puffs of air that escape that we perceive as voice (Hixon, Weismer, & Hoit, 2008) (see Figure 3-6).

Frequency, Intensity, and Quality of Voice

Frequency is the number of complete cycles (opening, closing) per second that the vocal folds vibrate per second. *Pitch* is the psychological perception (sensation) of frequency. Frequency is measured in **hertz (Hz)** and a frequency of 100 complete cycles per second (opening-closing) of the vocal folds would be 100 Hz. The rate at which the vocal folds vibrate during normal voicing of the "ah" sound is a person's *fundamental frequency* (f_0). Adult males typically have a fundamental frequency of about 120 Hz and adult females have a fundamental frequency of about 220 Hz.

Intensity, in reference to voice, is the force with which the vocal folds open and close and the amount of air that escapes between the open vocal folds (the puffs of air). *Loudness* is the psychological perception of intensity. Intensity is measured in **decibels (dB)**. A person's average intensity level is related to how loud other people perceive the person (some people are perceived as loud talkers and others as soft spoken). During normal conversation, we use subtle interactions of loudness, pitch, and duration of sounds to give our speech **intonation** (i.e., some variability, "vitality" or "life").

The auditory perceptual judgments of **voice quality** are highly subjective. Generally voice quality is affected by adequate vocal fold closure, efficient timing of closure, and the amount of muscle tone of the folds. Normal voice quality is difficult to describe and may be described more easily by saying what it is *not* rather than what it is. Nicolosi, Harryman, and Kresheck (2004) describe normal voice quality as nontense, nonbreathy, not having extraneous noise, and being easily produced and sustained throughout phonation. However, the voice that is produced at the level of the vocal folds is actually a rather raucous buzzing sound, somewhat like hearing the mouth piece of a saxophone being blown without the rest of the horn to alter the vibration of the reed by adding resonance.

THE RESONATORY SYSTEM

The structures important for normal speech and **resonance** are the facial structures, the articulators, the hard and soft palates, and the pharyngeal region. The anatomy and physiology of these may affect speech intelligibility. When anatomy is abnormal the secondary effect is abnormal physiology. However, it is possible to have intact structures and still have abnormal function resulting in disorders of resonance (e.g., when there is weakness in the muscles of the soft palate).

Embryological Development of the Upper Lip and Palates

The first trimester of pregnancy is crucial in facial and palatal development, with the lips and hard and soft palates forming. The upper and lower lips have formed by 8 weeks gestation and the shape of the upper lip is typically referred to as the "cupid's bow" (see Figure 3–7). Between the 8th and 12th weeks of gestation, the hard and soft palates of the roof of the mouth are formed and fused together, with the fusion occurring in an anterior to posterior direction (see Figure 3–8). We need to keep in mind how very small each of these structures is during the embryological development and the numerous potential influences that may interfere with normal facial and palatal development.

Hard and Soft Palates

The **maxilla** (upper jaw) contains the **hard palate**, which is a thin, bony, shelf-like structure that is covered by mucous tissue and separates the

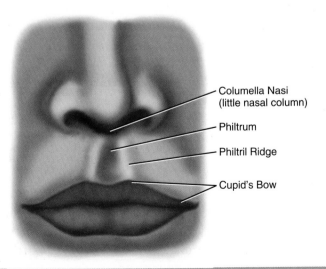

Columella Nasi
(little nasal column)

Philtrum

Philtril Ridge

Cupid's Bow

Figure 3–7

Landmarks of the lips.

© Cengage Learning 2013.

---

intensity

In reference to voice, the force with which the vocal folds open and close and the amount of air that escapes between the open vocal folds; *loudness* is the psychological perception of intensity.

decibels (dB)

A basic unit of measure of the intensity of sound; it is one-tenth of 1 bel (B); an increase in 1 bel is perceived as a 10-fold increase in loudness.

intonation

Variations in pitch on syllables, words, and phrases that produce *stress* to give emphasis and meaning to utterances.

voice quality

The auditory aspects of the function of the vocal folds that is affected by adequate closure, efficient timing of closure, and the amount of muscle tone of the vocal folds; normal voice quality is a described as nontense, no extraneous noise, nonbreathy, and easily produced and sustained throughout phonation.

resonance

The quality of the voice that results from the vibration of sound in the vocal tract (i.e., spaces and tissues of the pharynx, oral cavity, and nasal cavity).

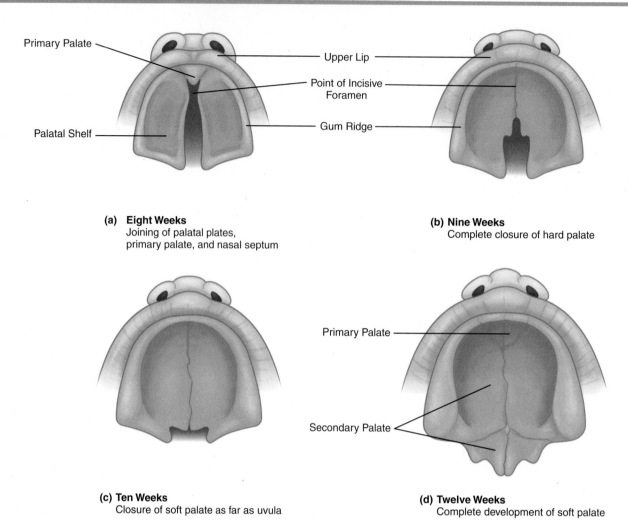

(a) **Eight Weeks**
Joining of palatal plates, primary palate, and nasal septum

(b) **Nine Weeks**
Complete closure of hard palate

(c) **Ten Weeks**
Closure of soft palate as far as uvula

(d) **Twelve Weeks**
Complete development of soft palate

Figure 3–8
Development of the hard and soft palates looking up toward the roof of the mouth.
© Cengage Learning 2013.

maxilla

The upper jaw that includes the hard palate and contains sockets for the upper teeth; forms much of the midfacial structure.

hard palate

The bony anterior two-thirds of the roof of the mouth that separate the oral cavity from the nasal cavity.

alveolar ridge (alveolar process, dental arch)

The upper portion of the mandible and the lower portion of the maxilla that contain sockets for the roots of the teeth.

oral cavity from the *nasal cavity* (see Figure 3–9). The hard palate is the anterior two-thirds of the roof of the mouth. The ridge surrounding the hard palate on three sides is referred to as the **alveolar ridge**, which is covered by the "gums" (*gingiva*). The anterior portion of the hard palate is the *premaxilla*, which holds the four front teeth. The rest of the hard palate is composed of the *maxillary* and *palatine bones* (two on each side of the midline). Down the center of the hard palate a slight ridge can be felt with the tip of the tongue, which is where the two halves of the hard palate have fused together during the first trimester of gestation. However, wherever there is supposed to be a fusion there is the possibility that fusion may not occur, which can result in a cleft. The hard palate provides points of contact for tongue placement to produce several sounds (e.g., the tongue tip makes contact with the alveolar ridge just behind the top front teeth to produce a /t/ or /d/). The posterior border of the hard palate is the location of the beginning of the **soft palate (velum)**.

The soft palate is the muscular structure that forms the posterior one-third of the roof of the mouth. At the posterior end of the soft palate

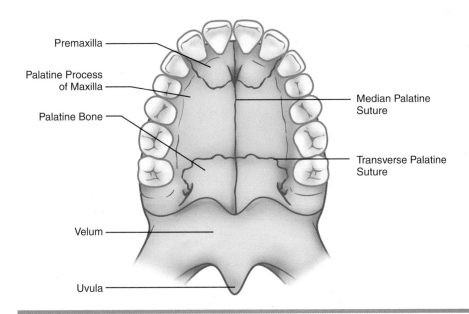

Figure 3-9

Bony structures of the hard palate.

© Cengage Learning 2013.

is the **uvula**, the cone-shaped structure that hangs from the back of the soft palate but does not have any known function. At rest, the soft palate is down and rests near the base of the tongue, which allows an open passageway for breathing through the nose. During speech, the soft palate raises and moves posteriorly (up and back) to make contact with the *posterior pharyngeal wall* (back of the throat) to separate the oral cavity from the nasal cavity for all oral sounds (vowels and consonants) except /m/, /n/, and "ng." Those three sounds are *nasal sounds* and are produced with the soft palate down. The terms *velopharyngeal mechanism* and *velopharyngeal system* refer to the *velum* and the *lateral* and *posterior pharyngeal walls* at the level of the velum (see Figure 3–10). The upward and backward movement of the soft palate to make contact with the posterior pharyngeal wall to close off the coupling of the oral and nasal cavities is referred to as **velopharyngeal closure**.

THE ARTICULATORY SYSTEM

The biological purpose of the mouth is not speech but eating, although most people do more talking than eating. We need to keep in mind that the actions of each articulator are determined by the neurological impulses sent from the brain to tell specific muscles when, how much, and how long to contract or relax. The **sensory** and **motor** systems of the brain are involved in every movement of an articulator. This is noteworthy for both SLPs and Auds because it emphasizes that our therapy to improve articulation (as well as all other aspects of communication) causes changes in neuronal firing and synaptic connections inside the brain.

The Skeletal Structures of Articulation

Numerous bones make up the face and skull, but SLPs are primarily concerned with the maxilla (see above) and **mandible**. The mandible

soft palate (velum)

The muscular tissue in the posterior one-third of the roof of the mouth that separates the oral cavity from the nasal cavity when raised and in contact with the posterior pharyngeal wall.

uvula

The cone- or teardrop-shaped structure that hangs from the back of the soft palate but does not have any known function.

velopharyngeal closure

The upward and backward movement of the soft palate to make contact with the posterior pharyngeal wall to close off the coupling of the oral and nasal cavities.

sensory

Pertaining to sensation or awareness of stimuli that are received in the central nervous system.

motor

Pertaining to motion or movement; nerve cells that initiate and regulate contracting and relaxing of muscle fibers.

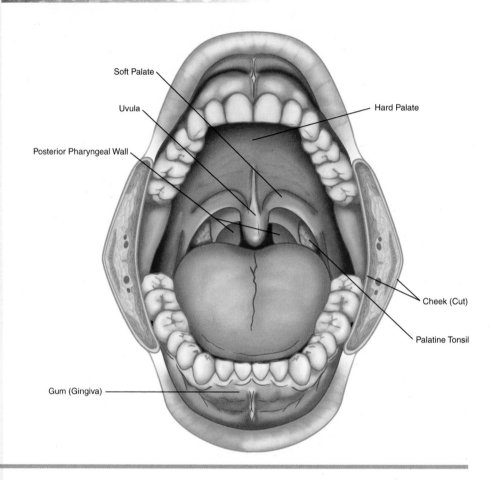

Soft Palate

Uvula

Posterior Pharyngeal Wall

Hard Palate

Cheek (Cut)

Palatine Tonsil

Gum (Gingiva)

Figure 3–10

Anterior view of the oral cavity.

© Cengage Learning 2013.

mandible

The lower jaw that is hinged to the temporal bone for opening and closing and contains sockets for the lower teeth.

is the lower jaw that is hinged to the temporal bones of the skull (*temporomandibular joins—TMJ*) for opening and closing the mouth. Like the maxilla, the mandible's alveolar ridge is covered by *gingiva* ("gums") and contains sockets for the lower teeth. The mandible is normally held in a closed position so that the lips are touching but the teeth are not in contact with the maxillary teeth. During speaking the mandible moves up and down only slightly in the production of many sounds, but a more open mouth position allows more sound to escape, creating a "megaphone" effect and a louder voice.

Facial Muscles

The facial muscles are connected to the numerous bones that make up the front and sides of the skull, including the *frontal bone* (forehead), *temporal bones* (sides of the skull behind and around the ears), *zygomatic bones* (cheek bones), maxilla, and mandible. Although we do not use all of our facial muscles for articulation, we use most of them for communicating our facial expressions, which may either agree or disagree with the words we are articulating.

Lips and Cheeks

labia

Pertaining to the lips.

The biological function of the lips (**labia**) is to hold food and liquid in the oral cavity during chewing, drinking, and swallowing, and the overlaid function is to help with the articulation of some speech sounds. The lips are particularly sensitive to touch so that nothing can enter the mouth (and possibly be swallowed) without a person's awareness. The muscular structure of the lips is the oval-shaped sphincter **orbicularis oris**. The lips are the second most important articulator and have several movements that involve speech: opening, closing, rounding, flattening, **protruding**, and **retracting**. The timing and extent of each of these movements help shape various sounds and allow sounds to exit the mouth.

The *masseter* and *buccinator* muscles make up the bulk of the cheeks, and the inner surfaces of the cheeks are covered with mucous membranes. Biting and chewing are the biological purposes of these muscles, and their overlaid function is to contribute to the production of oral sounds.

Tongue

The three biological functions of the **tongue** (**lingua** or **glossus**) are taste, movement of food in the mouth while chewing (**mastication**), and movement of food and liquid posteriorly for swallowing (**deglutition**). Taste is achieved through the taste buds, which give the tongue its characteristic rough texture. Speech requires the most rapid and complex muscular coordination in the entire body and the tongue is the primary articulator. The slightest movement can modify the air stream to produce the numerous consonants and vowels in our language, as well as the countless different sounds and dialects articulated by speakers of languages around the world (see Figure 3–11).

orbicularis oris

The muscle surrounding the opening of the mouth; the muscular structure of the lips.

protrude

In speech, the puckering of the lips forward or the movement of the tongue forward past the lips.

retract

In speech, the pulling back of the lips past their neutral, resting position or the movement of the tongue back into the oral cavity after protrusion or past the neutral, resting position.

tongue (lingua/lingual or glossus/glossal)

The primary articulator, whose movements creates consonants and vowels as well as perform biological functions.

mastication

The act of chewing food in preparation for swallowing and digestion.

deglutition

The act of swallowing.

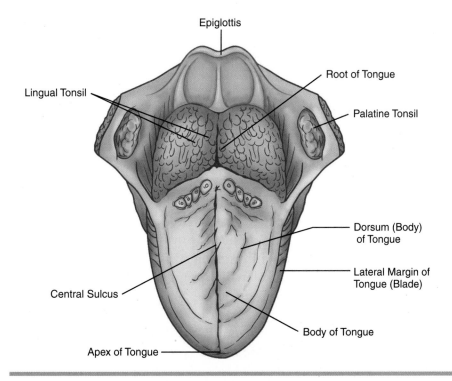

Figure 3–11

The tongue.

© Cengage Learning 2013.

The tongue is divided in the midline by the *central sulcus* and is made up of eight pairs of muscles on each side. Four of the muscle pairs help *position* (protrude, retract, elevate, depress, lateralize) the tongue in the mouth and four of the muscle pairs help *shape* (round, flatten, groove, hump) the tongue to refine the production of specific sounds. Any significant abnormalities in **range of motion**, strength, coordination, or rate of ability to move, position, or shape the tongue rapidly and precisely may noticeably affect speech intelligibility.

Tongue Thrust

Tongue thrust refers to the habitual pushing of the tongue against the inner surface of the front teeth (**incisors**) or the protrusion of the tongue between the upper and the lower teeth. Although the tongue is not thrust forward forcefully when producing *sibilant sounds* (e.g., /s, z/), the forward movement creates distortions of sibilants (i.e., a *frontal lisp*). Some children have a tongue-resting position with the tongue tip lightly pressing against the frontal incisors, and during swallowing they tend to push the tongue forward against the incisors (sometimes referred to as a *tongue thrust swallow* or *reverse swallow*), which may contribute to misalignment of teeth. Some clinicians take additional training in the area of **myofunctional therapy** to provide intervention for tongue thrust and have had considerable success helping children who have problems in this area. Some orthodontists refer children who have a tongue thrust to an SLP for management before proceeding with placement of appliances (braces).

Dentition

Development of the **dentition** begins in utero when tooth buds are forming. The **deciduous teeth** (primary or "baby teeth") usually begin to erupt between six and nine months of age, with the lower incisors erupting first and the upper incisors after that. Teeth continue to erupt over 18–24 months until all 20 (10 uppers and 10 lowers) are in place. *Shedding* (losing) of the deciduous teeth usually occurs between 6 and 13 years of age, with the front teeth being lost first (first-grade school photographs are often permanent records of the beginning of this process). During the shedding, permanent teeth erupt to replace the deciduous teeth. There are 32 permanent ("adult teeth"), with 16 in the upper dental arch and 16 in the lower dental arch (i.e., four incisors [two central and two lateral], two canines, four premolars, and six molars in each arch).

There are three basic dental **occlusions** (see Figure 3–12). Class I (*neutrocclusion*) is considered the normal relationship in which the upper incisors are slightly forward of the lower incisors and the molars of the upper and lower dental arches are in proper relationship and alignment. In class II **malocclusion** (*overbite*), the upper incisors are considerably anterior of the lower incisors. In class III malocclusion

range of motion/movement (ROM)

For speech, the limits the mandible can open and close, the lips can protrude and retract, and the tongue can protrude, retract, elevate, lower, and move side to side (*lateralize*).

incisors

The four front upper and lower teeth (central and lateral incisors).

myofunctional therapy

Treatment designed to correct a tongue thrust or habitual forward-resting position of the tongue against the front teeth.

dentition

The type, number, and arrangement of teeth in the maxilla and mandible, including the incisors, cuspids (canines), bicuspids (premolars), and molars.

deciduous teeth

The set of 20 teeth that appear during infancy and early childhood (10 uppers, 10 lowers), with the front teeth appearing (erupting) through the gums about 6 months of age; all 20 teeth normally have erupted by 18–24 months. Shedding (losing) the deciduous teeth occurs between 6 and 13 years of age.

occlusion

The process of bringing the upper and lower teeth into contact.

malocclusion

Misalignment of the maxillary teeth with the mandibular teeth.

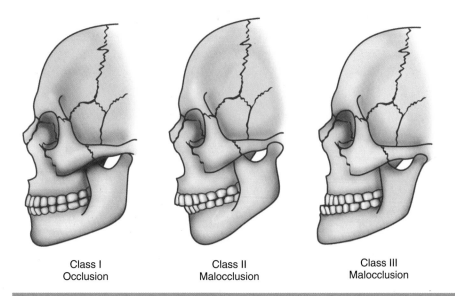

| Class I Occlusion | Class II Malocclusion | Class III Malocclusion |

Figure 3-12

Types of dental occlusions.

© Cengage Learning 2013.

(*underbite*) the upper incisors rest behind the lower incisors and the mandible juts forward. An **open bite** (not one of the three classes) describes an abnormal vertical space between the anterior maxillary and mandibular teeth that often allows the tongue tip to be seen when a person smiles.

It has long been known that there is not a strong relationship between dentition and articulation of speech because the articulatory mechanism (especially the tongue and lips) is highly adaptable (Bernthal, Bankson, & Flipsen, 2009). People rapidly and automatically make subtle adjustments of their articulators while talking, when chewing gum, or after receiving a local anesthetic at the dentist office. Most pipe smokers learn to articulate clearly with a pipe clenched tightly between their teeth. Although mild dental anomalies usually do not affect articulation of sounds and speech intelligibility, severe dental malocclusions or missing front teeth may contribute to or result in some articulation errors.

THE NERVOUS SYSTEM

The brain is a three-pound glob of matter, the consistency of Jell-O and the color of day-old slush. The brain contains about 100 billion **neurons** (cell bodies) and each neuron has thousands of connections to other neurons, giving us trillions of connections within the brain. Every fleeting thought, emotion, and movement is the result of chemical and electrical activity within our brains. Our brains understand many things, but what the brain does not understand is *how* the brain understands. How does the brain transform sight, sound, touch, taste, and smell into thoughts and emotions? Where in the brain does a thought begin and where does it go from there? What happens when the brain does not do what it is supposed to do? Humans will never fully understand the brain—and perhaps we are never meant to (see Figure 3–13).

open bite

An abnormal vertical space between the anterior maxillary and mandibular teeth that often allows the tongue tip to be seen when a person smiles.

neuron (gray matter)

The basic nerve cell of the nervous system, containing a nucleus within a cell body and extending an axon and multiple dendrites.

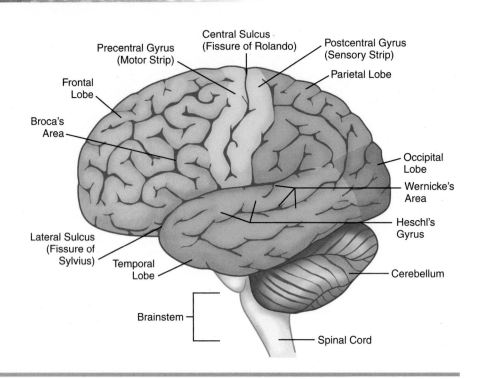

Figure 3-13

The brain, cerebellum, and brainstem.

© Cengage Learning 2013.

---

process/processing

In reference to neurological functioning, the activation of neurons (hundreds to millions at any instant) with their impulses sent through axons and dendrites to other neurons to bring about general and specific cognitive, linguistic, and motor activity.

axon (white matter)

The cellular extension of a neuron that carries impulses away from the cell body.

dendrite (white matter)

A branching extension of a neuron that carries impulses to the cell body.

synapse

The junction at which two neurons communicate with each other.

central nervous system (CNS)

The brain, cerebellum, brainstem, and spinal cord.

Before any of the speech systems are set in motion, the brain must **process** countless bits of information to decide what needs to be communicated and how. The motor and sensory systems then initiate every movement of the structures and muscles that will communicate the message. As SLPs and Auds we need to keep in mind that all of our therapy for hearing, speech, language, cognition, and swallowing disorders involves the brain. That is, whether we are working with a child or adult with a hearing impairment, an articulation disorder, language disorder, stuttering problem, neurological disorder, or any other communication or swallowing disorder, we are working with neurons, **axons**, **dendrites**, and **synapses** within the person's brain to change the way muscles contract and relax for specific behaviors to occur. More subtly, when we are helping people change their attitudes, thoughts, feelings, and reactions toward their communication problems (e.g., stuttering), we are working on new or different neuronal connections within the brain (see Figure 3–14).

The Central Nervous System

The **central nervous system (CNS)** is composed of the brain (*cerebrum*), cerebellum, brainstem, and spinal cord. All incoming and outgoing signals are generated and processed through the CNS. The skull rests on the *atlas*, the top vertebra in the spinal column, named after the mythical figure Atlas who carried the world on his shoulders. Essentially, our brain is our world.

The brain is divided into left and right **cerebral hemispheres** that look grossly the same; however, their functions differ significantly. Each hemisphere has four lobes (*temporal, frontal, parietal,* and *occipital*).

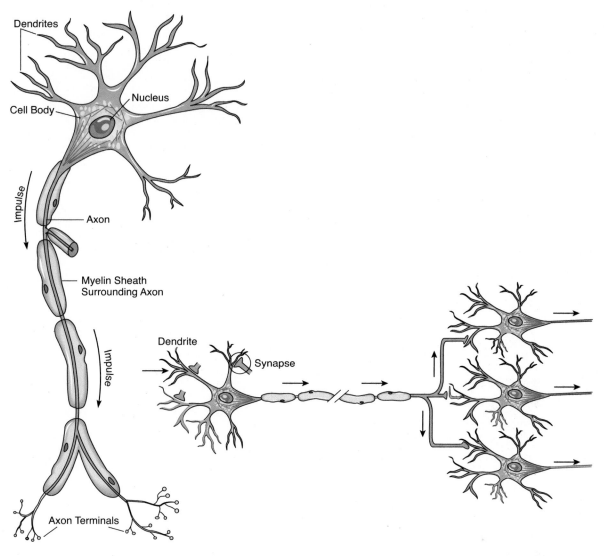

Figure 3-14

Neurons, axons, dendrites, and synapses.

© Cengage Learning 2013.

The left hemisphere is important for receptive and expressive language and speech, for processing rapidly changing information, and for perceiving and analyzing information in a sequential order (e.g., sounds in words and words in sentences). The left hemisphere is commonly referred to as the *dominant hemisphere* for speech, language, and motor functioning. Approximately 95% of right-handed people have dominant left hemispheres and approximately 80% of left-handed people have dominant left hemispheres for speech and language even though their right hemisphere is dominant for motor functioning (Nolte, 2008).

The right hemisphere is particularly important for *attention, orientation* (e.g., self-awareness, where the person is, time of day, etc.),

cerebral hemisphere

Either of the two halves of the brain that contains a frontal lobe, parietal lobe, occipital lobe, and temporal lobe.

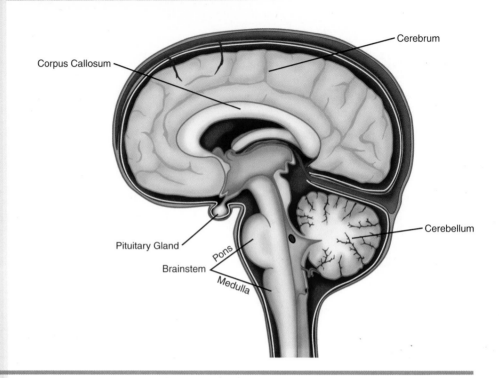

Figure 3-15

Corpus callosum. Midline view of the brain.

© Cengage Learning 2013.

---

cortex (gray matter)

The outer layer (approximately one-fourth to one-half inch) of brain tissue containing nerve cell bodies (neurons).

---

emotions, and *cognition* (Ponsford, 2004). The two hemispheres of the brain work together because they are connected by a large band of nerve fibers (*corpus callosum*) in the center of the brain (see Figure 3-15). Both hemispheres are needed to competently and completely analyze information from the various modalities (auditory, visual, tactile, taste, and smell), and to program an appropriate and timely response (Carter, 2009; Gazzaniga, 2004).

Most of the estimated 100 billion neurons in the brain are in the **cortex**—the outer one-fourth to one-half inch of brain tissue. The cell bodies in various areas of the brain have similar structures but diverse functions, which allow different brain areas to have various responsibilities. When the brain is damaged, millions or even billions of neurons, axons, dendrites, and synapses may not function normally or at all (see Figure 3-16).

The brain has a limited capacity to process incoming stimuli; therefore, it must focus its attention on relevant stimuli and ignore or inhibit much of the other stimuli. For example, in a noisy room filled with people we try to attend to one or two people talking while ignoring all other sounds and words that are reaching our ears. Likewise, we try to visually ignore all people and objects in the room that may distract us from the person we are visually focusing on. At the same time, we are ignoring almost everything touching our bodies, from our clothes to jewelry, yet attending to the glass we are holding. Nevertheless, our discussion of language processing focuses on auditory skills, keeping in mind that similar processing may be occurring in other modalities.

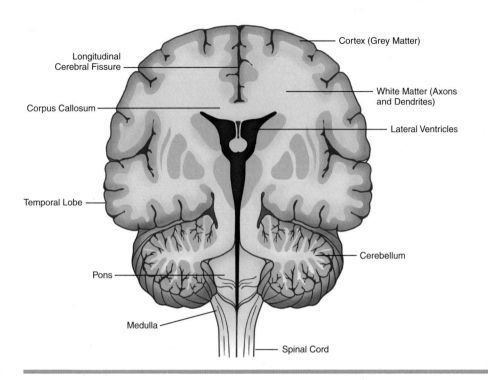

Figure 3-16

Corpus callosum. Cross section of the brain.

© Cengage Learning 2013.

Blood Circulation in the Brain (Cerebrovascular System)

Three arteries supply each hemisphere of the brain (see Figure 3-17). Although the brain weighs only about 3 pounds, it uses 20% to 25% of the blood that is pumped from the heart, depending on the activity level of the brain. This means, for example, that a 150-pound person will use 20% to 25% of his blood every minute for just 2% of his body. When the oxygen-rich blood is prevented from reaching the brain for several seconds (**anoxia**), a person will lose consciousness, and if blood and oxygen cannot reach the brain for just a few minutes, irreversible brain damage will result (e.g., in cases of *near-drowning*). The brain can function normally only with the help of the extensive vascular system supplying it with blood.

Temporal Lobes

The temporal lobes lie behind the frontal lobes, under the parietal lobes, and in front of the occipital lobes. The temporal lobes are essential for *auditory processing* of sounds and language processing. Nerve impulses from the ears are received by the *primary auditory cortex (Heschl's gyrus)* at the top margins of the temporal lobes. The right ear sends impulses to the left hemisphere's primary auditory cortex and the left ear sends impulses to the right hemisphere's primary auditory cortex; however, the information received in the right hemisphere must cross over by way of the corpus callosum to the left hemisphere's temporal lobe for language processing. The primary auditory cortex of both hemispheres perceives sounds as human speech or *environmental* sounds (e.g., animals, telephone ringing, and all other nonhuman sounds)

anoxia

Lack of oxygen in the brain usually caused by asphyxiation (e.g., near-drowning or loss of airway from choking) or inadequate blood circulation (e.g., heart attack) that results in unconsciousness and death of brain tissue.

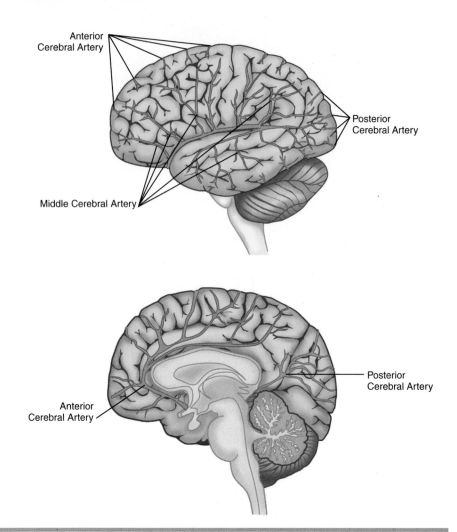

Figure 3-17

The major cerebral arteries (red—middle cerebral artery, blue—anterior cerebral artery, green—posterior cerebral artery).
© Cengage Learning 2013.

auditory comprehension

The ability to understand spoken language at the single word, phrase, simple sentence, complex sentence, paragraph, and conversational speech levels.

but does not interpret their meanings. The auditory information is then sent to an area of the cortex called *Wernicke's area* for interpretation and language processing. Wernicke's area lies just behind the primary auditory cortex but is only in the left temporal lobe in right-handed people, as well as the vast majority of left-handed people (recall the discussion of the dominant hemisphere).

Language Processing

Language processing is a complex phenomenon for the brain that involves not only Wernicke's area in the left hemisphere, but may involve all lobes of the brain at any given instant. SLPs and Auds typically are more concerned about auditory processing than visual or tactile processing. However, when we are in conversation with someone, our brains are processing information from all modalities being stimulated (including in some situations taste and smell, such as when talking about food).

Language processing and **auditory comprehension** involve numerous areas and functions within the brain and occur simultaneously (Bellis, 2002; Geffner & Ross-Swain, 2007). Auditory comprehension begins when meaning is attached to auditory information. However, to comprehend, **integrate**, and **formulate** language, all lobes in both hemispheres of the brain may be involved. Overall, we cannot separate auditory, visual, and tactile processing of information from cognition (Byrnes, 2007). We use language for cognition and we use cognition to comprehend, integrate, and formulate language. When language is impaired, cognition is impaired; when cognition is impaired, language processing is impaired.

Frontal Lobes

The frontal lobes are located behind the forehead and are the largest lobes of the brain. The *prefrontal cortex* (anterior two-thirds of the frontal lobes) is essential for cognition and, along with the right hemisphere of the brain, is involved in a variety of mental activities, including attention, reasoning, judgment, decision making, and problem solving. Our personalities, character, philosophies, religious beliefs, political orientation, and abilities to monitor and regulate our own behaviors, set goals and see them through (**executive functions**) are largely functions of the anterior portions of our frontal lobes (Casey, Gledd, & Thomas, 2000; Sowell, Dells, Stiles, & Jernigan, 2001). We develop our cognitive skills and ability to make thoughtful, wise decisions because of maturity of our brains, learning, and life experiences.

Behind the prefrontal cortex lie the motor areas (*premotor cortex* and *motor cortex*) that generate the impulses for voluntary movement. The left premotor and motor cortex of the brain control the right side of the body, and the right premotor and motor cortex control the left side of the body. The largest portions of the premotor and motor cortex are for movements of the face and hands. **Broca's area** in the premotor cortex of the left hemisphere controls motor movements of the articulators for speech. The motor cortex takes direction from the premotor cortex and is the primary pathway for carrying neural impulses to muscles throughout the body.

Motor Control of Speech

To communicate with Broca's area in the left frontal lobe of the brain, Wernicke's area in the left temporal lobe sends impulses over an axonal pathway (the *arcuate fasciculus*) to Broca's area. Broca's area plans, sequences, coordinates, and initiates the motor movements of the articulators. After this processing, the information is conveyed to the motor cortex in the left and right frontal lobes for execution. Simultaneous feedback by the *sensory cortex* in the left and right parietal lobes allows for fine adjustments of the articulators. Speech is a *sensorimotor* process that involves the parietal lobes for feedback about muscle activity (Kent, 2004; Duffy, 2005). The production of speech is an extraordinarily complex process that involves extensive interaction of different areas of the brain in rapid coordination (see Figure 3–18).

---

integrate/integration

In neurology, the process of combining information from various input modalities, attaching meaning and interpreting the information, storing (remembering), and making decisions about responding.

formulate/formulation

In language, the choice of words and grammatical structures in the construction of a meaningful verbal expression.

executive functions

A composite of the following activities related to goal completion: anticipation, goal selection, planning, initiation of activity, self-regulation or self-monitoring, and use of feedback to adjust for future responses.

Broca's area

The center for motor speech control (planning, sequencing, coordinating, and initiating) of the articulators located in the lower posterior portion of the left hemisphere's frontal lobe.

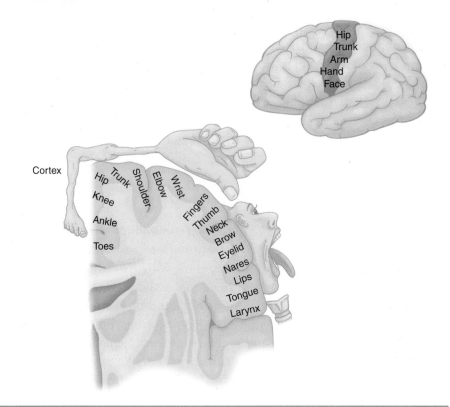

Figure 3-18

Homunculus (L. *homo*, man, + *uncula*, little), representing relative amounts of cortical areas devoted to motor movements.

© Cengage Learning 2013.

Parietal Lobes

The parietal lobes lie just behind the frontal lobes. The left parietal lobe receives sensations from the right side of the body and the right parietal lobe receives sensations from the left side of the body. The anterior portion of the parietal lobes is important in the *tactile* (touch) detection of objects touching the body. The largest portions of the parietal lobes are for sensations of the hands and face, including sensations of taste from the tongue. The remaining areas of the parietal lobes interpret what is detected and integrate bodily sensations such as temperature, touch, pressure, and pain (*somesthetic information*).

Occipital Lobes

The occipital lobes are in the back of the brain and lie posterior and inferior to the parietal lobes. Impulses from the retinas of the eyes travel along the optic nerve to the most posterior areas of the occipital lobes where visual images are received. The visual images are then processed in the *visual association cortex* (the rest of the occipital lobes) to interpret what is seen and enable the cerebrum to use the information. The occipital lobes also are involved with recognizing and interpreting spatial relationships, such as judging distance and seeing things in three dimensions.

Cerebellum, Brainstem, and Spinal Cord

The **cerebellum** lies just below the temporal and occipital lobes and communicates with the brain, brainstem, and spinal cord. The cerebellum is important in coordinating muscle groups for complex motor activity to

cerebellum

The CNS structure largely concerned with the coordination of muscles and the maintenance of balance and body equilibrium.

allow for smooth, accurate movements of the body, limbs, and articulators. The cerebellum is also essential in maintaining balance and equilibrium.

The two components of the **brainstem** (*pons* and *medulla oblongata* [*medulla*]) connect the brain to the spinal cord. All sensory and motor impulses sent to and from the brain pass through the brainstem. Most sensory and motor nerve fibers cross over at the level of the medulla in the brainstem, which is the reason the left hemisphere of the brain controls the right side of the body and the right hemisphere controls the left side of the body. The brainstem controls the face, mouth, and larynx, for the production of speech.

Twelve pairs of *cranial nerves* exit the pons and medulla and course to the mouth, face, neck, and shoulders (see Figure 3–19). The 12 pairs

brainstem

The structure (pons and medulla oblongata [medulla]) that connects the brain to the spinal cord; it is important in sensory and motor functions and contains neurons for the cranial nerves that exit the pons and medulla.

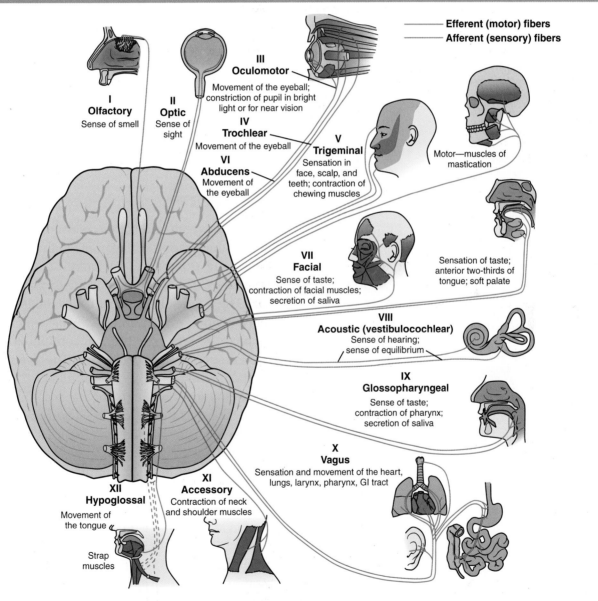

Figure 3-19

Brainstem and cranial nerves coursing to the head and neck.

© Cengage Learning 2013.

of cranial nerves have both motor and sensory pathways for impulses to be sent from the brain to the muscles and for impulses from the muscles to be sent back to the brain. Seven of the cranial nerves are important for speech: *trigeminal* (V) [face and jaws], *facial* (VII) [face and tongue], *vestibulocochlear* or *auditory* (VIII) [hearing and balance], *glossopharyngeal* (IX) [tongue and pharynx], *vagus* (X) [larynx, respiration, heart, gastrointestinal system], *accessory* (XI) [neck and shoulder], and *hypoglossal* (XII) [tongue and neck].

The **spinal cord** is a thick "cord" (approximately the diameter of a finger) of nerve fibers located in the passageway of the vertebral column. The spinal cord *conducts* (sends) sensory and motor impulses of the body to and from the brain and controls many body **reflexes**. Thirty-one pairs of spinal nerves originate from the spinal cord and send branches to innervate every muscle of the body below the face.

Peripheral Nervous System

The **peripheral nervous system (PNS)** is composed of the cranial nerves that exit from the brainstem and the spinal nerves that exit from the spinal cord (see Figure 3–20). The PNS allows the body to communicate sensory information to the brain and the brain to communicate motor information to the body.

CHAPTER SUMMARY

Respiration is the exchange of oxygen and carbon dioxide between the lungs and the environment. Inspiration (inhalation) is the process of drawing air into the lungs, and expiration (exhalation) is the process of breathing air out of the lungs. The diaphragm is the primary muscle involved with respiration. The trachea begins just below the larynx and continues down to where it divides into the lungs. The trachea branches into the left and right primary bronchi; the bronchi continue to divide into smaller branches until they enter the alveolar sacs. The alveolar sacs make up the lung tissue and do the real work of respiration.

The larynx is located at the superior end of the trachea. The thyroid cartilage is what we normally consider the "voice box." The true vocal folds are paired muscle tissue covered with mucous membranes with a pearly white appearance. Closure of the vocal folds helps prevent material from entering the trachea and lungs (their biological purpose), and vibration produces voice (their overlaid function). The vocal folds close (adduct) and open (abduct) to produce voice for one complete vibratory cycle. Pitch is the psychological sensation of the physical property of the frequency of a sound and is measured in hertz (Hz). Loudness is the psychological sensation of the intensity of a sound and is measured in decibels (dB).

The structures important for normal speech and resonance are the facial structures, the articulators, the hard and soft palates, and the pharyngeal region. The first trimester of pregnancy is crucial in facial and palatal development. The maxilla (upper jaw) contains the hard palate

---

spinal cord

A thick "cord" of nerve fibers that passes through the vertebral column that conducts sensory and motor impulses to and from the brain and controls many body reflexes.

reflex

An involuntary response to a sensory input, such as the corneal reflex in which both eyes blink in response to something irritating an eye; the gag reflex, caused by something touching the posterior wall of the pharynx; and the knee jerk (deep tendon) reflex, caused by a sharp tap just below the knee.

peripheral nervous system (PNS)

The cranial nerves that exit the brainstem and the spinal nerves that exit the spinal cord that allow the body to communicate sensory information to the brain and the brain to communicate motor information to the body.

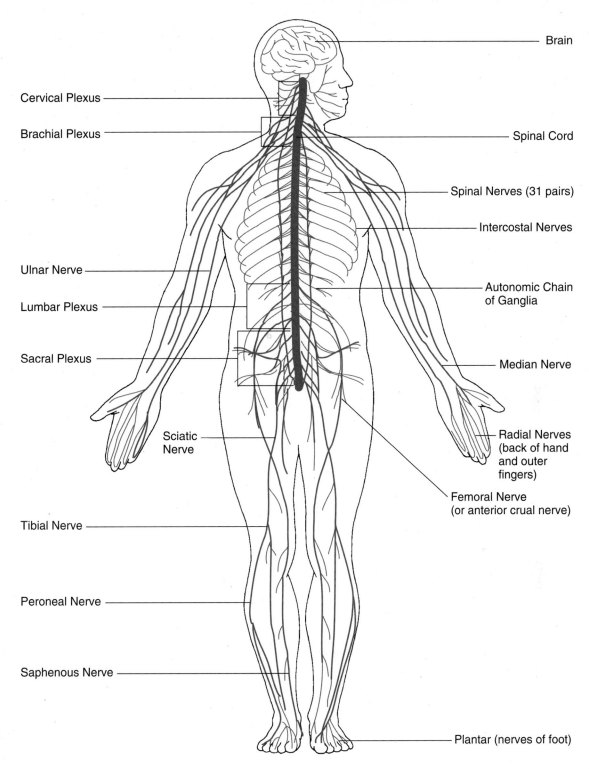

Brain

Cervical Plexus

Brachial Plexus

Spinal Cord

Spinal Nerves (31 pairs)

Intercostal Nerves

Ulnar Nerve

Autonomic Chain of Ganglia

Lumbar Plexus

Sacral Plexus

Median Nerve

Sciatic Nerve

Radial Nerves (back of hand and outer fingers)

Femoral Nerve (or anterior crual nerve)

Tibial Nerve

Peroneal Nerve

Saphenous Nerve

Plantar (nerves of foot)

Figure 3-20

The peripheral nervous system.

and is the anterior two-thirds of the roof of the mouth. The soft palate is the muscular posterior one-third of the roof of the mouth that separates the oral cavity from the nasal cavity when raised.

The structures important for articulation are the maxilla, mandible, lips, and tongue. The lips and tongue are the two most important articulators. It is the timing and extent of their movements that help shape various sounds and allow sounds to exit the mouth.

The central nervous system is composed of the brain (*cerebrum*), cerebellum, brainstem, and spinal cord. All incoming and outgoing signals are generated and processed through the CNS. The brain is divided into left and right cerebral hemispheres, with each hemisphere having a frontal, parietal, occipital, and temporal lobe. The left hemisphere is the dominant hemisphere for speech and language and the right hemisphere is very important for cognition.

STUDY QUESTIONS

Knowledge and Comprehension

1. Define inspiration and expiration.
2. Describe the true vocal folds and their functions.
3. Explain the anatomical relationship of the hard palate to the soft palate.
4. Why is it important to keep in mind that the physiology of each articulator is determined by the neurological impulses sent from the brain to the muscles?
5. What are the primary functions of the left hemisphere of the brain?

Application

1. How could difficulty inspiring a normal amount of air during a normal breath affect voice?
2. How could you explain respiration and phonation (voice) to an 8-year-old child who has a voice disorder, including some important anatomical (body) terms?
3. How could you explain to an adult client how the soft palate moves during speech?
4. Why could a person have severe speech, voice, and swallowing problems following damage to the brainstem?
5. How could damage to a person's frontal lobes severely affect his quality of life?

Analysis/Synthesis

1. Why is it important to be able to explain in nontechnical terms the processes of respiration and phonation to clients?

2. Why is it important to understand the movement of the soft palate during speech?

3. Discuss the concept that speech requires essentially perfect timing and coordination of muscle contraction and relaxation for precision of articulator movements.

4. Compare and contrast the functions of the left hemisphere with those of the right hemisphere.

5. Why are auditory comprehension and language processing essentially inseparable?

REFERENCES

Bellis, T. (2002). *Assessment and management of central auditory processing disorders in the educational setting: From science to practice* (2nd ed.). Clifton Park, NY: Delmar Cengage Learning.

Bernthal, J. E., Bankson, N. W., & Flipsen, P. (2009). *Articulation and phonological disorders* (6th ed.). Upper Saddle River, NJ: Pearson.

Byrnes, J. P. (2007). *Cognitive development and learning in instructional context* (3rd ed.), Boston, MA: Allyn and Bacon.

Carter, R. (2009). *The human brain book.* London: DK Publishers.

Casey, B., Gledd, J., & Thomas, K. (2000). Structural and functional brain development and its relation to cognitive development. *Biological Psychology, 54,* 241–257.

Duffy, J. R. (2005). *Motor speech disorders: Substrates, differential diagnosis, and management* (2nd ed.). Philadelphia, PA: Elsevier Mosby.

Gazzaniga, M. S. (Ed.). (2004). *The cognitive neurosciences* (3rd ed.). Boston, MA: Massachusetts Institute of Technology.

Geffner, D., & Ross-Swain, D. (2007). *Auditory processing disorders: Assessment, management and treatment.* San Diego, CA: Plural Publishing.

Hixon, T. J., Weismer, G., & Hoit, J. D. (2008). *Clinical speech science: Anatomy, physiology, acoustics, perception.* San Diego, CA: Plural Publishing.

Kent, R. D. (2004). The uniqueness of speech among motor systems. *Clinical Linguistics and Phonetics, 18*(6), 495–505.

Nicolosi, L., Harryman, E., & Kresheck, J. (2004). *Terminology of communication disorders: Speech-language-hearing* (5th ed.). Philadelphia, PA: Lippincott Williams & Wilkins.

Nolte, J. (2008). *The human brain: An introduction to its functional anatomy* (6th ed.). Philadelphia, PA: Elsevier Mosby.

Ponsford, J. (2004). *Cognitive and behavioral rehabilitation: From neurobiology to clinical practice.* New York, NY: Guilford Press.

Seikel, J. A., King, D. W., & Drumright, D. G. (2010). *Anatomy and physiology for speech, language, and hearing* (4th ed.). Clifton Park, NY: Delmar Cengage Learning.

Sowell, E., Dells, D., Stiles, T., & Jernigan, J. (2001). Structural and functional brain development and its relation to cognitive development. *Journal of International Neuropsychological Society, 7,* 312–319.

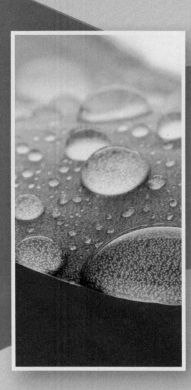

CHAPTER 4
Speech and Language Development

LEARNING OBJECTIVES

After studying this chapter, you will:

- Be able to discuss each of four theories of speech and language development.
- Be able to discuss the four general stages of speech development that children follow in any language or culture.
- Be familiar with multicultural considerations of speech and language development.

KEY TERMS

accent

babbling

behavioral theory

bilingual

blend

code switching

cognitive development

communicative competence

cooing

cultural–linguistic diversity (CLD)

culture

dialect

discourse

echolalia

English as a second language (ESL)

functor (function) words

holophrastic language

inner speech

jargon

language development

lexicon

mean length of utterance (MLU)

multicultural

narrative

nativistic theory

natural processes

neonate

KEY TERMS continued

operant (instrumental)
  conditioning

parallel speech

parentese

phonological processes

prelinguistic (preverbal)
  vocalizations

semantic-cognitive theory

social-pragmatic theory

speech development

standard dialect

stress

telegraphic speech (language)

utterance

vocal play

CHAPTER OUTLINE

Introduction
Theories of Speech and Language Development
  Behavioral Theory
  Nativistic Theory
  Semantic-Cognitive Theory
  Social-Pragmatic Theory
  Cultural and Linguistic Diversity Perspective
Speech Development
  Stage I: Birth–12 Months (Infancy)
  Stage II: 12–24 Months (Toddlerhood)
  Stage III: 2–5 Years (Early Childhood)
  Stage IV: 6–12 Years (Middle Childhood to Early
        Adolescence)
Language Development
  Stage I: Birth–12 Months (Infancy)
  Stage II: 12–24 Months (Toddlerhood)
  Stage III: 2–5 Years (Early Childhood)
  Stage IV: 6–12 Years (Middle Childhood to Early
        Adolescence)
Chapter Summary
Study Questions
References

INTRODUCTION

Speech and **language development** in infants and children is a complex and intricately interrelated process. For normal communication to develop there must be an integration of anatomy and physiology of the speech systems, neurological development, and sufficient interaction for infants and children to be encouraged and rewarded for communication attempts. Language development involves the development of both receptive language (i.e., what a child understands of what is said) and expressive language (i.e., the words, grammatical structures, and meanings that a child uses verbally) (Owens, 2012).

THEORIES OF SPEECH AND LANGUAGE DEVELOPMENT

Four general theories explain much of speech and language development: behavioral, nativistic, semantic-cognitive, and social-pragmatic. Although not necessarily considered a theory of language development, speech-language pathologists and audiologists need to be aware of cultural and diversity perspectives.

Behavioral Theory

B. F. Skinner is considered the father of modern **behavioral theory**. Behavioral theory may be applied to many aspects of human learning, including speech and language. The behavioral perspective maintains that language is a set of verbal behaviors learned through **operant (instrumental) conditioning**. Operant conditioning is a method of changing behavior in which a desired behavior is reinforced immediately after it spontaneously occurs.

Behaviorists believe that language behaviors are learned by imitation, reinforcement, and successive approximations toward adult language behaviors. They consider language to be determined not by self-discovery or creative experimentation, but by selective reinforcements received from speech and language models (usually parents and other family). Behaviorists focus on the external forces that shape a child's verbal behaviors into language and see the child primarily as a reactor to these forces (Hulit, Howard, & Fahey, 2011).

Two other concepts important in the operant model for speech and language development are *imitation* and *practice*. A young child imitates as best he can the sounds and words he hears his parents say. When a word is said by a child that *approximates* (sounds close to) the word the parents say, they accept and reinforce it. That is, they begin *shaping* the

---

speech development

The progressive evolving and shaping of individual sounds and syllables that are used as arbitrary symbols and applied in rule-governed combinations to produce words to communicate a person's wants, needs, thoughts, knowledge, and feelings.

language development

The progressive growth of a receptive and expressive communication system for representing concepts using arbitrary symbols (sounds and words) and rule-governed combinations of those symbols (grammar).

behavioral theory (behaviorism)

In reference to speech and language, a perspective of development that asserts that speech and language are behaviors learned through operant conditioning.

operant (instrumental) conditioning

A learning model for changing behavior in which a desired behavior is reinforced immediately after it spontaneously occurs.

word until the child, through practice, eventually can say the word as the parents do. James (1960, p. 165) provided a well-known illustration of operant conditioning of verbal behavior using selective reinforcement:

> A child says *mama* as his mother starts to pick him up. The mother, who is delighted that the child knows her name, gives him a big hug and kiss and says, *Mama, that's right—I'm mama!* The affectionate physical response from the mother is undoubtedly pleasurable and is likely, therefore, to increase the probability that the child will say *mama* again. In other words, the mother's response to the child's behavior was a reinforcer.

Clinical Application

For decades, clinicians have used a behavioral approach to study children's language by observing, describing, and counting specific language behaviors. This basic *stimulus–response* [S-R] paradigm first teaches children to imitate a sound and then reinforces the production with verbal praise (e.g., "Good job!" and "That was super!"). The children's productions are then shaped into increasingly closer approximations of the target sound, and when they are finally able to produce the sound correctly, the sound is practiced in a variety of sound and word combinations. This same approach is used for language structures and numerous other targets being developed for speech and language.

Parentese

Parentese (also called *motherese* and *baby talk*, but more professionally called *child-directed speech*) refers to how parents and other caregivers often talk to infants. Adults using parentese typically (1) use a high-pitched voice with greater pitch variation; (2) use one- and two-syllable words in short, simple sentences; and (3) speak at a slower rate with clearer articulation, sometimes emphasizing every syllable (Berko-Gleason, 2001).

Application Question

Have you ever used parentese when playing with an infant? How did your speech differ from its normal form? Why do you think this came naturally to you?

Nativistic Theory

The **nativistic theory** emphasizes that the acquisition of language is an innate, physiologically determined, and genetically transmitted phenomenon. That is, a newborn is "prewired" for language acquisition and a linguistic mechanism is activated by exposure to linguistic stimuli (speech and language) (Hulit, Howard, & Fahey, 2011). This theory considers that language is universal and unique among humans and that unless there are severe mental or physical limitations or severe isolation and deprivation, humans will acquire language. The nativistic perspective argues that caregivers (e.g., parents) do not teach children a

nativistic theory

A perspective of language development that emphasizes the acquisition of language as an innate, physiologically determined, and genetically transmitted phenomenon.

progressive understanding of language forms, and that young children are exposed to complex and inconsistent language and are usually not provided feedback about the correctness of their utterances (Pinker, 1984).

Clinical Application

When children do not use certain language structures that are appropriate for their age, they likely have not acquired them through their natural tendency and, therefore, a goal would be to target those language structures in therapy. Helping children learn how to combine words, phrases, and sentences lets them convey their messages to others. Instructing children about how to use language appropriately in different social situations and environments allows them to use appropriate pragmatics when communicating.

Semantic-Cognitive Theory

semantic-cognitive theory

A perspective of language development that emphasizes the interrelationship between language learning and cognition; that is, the meanings conveyed by a child's productions.

The **semantic-cognitive theory** emphasizes the interrelationship between language learning and cognition. Children demonstrate certain cognitive abilities as a corresponding language behavior emerges (Bloom & Lahey, 1978). The semantic meaning that a person wants to communicate determines the words and word order (syntactic form) the person uses—that is, meaning precedes form. For example, children know what they want to communicate (cognition) but do not always use the correct semantics or grammar. Also, children may not know the correct use of a word or understand that a two-word utterance can have many meanings.

Clinical Application

Clinicians use the semantic-cognitive theory by describing children's strategies for acquiring new information (i.e., cognitive skills). For example, the *complexity* of a sentence (the message), the *amount* of information in a sentence, and the *rate* (*c-a-r*) at which a sentence is said may significantly affect a child's understanding of a sentence. A child with delayed or disordered language may benefit from a clinician who is able to adjust one or all of these variables. That is, a clinician may be able to make a sentence simpler (less *complex*), with less information for the child to process (decreased *amount*), and slow the *rate* of speech so the child has a better opportunity to understand a message.

Social-Pragmatic Theory

social-pragmatic theory

A perspective of language development that considers communication as the basic function of language.

The **social-pragmatic theory** considers communication as the basic function of language. This perspective is first seen in infant–caregiver interactions in which the caregiver responds to an infant's sounds and gestures. The prerequisites for the social-pragmatic theory are: (1) the infant must have a caregiver in close proximity to see, hear, or touch;

(2) the caregiver must provide the infant with basic physical needs such as food, warmth, and exploring the environment; (3) the infant must develop an attachment to the caregiver; (4) the infant and caregiver must be able to simultaneously attend to the same objects or actions; and (5) the infant and caregiver engage in *turn-taking* in both verbal and nonverbal behaviors (McLaughlin, 2006). In ideal parent–child communication, all five of these prerequisites are occurring in most interactions. The social-pragmatic perspective emphasizes the importance of the communicative partner's role; the partner's interpretation of what is said defines the results of the speech act.

Clinical Application

Caregivers can facilitate language in a number of ways, including playing social games (e.g., peekaboo) that are stimulating and exciting to infants; taking turns in activities in which the caregiver speaks and expects the infant to respond in some manner; and reading books with young children (see Figure 4–1). Clinicians can assess and treat children's language impairments from a social-communicative and contextual perspective. The therapeutic goal is maximizing communicative competence.

Cultural and Linguistic Diversity Perspective

Regardless of the theory of language acquisition that is followed, children mature within the context of caregivers, whether they are parents, family members, or other individuals within the community.

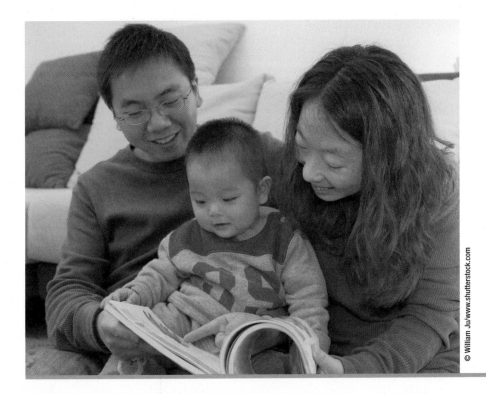

© William Ju/www.shutterstock.com

Figure 4–1

Parents and children reading together is an excellent application of the social-pragmatic perspective.

culture

The philosophies, values, attitudes, perceptions, religious and spiritual beliefs, educational values, language, customs, child-rearing practices, lifestyles, and arts shared by a group of people and passed from one generation to the next.

multicultural

A society characterized by a diversity of cultures, languages, traditions, religions, and values, as well as socioeconomic classes, sexual orientations, and ability levels; ideally, where individuals are respected and valued for their contributions to the whole of that society.

cultural–linguistic diversity (CLD)

A perspective of language development that emphasizes the similarities and differences of the people and the languages spoken around the world, and that stresses how one language or dialect is no better than another.

accent

Usually considered the speech pronunciation and inflections used by nonnative American English speakers (foreign accent).

dialect

A specific form of speech and language used in a geographical region or among a large group of people (*social* or *ethnic dialects*) that differs significantly from the standard of the larger language community in pronunciation, vocabulary, grammar, and idiomatic use of words.

standard dialect

The dialect of a language that is commonly spoken or established by individuals with considerable formal education.

These people provide a communicative environment for the maturing child that is reflective of the range of meanings, values, perceptions, and beliefs of the **cultures** of which they are a part. Like many other countries, the United States is considered **multicultural**. Speech-language pathologists and audiologists must understand and appreciate the **cultural–linguistic diversity (CLD)** of client populations in order to better serve them (Owens, 2012).

Cultural diversity is not determined by the origin of a person's ancestors or color of skin but by numerous other factors, including linguistic background, regional affiliations, educational levels, socioeconomic status, and religious beliefs. Any of these factors may influence speech and language development. Many children in America are in families who have recently immigrated to America. These families often continue to speak their native language at home and in their social environments. The children, therefore, typically develop the family's native language as their first language. Many children, however, may be exposed to both English and the family's native language in the home and community and learn to speak English with a distinct **accent**.

There are approximately 1,000 languages in the world spoken by at least 10,000 people (Crystal, 2010). Most of these languages have a variety of forms and **dialects** that vary in phonology, vocabulary, and grammar. One dialect is no better than another within a language. However, the concept of a **standard dialect** within a language is strongly associated with the higher educational levels of the native speakers and is used in educational environments. It is important to consider that standard dialects for the same language may vary significantly among nations. For example, America, England, Australia, New Zealand, and Singapore all use the English language but have significantly different standard dialects for their nations.

ASHA's Position on Dialects of Speech-Language Pathologists

ASHA (1998) provided a position statement and technical report on speech-language pathologists working in school settings who, themselves, have dialectical variations from the local community dialect. ASHA maintains that members may not discriminate against people who speak with a nonstandard dialect in educational programs, employment, or service delivery. However, clinicians must have the necessary diagnostic and clinical skills and be able to model required treatment targets. In addition, the clinician may not have limited English proficiency.

In the United States, the four major ethnic groups are: Hispanics (Latinos), African Americans, Asian and Pacific Island Americans, and Native Americans (American Indians and indigenous Alaskans). Together, these groups represent between 30% and 35% of the nation's approximate 313,000,000 people; however, for individual states, certain ethnic groups significantly exceed the national average. For example, in California slightly more than 50% of the population is now Hispanic (U.S. Bureau of the Census, 2011). All major ethnic groups have broad and specific linguistic and cultural differences that influence their speech and language development (see Battle, 2002, Roseberry-McKibbin, 2008, and ASHA Division 14, *Communication Disorders and Sciences in Culturally and Linguistically Diverse Populations*, for more information on various cultures).

Hispanic (Latino)

Children of immigrants constitute the fastest-growing portion of the child population of the United States and the overall Hispanic population is approximately 15.5% of the population (U.S. Census Bureau, 2011). It is important for clinicians to keep in mind the differences in Spanish morphology and syntax when making decisions about whether a child has a language difference or a language disorder. When a clinician hears a child from a different linguistic and cultural background use morphology and syntax that differs from General American English, it is important to consider whether the child's first language is interfering with his second language (i.e., English). Clinicians who speak Spanish fluently have a distinct advantage working with these children.

English as a Second Language

Native Spanish-speaking parents who are learning **English as a second language (ESL)** (English language learner [ELL]) must decide whether to raise their children as English speakers, Spanish speakers, or **bilinguals**. Families often base their choices about the language their children will learn on fear of discrimination, limited information about the benefits of bilingualism, and other negative sociocultural considerations (Hammer, Miccio, & Wagstaff, 2003). Immigrant parents want their children to succeed; therefore, a common assumption among family members is that they must choose English over their home language, which may for some children result in the loss of the home language. Unfortunately, many educators and professionals (likely including some speech-language pathologists) continue to discourage the use of a child's home or first language and recommend that children focus on learning English to the exclusion of the language of the home. Children who become fluent in both their home language and English can choose to use one language one moment and the other language the next moment (**code switching**), depending on whom they are talking to and what they are talking about.

African American

African Americans comprise almost 13% of the U.S. population and are the largest racial minority in the United States (U.S. Census Bureau, 2011). African American English (AAE) is a systematic, rule-governed,

English as a second language (ESL)

Learning English after a child's native (home) language has been established.

bilingual

Children who often speak the parents' native language in the home environment and speak American English in school or other environments.

code switching

An occurrence for bilingual individuals in which sounds, words, semantics, syntactic, or pragmatic elements from one language are included when speaking another language, either automatically or intentionally; also can be expanded to include nonstandard and standard dialects.

phonological, grammatical, syntactic, semantic, and pragmatic system of language (Terrell & Jackson, 2002). AAE is considered a dialect of General American English (GAE) (Seymour & Pearson, 2004). AAE has both verbal and nonverbal aspects, including the use of personal space, body postures and gestures, eye contact, vocal inflections, word choice, and word order. Not all African Americans use AAE and its use is on a continuum that ranges from African Americans who do not use the dialect to those who use most AAE features in all communicative contexts (Wyatt, 2001).

Asian and Pacific Island American

Approximately 3.5% of the U.S. population is Asian and about 1.0% is Native Hawaiian or Pacific Islander (U.S. Census Bureau, 2011). Millions of people from Asian countries (e.g., China, Taiwan, Hong Kong, Japan, Korea, Singapore, Malaysia, Indonesia, India, and Pakistan) and the Pacific Island countries (e.g., Philippines, Guam, Fiji, Samoa, and Hawaii) have immigrated to America over the past 200 years. In addition, since 1975 more than 1 million refugees from Southeast Asia (e.g., Vietnam, Cambodia, Laos, and Thailand) have come to the United States. Asian and Pacific Island countries have diverse and unique languages, cultures, religious beliefs, folk beliefs, worldviews, values, and attitudes toward education and child rearing. Each of these factors, plus the complicated interactions of factors, can profoundly affect the speech-language pathology services we try to provide (Cheng, 2002).

The attitudes of Asian and Pacific Island Americans toward disabilities can be traced in part to folk beliefs, spiritualism, and superstitions. Attitudes range from beliefs that a disability is the result of wrongdoing of an ancestor to an imbalance of inner forces, gods, spirits, or demons. Some cultures believe that a disability is a gift from God, and the person with a disability is then protected and sheltered by the family and community. On the other hand, some cultures view individuals who have obvious disabilities as cursed and ostracize them from society. Treatment of disabilities varies widely among cultures, and Western methods may be counter to Asian religious and cultural beliefs. (For a fascinating and enlightening account of a Hmong child from Laos with cerebral palsy and her parents' struggles with Eastern versus Western medicine and rehabilitation, read Fadiman's 1997 book *The Spirit Catches You and You Fall Down.*)

Native American (American Indians and Indigenous Alaskans)

Native Americans (American Indians and indigenous Alaskans) comprise about 1% of the total U.S. population (U.S. Census Bureau, 2011). Native American societies and cultures vary significantly from one another, as do their languages. Many Native American languages have been lost and some have relatively few speakers (Harrison, 2010). Similar to other ethnic groups, Native Americans have experienced hardships through loss of their ancestral lands, conflicts with mainstream values, and stereo-typing that has resulted in confusion of who they are as a people.

American Indians often bypass professionals and instead choose to use a *medicine man/woman* (a person believed to be able to heal others by making use of supernatural powers) or *shaman* (a spiritual leader who is believed to have special powers such as prophecy and the ability to heal) and healing ceremonies to work through a variety of problems. The *worldviews* (an individual's or group's perception of reality and framework of ideas, beliefs, and attitudes about the world, life, and themselves) of some Native Americans may be considerably different from those of clinicians and may affect understanding of and compli-ance with therapy (Ryback, Eastin, & Robbins, 2004).

The Influence of Poverty on Language Development

Complicating our work with children from culturally and linguistically diverse backgrounds are the effects of poverty. Many bilingual chil-dren in the United States live in low-income families, which increases their risk for language and learning problems, partly because they tend to have limited exposure to both oral and written language (Oller & Pearson, 2002; Rosin, 2006). English language proficiency is an impor-tant factor for family economic security and child well-being in at least three ways: (1) limited English language proficiency among both parents and children is associated with poor educational outcomes among chil-dren; (2) parents' limited English language proficiency can hamper their ability to communicate effectively with their children and help with their children's English language-related homework; and (3) children for whom English is their second language often have academic and social difficulties in school (Shields & Behrman, 2004; Kindler, 2002).

Children born into poverty are often raised in environments similar to the environments in which their mothers and fathers were raised; that is, with poor nutrition, inadequate stimulation, emotional neglect, and physical danger. There is a culture of poverty, and even children who are born with the potential to develop normal language and communication skills may never realize their potential because of their cultural influences (Kishiyama, Boyce, Jimenez, Perry, & Knight, 2009; Pence & Justice, 2008).

Clinical Application

Clinicians routinely work with children with culturally and linguistically diverse backgrounds to maximize their speech and language develop-ment (Roseberry-McKibbin, 2006). In reality, it is not possible for clini-cians to have a ready knowledge of each of the hundreds of individual cultures, religious beliefs, folk beliefs, values, and attitudes of the numer-ous cultures and populations with whom we work. However, it is impor-tant for clinicians to become familiar with and develop some functional level of understanding and appreciation of the various cultures of clients and family members with whom they work. As Salas-Provance (2012) emphasizes about working with Native American clients, clinicians need to focus on the people in front of them and not on our expectations of what these people should or should not be. Rapport is achieved by being open, warm, and genuine, and being aware that as clinicians we make mistakes because of our cultural ignorance, and by stating so before mistakes occur. Reading books and other literature on multicultural issues can help clinicians continually expand their multicultural knowledge and understanding (ASHA, 2004).

SPEECH DEVELOPMENT

Child development, including speech development, refers to an increase in complexity—a change from the relatively simple to the more complex and refined. The process involves a sequential progression along an expected continuum that is similar for all children of any culture or language. The rate of development, rather than the sequence, shows great variability among children (Owens, 2012). Speech and language development are intricately interrelated; however, for learning purposes it can be helpful to view them separately.

Speech development may be divided into four stages based on the ages of children and their biological development. Stage I is birth to 12 months; stage II is 12 to 24 months; stage III is 2 to 5 years; and stage IV is 6 to 12 years. Keep in mind that these stages always overlap and that a child emerges into a new stage while merging out of an earlier stage; that is, stages are never discrete (Allen & Marotz, 2007).

Stage I: Birth—12 Months (Infancy)

The foundations for all future speech and language development are built between birth and 6 months of age. From the earliest days of life, newborns absorb information through all of their senses, learning from what they see, hear, touch, taste, and smell. Stage I can be divided into **prelinguistic (preverbal) vocalizations**, birth–6 months and 6–12 months. The months are approximate beginnings and endings for acquisition of both speech and language skills.

Birth–6 Months: Prelinguistic (Preverbal) Vocalizations

Prelinguistic (preverbal) vocalizations are the sounds produced by an infant before the production of true words (e.g., crying, **babbling**, **cooing**, and **echolalia**). The first preverbal vocalization is, ideally, a robust cry at the moment of birth. This cry is important because it begins with a quick and forceful inhalation of air that fills the lungs and closes a valve in the newborn's heart to allow blood to be directed for the first time from the heart to the lungs for oxygenation. The cry is also a **neonate's** first communication—that it is alive and breathing.

---

prelinguistic (preverbal) vocalizations

The sounds produced by an infant before the production of true words and language (e.g., crying, cooing, babbling, and echolalia).

babbling

The production of a consonant and vowel in the same syllable, either reduplicated *(ba-ba, gaa-gaa)* or nonreduplicated *(baa-da-gi)*, that tends to appear at about 6 or 7 months of age.

cooing

The production of vowel-like sounds (usually /u/ and /oo/ with occasional brief consonant-like sounds similar to /k/ and/g/), usually produced by infants when feeling comfort or pleasure and interacting with a caregiver.

echolalia

An infant's immediate and automatic reproduction or imitation of speech heard from the sounds made by others in the environment; the words infants imitate are not yet meaningful to them.

neonate

A child within the first 28 days after birth.

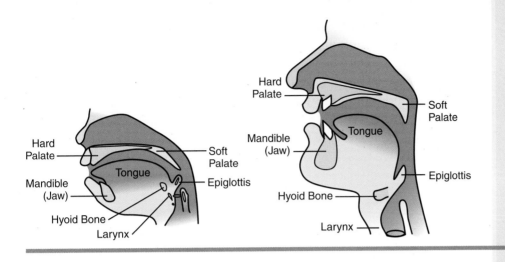

Figure 4-2

Vocal tracts of infants and adults.

© Cengage Learning 2013.

By 2 to 4 months of age infants have begun making cooing and gooing sounds. The consonants infants typically produce are /g/ and /k/, and the vowels are /u/ and /oo/. These sounds are produced in the back of the oral cavity and are easier to produce than other sounds that require more precise movements of the mandible, lips, and tongue in the anterior region of the mouth. The cooing sounds of infants are not intentional forms of communicating with caregivers, although these vocal behaviors usually elicit attention from caregivers followed by closeness, cuddling, and soft, caring speech.

An infant's *vocal tract* (pharyngeal, oral, and nasal cavities) is significantly different from an adult's vocal tract in terms of its size, shape, and location of structures. These differences also play an important role in the sounds an infant can produce (see Figure 4-2). Before about the sixth month of life, an infant does not have control of the movement of the soft palate and, therefore, makes random oral and nasal sounds.

6–12 Months: Prelinguistic (Preverbal) Vocalizations

Between about 6 and 8 months of age infants can produce a variety of vowels and several consonants, although not in a voluntary, intentional manner. They begin to babble and engage in **vocal play** using longer strings of syllables that extend babbling (e.g., *gaga, googoo, baa-da-gi-daa-um-ma*). During vocal play, infants also playfully produce squeals, grunts, screams, growls, and the always entertaining "raspberries." Some children seem to fixate on one particular sound or noise for a few days before moving on to another. If an infant does not babble or begin vocal play by about the eighth month of life, the infant's hearing should be checked by an audiologist. Infants who do not hear well do not receive the enjoyment and motivation of hearing their own babbling and vocal play and, therefore, usually begin decreasing their vocalizations.

After about the sixth month infants have gained some control of the soft palate and can more consistently produce either oral (e.g., *dada*) or nasal (e.g., *mama*) sounds. Over the next several months, an infant's

vocal play

The longer strings of syllables that extend babbling (e.g., *baa-da-gi-daa-um-ma*).

vocal tract begins to more closely resemble the vocal tract of an adult in terms of location and shape of structures, which further changes the acoustic characteristics of the child's sounds. During this time, infants are playing and experimenting with their newly developing ability to make sounds voluntarily. They make sounds when they are happy and are happy when making sounds. They express emotions such as pleasure and displeasure by making different sounds. During the latter part of the first year of life, infants are producing long strings of syllables (consonant–vowel combinations) with different stress and intonation patterns.

Between 8 and 12 months of age, infants are preparing for two major developmental milestones—talking and walking. They are becoming increasingly social and like being the center of attention. Their increasing ability to imitate sounds of adults (*echolalia*) extends their social interactions and helps them develop new skills. During this time the upper and lower front teeth begin to erupt, which also is the time that many mothers wean their infants from nursing and begin feeding them baby (*pureed*) foods. Learning to eat pureed foods may help develop the tongue control that is necessary for developing speech. Better control of the tongue, lips, mandible, and soft palate helps infants develop more precise, rapid, and independent movements needed for articulation.

During this age, infants babble or jabber deliberately to initiate social interaction and shout to attract attention. They babble in sentence-like sequences with inflections as though they are actually talking (sometimes referred to as **jargon**). About 90% of the sounds produced by infants between 11 and 12 months of age are stops (/p, b, t, d, k, g/), nasals (/m, n/), glides (/w, j, h/), and the fricative /s/. It is also during this time that infants begin to say "da-da" and "ma-ma," which parents take as their infant talking to them. Infants are learning that their sounds can control others.

jargon

Strings of syllables produced with stress and intonation that mimic real speech but are not actual words.

Stage II: 12–24 Months (Toddlerhood)

The term *toddlerhood* refers to children learning to stand and walk when they are clumsy and may "toddle" over. We can extend that thought to children's early attempts to speak when they are clumsy with their communicative abilities. Toddlers begin this period of life with the limited abilities of an infant and end with the relatively sophisticated skills of a young child. The first true word emerges about the 12th month of life, and by the 24th month toddlers are typically using two-word sentences to communicate. The ability to stand upright and eventually walk occurs about 12 months of age and allows toddlers to explore their available environments, which significantly expands their world and experiences.

By about 12 months of age, infants express their needs and wants through vocalization and gestures. An infant's first words mark the beginning of a transition from preverbal to verbal communication (Pence-Turnbull & Justice, 2012). The designation of "true" word is not always easy to agree upon. From a parent's point of view, the first time an infant says "mama" or "dada" the infant is using intentional and meaningful speech (true words to the parents). However, a vocalization is considered a true word only if it meets three specific criteria (Locke, 1993):

1. A word must be uttered with a clear intention and purpose. For example, when an infant or toddler is petting a cat and says "kitty," it is a clear intention and purpose that it is in reference to the cat. If a parent tells the child to say "kitty" and the child does, it is considered an imitation or repetition rather than a true word.

2. A true word must be recognizably close to an adult's pronunciation of the word. For example, if a child says "itty-itty" for "kitty-kitty," most adults would recognize the child's word as a good attempt at saying the word correctly. However, if a child uses a consistent but not close approximation (e.g., *ga-ku-me*) for "kitty," it would not be considered a true word.

3. A true word is used consistently by a child in various contexts. For example, if a child only uses *itty* for the family cat but does not use *itty* for other cats, for pictures of cats, or upon hearing a cat's meow, then the use of *itty* would not have a symbolic reference in addition to its specific reference to the family cat.

Phonologically, children's first true words are typically characterized by simple syllables, such as consonant–vowel (CV), vowel–consonant (VC), vowel–consonant–vowel (VCV), or consonant–vowel–consonant–vowel (CVCV) combinations. The sound combinations are usually stops, nasals, and glides—the same combinations used in the late babbling period (/k, g, t, d, p, b, m, n, w, h/). The preferred vowels tend to be /i, a, u/. However, from a speech development perspective, words such as *mommy, daddy, ba* (ball), *ca* (car), *goggy* (doggy), *iddy* (kitty), and *uss* (juice) are more likely to be considered true words than the first productions of *mama* or *dada*. By toddlerhood, children have emerged from prelinguistic vocalizations into linguistic communication. It is important to remember that after toddlers say their first true words, most of their vocalizations continue to be babbling. That is, during vocalizations there is a mixture of true words and babbling, with babbling eventually decreasing and being replaced with true words.

By about 18 months of age children usually can say approximately 50 words that are intelligible to parents and most other people. Even though children may produce a variety of CVC words, the final consonant is still often omitted, with the actual production of the word being a CV combination and the listener "filling in" the final consonant. The final consonant in a CVC word usually begins to emerge around 18 months and is typically the /t/ sound (e.g., *cat*). Three-syllable words are often reduced to two syllables; for example, *banana* (ba-nan-a) becomes *nana,* where the unstressed syllable of the word (e.g., *ba-*) is omitted and the **stressed** syllables (*-nana)* become the child's production of the word.

Between 18 and 24 months of age, children begin to use two-word sentences that are generally intelligible, particularly if the context is

stress

Variations in intensity, frequency, and duration on one syllable more than another in a word, which usually results in the syllable sounding both louder and longer than other syllables in the same word.

known, for example, "More juice," "Daddy go," and "Where mommy?" By 24 months of age, children are more consistently producing a variety of final consonants, including /t, p, k, n/ and sometimes /r/ and /s/. As children are developing intelligible sequences of sounds and words, they are developing the rules for combining phonemes to produce intelligible words that convey information. By 2 years of age, most children are approximately 25–50% intelligible to adults (Locke, 1993).

Stage III: 2–5 Years (Early Childhood)

The differences between a 2-year-old and a 5-year-old child are like night and day. A 2-year-old's speech is usually understandable when the context is known. However, by 5 years of age, most children develop adult-like speech that is approximately 90% intelligible to both familiar and unfamiliar listeners. Although these years are considered early childhood, they may be more specifically classified as early-early childhood (2-year-olds), middle-early childhood (3- and 4-year-olds), and late-early childhood (5-year-olds).

2-Year-Olds (Early-Early Childhood)

Two-year-olds no longer rely on pointing and gestures as primary forms of communication. They use their limited speech and language to communicate their wants, needs, thoughts, and feelings—and they feel strongly about many things. Many of the speech sounds have emerged or are well established and they are usually about 75% intelligible in their two- to three-word sentences. Two-year-olds can use their voice and articulators to produce unstressed syllables in the initial position of words (e.g., they can produce both the unstressed *ba* and the stressed *nana* in the word *banana*). Secord and Donohue (2002), in their *Clinical Assessment of Articulation and Phonology,* used the developmental age norms shown in Table 4–1.

| TABLE 4-1 | Clinical Assessment of Articulation and Phonology |

	STOPS						NASALS			GLIDES			FRICATIVES								AFFRICATES		LIQUIDS		
Age of Mastery*	p	b	t	d	k	g	m	n	ŋ	w	j	h	f	v	s	z	ʃ	ʒ	ɔ	ð	ʧ	ʤ	l	ɾ	ɚ
75%	2	2	2	2	2	2	2	2	2	2	2	2	3	3	3	3	3	6	5	3	3	3	3	4	3
95%	2	3	3	2	3	3	2	2	4	2	4	2	4	5	5	5	5	6	8	7	5	5	5	6	6

*Age when 75% or 95% of children mastered the sound.
Based on data from Secord and Donohue (2002).

3- and 4-Year-Olds (Middle-Early Childhood)

Vowel development is mostly completed by 3 years of age. Several consonants are considered established by age 3 (e.g., /m, n, p, b, d, k, g, h, f, w/), some of which children have been using since the babbling stage but not in a voluntary, intentionally produced manner. In general, sounds typically acquired by children by the end of 3 years of age are *early developing sounds* and sounds typically acquired after 3 years of age are *later developing sounds* (Bauman-Waengler, 2009). Children this age typically speak in three- to four-word sentences that are approximately 90% intelligible.

Four-year-old children are at least 95% intelligible, even though several sounds and most blends have not yet emerged or fully developed. It is not surprising, however, that children's speech is about as clear and well articulated as the adults' around them. Adult listeners fill in the sounds omitted or mispronounced by children to easily understand their speech. It is interesting, if not somewhat surprising, how easily children learn to understand the often-slurred speech of other children and even adults. Adults say many things for which listeners must fill in the sounds to make complete words and sentences, for example, "g'nai" (Good night) or "djaeet?" (Did you eat?).

5-Year-Olds (Late-Early Childhood)

Most speech sounds have emerged or are fully developed by age 5, although some sounds may not yet be completely and consistently established for some children until age 6 to 8 years of age (e.g., /r, l, s, z, sh, ch, dz, j, v/ "ng", "th", and **blends**) (see Figure 4–3). Many children this age begin to lose their front teeth, which affects the production of some sounds that may be emerging or already acquired (e.g., /s, z/). Speech is at least 95% intelligible even though some consonants and blends are not yet fully developed (e.g., /r, l/, /tr, spl, skw/).

Phonological Processes

Children younger than about 4½ years of age may not have sufficient ability to fully coordinate the movements of the vocal folds, soft palate, and each of the articulators. As a consequence, certain sounds, sound combinations or transitions from one sound to another may be too difficult for them. Young children may, therefore, simplify the production of some words (Williamson, 2010). These simplifications are common in the speech development of children across languages and are called **natural processes** or **phonological processes**. There are three common natural processes: (a) *syllable structure processes* describe changes that affect the structure of the syllable; (b) *substitution processes* for sound modifications in which one sound class (e.g., plosive) is replaced by another; and (c) *assimilatory processes* in which a sound is influenced by a neighboring sound in a word (Bauman-Waengler, 2009).

Five-year-olds are often still confused or have not learned the numerous changes in vowel productions with variations of words (e.g., n*a*ture

blend (consonant cluster)

A blend or consonant cluster occurs when two or more sounds appear together with no vowel separation (e.g., /tr, sp, bl, str, spl, str, skw/).

natural processes

The processes that are common in the speech development of children across languages.

phonological processes

The simplification of sounds that are difficult for children to produce in an adult manner; phonological processes help explain errors of substitution, omission, and addition that children may use to simplify the production of difficult sounds.

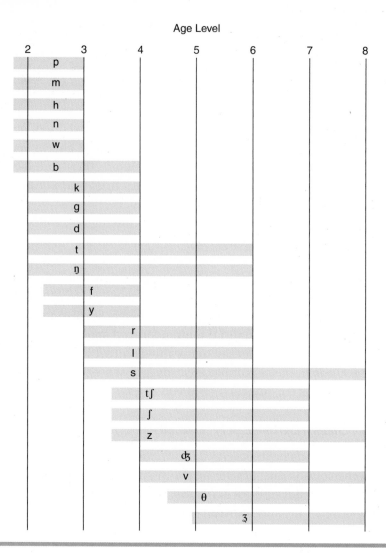

Figure 4–3

Sander's 1972 customary ages of production of English consonants.

Source: Sander, E. K. (1972). When are speech sounds learned? *Journal of Speech and Hearing Disorders, 37,* 62. Copyright 1972 by American Speech-Language-Hearing Association. Reprinted with permission.

versus n*a*tural and expl*a*in versus expl*a*nation). They are able to appropriately place stress on syllables in multisyllabic words (e.g., *happi*ness and *uncomfor*table) and on compound words (e.g., *WHITEhouse,* a noun) versus adjective–noun combinations (e.g., *white HOUSE*).

Stage IV: 6–12 Years (Middle Childhood to Early Adolescence)

When children enter stage IV, they are still very much children but they end as preteens, with the early signs of adolescence developing. At the beginning of stage IV many children have already been in nursery or preschool for a few years and are now entering kindergarten. At the end of this stage, they will be in junior high school.

Most children who are 6, 7, and 8 years of age are 95–100% intelligible, even though some later developing sounds and blends may still not be articulated clearly. Children who are 9, 10, 11, and 12 years old have mastered speech. They communicate easily and freely with people of all ages and adjust their communication to the age of the individual they are talking to; for example, they use early childhood speech with young children, slang and profanity with peers, and mature speech with older adults. This is an important step in pragmatics.

LANGUAGE DEVELOPMENT

For normal communication to develop, there must be an integration of three elements: (1) biological structures and functions must develop within normal limits; (2) cognitive functioning must be sufficient for language skills to emerge and be cultivated; and (3) social interaction (usually with parents or other caregivers) must be sufficient for infants and children to be encouraged and rewarded for communication attempts. As with speech development, language development may be divided into four stages based on the chronological ages of children: Stage I is birth to 12 months (further divided into birth to 6 months and 6 to 12 months); stage II is 12 to 24 months; stage III is 2 to 5 years; and stage IV is 6 to 12 years. Although the ages of the stages are discrete, the developmental levels are not; children merge into the next stage of development.

Stage I: Birth–12 Months (Infancy)

Language development begins in the earliest weeks and months of life. The five senses (sight, hearing, touch, taste, and smell) are the sources of stimuli from the environment that the infant responds to. Every new stimulus helps create new neural pathways and connections in the brain. When the environment is stimulating the language centers of the brain (as well as all other areas of the brain) are "primed" with millions (billions) of connections of neurons and synapses that can eventually be used to form concepts for language.

Sensory and Emotional Deprivation

Infants who have been deprived of sensory stimulation during their early months of life and into toddlerhood have difficulty ever developing normal cognitive–linguistic abilities, as well as emotional and social bonds. In some parts of the world, infant and child sensory deprivation is common. Some orphanages "warehouse" infants and children, keeping them in cribs for years with minimal nourishment and lack of emotional caring and socialization; the only stimulation is primarily self-stimulation. They learn that their whimpering and cries do not bring them attention or comforting.

Some of these infants and children are rescued and adopted by families from other countries. The adoptive parents often feel that all these infants or children need is "a lot of love and they will come around." However, when neural circuits for attachment and loving care are not established during infancy, it is difficult for them to be cultivated later in life for normal emotional and social bonding (attachment) to develop. For more information about development of emotions, read Goleman's (1995) *Emotional Intelligence: Why It Can Matter More Than IQ.*

Birth–6 Months: Prelinguistic (Preverbal) Vocalizations

The primary sensory systems of infants are vision, hearing, taste, and smell. Tactile sensation is less developed, which goes along with their relatively poorly developed motor system. As their first year progresses, they begin integrating their senses by coordinating the use of their hands, mouth, and eyes to explore their own bodies, toys, and surroundings. After visually inspecting objects, they like to put them in their mouths because taste and smell are two of their strongest senses during this time.

The reflexive crying and vegetative grunts and other such sounds may communicate something to parents, but they are often just educated guesses as to what the infant wants or needs. The infant's body and limb movements are generally random without much specific intention, other than to withdraw from an unwanted stimulus or to move toward a wanted stimulus. The cooing and gooing sounds made by infants begin as reflexive and later develop into more intentionally produced sounds. When the sounds become intentionally produced to draw or hold a parent's attention, infants may be using their first verbal expressive language.

6–12 Months: Prelinguistic (Preverbal) Vocalizations

The early months of life created neural pathways that now become knowledge about the environment—the objects and people in it. Infants have an affinity for certain objects, toys, and sounds, as well as the familiar people they see and voices they hear. They also learn how to obtain what they want by whimpering or crying until food or a favorite toy is given to them, or smiling and giggling to keep an adult's attention (all ways of communicating). During the first year of life, infants form attachments (emotional bonds) to people and seek stimulation and comfort from them (Peluso, et al., 2004).

In the latter half of their first year, infants are using their facial expressions and body language to communicate turn-taking (e.g., giving or taking a toy) and parents begin to feel that their child is becoming a true partner in their interactions. Infants this age may be trying to communicate more than what parents and other caregivers think they are because the adults in the environment are not able to consistently and accurately interpret the infants' verbal (jargon) and nonverbal (facial expressions, body and limb movements) messages.

Language Development of Visually Impaired Children

Most students of speech-language pathology probably think more about the effects of a hearing impairment on a child's speech and language development than the effects of a visual impairment. The American Foundation for the Blind recommends the term *blind* be used to refer to individuals with no usable sight. Individuals with even minimal usable vision are referred to as *visually impaired, partially sighted,* or *low visioned.* Congenital blindness is rare compared to visual impairments, and both of these are rare compared to congenital hearing impairments. The following discussion will refer to children who are severely visually impaired or blind.

The language development of children who are severely visually impaired or blind is neither delayed nor deviant; rather, an alternative route of language acquisition is followed. Children with severe visual impairments rely on auditory and tactile resources more fully than do children with normal sight. Infants with severe visual impairments cannot make eye contact or use eye gaze to interact with parents, so they must rely on auditory and tactile cues. They need active encouragement to vocalize, which serves as an emotional link to the parents and an important sensory experience for the infant (Perez-Pereira & Conti-Ramsden, 1999).

The onset of meaningful speech occurs slightly later for children with severe visual impairments than for children with normal vision. Children with severe visual impairments tend to have a narrow use of words rather than generalizing or overextending them (e.g., anything round is a ball), as is typical of normally visioned children. Objects that cannot be directly touched are named or requested less often by children who are severely visually impaired. They usually are slower to develop some basic concepts that require vision, such as *clean, dirty, open, shut, in, out, up,* and *down.*

Action words may be used only to refer to things they are doing and not to the actions of others (actions they cannot see). They are slightly delayed in using two- and three-word combinations, but by the end of the third year the average number of morphemes they use in an **utterance** is comparable to sighted children. Visually impaired children tend to echo phrases of others before they can use the syntax voluntarily. They have difficulty understanding and using words such as *here, there, this,* and *that,* although by age 7 they usually have these words mastered (Landau & Gleitman, 1985).

Severely visually impaired children tend to use rising voice intonation to maintain a person's attention and interaction, and sighted children typically use eye contact. Visually impaired children tend to talk louder than necessary because they cannot judge the distance of their listener. They tend to nod their heads less often but smile more often. Some facial expressions may not match their sound and word meanings.

Overall, language development in children who have severe visual impairments or are blind cannot always be judged accurately by comparing them to normally sighted children. However, children with visual impairments may have all of the same phonological, morphological, syntactic, semantic, and pragmatic problems of other children, plus unique developmental differences. Therapeutically, the challenge for speech-language pathologists with these children is that we cannot use the visual modality that we so often rely on, particularly for teaching articulator placement for correct sound production and language therapy.

utterance

A unit of vocal expression preceded and followed by a pause or silence; may be a single sound, word, phrase, or sentence.

Application Question

Have you ever considered what it would be like to work with visually impaired children? Would you consider someday working with this population? What do you imagine some challenges would be working as a clinician with children who have both hearing and visual acuity impairments?

Stage II: 12–24 Months (Toddlerhood)

Toddlerhood allows children to explore their environment more independently because of their increased *ambulatory* (walking) and general motor skills. If something will not come to the toddler, the toddler may be able to go to it. Every new perception and sensation that enters the toddler's brain may be stored for further language development.

Toddlers like to attach words to the new things they are exploring and, therefore, have dramatic increases in receptive and expressive language abilities. Toddlers can understand more than they can express, particularly when spoken to at a moderate rate and with one- or two-syllable words that are in short (three- to five-word) sentences. It is important to understand that the early expressive language of young children is built on what they have experienced and know of their world; that is, children must first experience objects, events, or relationships and understand the words that relate to them before they can use the words meaningfully in expressive language.

Between 12 and 18 months of age children usually have an expressive vocabulary (**lexicon**) of approximately 50 words. They use one word to convey an entire thought; that is, they use one-word sentences (**holophrastic language**) such as "uus" for "I want some juice." The most typical forms of early words are common nouns such as *ball (ba)*, *milk, doggie, mommy, baby,* and *car (ca).* Toddlers learn to use action words, such as *go, bye-bye,* and *look;* modifiers, such as *red, pretty,* and *hot;* and personal–social words, such as *no, want,* and *please (pweez).* Between 12 and 26 months normally developing children begin using one-word utterances with a rising inflection to ask yes-or-no questions; for example, they may say "juice?" as in "Am I going to get some juice now?"

By 18 to 24 months of age, children begin to use two-word utterances, which significantly decrease the ambiguity of a child's communication. For example, when a child says "Mommy" there are any number of possible references; however, when the child says "Mommy home," "Mommy go," or "Mommy hurt," the listener has a better idea of the child's meaning. **Communicative competence** increases significantly with two-word utterances. A toddler can more easily communicate requests ("More milk."), negation ("No more!"), and commentary ("Me home!"). Children this age also begin to use grammatical morphemes such as articles (*a, the*), copulas (*is, be*), and auxiliary verbs (*have, can*) to make their utterances longer and more complex.

Brown (1973) investigated the **mean length of utterance (MLU)** of young children's language by counting the number of morphemes (not individual words) they used in single utterances. Brown viewed language as developing in five stages, with an increase of one morpheme per stage (see Table 4–2).

Stage III: 2–5 Years (Early Childhood)

Following toddlerhood, the next few years of life help prepare children cognitively and communicatively for beginning school. Between 2 and 5 years of age, dramatic changes occur in all aspects of children's development. Although these years are considered early childhood, they may

lexicon

Refers to all morphemes, including words and parts of words, that a person knows.

holophrastic language

The use of a single word to express a complete thought.

communicative competence

A child's grammatical knowledge of phonology, morphology, syntax, semantics, and pragmatics.

mean length of utterance (MLU)

The average number of morphemes in a young child's individual utterances; generally equivalent to a child's chronological age.

TABLE 4-2	Brown's Stages of Language Development		
STAGES	**CHARACTERIZED BY**	**FEATURES**	**EXAMPLES**
Stage I MLU: 1.0–2.0 Age 12–26 months	First words; semantic roles expressed in simple sentences	Single-word utterances; Combining semantic roles.	Naming significant objects, persons, and events in their daily experiences (*cup, spoon, Mommy, Daddy,* etc.) Agent + Action, Action + Object, Action + Location, Entity + Location, Entity + Attribute, Demonstrative + Attribute.
Stage II MLU: 2.0–2.5 Age 27–30 months	Modulation of meaning	Emerging of grammatical morphemes	Present progressive (*-ing*), prepositions (*in, on*), plural(*-s*), Irregular past (e.g., *ran, ate*), possessive (*-'s*), articles (*a, the*), regular past (*-ed*), third person regular, third person irregular, auxiliary and copula verbs (*is, are, was, were*).
Stage III MLU: 2.5–3.0 Age 31–34 months	Development of sentence form	Noun phrase elaboration and auxiliary development	Noun phrases elaborated in subject and object positions (*Big boy running fast, Billy ate my cookie*). Auxiliary verbs allow more mature interrogatives and negatives.
Stage IV MLU: 3.0–3.75 Age 35–40 months	Emergence of complex sentences	Embedding sentence elements	Object noun phrase complements (*I know you are my friend*); bedded with questions (*I know who is hiding*); relative clauses (*I helped boy who is nice*).
Stage V MLU: 3.75–4.50 Age 41–46 months	Emergence of compound sentences	Conjoining sentences	Conjoining two simple sentences (*I have a book and you have a toy*).

Adapted from *A First Language: The Early Stages* by R. Brown, 1973. Cambridge MA: Harvard University Press. In McLaughlin, 2006.

be more specifically classified as early-early childhood (2-year-olds), middle-early childhood (3- and 4-year-olds), and late-early childhood (5-year-olds).

2-Year-Olds (Early-Early Childhood)

Two-year-olds understand much of what is said to them when spoken in simple, clear sentences. They love being read to, especially if allowed to turn the pages and point to different objects in pictures. Remarkable growth occurs in their abilities to understand what they hear and to communicate their many thoughts and experiences in simple sentences. They understand more than they can express; however, they like to

parallel speech

Naming, describing, and explaining what the child is experiencing and probably feeling, almost as if the caregiver is the child; a technique used by some parents, as well as clinicians, to help children develop receptive and expressive language.

inner speech (internal discourse, stream of consciousness)

The nearly constant internal monologue a person has with himself at a conscious or semi-conscious level that involves thinking in words; a conversation with oneself.

cognitive development

The progressive and continuous growth of perception, memory, imagination, conception, judgment, and reasoning; it is the intellectual counterpart of a person's biological adaptation to the environment.

functor (function) words

Words whose grammatical functions are more obvious than their semantic content and that serve primarily to give order to a sentence, such as articles, conjunctions, determiners, prepositions, and modal and auxiliary verbs.

telegraphic speech (language)

Condensed language in which only the essential words are used, such as nouns, verbs, and adjectives; often used by 3-year-old children and college students taking lecture notes.

narrative

The orderly, sequenced relating of accounts or events.

communicate whatever fleeting thoughts they have. By the end of their second year, 2-year-olds have vocabularies of approximately 300 words; nevertheless, their favorite word tends to be "No!" They often have definite opinions about what they like and do not like, what they want and do not want—and what they want, they want *right now*. When they do not get what they want, they may communicate their displeasure with temper tantrums.

3- and 4-Year-Olds (Middle-Early Childhood)

Three-year-old children understand most of what is said to them; if one or two words are not familiar to them, they can usually figure them out from the context. Their receptive vocabularies are growing faster than their expressive vocabularies. Children this age begin to learn that more than one word can mean the same thing (*little, small, tiny*), but they tend to use one word rather than alternative words to express themselves. Children brought up in homes in which parents or other caregivers use a variety of synonyms benefit from the increased language exposure. This is an important reason for parents and caregivers to engage in **parallel speech**—that is, naming, describing, and explaining what the child is experiencing and probably feeling, almost as if the caregiver is the child. For example, "Mommy is turning on the bathroom light now. Now it is really bright in the bathroom. Mommy is turning on the faucet to wash your hands. The water is cold at first but it will warm up and feel good when I'm washing your hands." Parallel speech provides language and concepts for a child when the child does not have the language or concepts for **inner speech**. Parallel speech can help the child's speech, language, and **cognitive development**.

By the end of their third year children may have a 1,000-word vocabulary that they use in their typical 3-word sentences. Sentences used by 3-year-old children often omit the **functor (function) words**, such as articles (*a, the*), conjunctions (*and, but*), determiners (*this, that*), prepositions (*in, on*, etc.), and auxiliary verbs (*have, had*). This omission results in **telegraphic speech (language)**; that is, only the essential nouns, verbs, and adjectives are used. This is also a time when learning grammar and syntactical rules becomes increasingly important to convey meaning (Eisenberg, Guo, & Germezia, 2012). Children learn basic word order to convey simple messages, such as subject/verb/direct object (*"Mommy spill juice."*); subject/verb/indirect object (*"Girl go home."*); and subject/verb/subject complement (*"Boy run fast."*). Later they learn that when the subject and the auxiliary or helping verb are reversed in order, the sentence is changed into a question (*"Is the boy running fast?"*).

Three- and four-year-old children have developed several *grammatical morphemes*, such as *–ing* (eating), *-s* (shoes), *-'s* (baby's), *-ed* (jumped), and others. They begin using **narratives** for relating events and making up stories, but often without including the essential *who, what, when, where,* and *how* information, leaving listeners uncertain or confused. **Discourse** becomes part of 4-year-olds' communication abilities, with children relating long and intertwined stories.

Conversations demonstrate an organizational structure based on such elements as *initiation of topics, turn-taking,* and *topic maintenance* (staying on a topic) and *repairs* (rewording or restating an utterance that was not understood); that is, good pragmatics. Normal conversation adheres to the *cooperation principles* (Grice, 1975). That is, each participant must (1) include an appropriate *quantity* of information that is (2) of adequate *quality* and truthfulness, is (3) *relevant* to the established topic, and is (4) delivered in a *manner* that is clear and understandable. Through interactions with adults, young children learn these conversation or cooperation principles, and some become adept with conversation, also contributing to pragmatic skills.

5-Year-Olds (Late-Early Childhood)

Five-year-olds have the foundations of language from which all other language development is built. Children this age have learned to use functor words and grammatical morphemes, but still most of their sentences are declarative sentence forms or basic questions. Children begin refining and using more adult sentence structure that can better communicate the increasing subtleties of their messages. Children primarily use the contracted forms of many words (*can't, won't, don't, wouldn't, shouldn't, couldn't,* etc.) but have not learned the uncontracted forms (*cannot, will not,* etc.). It is sometimes surprising to clinicians that even children who do not have language development problems do not know the uncontracted forms and need to be taught the words.

Stage IV: 6–12 Years (Middle Childhood to Early Adolescence)

6-, 7-, and 8-Year-Olds

Middle childhood is a continual evolution of more complex and elaborate forms of language use. Children are increasingly using compound and complex sentences, passive sentences, and a variety of morphemes that may be used with *root* (base) words. Language is their tool for learning, and when they have language problems, they have learning problems.

9- and 10-Year-Olds

Nine- and 10-year-old children continue to develop increased language complexity as well as social and pragmatic skills. During these years, children gradually develop more awareness and insight into the effects of their language on others. Children are now "reading between the lines" of what others say. They often do not take statements at face value but increasingly interpret them from a personal perspective, asking, "What do you mean by *that*?" to even the most innocuous statements or questions, particularly from parents.

By the preteen years children ideally have developed their receptive and expressive language abilities to prepare them for high school

discourse

An extended verbal exchange on a topic (i.e., a conversation or long narrative).

and more advanced education if they choose. Their communication abilities will likely determine much of their educational success, social success, and future employment success. Speech and language are learned to communicate our wants, needs, thoughts, knowledge, and feelings with increasing accuracy and ease.

11- and 12-Year-Olds

During early adolescence children continue to develop language. However, as language demands at school are increasing in areas of both comprehension and expression, children who have borderline skills have increasing problems with academics and interactions with others. Adolescence is a peak period for learning and using *figurative language*, including idioms, metaphors and similes, and verbal humor that is often based on ambiguities and double meanings (being able to take a word or statement more than one way). Slang and jargon (which seem to be the foundation of many teenagers' social communication) are based primarily on figurative language. Competence in figurative language is important (if not essential) for peer acceptance and the social lives of teenagers.

CHAPTER SUMMARY

From the earliest days of life newborns absorb information through all of their senses. Speech development allows children to begin communicating with caregivers about their wants, needs, and feelings. The first 6 months of life lay the foundations for speech and language development. Speech development continues well after the beginning of the early school years. Language development is a long and complex process that all children must go through to develop communication skills in whatever native language they learn. The stages of language development are predictable, but each child has an individual rate of development. By knowing the language expectations of the various stages, parents and clinicians may have impressions of a child's development and whether it is at or near what is expected for the child's chronological age.

STUDY QUESTIONS

Knowledge and Comprehension

1. What is babbling and at what age does it normally begin?
2. What are three criteria for an infant's vocalization to be considered a true word?
3. By what age are most children using adult-like speech?
4. What three elements must be integrated to develop normal communication?
5. What is the *mean length of utterance*?

Application

1. How could knowing the age ranges and sequence of speech and language development help clinicians determine whether a child is developing speech and language at a normal rate?

2. Why should parents be concerned and what should they do if their infant does not begin to babble within the normal age range?

3. What can parents and other caregivers do regularly that can help children's speech and language development?

4. What could be the effects of a child not having a stimulating language environment?

5. Discuss the importance of children developing the ability to communicate their wants, needs, thoughts, information, and feelings to other children and to adults.

Analysis/Synthesis

1. How could knowing various theories of speech and language development help you understand a child's speech and language problems?

2. What is the relationship between speech development and language development?

3. Discuss the possible effects of an infant's severe hearing impairment on the development of speech and language.

4. Discuss the importance of a child developing narrative and discourse language abilities.

5. Discuss the cooperation principles and their importance in a child's language development.

REFERENCES

Allen, K. E., & Marotz, L. R. (2007). *Developmental profiles: Pre-birth through twelve.* Belmont, CA: Wadsworth Cengage Learning.

American Speech-Language-Hearing Association. (2004). Knowledge and skills needed by speech-language pathologists and audiologists to provide culturally and linguistically appropriate services. *The ASHA Leader, 24 (Supplement).*

Battle, D. (2002). *Communication disorders in multicultural populations* (3rd ed.). Boston, MA: Butterworth-Heinemann.

Bauman-Waengler, J. (2009). *Introduction to phonetics and phonology: From concepts to transcription.* Boston, MA: Pearson.

Berko-Gleason, J. (Ed.). (2001). *The development of language* (5th ed.). Boston, MA: Allyn and Bacon.

Bloom, L., & Lahey, M. (1978). *Language development and language disorders.* New York, NY: John Wiley.

Brown, R. (1973). *A first language: The early stages.* Cambridge, MA: Harvard University Press.

Cheng, L. (2002). Asian and Pacific American cultures. In D. E. Battle (Ed.). *Communication disorders in multicultural populations* (3rd ed.). Boston, MA: Butterworth-Heinemann.

Crystal, D. (2010). *The Cambridge encyclopedia of language* (3rd ed.). Cambridge, MA: Cambridge University Press.

Eisenberg, S. L., Guo, L., & Germezia, M. (2012). *How grammatical are 3-year-olds? Language, Speech, and Hearing Services in the Schools, 43,* 36–52.

Fadiman, A. (1997). *The Spirit Catches You and You Fall Down.* New York, NY: Farrar, Straus and Giroux.

Goleman, D. (1995). *Emotional intelligence: Why it can matter more than IQ.* New York, NY: Bantam Books.

Grice, H. P. (1975). Logic and conversation. In P. Cole & J. Morgan (Eds.), *Syntax and semantics: Speech acts.* New York, NY: Academic Press.

Hammer, C., Miccio, A. W., & Wagstaff, D. (2003). Home literacy experiences and their relationship to bilingual preschoolers' developing English literacy abilities: An initial investigation. *Language, Speech, and Hearing Services in Schools, 34,* 20–30.

Harrison, K . D. (2010). *The last speakers: The quest to save the world's most endangered languages.* Washington, D.C.: National Geographic Society.

Hulit, L. M., Howard, M. R., & Fahey, K. R. (2011). *Born to talk: An introduction to speech and language development* (5th ed.). Boston, MA: Allyn and Bacon.

James, S. (1960). *Normal language acquisition.* Boston, MA: Little Brown.

Kindler, A. (2002). *Survey of the states' limited English proficient students and available educational programs and services.* Washington, DC: National Clearinghouse for English Language.

Kishiyama, M. M., Boyce, W. T., Jimenez, A. M., Perry, L. M., & Knight, R. T. (2009). Socioeconomic disparities affect prefrontal function in children. *Journal of Cognitive Neuroscience, 21*(6), 1106–1115.

Landau, B. & Gleitman, L. R. (1985). *Language and experience: Evidence from the blind child.* Cambridge, MA: Harvard University Press.

Locke, J. L. (1993). *The child's path to spoken language.* Cambridge, MA: Harvard University Press.

McLaughlin, S. F. (2006). *Introduction to language development* (2nd ed.). Clifton Park, NY: Delmar Cengage Learning.

Oller, D. K., & Pearson, B. (2002). Assessing the effects of bilingualism: A background. In D. K. Oller & R. Eilers (Eds.), *Language and literacy in bilingual children.* Clevedon, England: Multilingual Matters.

Owens, R. E., Jr. (2012). *Language development: An introduction* (8th ed.). San Antonio, TX: Pearson/Allyn & Bacon.

Peluso, P. R., Peluso, J. P., Kern, R. M., White, J. A. (2004). *A comparison of attachment theory and individual psychology: A review of the literature. Journal of Counseling and Development, 83*(2), 139–145.

Pence-Turnbull, K. L., & Justice, L. M. (2012). *Language development from theory to practice* (2nd ed.). Upper Saddle River, NJ: Pearson Prentice Hall.

Perez-Pereira, M., & Conti-Ramsden, G. (1999). *Language development and social interactions in blind children*. Hove, England: Psychology Press.

Pinker, S. (1984). *Language, learnability, and language development*. Cambridge, MA: Harvard University Press.

Roseberry-McKibbin, C. (2006). *Language disorders in children: A multicultural and case perspective*. Boston, MA: Allyn and Bacon.

Roseberry-McKibbin, C. (2008). *Multicultural students with special language needs: Practical strategies for assessment and intervention* (3rd ed.). Oceanside, CA: Academic Communication Associates.

Rosin, P. (2006). Literacy intervention in culturally and linguistically diverse worlds: The Linking Language and Literacy Project. In L. M. Justice (Ed.). *Clinical approaches to emergent literacy intervention*. San Diego, CA: Plural Publishing.

Ryback, C., Eastin, C. L., & Robbins, I. (2004). Native American healing practices and counseling. *Journal of Humanistic Counseling, Education, and Development, 43*(1), 25–33.

Salas-Provance, M. (2012). Counseling in a multicultural society: Implications for the field of communicative disorders. In L. V. Flasher & P. T. Fogle, *Counseling skills for speech-language pathologists and audiologists*. Clifton Park, NY: Delmar Cengage Learning.

Sander, E. K. (1972). When are speech sounds learned? *Journal of Speech and Language Disorders, 37*, 62.

Secord, W. A., & Donohue, J. S. (2002). *Clinical assessment of articulation and phonology*. Greenville, SC: Super Duper.

Seymour, H. N., & Pearson, B. (2004). Evaluating language variation: Distinguishing dialect and development from disorder. *Seminars in Speech and Language, 25*(1), 18–26.

Shields, M. K., & Behrman, R. E. (2004). Children of immigrant families: Analysis and recommendations. *The Future of Children, 14*(2), 4–15.

Terrell, S. L., & Jackson, R. S. (2002). African Americans in the Americas. In D. E. Battle (Ed.), *Communication disorders in multicultural populations* (3rd ed.). Boston, MA: Butterworth-Heinemann.

U.S. Census Bureau. (2011). *Statistical abstract of the United States: 2012* (130th ed.). Washington, DC: U.S. Census Bureau.

Willamson, G. (2010). *Phonological processes: Natural ways of simplifying speech production*. London, England: Speech Therapy Information and Resources.

Wyatt, T. A. (2001). *The role of the family, community, and school in children's acquisition and maintenance of African American English: Sociocultural and historical contexts of African American English*. Amsterdam, Netherlands/Philadelphia, PA: John Benjamin Publishing.

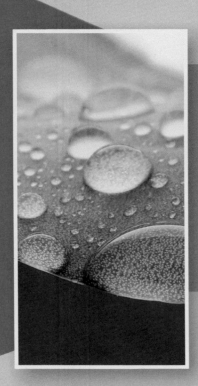

CHAPTER 5
Articulation and Phonological Disorders in Children

LEARNING OBJECTIVES

After studying this chapter, you will:

- Be able to discuss vowels and consonants and how they are produced.
- Be able to discuss the etiologies of articulation and phonological disorders.
- Understand the essentials of articulation disorders.
- Understand the essentials of phonological disorders.
- Understand the essentials of childhood motor speech disorders.
- Be able to discuss the assessment of articulation and phonology.
- Be able to discuss the general principles of therapy for articulation and phonological disorders.
- Be familiar with multicultural considerations of children with articulation and phonological disorders.
- Appreciate the emotional and social effects of articulation and phonological disorders on children.

KEY TERMS

addition

allophone

anoxia

auditory discrimination training (ear training)

bilabial

cerebral palsy

childhood apraxia of speech (CAS)

cognate

diadochokinetic (diadochokinesis, diadochols)

diphthong

distinctive feature

distortion

dysarthria

failure to thrive

frenum/frenulum

fricative

functional

gavage feeding

generalization

glide

KEY TERMS continued

hypertonicity

hypotonicity

idiopathic

infantile hypoxia

International Phonetic Alphabet (IPA)

labiodental

letter

linguadental (interdental)

linguapalatal

linguavelar

low birth weight

manner

multifactorial

nasal

nasogastric (NG) tube

omission

organic

perinatal

perseverate/ perseveration

phonetics

place

positive reinforcement (positive feedback, reward)

premature

sensorimotor

sibilant

significant

social reinforcer

spontaneous (connected, running) speech sample

stimulability

stop

substitution

symmetry (symmetrical)

voice

INTRODUCTION

Articulation and phonological disorders are the most common communication disorders of children. As defined previously, an articulation disorder is an incorrect production of speech sounds because of faulty placement, timing, direction, pressure, speed, or integration of the movements of the mandible, lips, tongue, or soft palate. A phonological disorder is defined as errors of several phonemes that form patterns or clusters and are the result of a child simplifying speech sounds and sound combinations that are used by normal speaking adults. Articulation and phonological disorders may occur as isolated problems or as part of other delays or disorders, including language disorders, developmental delays, neurological disorders such as cerebral palsy or brain injuries, and *orofacial* (oral-facial) anomalies such as cleft lip and cleft palate. However, before articulation and phonological disorders can be discussed, it will be helpful to have more of an understanding of General American English (GAE) speech sounds, followed by some causes of articulation and phonological disorders.

GENERAL AMERICAN ENGLISH

American English has as its foundation British English; however, the glossary of this book provides many Latin and Greek derivatives of our professional terminology, and some can be traced back hundreds to thousands of years. General American English or "American English" speech is spoken by millions of people throughout the United States and is considered not to have a regional dialect associated with it. This is the speech normally used by radio and television broadcasters, and when used a person is less likely to be asked, "Where are you from?" General American English is considered the speech of most people in the western regions of the United States (Edwards, 2003).

Speech-language pathologists, audiologists, linguists, and phoneticians make a distinction between a **letter** and a phoneme. A letter is an arbitrary written or printed symbol or character representing a speech sound. A phoneme is the shortest arbitrary unit of sound in a language that can be recognized as being distinct from other sounds in the language. In the English language there are 26 letters but 45 speech sounds (phonemes) because as the language developed, sounds were added after the 26-letter alphabet was established. Other languages may have significantly more or fewer letters in their alphabets and more or fewer phonemes.

The "name" of a letter may not have any resemblance to the sound associated with the letter. For example, we have the letter "h," which we pronounce as "eytch," but the sound is made by opening the vocal folds

letter

An arbitrary written or printed symbol or character representing a speech sound.

and forcing air through with no vibration (as in whispering), while holding the mandible in a slightly open position and with the articulators not creating any restriction of the air. Also, the alphabet has the letter "c," but the sound of the letter is either /s/ or /k/, as in *city* or *cup*. The many variations of spellings of the same sound cause confusion for children learning to spell (e.g., the sound /f/ may be spelled *f* [*for*], *ff* [*off*], *ph* [phone], or *gh* [*rough*]).

In the study of phonology, SLPs use **phonetics** to describe the individual sounds in a language and use the **International Phonetic Alphabet (IPA)** transcription symbols in an attempt to identify specific sounds for any language or dialect (see Table 5–1). The IPA includes 25 consonants (compared to 21 letters in the alphabet), 15 vowels (compared to 5 in the alphabet), and 5 **diphthongs** (not represented by single letters in the alphabet), giving a total of 45 phonemes (compared to 26 letters) (Small, 2012). (Note: Phoneticians do not necessarily agree on the precise number of consonant and vowel phonemes.) However, although a single phonetic symbol may be used for a phoneme, in reality there are slight variations in the way different people produce individual phonemes, and there can be variations of a phoneme depending on whether it is in the *initial, middle (medial)*, or *final* position of a word, or what sounds precede or follow an individual phoneme. These slight variations in individual phonemes are referred to as **allophones**.

Vowels

Vowels, as defined in Chapter 1, are voiced speech sounds from the unrestricted passage of the air stream through the mouth without audible stoppage or friction. Vowels can be described by the placement of the tongue during their production. The *vowel quadrilateral diagram* is a four-sided figure (usually shown as a trapezoid) that represents tongue positions and movements. The corners are labeled *high front, high back, low front*, and *low back*. Figure 5–1 shows a vowel quadrilateral with key words representing the sound of each vowel (note: there can be some variation of vowels in words depending on dialects and accents). You can experiment with producing different vowels by keeping the mandible slightly open and the lips in a neutral position, and then slowly moving the tongue forward and backward, raising and lowering it, and flattening and then humping it up in back. Then keeping the tongue in a neutral position and the mandible slightly open, slowly protrude and retract the lips while voicing.

Consonants

As defined in Chapter 1, consonants are speech sounds articulated by either stopping of the outgoing air stream or creating a narrow opening of resistance using the articulators. Consonants are commonly described by their **distinctive features**; that is, the smallest individual differences required to differentiate one phoneme from another. The three

---

phonetics

The study of speech-sound production and the special symbols that represent speech sounds.

International Phonetic Alphabet (IPA)

Specially devised signs and symbols designed to represent the individual speech sounds of all languages.

diphthong

A combination of two vowels in which one vowel glides continuously into the second vowel; in American English: /eɪ/, /aɪ/, /oʊ/, and /aʊ/.

allophone

Slight variation in the way different people produce individual phonemes that can be affected by the initial, middle, or final position of a word, or what sounds precede or follow an individual phoneme.

distinctive feature

The smallest individual differences required to differentiate one phoneme from another in a language.

TABLE 5-1   International Phonetic Alphabet Symbols

CONSONANTS		VOWELS	
SYMBOL	**COMMONLY HEARD IN**	**SYMBOL**	**COMMONLY HEARD IN**
p	*p*ick	i	*ea*t
b	*b*ook	ɪ	*i*t
t	*t*ake	ɛ	*e*gg
d	*d*ay	æ	*a*pple
k	*c*at	ʌ	*o*ven
g	*g*et	ə (schwa)	*a*mong
f	*f*ish	a	f*a*ther*
v	*v*ase	ɔ	f*a*ther*
θ	*th*ink	ɑ	h*o*p
ð	*th*at	o	*o*cean
s	*s*it	u	*u*se
z	*z*oo	ʊ	f*oo*t
ʃ š	*sh*oe	ɜ	g*ir*l*
ʒ' ž	mea*s*ure	ɝ	b*ir*d*
h	*h*ome		
ʧ č	*ch*ip	**ENGLISH DIPHTHONGS**	
ʤ ǰ	*j*ob	**SYMBOL**	**COMMONLY HEARD IN**
m	*m*oon	eɪ	*a*te
n	*n*o	aɪ	*I'm*
ŋ	ri*ng*	oʊ	*oa*ts
j y	*y*es	aʊ	*ou*ch
w	*w*eek	ɔɪ	*oi*l
(r)	*r*ed	u	*u*se
l	*l*ake		
ʍ*	*wh*at		

*May be regional or individual pronunciations.
Based on Tables 2–1 and 2–2 in Yavas, M. (1998). *Phonology development and disorders*. Clifton Park, NY: Delmar Cengage Learning.

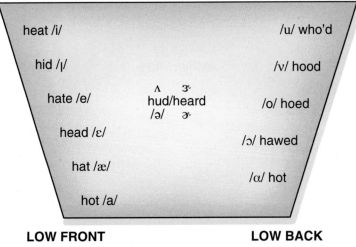

HIGH FRONT   **HIGH BACK**

heat /i/   /u/ who'd

hid /ɪ/   /ʊ/ hood

hate /e/   ʌ   ɝ   /o/ hoed
    hud/heard
    /ə/   ɚ

head /ɛ/   /ɔ/ hawed

hat /æ/   /ɑ/ hot

hot /a/

LOW FRONT   **LOW BACK**

Figure 5–1

Vowel quadrilateral with key words and phonetic symbols.

© Cengage Learning 2013.

major distinctive features are place, manner, and voice (see Table 5–2). Speech sounds may be **voiced**, with the vocal folds vibrating (e.g., /b, d, g, z, v/ and all vowels), or *unvoiced,* with no vocal fold vibration (e.g., /p, t, k, s, f/). When sounds are articulated in the same place and differ only in being voiced or unvoiced, they are referred to as **cognates** (e.g., /b-p, t-d, k-g, s-z, f-v/). Table 5–2 shows the classification of consonants by place, manner, and voice.

    Place refers to the location in the mouth where two articulators come together (constrict) to produce specific sounds. Places may include the lips, teeth, alveolar ridge, tongue, and hard and soft palates. The place where articulator constriction occurs is used to classify consonants:

- *Bilabial* consonants are produced when there is contact between the two lips (/p, b, m/) or the two lips *approximate* (/w/).
- *Labiodental* sounds are produced with the upper incisor teeth in contact with the lower lip (/f, v/).
- *Linguadental* consonants are produced when the tongue tip is placed between the upper and the lower incisor teeth (i.e., *linguadental* voiced and unvoiced /th/).
- *Alveolar* consonants are produced when the tip of the tongue (*apex*) is in contact with the alveolar ridge of the maxilla, just behind the upper incisor teeth (i.e., *lingua [tongue]-alveolar* /t, d, s, z, n, l/). This point of contact produces more sounds than any other; however, it is the pressure of the tongue tip against the alveolar ridge and the length of time the tongue tip and alveolar ridge are in contact that allow us to produce the various sounds.
- *Palatal* consonants are produced when the blade or body of the tongue is near the hard palate (i.e., *linguapalatal* /ʃ/ [sh], /tʃ/ [ch], /dʒ/, /j/, and /r/).
- *Velar* consonants are produced by the back of the tongue (root) approaching the soft palate (velum) (i.e., *linguavelar* /k/, /g/, and /ŋ/).

voice

The distinctive feature that refers to a sound produced either with the vocal folds vibrating (*voiced*) or not vibrating (*unvoiced*).

cognate

Two sounds that differ only in voicing (e.g., /p/ - /b/).

place

The location in the mouth where two articulators come together (make contact or near contact to constrict the air) to produce specific sounds; places may include the lips, teeth, alveolar ridge, tongue, and hard and soft palates.

TABLE 5-2   Classification of Consonants by Distinctive Features: Place, Manner, and Voice

PLACE OF ARTICULATION	PHONETIC SYMBOL AND KEY WORD	MANNER OF ARTICULATION	VOICE
Bilabial	/p/ (pay)	Stop	−
	/b/ (bay)	Stop	+
	/m/ (may)	Nasal	+
Labial	/ʍ/ (which)	Glide (semivowel)	−
	/w/ (witch)	Glide (semivowel)	+
Labiodental	/f/ (fan)	Fricative	−
	/v/ (van)	Fricative	+
Linguadental	/θ/ (thin)	Fricative	−
(interdental)	/ð/ (this)	Fricative	+
Lingua-alveolar	/t/ (two)	Stop	−
	/d/ (do)	Stop	+
	/s/ (sue)	Fricative	−
	/z/ (zoo)	Fricative	+
	/n/ (new)	Nasal	+
	/l/ (Lou)	Lateral	+
Linguapalatal	/ʃ/ (shoe)	Fricative	−
	/ʒ/ (rouge)	Fricative	+
	/tʃ/ (chin)	Affricative	−
	/dʒ/ (gin)	Affricative	+
	/j/ (you)	Glide (semivowel)	+
	/r/ (rue)	Rhotic	+
Linguavelar	/k/ (back)	Stop	−
	/g/ (bag)	Stop	+
	/ŋ/ (bang)	Nasal	+
Glottal (laryngeal)	/h/ (who)	Fricative	−
	—	Stop	+ (−)

Source: Gelfer, M. P. (1996). *Survey of communication disorders: A social and behavioral perspective.* New York: McGraw-Hill. Reproduced with permission of the McGraw-Hill Companies.

- The *glottal* consonant is produced at the level of the vocal folds by having the vocal folds in an open position and briefly exhaling air (/h/).

Manner is the way in which the air stream is modified as a result of the interaction of the articulators (Bauman-Waengler, 2012). One manner of articulation, *stop-plosives*, consists of consonants that are produced when a complete occlusion between two articulators occurs, for example, /p/, /b/, /t/, /d/, /k/, and /g/. Another manner is **fricatives**, which are produced when air is forced through a narrow constriction between two articulators, such as /f/ and /v/. **Sibilants** are a subcategory of fricative and are produced with a hissing noise, such as /s/, /z/, /ʃ/ [sh], and /ʒ/. *Affricates* are produced as a stop-plosive that releases into a fricative /tʃ/ and /dʒ/. Nasals are produced by lowering the velum so the air passes into the nasal passages resulting in /m/, /n/, or /ŋ/. *Approximates* are produced when the articulators are near one another but do not close enough to cause friction, such as /w/, /j/, /r/, and /l/.

The lips are important in producing several sounds, especially the **bilabial** (two lips) **stops** /p/ and /b/, where both lips touch and then release for sound to escape; the **nasal** sound /m/, where the lips are closed and the sound passes behind the soft palate and through the nasal passage; the bilabial **glide (semivowel)** /w/, where the lips are rounded and slightly protruded then relaxed; and the **labiodental fricatives** /f/ and /v/, where the upper front teeth are in contact with the lower lip (compare to other fricatives: e.g., /θ/ [th], /ð/ [th], and /s/, /z/).

In English, the tongue is particularly important when producing the **linguadental (interdental)** voiced and unvoiced /th/ sounds, where the tongue tip is placed lightly between the top and the bottom front teeth; the **lingua-alveolar** voiced and unvoiced /d/ and /t/ sounds, where the tongue tip makes contact with the alveolar ridge just behind the upper front teeth; the **linguapalatal** /ʃ/ [sh] and /tʃ/ [ch] sounds, where the top center of the tongue is near the hard palate; and the **linguavelar** /k/ and /g/ consonants, where the back of the tongue moves near the soft palate.

Blends (consonant clusters)

Blends (consonant clusters) are combinations of two or three consonants where each consonant can be heard. There are four major categories of consonant blends: *l*-blends (e.g., _bl_ack, _cl_ean, _fl_at), *r*-blends (e.g., _br_own, c_r_edit, _dr_eam), *s*-blends (e.g., _st_ate, _sm_ooth, _sp_in, _sw_im, _scr_am, _squ_are, _spl_ash, _spr_ing, _str_aw), and middle/end blends (pas_t_ure, ex_pl_ain, fo_ld_, mi_lk_). (Note: When two consonants are together but one is silent, it is not considered a blend [e.g., half], or when two consonants are combined to form one sound it is not considered a blend [e.g., children].) Blends are typically later developing sounds for children.

Figure 5–2 shows the relationship between the articulators and their corresponding places of articulation for consonants. Figure 5–3 illustrates the general places of articulation for the primary consonants in American English.

---

manner

The way in which the air stream is modified as a result of the interaction of the articulators; direction of airflow (e.g., oral or nasal sounds), or the degree of narrowing of the vocal tract by the articulators in the various places.

fricative

A sound formed by forcing the air stream through a narrow opening between articulators (tongue-teeth /θ/, /ð/ [th]; lips /f/, /v/; tongue-alveolar ridge /s/, /z/, and tongue-hard palate /ʃ/).

sibilant

A fricative sound whose production is accompanied by a "hissing" sound (/s/, /z/, /ʃ/ [sh], and /ʒ/).

bilabial

Referring to the two lips or bilabial sounds, /p/ and /b/.

stop

A sound made by building up air pressure in the mouth and then suddenly releasing it; the airflow can be blocked momentarily by pressing the lips together (bilabial—/p, b/) or by pressing the tongue against either the gums (lingua-alveolar—/t, d/) or the soft palate (linguavelar—/k, g/).

nasal

A sound resulting from the closing of the oral cavity, preventing air from escaping through the mouth, with a lowered position of the soft palate and a free passage of air through the nose (/m/, /n/, and /ŋ/ [ng]).

glide (semivowel)

A type of consonant that has a gradual (gliding) change in an articulator (lips or tongue) position and a relative long production of sound; /w/, /j/.

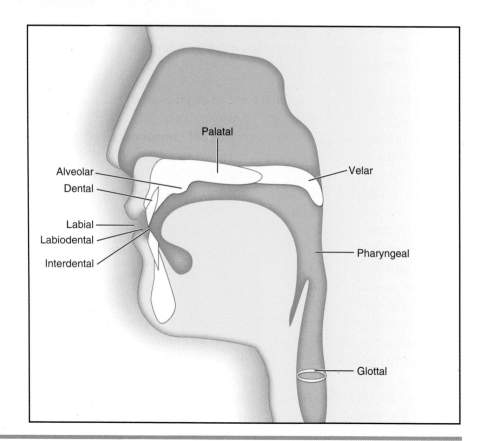

Figure 5-2

The relationship between the articulators and their corresponding places of articulation.

© Cengage Learning 2013.

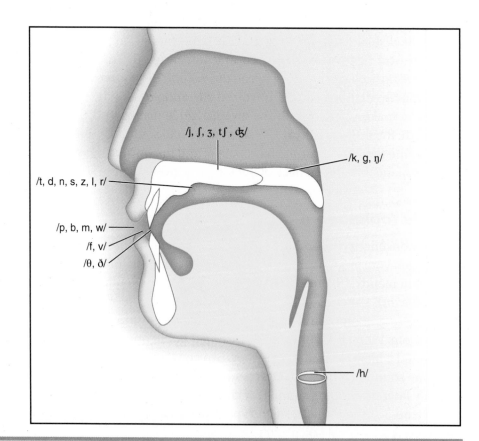

Figure 5-3

General places of articulation for the primary consonants in American English.

© Cengage Learning 2013.

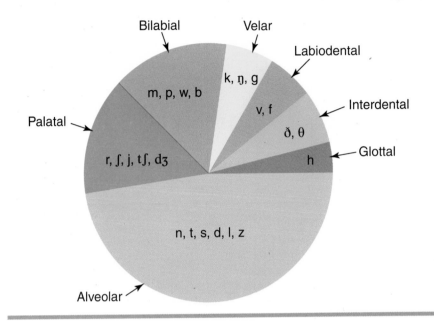

Figure 5-4

Pie chart showing the relative frequency of occurrence of consonants produced at different places of articulation.

Based on data from Dewey, 1923.

Dewey (1923) studied the frequency of occurrence of English consonants by using 100,000 words taken from newspapers, fiction books, speeches, letters, scientific articles, and magazines. A pie chart shows the relative frequency of occurrence of consonants produced at different places of articulation (Figure 5-4). The rank order of frequency of occurrence for place of articulation, from most to least frequent, is alveolar (almost 50% of consonants), palatal, bilabial, velar, labiodental, interdental, and glottal. Also, the individual consonants are listed in rank order of frequency of occurrence. For example, /n/ is the most frequent alveolar consonant (it is the most frequent of *all* consonants). Knowing the frequency of occurrence for place of articulation of consonants is important clinically; for example, by helping children who have difficulty with alveolar sounds, we can help them improve the articulation of almost half of all consonants they speak. Bilabial sounds and labiodental sounds are often relatively easy to remediate; therefore, by helping children improve the articulation of the alveolar, bilabial, and labiodental sounds, approximately 75% of consonants will be correctly articulated.

ETIOLOGIES OF COMMUNICATION DISORDERS

There are three general etiologies, or causes, of communication disorders (articulation, phonology, and language) in children: normal variation, environmental problems, and physical impairments or differences. In many cases, a combination of etiologies affects a child. Often the cause or causes of a communication disorder remain elusive, even with a careful case history, review of all educational and medical records, and extensive testing of the client.

labiodental

The /f/ and /v/ sounds, where the upper front teeth are in contact with the lower lip.

linguadental (interdental)

Voiced and unvoiced /th/ sounds with the tongue tip placed lightly between the top and the bottom front teeth.

linguapalatal

The /ʃ/ [sh] and /ʒ/ [zh] sounds, where the top center of the tongue is near the hard palate.

linguavelar

The /k/ and /g/ consonants, where the back of the tongue moves near the soft palate.

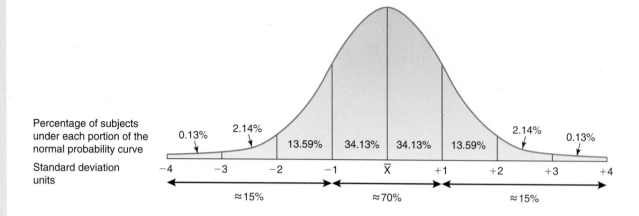

Figure 5–5

Normal distribution.

Adapted from Nicolosi, Harryman, & Kresheck, 2004.

Normal Variation

If we consider the basic bell-shaped curve that reflects the normal distribution of any trait or ability, it helps us realize that most children (approximately 70%) are within the normal range of speech and language development and that relatively few are outside of the normal range by one, two, or three standard deviations (see Figure 5–5). This is an important concept for SLPs and Auds because it is possible to lose the perspective of normalcy if we are not around normal-speaking children enough to keep our ears and perception finely tuned to what is within the normal range and what is outside of it. As clinicians, we work with individuals who are one, two, or more standard deviations below the mean in hearing, speech, language, and cognitive functioning. If a clinician works with many children who have moderate to severe impairments (two or three standard deviations below the mean) and then evaluates a child who is just one standard deviation below the mean, the clinician may feel and report to the parents that the child is doing "just fine" or even "great." However, when compared to normal children of the same age rather than to children with **significant** communication problems, the child is not doing "just fine" or "great."

All parts of our bodies and their functioning may be considered inside or outside normal variation. A body structure or system outside of normal variation could cause or contribute to communication impairments. However, another structure or system may compensate to prevent communication impairments from manifesting. A classic example is a moderate or even severe dental malocclusion that would appear to significantly affect an individual's speech intelligibility; however,

significant

A term often used to specify the impairment level a child must exhibit before he is considered to have a speech or language disorder; no "gold standard" is available to use to define this term as it applies to speech and language disorders. In statistics, the probability that a given finding (e.g., an individual test score) may have occurred by chance; usually a finding that occurs fewer than 5 times in 100 by chance alone ($p < .05$).

because of the remarkable adaptability of the tongue, an individual may have normal or near-normal speech intelligibility.

"Functional" versus "Organic" Disorders

SLPs and Auds have long debated the distinction between **functional** and **organic** communication disorders. They are considered labels of convenience because communication disorders may be neither all organic nor all functional. That is, "functional" disorders may have some organic elements, and "organic" disorders may have some functional elements.

The terms *speech impediment* or *defect* and *tongue-tie* have long been used by lay people (individuals not educated in speech-language pathology or audiology, including parents, teachers, nurses, and physicians) in reference to individuals of all ages who have some speech impairment. These terms suggest that there is a structural cause of a speech problem even though there is no apparent structural (organic) problem that can be found when an evaluation is conducted. The terms *speech impediment* or *defect* and *tongue-tie* are considered obsolete terms for *speech disorder* or *speech impairment (problem)*.

functional

An incorrect production of standard speech sounds for which there is no known anatomical, physiological, or neurological basis.

organic

The inability to correctly produce standard speech sounds because of anatomical, physiological, or neurological causes.

Tongue-tie (ankyloglossia)

"Tongue-tie" is a term that has been applied to a variety of communication problems, including impaired articulation, stuttering, and shyness. However, tongue-tie (*ankyloglossia*) is caused by a restrictive lingual **frenum** or **frenulum** that is abnormally short or is attached too close to the tip of the tongue (see Figure 5–6). This causes difficulty elevating and protruding the tongue tip, which affects production of some sounds (e.g., /t, d, l, th/).

frenum/frenulum

A fold of mucous tissue connecting the floor of the mouth to the midline underside of the tongue.

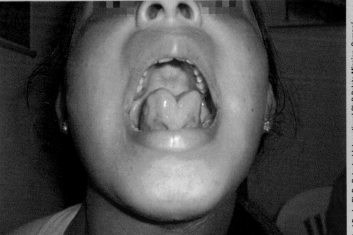

Paul Fogle, Ph.D., Rotaplast International Cleft Palate Mission, Cumaná, Venezuela, 2008

Figure 5–6
Restrictive lingual frenum (tongue-tie).

Environmental Problems

Even though a person may have the best of genetic potential at the moment of conception, the embryo and fetus's prenatal environment may seriously affect the realization of that potential. Furthermore, when genetic potential is good and the embryo or fetus develops in an ideal prenatal environment, the postnatal environment may seriously or even profoundly diminish a person's potential in life.

Prenatal Environment

In a way, the prenatal environment begins at the moment of conception and is affected by the combination of genetic material. It is also influenced by both the mother's and the father's physical health at that moment and thereafter by the mother's self-care and general health throughout the pregnancy. Unfortunately, even women who take excellent care of themselves during their pregnancies may have health problems that predispose a child to developmental delays and disorders; examples include pre-pregnancy obesity, type II diabetes mellitus, insufficient amounts of folic acid in the diet, the need to take seizure medication, and the human immunodeficiency virus (HIV) found in those with AIDS. During the embryo's first trimester of life, it is most susceptible to medical complications.

Apgar Scores

Apgar scores (named after Virginia Apgar, an American obstetric anesthesiology specialist, 1909–1974) evaluate an infant's physical condition at 1 minute and again at 5 minutes after birth. The attending pediatrician rates five factors: skin color, heart rate, respiratory effort, muscle tone, and reflex irritability. The rating procedure now utilizes an acronym based on Virginia Apgar's name: A (appearance), P (pulse), G (grimace), A (activity), and R (respiration). Each factor is scored with a low value of 0 to a normal value of 2, and the scores are totaled for each evaluation; for example, a newborn may have an Apgar of 8 at 1 minute and of 10 at 5 minutes. Most newborns have a score of 7–9 at 1 minute. Scores of 5–6 are borderline, and scores of 4 or less mean the newborn requires immediate assistance with breathing and possible transfer to a *neonatal intensive care unit* (NICU) (Apgar, 1953). Infants with low Apgar scores may be considered high risk for various developmental delays and disorders that may not be noticeable until the child begins to walk, develop speech and language, or has difficulty reading and learning. Most mothers and fathers do not know their children's Apgar scores and, therefore, may not make the connection that the early minutes after birth may set the stage for the child being at risk for developmental problems through the years and challenges throughout adulthood.

Syndromes

Various syndromes can cause or contribute to communication delays and disorders. A few examples of syndromes that may significantly affect communication development include (1) *Down syndrome*, the most common chromosomal disorder, which is characterized by a small head, flat face, upward slanting eyes, and short fingers; (2) *fetal alcohol syndrome* (FAS), characterized by prenatal and postnatal growth retardation, facial abnormalities, heart defects, joint and limb abnormalities, and intellectual impairment; (3) *Asperger's syndrome*, which is a pervasive developmental disorder similar to autistic disorder, characterized by severe impairment of social interactions and by restricted interests and behaviors, although speech, language, and cognitive development may be near normal. Many syndromes, including those mentioned here, also include mild to severe speech, language, and cognitive delays or disorders.

Maternal Substance Abuse

The most likely etiology of prenatal problems of all kinds is the mother's abuse of illegal drugs, alcohol, and nicotine (Center on Addiction and Substance Abuse, 2005). Approximately 35% to 40% of women in the United States abuse illegal drugs, alcohol, or nicotine sometime during pregnancy. In addition, approximately 75% of pregnant women who abuse one substance abuse other substances that could be harmful to the unborn child. Maternal substance abuse resulting in neurological and other damage to newborns is perhaps the only cause of communication and other impairments that is 100% preventable.

When maternal substance abuse is the cause of or a contributor to a child's communication problems, the child's potential for developing normal or merely functional communication abilities and skills for independent living may be significantly reduced, even with the best long-term professional involvement. The long-term consequences for these children are not always clear and ongoing therapy is usually necessary. Figure 5–7 presents risks of prenatal drug exposure for physical and communicative development.

Low Birth Weight and Prematurity

In the United States, approximately 8.5% of infants have **low birth weight** (Rossetti, 2001); this percentage may be significantly higher in less-developed countries. Seventy percent of low birth weight infants (weight less than 5.5 pounds or 2,500 grams) are **premature**. In the United States, 97% of newborns weigh between ≈5.5 pounds (2,500 grams) and ≈10 pounds (4,500 grams), with an average of ≈7.5 pounds (3,500 grams) (Mosby, 2009). Unlike normal birth weight infants, premature and low birth weight infants have fragile and underdeveloped vascular systems, including in their brains. Infants may have strokes in utero (primarily *hemorrhagic* strokes where a blood vessel in the brain ruptures and blood leaks or flows into the brain tissue). Prematurity and low birth weight put an infant at risk for communication problems, including learning disabilities that may not be evident until early elementary school when the child is learning to read (Grunau, Kearney, & Whitfield, 1990).

low birth weight

An infant whose weight at birth is less than 5.5 pounds (2,500 grams), regardless of gestational age.

premature (infant)

Any infant born before the gestational age of 37 weeks; often associated with low birth weight that results in high risk for incomplete organ system development, causing poor temperature regulation, respiratory disorders, and poor sucking and swallowing reflexes.

Physical Risks
- Small head circumference
- Low birth weight from prematurity or intrauterine growth retardation
- Small strokes or heart attacks (intrauterine cerebral and cardiac infarctions) before birth
- Congenital malformations of the heart, genitourinary tracts, and limbs
- AIDS and other infections

Behavioral Risks
Infancy
- Irritability
- Hypertonicity or hypotonicity
- Hyperactivity
- Tremulousness
- Deficiencies in organization of state and interactive abilities
- Seizures

Childhood
- Reduced self-regulation
- Distractibility (ADD or ADHD)
- Reduced pretend play
- Flat affect
- Attachment problems

Figure 5-7

Risks of prenatal drug exposure for physical and communicative development.

Adapted from Sparks, 1993.

perinatal

Pertaining to the time and process of giving birth or being born.

infantile hypoxia

In newborns and infants, inadequate oxygenation of the blood leading to *tachycardia* (rapid heart rate) and rapid, shallow breathing that quickly affects the brain and other organs and systems; severe hypoxia can result in cardiac failure.

anoxia

A complete lack of oxygen to the brain that is relatively rare but causes devastating neurological disorders.

Perinatal Environment

Perinatal (time of birth) problems occur because of complications at birth and often result in multiple severe handicaps. **Infantile hypoxia**, a partial or significantly diminished supply of oxygen to the brain that results in neurological damage, is the most common perinatal complication. **Anoxia**, a complete lack of oxygen reaching the brain, is a relatively rare but devastating cause of neurological disorders. When hypoxia or anoxia occurs, the cerebral cortex is most severely damaged because it is furthest from where the blood enters the brain. In many cases, the brainstem and midbrain may be relatively well preserved, allowing the major body systems and organs to function; however, the cortical damage may cause severely impaired communication, cognition, and swallowing abilities.

Postnatal Environment

Our environment influences or determines the sounds we produce for individual words and the words we use to express ourselves. In most cases, children are about as intelligible as the parents who have helped them learn speech and language. Some home and community environments for children are not conducive to good speech and language development. When a child has limited environmental stimulation (deprivation),

Chanel

Chanel was 2 years old when her parents contacted me to evaluate their daughter who was not yet saying her first intelligible words. The case history revealed that the child had been adopted as a newborn in another state and was a **failure-to-thrive** infant. Chanel had inefficient sucking and swallowing reflexes, and the parents went through extraordinary measures to provide sufficient nutrition for the infant, including **gavage feeding** for 7 months. Metabolically, Chanel was unable to accept food. The parents eventually were able to contact the obstetrician who delivered the infant and learned that the mother "may have" used illegal drugs during the pregnancy, which likely was the etiology of Chanel's failure to thrive and other developmental problems.

I worked with the child three times a week in the family home on a blanket on the living room floor demonstrating to the mother and grandmother, who were always present, how to maximize speech and language development throughout the day and techniques to improve muscle tone of the various speech systems (the child had been diagnosed by a pediatrician as having cerebral palsy). I eventually discontinued working with Chanel when she entered a public preschool program for severely handicapped children where she would receive more extensive therapy throughout the day; however, I maintained intermittent contact with the parents to follow the child's progress.

At 8 years of age, Chanel was the size of a 2-year-old. She underwent a magnetic resonance imaging (MRI) examination, which revealed that during the birthing process she had sustained an *occlusive stroke* (blockage of an artery in the brain) that had cut off all of the blood supply to the pituitary gland (the "master gland" that controls growth and the secondary production of other hormones and functioning of organ systems). The stroke that caused the lack of pituitary functioning also severely complicated the developmental problems she had from the mother's use of illegal drugs during the pregnancy. Over the years, Chanel developed slow but steady communication abilities, including a simple sign language system. As clinicians we sometimes work with children who have extraordinary and complicated medical problems. ■

failure to thrive

The abnormal retardation of growth and development of an infant resulting from conditions that interfere with normal metabolism, appetite, and activity.

gavage feeding

The use of a **nasogastric (NG) tube** to provide sufficient nutrition and hydration for newborns who have a failure-to-thrive condition, with infant milk or specialized formulas (e.g., PediaSure®) inserted into the tube.

nasogastric (NG) tube

A medical device consisting of a long flexible tube that is passed through the nose, down the esophagus, and into the stomach for the delivery of liquids, nutrition, and medications.

especially interaction with adults, then fewer synaptic connections may be made in the brain. This can significantly affect development of speech, language, and cognition. However, in most cases of limited environmental stimulation, there are only gaps in speech and language development compared to children who have normal experiences. Cases of extreme environmental and sensory deprivation are rare.

CASE STUDY

Genie

On November 4, 1970, a 13-year-old girl was taken into custody by officials in Los Angeles, California. The child had been kept in such isolation by her parents that she never learned to talk. Genie was locked in a closet and tied to a potty chair most of her life. Completely restrained, she was forced to sit alone with little to look at and no one to talk to for more than 10 years. When she was discovered by a social worker, she was functioning as an infant and uttering only infantile noises. Genie was placed at a children's hospital for care, training, and education. By May 1971 she was beginning to imitate and repeat single words, although not clearly. By the end of spring, the 13-year-old child could say more than 100 words. When given a new item, she looked at it carefully, often putting it to her mouth (much like an infant), as though she was investigating it because she had little or no experience with common, everyday objects.

Genie was eventually placed with a foster family, the psychologist who had been working with her at the children's hospital and his wife, who was a graduate student in human development. Genie's foster parents became her full-time teachers. Genie eventually developed simple language to help her describe what her life had been like for 10 years in the tiny room. Her foster parents began to feel that Genie was successfully learning a first language even though she had passed the early years of normal language development. Because Genie was more inclined to use gestures to communicate than to use speech, her therapists decided to bring in a teacher who taught sign language. Over the next few years, it became clear that Genie was able to learn vocabulary and to sign or say words but she was not able to use words in sequence to form grammatical language. Genie was eventually placed in an adult foster care home in southern California where she continues to live. (For more information on the language intervention attempts with Genie, see Curtis, 1977.) ■

Application Question

What are five things parents can do to help provide a rich communication environment for their children?

Hearing Impairments

Among the variables that influence speech and language development, perhaps none is as crucial as hearing (Martin & Clark, 2012). One of the most important factors in the development of speech and language is an intact auditory system sensitive to the frequency range within which most speech sounds occur (500 to 4,000 Hz). Hearing impairments almost always result in delays and disorders of speech and language. When infants cannot hear at normal intensity levels (*conductive hearing loss*) or the sounds are distorted or misperceived from a damaged or poorly functioning cochlea or auditory pathway to the brain (*sensorineural* or *central hearing loss*), articulation and language development will likely be impaired. (See Chapter 14, Hearing Disorders in Children and Adults, for a more complete discussion of this topic.)

Physical Impairments or Differences in the Central and Peripheral Nervous Systems

Infants may be born with neurological disorders (e.g., cerebral palsy) and children at any age can acquire a neurological disorder from a traumatic brain injury that results in communication and cognitive impairments (see Chapter 13, Special Populations with Communication Disorders). Communication disorders also can be caused by diseases such as *bacterial* or *viral meningitis*.

Integration of Factors

For most children with communication problems, we cannot determine a single factor as a cause. In most cases, several factors (**multifactorial**) may come into play. For some children genetic and congenital syndromes contribute; for others, they do not. Some children have sensory problems and others have normal acuity and perceptual abilities. Some children come from home environments in which there is a lack of speech and language stimulation and good *modeling* (verbally or physically demonstrating a good example of a behavior, such as production of a sound or correct grammar), but many others come from normal home environments or even language-enriched environments.

> Even if the contributing causes of communication disorders can be determined, we cannot alter a child's genetic make-up or eliminate a syndrome. We often can help a child's auditory acuity problems with hearing amplification, but we have to work within a child's auditory perceptual abilities and limitations. We cannot change a child's impoverished home life, and seldom can we do much to change the parents' language stimulation and modeling skills (some parents would benefit from speech and language therapy themselves). Most of the time clinicians are left to work with children's communication disorders no matter the cause or current contributing factors. We do the best we can with what we are presented with and, perhaps surprisingly, often we help children in remarkable ways.

multifactorial

Referring to the likelihood of two or more causes contributing to the etiology or development of an impairment or disorder, including genetic influences.

ARTICULATION DISORDERS

Articulation involves very rapid and accurate direction of movement, placement, timing, pressure, and coordination of the mandible, lips, tongue, and soft palate. Therefore, an articulation disorder is the incorrect *production* (pronouncing) of speech sounds because a child is (1) not moving an articulator in the correct direction, (2) not placing it in the correct position in the mouth (e.g., the tongue tip not being placed on the alveolar ridge properly), (3) not having precise timing and speed of movement of the articulators (down to milliseconds), (4) having inadequate pressure or too much pressure of one articulator against another, or (5) having difficulty coordinating the movements of the articulators.

The term *articulation disorder* implies that a child has a motor component to the disorder that affects an ability to clearly articulate specific sounds and syllables in words. Articulation disorders are often developmental disorders in which sounds are produced incorrectly or inadequately compared to normative standards for a child's age. Articulation disorders may occur as an isolated problem or as part of other delays or disorders, including language disorders, cognitive impairments, neurological disorders such as cerebral palsy or brain injuries, and orofacial anomalies such as cleft lip and cleft palate.

Four primary types of articulation errors can be made on any one sound: **s**ubstitutions, **o**missions, **d**istortions, and **a**dditions (S.O.D.A.). Articulation errors can occur in the initial, medial, or final position of words. A sound **substitution** is the replacement of one *standard speech sound* by another (a standard speech sound can be represented by a phonetic symbol). When a child has a sound substitution she has produced a wrong sound in place of the correct sound, such as "thoup" for *soup* (a *frontal lisp*), "shoup" for *soup* (a *lateral lisp*), or "wed" for red (/w/ for /r/). Sound substitutions are probably the most common type of articulation errors children have. A sound **omission** is the absence of a speech sound where one should occur in a word; for example, "k-on" for *crayon*, or "ba" for *box*. Some children will have both a substitution and an omission in the same word, for example, "sketty" for spaghetti, where there is an omission of the /p/ and schwa sound /ə/, and substitution of /k/ for /g/. A sound **distortion** is a sound that does not have a phonetic symbol to represent the sound that is produced in place of the intended sound, such as a lateral lisp that is not a clear "sh" sound, or a distorted /r/ sound that cannot be clearly represented by a phonetic symbol. Sound distortions are commonly heard in children who have neurological disorders such as cerebral palsy or traumatic brain injuries when the articulators are weak and cannot make rapid or precise movements. An **addition** is the insertion of a sound or sounds that are not part of the word itself, such as *animamal* for *animal*.

PHONOLOGICAL DISORDERS

As discussed previously, a phonological disorder (also referred to as *developmental phonological disorder* or *phonological impairment*) can be defined as errors of several phonemes that form patterns and are the result of a child simplifying individual sounds and sound combinations. Children with phonological disorders may be able to physically produce all of the speech sounds that are appropriate for their age. Their difficulty relates to the use of particular sounds in particular contexts within words. Phonology is a subsystem of *linguistics*, the scientific study of language, and phonological disorders involve a child's lack of knowledge and development of the phonological (sound) system of a language.

substitution

The replacement of one standard speech sound by another, e.g., /th/ for /s/.

omission

The absence of a speech sound where one should occur in a word, e.g., *k-on* for *crayon*.

distortion

A sound that does not have a phonetic symbol to represent the sound that is produced in place of the intended sound (e.g., a lateral lisp that is not a clear "sh" sound, or a distorted /r/ sound that cannot be clearly represented by a phonetic symbol).

addition

The insertion of a sound or sounds not part of the word itself, such as *animamal* for *animal*.

This difficulty with the acquisition of the sound system is intricately connected to a child's overall growth in language.

A child with a phonological disorder has not learned all of the linguistic rules to properly produce and combine sounds into syllables, even though the motor movements can be executed adequately. Examples of phonological errors are when a child uses a /t/ for /s/ but uses /s/ for /sh/ and /sh/ for /ch/ (Gordon-Brannan & Weiss, 2007). However, it is possible that a child may have a combination of a phonological disorder and an articulation disorder; they are not mutually exclusive. In such cases it is difficult to determine where one disorder leaves off and the other begins. The two problems compound one another, resulting in a child not knowing the sound system and not being able to easily and accurately move the articulators. A child's therapy often focuses on both articulation and phonology.

When a child has not acquired certain phonemes by a particular age that would be expected and there are patterns to her speech errors, the child may be said to be exhibiting *phonological processes*. For example, if a child has the pattern of omitting final consonants in words, she is said to have a *final consonant deletion process*. There are approximately 35 phonological processes that may affect a child's speech intelligibility; however, approximately 10 are considered common phonological processes (see Table 5–3).

EVALUATION OF ARTICULATION AND PHONOLOGY

When a child's articulation and phonology are going to be evaluated, initial interactions with a clinician typically involve rapport building, with the hope that the child will like and trust the clinician enough to be willing to cooperate during the structured evaluation portion. The clinician will visit with the child, ask about home, school, and other involvements of the child, and show genuine interest in the child. The clinician may have some age-appropriate toys and games for the child to play with to help make the time more enjoyable. However, throughout this apparently unstructured time with the child, the clinician is making mental notes of the child's respiratory, phonatory, resonatory, and articulatory systems to develop an impression of whether there may be an anatomical or physiological cause for the child's delayed or disordered speech. Other observations important to make are the child's general speech intelligibility and receptive and expressive language abilities. (Note: Sometimes a child's articulation or phonological problems may be the first sign of language or cognitive problems. Sometimes parents will refer a child for a speech evaluation when there may be significant problems in other areas of the child's development.) The clinician may tape-record the interaction for a later analysis of a **spontaneous (connected, running) speech sample** (usually 50 to 100 utterances)

spontaneous (connected, running) speech sample

A sample of a child's oral discourse in conversation or while describing a picture, usually 50 to 100 consecutive utterances.

TABLE 5-3 Common Phonological Processes in Typical Speech Development

PHONOLOGICAL PROCESS	DESCRIPTION	EXAMPLE
Context sensitive voicing	A voiceless sound is replaced by a voiced sound.	pig → big, car → gar
Final consonant devoicing	A final voiced consonant in a word is replaced by a voiceless consonant.	red → ret, bag → bak
Final consonant deletion	The final consonant in many words is omitted.	home → hoe, cat → ca
Velar fronting	A velar consonant is replaced with a consonant produced at the front of the mouth.	kiss → tiss, give → div
Palatal fronting	The sibilant consonants /ʃ/ and /ʒ/ are replaced by alveolar sibilants made on the alveolar ridge.	ship → sip, measure → mezza
Consonant harmony	The pronunciation of the whole word is influenced by a single sound in the word.	dog → gog hat → tat
Weak syllable deletion	Unstressed or weak syllables are omitted.	telephone → teffone, banana → _nana
Cluster reduction	Part of a consonant cluster is omitted.	spider → pider, friend → fend
Gliding of liquids	The liquid consonants /l/ and /r/ are replaced with /w/ or /j/ (y).	real → weal, leg → yeg
Stopping	A fricative or affricate is replaced by a stop consonant.	funny → punny jump → dump

Adapted from Bowen (1998) and Grunwell (1997).

(see Figure 5–8). Several areas of speech may be analyzed from the spontaneous speech sample, including the following:

- Correctly produced sounds
- Errored speech sounds
- Number of sound errors
- Types of errors
- Consistency of errors between the speech sample and the articulation test
- Intelligibility in conversation
- Speech rate
- Prosody

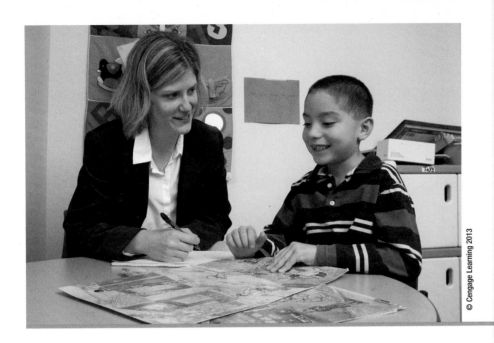

© Cengage Learning 2013

Figure 5-8
Collecting a spontaneous speech and language sample.

During the speech sample the clinician listens for the child's level of speech intelligibility in single words, short phrases, sentences, and conversation and makes note of her intelligibility (e.g., ≈80% accurate [intelligible] with single words, ≈70% with phrases and sentences, and ≈60% in conversation). When a child has inconsistent errors on a particular sound (i.e., sometimes says it correctly and sometimes does not), it may mean that the sound is *emerging* and that with a little therapy the sound may be *established*. Speech-language pathologists and audiologists may be considered "trained listeners"; therefore, a child may be somewhat more intelligible to clinicians than to people who may have only occasional opportunities to hear the child speak.

The clinician will assess the child's articulatory system during an *oral-mechanism* or *oral-peripheral examination*. This somewhat methodical examination notes the anatomy (structure) of the mandible, lips, tongue, and hard and soft palates to determine whether they are within normal limits in size and **symmetry** for the child's chronological age. The physiology (function) of each articulator will be assessed for range of motion (ROM), strength, coordination, and rate of movement to determine whether they are within normal limits for the child's age (see Figure 5-9). A child may have articulators within normal limits in structure and they may function within normal limits during *nonspeech* tasks (e.g., *protruding, retracting, elevating, depressing,* and *lateralizing* the tongue), but the child may not be able to coordinate all of the speech systems together—respiratory, phonatory, resonatory, and articulatory. In many cases, however, it is just the articulators (mandible, lips, and tongue) that children have difficulty coordinating during the rapid, precise movements needed for good articulation.

Clinicians usually have several tasks to formally and informally evaluate a child's speech; that is, structured and unstructured evaluation tasks.

symmetry (symmetrical)

Both sides (e.g., the lips) in balanced proportions for size, shape, and relative position.

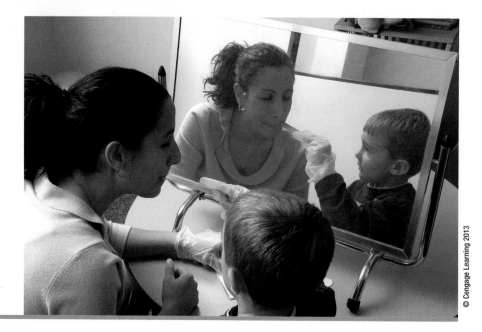

Figure 5–9

A clinician during an oral-mechanism examination (showing the child what she wants him to do).

© Cengage Learning 2013

Clinicians administer *standardized (norm-referenced) assessments* (formal tests) of articulation to collect samples of children's speech productions of individual sounds in the initial, medial, and final positions of words. The clinician asks the child to name or describe a set of test pictures, while carefully listening to the child's production of the individual sounds in the words. When evaluating a child's articulation of sounds in words, clinicians make notations on the test *protocol* (test form) to indicate the correct production of sounds and which sounds are in error in a word, in what way they are in error, and in what positions of a word they are in error. For example:

SOUND	INITIAL	MEDIAL	FINAL
p	p	b	– (omitted)
t	t	t	–
r	w	w	w
s	ʃ/s	ʃ/s	dist. (distorted)
br	b–	b–	

Note: Not all sounds occur in all three positions of words, particularly blends.

stimulability

The evaluation of a child's ability to produce a correct (or an improved) sound in imitation after the clinician models the sound for the child or after the child is given specific instructions on the articulatory placement or manner of production.

When a child has an errored sound, it is often reasonable to check the child's **stimulability** for the sound before beginning therapy. Stimulability refers to the child's ability to produce the correct (or an improved) sound in imitation after the clinician models it for the child or after the child is given specific instructions on the articulatory placement or manner of production. If a child is stimulable for a sound, the prognosis is often good that the child will be trainable for the sound without the need for extensive therapy.

In writing a report about a child's articulation errors, a clinician may make a statement such as "Jennifer demonstrated 6 sound errors in the initial position, including /s/, /z/ /r/, and initial /s/ blends, /sl/ and /st/; sound errors in the medial position, including /s/, /z/, /r/, /f/, /θ/, and /ʤ/; and 8 sound errors in the final position, including /s/, /z/, /r/, and /ʤ/, and omission of the final consonants /s/, /z/, /t/, and /d/."

A clinician who has completed an evaluation of articulation may determine that a child's speech problems go beyond the motor learning and skills for articulation. In such cases the clinician may choose to further assess the child's phonological development. Phonological evaluation may involve either tests specifically designed to assess phonology or special ways of analyzing standard articulation tests. Phonological evaluations measure performance of *sound processes* (i.e., the sound system) of a language. Results gathered from a test of phonology are reported as *phonological process errors* with a statement such as, "Michelle demonstrated errors in cluster reduction (e.g., friend → fɛnd) and final consonant deletion (bed → bɛ)."

Multicultural Considerations

The United States has a large population of immigrants from other countries, and many of the children in public schools have learned English as a second language (ESL) and are bilingual. Bilingual children often speak the parents' native language in the home environment and speak American English in school or other environments. This is frequently seen in the Hispanic culture. Spanish is the second-most-common language in the United States, with approximately 58% of the Spanish-speaking population speaking the Mexican dialect. There are also several large Asian immigrant populations in the United States, including Japanese, Mandarin Chinese, Cantonese, and Vietnamese (U.S. Census Bureau, 2010). When English is acquired after the native language, the sound system of the first language can significantly influence the pronunciation of the second language (Bauman-Waengler, 2009; Shipley & McAfee, 2009; Wyatt, 2002).

Many clinicians attempt to assess ESL children using tests standardized on native American English speakers. Two general problems may arise when clinicians use these norm-referenced tests with children who use English as a second language: (1) overinterpreting the scores obtained on the tests, and (2) using norms from a population other than the child being tested, which can cause incorrect interpretation of the child's abilities (Shipley & McAfee, 2009; Wyatt, 2002). Clinicians are confronted daily with children of all ages whom they cannot assess in their first or native language. Pena-Brooks & Hegde (2007) state that clinicians need to acquire special expertise in assessing and treating children who speak one of the following:

- A language other than English
- English as a second language acquired some time after the acquisition of their primary language
- A dialectical variety of American English (e.g., African American English)
- A different form of English (e.g., Australian English)

THERAPY FOR ARTICULATION AND PHONOLOGICAL DISORDERS

When working with any type of disorder with any age group, clinicians need to be three people rolled into one. First, we need to be *scientists*. We need to have a good understanding of the anatomy and physiology of the speech systems (respiratory, phonatory, resonatory, and articulatory), as well as the nervous system. We also need a thorough understanding of speech and language development to know when a client is within normal limits for each area of development. We need to base our therapy on well-researched data, considering each client as a *single-subject research design*. That is, we need to *develop a hypothesis* (e.g., the child has an articulation disorder), *test the hypothesis* (collect the data—the evaluation results), *analyze the data* (determine what the evaluation results mean), and *develop a treatment plan* based on the best available evidence.

Second, we must be *humanists*. We work with people, and a good understanding of people is essential to be an effective clinician. Beyond an understanding of the psychology of people, we need to be empathic and try to understand clients from their own point of view—that is, try to understand what they are thinking, feeling, and experiencing. We need to be congruent—genuine. We need to be in touch with our thoughts and feelings and to communicate them in the most appropriate (and often sensitive) way that we can. We need to have unconditional positive regard for the people we try to help. We need to convey a sense of acceptance and respect for all people.

Third, we must be *artists*. The artistic aspects of our work include being flexible and creative. Timing is often a crucial factor in our therapy; that is, saying the right thing at the right time and doing the right thing at the right time. Without the art, we may be functioning more as technicians. As clinicians, we need to "think on our feet." No textbook or therapy manual can tell us what to say and do at any given moment; it is our clinical skills, savvy, and intuition that help us from moment to moment go beyond robotic therapy to creative therapy that both the client and the clinician enjoy and benefit from.

All three of these "beings" take years of education, training, and experience to develop. Most clinicians begin their direct clinical experience with children who have articulation and phonological disorders. From there, clinicians usually begin gaining experience with children who have language disorders. Many training institutions help clinicians develop their clinical skills in an orderly sequence. Speech-language therapy is all about communication; we want our clients to develop their skills to be better communicators, and we want to develop our own skills to be better communicators and clinicians.

Therapy Approaches

Articulation therapy (sometimes referred to as *phonetic [motor] treatment*) focuses on the mechanics of producing the speech sounds. There are several treatment approaches, and there is considerable commonality among the approaches. However, some approaches incorporate **auditory discrimination training** or **ear training** (teaching a child to distinguish individual sounds from other sounds) and others do not; some begin production at the *sound isolation level* (teaching a child to produce a phoneme by itself before adding vowels) and others at the syllable level or even the word level; some include practice of the target speech sounds in nonmeaningful combinations (*"nonsense syllables,"* e.g., "bap"), and some practice only meaningful syllables and contexts (Gordon-Brannan & Weiss, 2007).

Articulation and phonology therapy with children require the clinician to listen very closely to a child's every production of a target sound and provide immediate feedback for the child to know when the sound is improving. The clinician may have the child imitate what the clinician says, have the child name pictures, read individual words or sentences, or use other methods to *elicit* (have the child produce) the targeted sound. Clinicians provide *corrective feedback* (letting the child know that a sound was produced correctly or incorrectly) and give generous **positive reinforcement** or **social reinforcers** for correct productions, such as *verbal praise* (e.g., "Good job!", "Great!", "Excellent!", "Perfect!", "Way to go!", "That's it!", "You got it!", "I knew you could do it!", "That was your best one!", "Yes! High five!").

The position of a word where an error is made is important in the analysis of a child's articulation. Most sounds in English can be produced in the initial, medial, or final position of words. For this reason, most articulation tests assess each consonant separately in those three positions (e.g., *pan, puppy, mop; soap, messy, bus*). A child may have an errored production of the sound in the middle and final positions of words but not in the initial position.

Many children with relatively minor articulation problems can have several sounds in error, and these children often benefit from "traditional" articulation therapy approaches (Bernthal, Bankson, & Flipsen, 2009; Gordon-Brannan & Weiss, 2007). In articulation therapy, the focus is on individual sounds in isolation and nonsense syllables, *phonetic drills* (practicing numerous repetitions producing specific sounds), and small increments of change. Articulation approaches tend to emphasize working with articulator movements to produce a sound correctly.

The general goals of traditional treatment approach are as follows:

- To become aware of characteristics of the standard phoneme (auditory discrimination).

- To recognize characteristics of misarticulations and how they differ from the target sound.

auditory discrimination training (ear training)

The ability to distinguish sounds from one another; involves a comparison of heard sounds with other sounds; a technique used in articulation therapy that stresses careful listening to differentiate among speech sounds.

positive reinforcement (positive feedback, reward)

A technique used to encourage a desired behavior by presenting something the person wants soon after the desired behavior is made.

social reinforcer

A word, phrase, or short statement said with warmth and enthusiasm as a reward and encouragement for an accurate response or good attempt at a specific task or target.

- To produce the standard sound at will, and to stabilize or strengthen the use of the target sound in isolation, syllables, words, phrases, and sentences.

- To use the standard sound in spontaneous speech of all kinds and under all conditions; that is, to *achieve carryover*.

The above goals may be condensed into two main components of articulation therapy: *perceptual training* and *production training*. Clinicians tend to follow an often-used sequence for remediating articulation errors (Bernthal, Bankson, & Flipsen, 2009; Gordon-Brannan & Weiss, 2007): (1) establish or improve auditory discrimination of the target sound so that the child can easily recognize the sounds said by others as correct or incorrect, as well as recognize the accuracy of his own productions; (2) produce the sound in isolation by imitating the clinician; (3) produce the sound in various consonant-vowel, vowel-consonant, and consonant-vowel-consonant combinations; (4) establish the sound first in the initial position, then the final position, and then the medial position of single syllable, *bisyllable* (two syllable), and *multisyllable* words; (5) establish the sound in simple phrases and sentences; (6) establish the sound in controlled discourse (e.g., storytelling); and (7) develop **generalization** of the sound to spontaneous conversation. These seven steps may be condensed into three basic steps: (1) listen, (2) experiment, and (3) practice (see Figure 5–10). The challenge, however, has always been the consistent generalization (*carryover*) to spontaneous conversational speech of the newly acquired and correctly articulated sounds.

generalization

The transfer of learning from one environment to other environments; usually considered the therapy or classroom to a natural environment, such as the home.

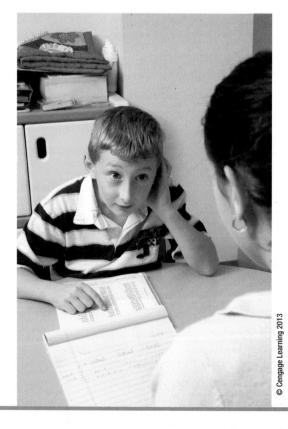

© Cengage Learning 2013

Figure 5–10

"Traditional" speech therapy often involves extensive drill of correct production of a sound in words.

Hunter

Hunter was a 7-year-old boy seen for therapy by a speech-language pathologist in private practice because of his difficulty being understood by friends, family, and even his parents. His parents had resorted to using a simple sign language system to better understand his communications. An evaluation of his speech systems revealed that his respiratory, phonatory, and resonatory systems functioned within normal limits for the development of normal speech. His articulatory system (mandible, lips, and tongue) were within normal limits in structure and symmetry, as well as for function (range of motion, strength, coordination, and rate of movement). Analysis of his speech errors did not reveal a phonological disorder. Neurologically, Hunter appeared intact; he was an excellent student with no apparent attention or behavioral problems, and he was motivated to improve his speech. The cause of his articulation problems could not be determined. However, following a traditional articulation therapy approach over time helped Hunter to become 95%–100% intelligible to his family, friends, and strangers. ∎

Phonology therapy applies a different approach compared to articulation therapy. The basic treatment principles for phonological therapy include: (1) intervention begins at the word level; (2) treatment focuses on the phonological system of the child; and (3) groups of sounds or sound classes, rather than individual speech sounds are targeted (Bauman-Waengler, 2007). There are several phonological approaches; however, the *distinctive features approach* is frequently used by clinicians. The general goals of the distinctive features approach are to teach children how to produce specific distinctive features in the context of phonemes and to teach the rules for correct use of a particular distinctive feature (see Table 5–2). Therapy is often begun at the isolation level, that is, the phoneme without a vowel, followed by progressively more advanced levels: syllables, words, phrases, sentences, stories, and finally spontaneous conversation.

Application Question

Why could it be helpful to begin therapy with auditory discrimination training with a child?

MOTOR SPEECH DISORDERS

According to the ASHA, 2010 *Schools Survey Report*, in 2001 (the most recent data available on motor speech disorders in children) approximately 80% of school-based clinicians reported that their caseloads include an average of four children with a motor speech disorder, either childhood apraxia of speech (CAS) or dysarthria. As defined in Chapter 1, a motor speech disorder is impaired speech intelligibility that is caused by a neurological impairment that affects the motor (movement) planning or the strength of the articulators needed for rapid, complex movements in smooth, effortless speech. Motor speech disorders are often considered *sensorimotor* disorders because both sensory and motor

sensorimotor

The combination of input of sensations and output of motor activity; motor activity reflects what is happening to the sensory systems.

CASE STUDY

Jonathan: A Multihandicapped Child

Jonathan was a 16-year-old student who was medically diagnosed with Alstrom syndrome, which is a rare disease in which a child progressively loses visual and hearing acuities and has other organ and system disorders, including infantile obesity, baldness, and diabetes type 2. Jonathan's vision was monochromatic—everything he saw was the same color. He eventually learned to read *Braille*. Even with the use of hearing aids, he had a mild hearing loss. His auditory processing skills and memory were both in the average range. Jonathan was unable to identify or produce vowel sounds in isolation. He also had difficulty accurately identifying words in which he had to distinguish between /f/ and /th/ and /m/ and /n/, which correlated with his hearing impairment. Jonathan tended to "fill in the blanks" with what he thought he had heard instead of asking for clarification. This caused him to make numerous mistakes and inappropriate comments to his teachers and peers.

Jonathan had decreased range of motion of his mandible, lips, and tongue, which affected his overall speech intelligibility. He had difficulty placing his tongue in the positions requested by the clinician, so he was allowed to put on a latex glove and feel the clinician's mouth when unable to understand what was wanted for a specific task. He was enrolled in articulation and phonological processing therapy to work on speech intelligibility. His speech clinician began at the single-sound level, and after 3 years, Jonathan was able to segment sounds (recognize individual sounds in words) and spell lengthy words. Vowels remained the most difficult for him to recognize because of his hearing impairment. Extensive modeling and repetitions were needed in therapy to help him achieve the smallest goals. This case study reflects the complexity of working with multihandicapped children. ■

Source: Vic Trierweiler, M.A., CCC-SLP, California School for the Blind, Fremont. Used with permission.

---

childhood apraxia of speech (CAS)

A childhood motor speech disorder in the absence of muscle weakness that affects planning, programming, sequencing, coordinating, and initiating motor movements of the articulators that interferes with articulation and prosody.

perseverate/ perseveration

Automatic and involuntary repetition of a behavior, including repetition of a sound, syllable, word, or phrase when speaking.

neurological systems are involved. These children often have other developmental language and cognitive problems that make evaluation and treatment more challenging.

Childhood Apraxia of Speech

Childhood apraxia of speech (CAS) involves disruptions of planning (programming), sequencing, coordinating, and initiating motor movements of the articulators, which affect articulation and *prosody* (voice inflections such as stress, intonation, and rhythm) (Yorkston, Beukelman, Strand, & Hakel, 2010). CAS causes difficulty moving the articulators into their correct positions to produce sounds; words with more sounds and syllables may create more difficulty for a child. Children with apraxia sometimes **perseverate** (i.e., repeat) sounds, syllables, or words in a somewhat disfluent manner. Childhood apraxia of speech has many similarities to apraxia of speech in adults. ASHA (ASHA, 2007) defines childhood apraxia of speech as:

> A neurological childhood speech-sound disorder in which the precision and consistency of movements underlying speech are impaired in the absence of neuromuscular deficits (e.g., abnormal reflexes, abnormal tone). CAS may occur as a result of known neurological impairment, in association with complex neurobehavioral disorders of known or unknown origin, or as an **idiopathic** neurogenic speech-sound disorder. The core impairment in planning and/or programming spatiotemporal parameters of movement sequences results in errors in speech sound production and prosody.

idiopathic

A disease or disorder of unknown etiology.

Unlike acquired apraxia of speech in adults where damage to Broca's area in the left hemisphere of the brain is the generally accepted site of lesion (see Chapter 11, Neurological Disorders in Adults), the neuropathology for CAS has not been well documented, which creates some controversy among some theorists and clinicians about the legitimacy of the disorder and has been discussed by various authors (Forrest, 2003; Maassen, 2002; Moriarty, Gillon, & Moran, 2005). It is not as easy to diagnose a child as it is to diagnose an adult as having apraxia of speech, although many characteristics of the disorders and the principles of evaluation and treatment are similar for children and adults.

Although there may be tentativeness to the diagnostic term, there is clinical value in differentiating the speech characteristics of CAS from articulation and phonological disorders. However, to complicate these diagnoses and the development of appropriate therapy strategies, children may have a combination of articulation problems, phonological problems, and apraxia of speech (Gordon-Brannan & Weiss, 2007; Velleman, 2003).

Speech Characteristics of Childhood Apraxia of Speech

Characteristics of CAS were first described by Morley in 1957 and have been discussed in the literature since that time. We need to keep in mind that speech involves all speech systems—which includes planning, sequencing, coordinating, and initiating respiratory, phonatory, and resonatory movements, as well as articulatory movements. Some children may perform adequately on isolated articulator movements (e.g., rapid protrusion and retraction of the tongue) but when the complex interactions of the speech systems are added to produce speech, the articulatory system is overtaxed and difficulty becomes apparent. A variety of articulatory errors and speech characteristics have been ascribed to children

Personal Story

Karen: A Child with Developmental Childhood Apraxia of Speech

diadochokinetic (diadochokinesis, diadochols)

In speech, the ability to execute rapid repetitive or alternating movements of the articulators; *diadochokinetic rate* is the speed at which the movements can be performed.

Karen was a very sweet 7-year-old girl who had severe CAS. She received speech therapy at her school; however, her parents felt that she needed more help and called me. I saw Karen twice a week in her home. We typically worked in her bedroom sitting on small chairs in front of the large mirror on her little makeup table. Her mother was often present to watch us work, and the door was always open so she could peek in or come in at any time. Karen was almost unintelligible and had difficulty with even rudimentary oral movements such as placement of her tongue in her mouth and slow **diadochokinetic** movements of her mandible and lips—so that is where we began therapy. I was aware of the conflicting data about the use of oral-motor exercises in therapy; however, for this child I felt it was important to begin at that level. It paid off. The development of oral-motor coordination laid the foundation for the much more complex coordination of respiration, phonation, resonation, and articulation for speech. The combination of school therapy and private therapy helped this child to develop intelligible speech over time. ■

who may be diagnosed with CAS (Bauman-Waengler, 2000; Campbell, 2003; Downing & Chamberlain, 2006; Gordon-Brannan & Weiss, 2007):

- More errors are made in the sound classes involving more complex oral movements (e.g., consonant clusters, fricatives, and affricates).
- Errors increase with increasing length of word or utterance, and articulation breaks down more in sentences and conversation than in single words.
- A large percentage of omission errors occur (e.g., omission of individual sounds in mono- and bisyllabic words but omission of syllables in multisyllabic words).
- Vowel and diphthong errors occur.
- Well-practiced utterances are produced or imitated more easily than unfamiliar utterances.
- Groping behavior and silent posturing of the articulators occur when the child attempts to articulate some words (e.g., abnormal movements of the articulators in an attempt to find the desired position for a specific sound).
- Prosodic impairments occur (e.g., inappropriate stress on sounds and syllables).

- There is a lack of progress in articulation and phonological therapy over a long period (e.g., many children are highly unintelligible and may be seen for several or many semesters of therapy with one or more clinicians with minimal progress).

Overall, a broad cluster of symptoms represents CAS. ASHA's Ad Hoc Committee on Childhood Apraxia of Speech (2007) narrowed the core symptoms down to (1) inconsistent errors on consonants and vowels when a child is asked to repeatedly produce individual words (i.e., the child makes different errors during different productions of the same word), (2) abnormal transitions between sounds and words (i.e., the child has difficulty with sequencing sounds and syllables, has abnormal breaks between consonants and vowels, and has increasing difficulty as the number of sounds and syllables increase in a word), and (3) inappropriate prosody during production of individual words and phrases (i.e., stress and intonation are abnormal). Bauman-Waengler (2000) says that not all symptoms must be present for a child to have apraxia of speech. Furthermore, no one characteristic or symptom must be present within a child's constellation of symptoms for a child to have CAS.

Childhood Dysarthria

Dysarthria may be caused by damage to either the central nervous system (brain and brainstem) or the peripheral nervous system (cranial nerves that supply the articulators [V, VII, IX, XI, and XII], and branches off of the vagus [X] cranial nerve that supply the larynx and diaphragm). For example, the speech disorder related to **cerebral palsy** is dysarthria caused by damage to the central nervous system (see Chapter 13, Special Populations with Communication Disorders).

Symptoms of dysarthria vary depending on the location and extent of the neurological damage. Dysarthria in children has many similarities to dysarthria in adults, with various combinations of **hypotonicity** and **hypertonicity** in the muscles that control respiration, phonation, resonation, and articulation. Dysarthria may affect each of the speech systems. Interaction of the systems causes a child's speech to be more severely impaired than if just the articulatory system is impaired. Dysarthria usually affects the range of motion, strength, coordination, and rate of movement of the muscles used for speech, often resulting in sound distortions that have no phonetic symbol that clearly represents the error.

Speech Characteristics of Childhood Dysarthria

Dysarthric speech is sometimes referred to as "hot potato speech" because it sounds somewhat like a person trying to talk with hot potatoes in his mouth–speech sounds "mushy." The following are some common characteristics of childhood dysarthria seen in each of the speech

dysarthria

A group of motor speech disorders caused by *paresis* (weakness), *paralysis* (complete loss of movement), or incoordination of speech muscles as a result of central and/or peripheral nervous system damage that may affect respiration, phonation, resonation, articulation, and prosody; dysarthric speech sounds "mushy" because of distorted consonants and vowels.

cerebral palsy (CP)

A developmental neuromotor disorder that is caused by damage to the central nervous system *prenatally* (before birth), *natally/perinatally* (during birth), or *postnatally* (during childhood) and results in a nonprogressive, permanent neuromuscular disorder; dysarthria affecting all speech systems is the most common speech problem.

hypotonicity

Weakness or absence of muscle tone or tension in a muscle or muscle group (e.g., laryngeal muscles, velar muscles).

hypertonicity

Excessive tone or tension in a muscle or muscle group (e.g., chest muscles, articulatory muscles).

Application Question

Like all other health care and educational specialists, speech-language pathologists and audiologists sometimes cannot determine the exact cause or make a clear diagnosis of a disorder. How comfortable will you be with some ambiguity in the cause, diagnosis, or specific course of treatment for a child's or an adult's communication disorder?

Personal Story — Mandy

Mandy was a beautiful and perfectly normal girl until she was 8 years old and was hit by a drunk driver as she was crossing a street near her home. She sustained a broken leg, abrasions, and a head trauma that affected her cerebellum. The brain damage affected her balance and her speech, which was moderately dysarthric. Although Mandy received speech therapy at her school, the parents wanted additional therapy for their daughter and contacted me. I worked with Mandy in her home at the kitchen table twice a week for about 12 months. I coordinated my therapy with what the SLP was working on at her school. My goal in therapy was to maximize her speech intelligibility, which required (1) improving her respiratory support for adequate inhalation and controlled exhalation for speech; (2) increasing her loudness and duration of voicing with variations in pitch when speaking; and (3) increasing her range of motion, strength, coordination, and rate of movement of each of the articulators. Prosody was focused on once she made significant gains in the other areas. When therapy was eventually ended, Mandy's speech was 95%–100% intelligible, although not all speech sounds were precise and she had her most difficulty when she was sleepy or fatigued. ■

systems (Morgan, Mageandran, & Mei, 2010; Yorkston, Beukelman, Strand, & Hakel, 2010):

- *Respiratory*—Low intensity and speech that is limited to short phrases because of decreased respiratory support.
- *Phonatory*—Breathy phonation because of unilateral or bilateral vocal fold paresis or paralysis.
- *Resonatory*—Hypernasality because of weak or absent movement of the soft palate, causing velopharyngeal incompetence.
- *Articulatory*—Distorted, imprecise consonants because of weakness and incoordination of the mandible, lips, and tongue.

EMOTIONAL AND SOCIAL EFFECTS OF ARTICULATION AND PHONOLOGICAL DISORDERS

Children of all ages with mild or moderate articulation or phonological disorders may hear negative comments about their speech and be the target of teasing, ridiculing, mocking imitation, labeling ("He talks like a baby."), and even exclusion and ostracism from conversations, games, parties, and clubs. Children who have such experiences are emotionally hurt, embarrassed, and frustrated with themselves for not being able to speak normally. They often suffer in silence. They may develop negative attitudes about themselves, such as feeling different, inadequate,

Mike's Apraxia

Personal Story

During the first 2 years after earning my master's degree, I worked in what was then called an "aphasia classroom" with adolescents who had "childhood aphasia" (a term no longer used). The class was limited to eight students. One student was Mike, who had been a normal (actually, above normal) boy before a sledding accident when he was on a snow trip with his Boy Scout troop. Mike had been a good student and a good Scout, and he loved playing Little League baseball. During the sledding accident, he hit his head on a tree and received a traumatic brain injury.

Mike's TBI resulted in moderate to severe aphasia and profound apraxia. He was extremely frustrated and angry about his impairments and newly acquired limitations. He tried to play baseball but no longer had the motor skills to play well. He now had learning disabilities, whereas learning used to come easy for him. His greatest frustration, however, was not being able to speak intelligibly. In the classroom my job was to teach academic subjects at the level at which each child could learn and to provide speech, language, and cognitive therapy.

Mike continued being as active in Boy Scouts as he could, but he was sometimes teased by the other boys. His mother asked if I would be willing to come to one of his evening Scout meetings to talk to the Scoutmaster and the other Scouts about Mike's problems. I was happy to do that. On the evening of the meeting, Mike proudly wore his full Scout uniform. He knew I was going to be talking about him. The Scoutmaster and other Scouts listened attentively and asked some very good questions as I tried to explain Mike's complex problems in layperson's terms. I could see that they were beginning to understand Mike's problems and were developing some empathy. Mike's mother and the Scoutmaster felt that the evening was a success. As clinicians, we need to learn how to explain our many professional terms and complex concepts in layperson's terms and be willing to go beyond our therapy rooms or classrooms to meet some of the most important needs of the children we help. ■

disliked, and socially incompetent. Children with more severe articulation and phonological disorders likely experience the most severe emotional and social consequences. Parents report that approximately 55% of their children with speech disorders also exhibit social competence problems, and 70% of the children have behavioral problems 10 years after they were initially diagnosed in preschool as having communication impairments (Aram & Hall, 1989; Rice, Hadley, & Alexander, 1993).

Communication skills are essential for students to be successful in school. Children with speech disorders may limit their willingness to speak up in class and avoid peer interactions for fear of being teased and embarrassed. Also, their articulation and phonological problems may be only part of their overall difficulties communicating. Of preschoolers, 75% to 85% with articulation and phonological disorders also experience disorders of language, and 50% to 70% of school age children with speech disorders also have academic difficulties in all grade levels, particularly with reading, writing, spelling, and mathematics (Bernthal, Bankson, & Flipsen, 2009; Gordon-Brannan, & Weiss, 2007). In order to help children become better communicators and successful in school and life, speech-language pathologists need to be willing and able to help children with their academic, emotional, and social struggles (Flasher & Fogle, 2012).

CHAPTER SUMMARY

General American English ("American English") is spoken by the majority of Americans and is considered not to have a regional dialect. SLPs use phonetics to describe the individual sounds in a language and use the International Phonetic Alphabet (IPA) transcription symbols to identify specific sounds for any language or dialect. Vowels are voiced speech sounds from the unrestricted passage of the air stream through the mouth without audible stoppage or friction. Consonants are speech sounds articulated by either stopping the outgoing air stream or creating a narrow opening of resistance using the articulators. Consonants are commonly described by their distinctive features—voice, manner, and place.

The three general etiologies of communication disorders in children are: normal variation, environmental problems, and physical impairments or differences. In many cases, there may be a combination of etiologies affecting any one child. Often the cause or causes of a communication disorder cannot be determined. Hearing impairments almost always result in delays and disorders of speech and language.

Four primary types of articulation errors can be made on any one sound: substitutions, omissions, distortions, and additions (S.O.D.A.). A phonological disorder involves errors of several phonemes that form patterns and is the result of a child simplifying individual sounds and sound combinations. An evaluation of a child's speech involves assessing all of the speech systems, focusing on the articulatory system, administering a standardized articulation and sometimes a phonological test, and analyzing the test results. Articulation therapy focuses on the mechanics of producing the speech sounds.

Childhood apraxia of speech is a motor speech disorder in the absence of muscle weakness that affects the planning, programming, sequencing, coordinating, and initiating motor movements of the articulators that interferes with articulation and prosody. Childhood dysarthria is a group of motor speech disorders caused by weakness, paralysis, or incoordination of speech muscles as a result of central and/or peripheral nervous system damage that may affect respiration, phonation, resonation, articulation, and prosody; dysarthric speech sounds "mushy" because of distorted consonants and vowels. As clinicians, we need to be aware of and concerned about possible emotional and social effects of articulation and phonological disorders on children.

STUDY QUESTIONS

Knowledge and Comprehension

1. Explain each of the three distinctive features (voice, manner, and place) that determine the production of sounds.

2. What are the three primary etiologies of articulation, phonological, communication, and cognitive problems?

3. How can hearing loss affect development of communication?

4. Explain substitution and distortion, and provide two examples of each.

5. Define and describe childhood apraxia of speech.

Application

1. Why is it important to consider a child's articulation errors in all three positions of words, that is, initial, medial, and final positions of words?

2. Why might you consider the frequency of sounds in our language when trying to determine which sounds to target with children who have developmental articulation delays?

3. How can clinicians maintain a perspective of normal children to help them better recognize and treat children with communication delays and disorders?

4. What could a clinician be informally assessing during the unstructured rapport-building time?

5. Which speech systems would you want to evaluate if you suspected childhood dysarthria? Why?

Analysis/Synthesis

1. When analyzing speech sounds, why might it be helpful to first consider whether a sound is voiced or unvoiced (voicing), then whether it is oral or nasal (manner), and finally, the location (place) in the oral cavity where the articulators make contact?

2. Why is it important for speech-language pathologists and audiologists working in the school systems to have a good background in syndromes and developmental and medical complications of children?

3. How could auditory discrimination problems cause articulation problems?

4. Why is a spontaneous speech sample important in determining a child's level of speech intelligibility?

5. Why would errors increase as the length of a word or utterance increases and articulation break down more in sentences and conversation than in single words for children who have apraxia of speech?

REFERENCES

American Speech-Language-Hearing Association. (2007). *Childhood apraxia of speech* [Position Statement]. Available from www.asha.org/policy.

American Speech-Language-Hearing Association. (2010). *School Survey report: Caseload characteristics.* Rockville, MD: ASHA.

Apgar, V. (1953, July/August). A proposal for a new method of evaluating the newborn infant. *Current Research in Anesthesiology and Analgesia,* 260.

Aram, D. M., & Hall, N. E. (1989). Longitudinal follow-up of children with pre-school communication disorders: Treatment implications. *School of Psychology Review, 19,* 487–501.

Bauman-Waengler, J. (2012). *Articulatory and phonological impairments: A clinical focus* (4th ed.). San Antonio, TX: Pearson/Allyn & Bacon.

Bernthal, J. E., Bankson, N. W., & Flipsen, P. (2009). *Articulation and phonological disorders* (6th ed.). San Antonio, TX: Pearson/Allyn & Bacon.

Bowen, C. (1998). *Developmental phonological disorders: A practical guide for families and teachers.* Melbourne, Australia: ACER Press.

Campbell, T. F. (2003). *Childhood apraxia of speech: Clinical symptoms and speech characteristics: Proceedings of the childhood apraxia of speech research symposium.* Carlsbad, CA: Hendrix Foundation, 37–40.

Center on Addiction and Substance Abuse. (2005). *Substance abuse and the American woman.* New York, NY: Columbia University.

Curtis, S. (1977). *Genie: A psycholinguistic study of a modern-day "wild child."* New York: Academic Press.

Dewey, G. (1923). *Relative frequency of English speech sounds.* Cambridge, MA: Harvard University Press.

Downing, R. S., & Chamberlain, C. E. (2006). *The source for childhood apraxia of speech.* East Moline, IL: LinguiSystems.

Edwards, H. T. (2003). *Applied phonetics: The sounds of American English* (3rd ed.). Clifton Park, NY: Delmar Cengage Learning.

Flasher, L. V., & Fogle, P. T. (2012). *Counseling skills for speech-language pathologists and audiologists* (2nd ed.). Clifton Park, NY: Delmar Cengage Learning.

Forrest, K. (2003). Diagnostic criteria of developmental apraxia of speech used by clinical speech-language pathologists. *American Journal of Speech-Language Pathology, 12*(3), 376–380.

Gelfer, M. P. (1996). *Survey of communication disorders: A social and behavioral perspective.* New York, NY: McGraw-Hill.

Gordon-Brannan, M. E., & Weiss, C. E. (2007). *Clinical management of articulatory and phonological disorders.* Philadelphia, PA: Lippincott, Williams & Wilkins.

Grunau, R., Kearney, S., & Whitfield, M. (1990). Language development at 3 years in pre-term children of birth weight below 1000 grams. *British Journal of Disorders of Communication, 25,* 173–182.

Grunwell, P. (1997). Natural phonology. In M. Ball & R. Kent (Eds.), *The new phonologies: Developments in clinical linguistics.* Clifton Park, NY: Delmar Cengage Learning.

Maassen, C. (2002). Issues contrasting adult acquired versus developmental apraxia of speech. *Seminars in Speech and Language, 23*(4), 257–267.

Martin, F. N., & Clark, J. G. (2012). *Introduction to audiology* (10th ed.). San Antonio, TX: Pearson/Allyn & Bacon.

Morgan, A. T., Mageandran, S. D., & Mei, C. (2010). Incidence and clinical presentation of dysarthria and dysphagia in the acute setting following pediatric traumatic brain injury. *Child: Care, Health, and Development, 36*(1), 44–53.

Moriarty, B., Gillon, G., & Moran, C. (2005). Assessment and treatment of childhood apraxia of speech (CAS): A clinical tutorial. *New Zealand Journal of Speech-Language Therapy, 60,* 18–30.

Morley, M. E. (1957). *The development and disorders of speech in children.* London, England: Livingston.

Mosby. (2009). *Mosby's dictionary of medicine, nursing, & health professions* (8th ed.). St. Louis, MO: Mosby Elsevier.

Pena-Brooks, A., & Hegde, M. N. (2007). *Assessment and treatment of articulation and phonological disorders in children.* Austin, TX: Pro-Ed.

Rice, M. L. , Hadley, P. P., & Alexander, A. L. (1993). Social biases toward children with specific language impairment: A correlative causal model of language limitations. *Applied Pyscholinguistics, 13,* 443–472.

Rossetti, L. (2001). *Communication intervention: Birth to three.* Clifton Park, NY: Delmar Cengage Learning.

Shipley, K. G., & McAfee, J. G. (2009). *Assessment in speech-language pathology: A resource manual* (4th ed.). Clifton Park, NY: Delmar Cengage Learning.

Small, L. H. (2012). *Fundamentals of phonetics: A practical guide for students* (2nd ed.). San Antonio, TX: Pearson/Allyn & Bacon.

U.S. Census Bureau. (2010). *Census summary file 3: 2010 census population and housing technical documentation.* Available at http://www.census.gov/newsroom/minority_links/asian.html.

Velleman, S. (2003). *Childhood apraxia of speech: Resource guide.* Clifton Park, NY: Delmar Cengage Learning.

Wyatt, T. A. (2002). Assessing the communicative abilities of children from diverse cultural and language backgrounds. In D. E. Battle (Ed.), *Communication disorders in multicultural populations* (3rd ed.). Boston, MA: Butterworth-Heinemann.

Yavas, M. (1998). *Phonology development and disorders.* Clifton Park, NY: Delmar Cengage Learning.

Yorkston, K. M., Beukelman, D. R., Strand, E. A., & Hakel, M. (2010). *Management of motor speech disorders in children and adults* (3rd ed.). Austin, TX: Pro-Ed.

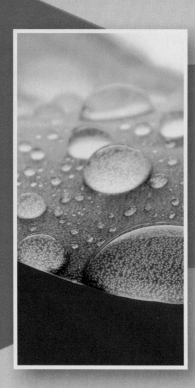

CHAPTER 6
Language Disorders in Children

LEARNING OBJECTIVES

After studying this chapter, you will:

- Be able to define language disorder.

- Be able to discuss language disorder versus language difference.

- Understand the various problems seen in children with specific language impairments.

- Understand the characteristics of language-learning disabilities.

- Be able to discuss the basic process of assessing a child's language.

- Be able to discuss the basic process of therapy for language disorders.

- Be familiar with multicultural considerations of children with language disorders.

- Appreciate the emotional and social effects of language disorders on children.

KEY TERMS

attainable treatment

chronological age

circumlocution

client-specific measurements (clinician devised assessments)

context

developmental coordination disorder

diagnosis

effective treatment

elicit

evidence-based treatment (best practices)

fine motor skills

functional treatment

goal (target behavior)

gross motor skills

heterogeneous

incidence

KEY TERMS continued

language arts
language comprehension
language-learning disability
language sample
learning disabilities (LD)
mean length of utterance (MLU)
measurement
metalinguistics
normative data (norms)
operationally defined goal

prevalence
reliable/reliability
replicate
screening
specific language impairment (SLI)
standardized test (norm-referenced test)
utterance
valid/validity

CHAPTER OUTLINE

Introduction
Definitions of Language Disorder
    Language Disorder versus Language Delay
    Language Disorder versus Language Difference
    Prevalence and Incidence of Language Disorders
    Severity Levels of Language Disorders
Specific Language Impairment (SLI)
    Receptive Language
    Expressive Language
    Multicultural Considerations
Language Disorders and Learning Disabilities
    Motor Skills
    Adolescents with Language-Learning Disabilities
Assessment of Language
    Referral and Screening
    Case History and Interview
    Developing Rapport and Observing the Child Informally
    Evaluating Receptive Language
    Evaluating Expressive Language
    Diagnosis
    Multicultural Considerations
Therapy for Language Disorders
    Selecting Goals (Target Behaviors)
    Organization and Structure of Therapy Sessions
    Multicultural Considerations
Emotional and Social Effects of Language Disorders
Chapter Summary
Study Questions
References

heterogeneous

Consisting of dissimilar or diverse individuals or constituents.

INTRODUCTION

Children with language impairments are a **heterogeneous** group who vary in numerous ways. Their language problems may be exacerbated as they progress in age and educational level. For a preschooler, a "mild" language disorder may create greater challenges as he progresses in school and is expected to understand increasingly difficult information presented by teachers and to verbally express himself with more complex language. These problems are again magnified when the child is expected to learn to read and then read to learn, as well as to be able to express himself proficiently in writing.

DEFINITIONS OF LANGUAGE DISORDER

The ASHA's Ad Hoc Committee on Service Delivery in the Schools (1993, p. IV) presented the following definition of language disorder:

> A language disorder is impaired comprehension and/or use of spoken, written (graphic), and/or other symbol systems. The disorder may involve (1) the form of language (phonology, morphology, and syntax), (2) the content of language (semantics), and/or (3) the function of language in communication (pragmatics) in any combination (p. 40).

The ASHA definition identifies the scope of practice for speech-language pathologists in reference to language disorders: we work with both receptive and expressive language disorders that may involve the form, content, and/or function of language in both the spoken and the written modalities. Although researchers and clinicians may discuss components of language separately (i.e., phonology, morphology, syntax, semantics, and pragmatics), in actuality all components interact at one time, with each component affecting the others (Reed, 2012).

Owens (2008) defines a language disorder (impairment) as a heterogeneous group of developmental and/or acquired disorders, delays, or both that are principally characterized by deficits, immaturities, or both in the use of spoken or written language for purposes of comprehension, production, or both that may involve the form, content, and/or function of language in any combination. This definition emphasizes the vast differences in the language problems of children and adolescents and that the impairments may manifest at any time (e.g., acquired language disorders from traumatic brain injuries).

Language disorders may be more apparent in some contexts and learning tasks than in others. The deficits or delays may exist in some or all modes of communication, such as listening, speaking, reading, or writing. Language disorders may be classified according to the areas of language that are impaired: *form* (phonology, morphology, and syntax), *content* (semantics), and *use* (pragmatics); their severity (mild, moderate, severe, profound); and whether they affect comprehension (receptive language), production (expressive language), or both.

Other terms may be used in place of *disorder,* such as impairment or disability. The terms *language disorder* and *language impairment* are often used interchangeably. However, the term *language disability* suggests that a child's language difficulties significantly affect communication and daily activities in both home and school. In addition, various terms may be used by different school districts or states, for example, *specific language disorder, language-learning disability,* or other combinations of these words (the designation used is often determined by children's age, as well as funding available for the provisions of services to children). The term *primary language impairment* suggests a significant impairment of language when there is no other disability, such as cognitive impairment or traumatic brain injury. A *secondary language impairment* accompanies more pervasive disabilities, such as developmental (intellectual) disabilities or developmental delays (see Chapter 13, Special Populations with Communication Disorders).

Language Disorder versus Language Delay

The term *language delay* implies that children may have a slow start at developing language but that they will eventually catch up with their peers (Hegde & Maul, 2006). Parents often refer to these children as "slow talkers" and "late bloomers." Although some children who exhibit early mild language delays eventually develop normal language skills, they are more likely to have residual language impairments and related disabilities throughout childhood (Johnson, Beitchman, Young, Escobar, Atkinson, & Wilson 1999). Children with language disorders do not eventually catch up with their peers; more commonly, the gap in language skills between children developing normally and those with language disorders widens over time (Pence & Justice, 2008).

Language Disorder versus Language Difference

Children's culturally and linguistically diverse backgrounds may significantly affect their expressive communication. However, expressive language affected by cultural and linguistic diversity is not a disorder—it is a *difference.* As discussed in Chapter 4 under Cultural and Linguistic Diversity Perspective, American English includes a variety of social dialects, such as variations of phonology, morphology, syntax, semantics, and pragmatics. No one dialect is better than another within the language.

When determining whether a particular child's language is disordered or different, we must consider two norms: the referenced norms of General American English (GAE) and the cultural norms or expectations of the child. Clinicians who work with children who are bilingual, are learning English as a second language (ESL), or who speak an English dialect that differs from the mainstream dialect need to be careful during their assessments. Many standard language tests are not sensitive enough to differentiate between children who are typically developing and those who have a language impairment (Dollagham & Horner, 2011). For example, the grammatical morphology of children who are learning ESL may look similar to that of children with language impairment, particularly their omission of grammatical morphemes (Hegde & Maul, 2006; Paradis, 2005; Roseberry-McKibbin, 2001).

Prevalence and Incidence of Language Disorders

Prevalence refers to the number of individuals diagnosed with a particular disorder at a given time. **Incidence** is the rate at which a disorder appears in the normal population over a period of time, typically one year. The prevalence of language disorders is more clinically relevant and, therefore, more commonly reported than is the incidence.

The few large studies available (more than 1,000 children) report that 7% to 8% of children entering kindergarten are recognized as having specific language impairment (SLI) with no other complicating conditions and that approximately 2% more boys than girls have SLI (Erwin, 2001). In terms of actual numbers, more than 1 million children in American schools receive special education services for primary speech or language disorders, and another approximately 700,000 school children receive services for secondary language impairments resulting from cognitive impairments, developmental delays, autism spectrum disorders, and traumatic brain injuries (U.S. Department of Education, 2008).

Severity Levels of Language Disorders

Severity levels for communication disorders (both speech and language) and cognitive disorders range from mild to profound. However, any one child may have different severity levels depending on the communication input or output modality (e.g., auditory or visual input or verbal, gestural, or graphic output). As mentioned earlier, depending on the communication demands, a child may appear to have mild problems when his receptive and expressive language functioning are only minimally challenged. However, when the challenges are more taxing, his true levels of difficulty may become apparent. For example, a child may have only moderate problems with auditory receptive and verbal expressive language but severe problems learning how to read and write. Paul (2011) provides a description of severity ratings that are clinically, educationally, and socially useful (see Figure 6–1).

prevalence

The number of individuals diagnosed with a particular disorder at a given time.

incidence

The rate at which a disorder appears in the normal population over a period, typically 1 year.

Mild	Mild language disorders have some effect on a child's ability to perform in social or educational situations but do not preclude participation in normal, age-appropriate activities in school or community.
Moderate	Moderate language disorders involve a significant degree of impairment that necessitates some special accommodations for the child to participate in mainstream community and educational settings.
Severe	Severe language disorders usually make it difficult for a child to function in community and educational activities without extensive support.
Profound	Profound language disorders imply that a child has little or no ability to use language to communicate and is unable to function in community and educational activities.

Figure 6–1

Variations in severity of language disorders.
Adapted from Paul, 2011.

SPECIFIC LANGUAGE IMPAIRMENT (SLI)

As noted previously, **specific language impairment** (sometimes called *primary language disorder*) refers to significant receptive and/or expressive language impairments that cannot be attributed to any general or specific cause or condition (Pence & Justice, 2008; Tomblin, Zhang, Buckwalter, & O'Brian, 2003). These children have hearing within normal limits (although many have histories of middle ear infections), there are no obvious perceptual or neurological disorders, and their nonverbal intelligence is within normal limits. Specific language impairments are characterized more by the absence of other disorders than by some clearly identifiable set of observable traits (Bishop, 2006; Leonard, 2000; Owens, 2008). SLI is the most frequent reason for administering early intervention and special education services to preschool and early primary school children (Pence-Turnbul & Justice, 2012).

.   Children who are considered "slow talkers" by parents often have some "red flags" that can alert parents and clinicians to a young child's potential specific language impairments (Bishop, 2006; Hegde & Maul, 2006; Leonard, 2000):

- Slow development of speech sounds
- Does not say "Mama" or "Dada" by 12–18 months of age
- Significant late appearance of the first true word (i.e., after approximately 18 months of age)
- Significant late use of two-word combinations (i.e., after approximately 30 months of age)

specific language impairment (SLI)

Significant receptive and/or expressive language impairments that cannot be attributed to any general or specific cause or condition.

- Restricted vocabulary in both comprehension and production
- Reliance on gestures for getting needs met
- Infrequent use of verbs and poor development of verbs
- Lack of yes-or-no responses to questions
- Difficulty initiating interactions with age peers
- Difficulty with turn-taking during conversations
- Difficulty rhyming words
- Difficulty naming letters

Most children under 3 years of age who may have mild to moderate SLI are not recognized as having a significant problem by their parents, although the parents may voice concern to their pediatrician regarding the child's development. Pediatricians often take a "wait and see" approach and encourage parents to be patient, saying that they can expect their "late talker" or "late bloomer" to be a "chatterbox" sometime soon. After another 6 to 12 months pass, the parents' concerns *may* be reinforced by their pediatrician, who then *may* suggest the parents seek an evaluation of the child's speech by a speech therapist. Some pediatricians will again encourage the parents to be patient, particularly if the child is a boy because boys are generally expected to develop language slower than girls. This 6- to 12-month delay (or longer) in seeking services from an SLP can result in important time being lost that could have been used to help the child's speech and language development.

Physicians' Education of Speech-Language Pathology and Audiology

Physicians (e.g., general practitioners, pediatricians, otolaryngologists, and neurologists) in their education and training do not take specific course work on speech and language development or speech and language disorders of children and adults. Some of their textbooks may include cursory discussions of the many disorders that speech-language pathologists and audiologists assess and treat, but physicians do not have specific texts that discuss in detail the theory or SLP or Aud assessment and treatment of any disorders. Because of this lack of education and knowledge about our work, many physicians do not refer patients to us that we could help, leaving patients without the habilitation or rehabilitation we could provide and the gains they could make to improve their quality of life. As professionals, we need to educate physicians about what speech-language pathologists and audiologists can do to benefit patients.

Seldom can we clearly determine the cause of a child's specific language impairment, and it is unlikely that specific language impairment has a single cause. However, genetic makeup may exert a strong influence in determining which children develop SLI. Most researchers agree it is a complex disorder that may have multiple genetic influences that interact with environmental factors (Bishop, 2006). In some children with SLI, there may be subtle impairments of cognitive skills such as auditory perception, memory, and sequencing, although the relationship between cognition and language is not fully established (Choudhury & Benasich, 2003).

Receptive Language

Receptive language (**language comprehension**) is a process by which a listener infers the meaning of a message based on the **context** of the information and long-term stored memory that relates to what is being heard. Children with SLI commonly have difficulty with receptive language. In general, they have impaired ability to understand and integrate information, whether presented verbally or nonverbally. Their slow processing of auditory information can contribute to their difficulty understanding; that is, spoken words may be "coming at them too fast" and they are not able to keep up with a normal rate of conversation (Pence-Turnbull & Justice, 2012). Children with SLI may have difficulty understanding direct questions (e.g., "Do you want to go to McDonald's for lunch?") and even more difficulty understanding indirect questions (e.g., "McDonald's for lunch might be good."). Poor comprehension of individual words and the subtleties of language make it difficult for children to understand connected speech and contribute to their weak expressive vocabularies and impaired expressive language.

Children in primary and junior high school with SLI continue to have weak receptive vocabularies for their ages. They understand direct statements and requests easier than those that are indirect. They are often quite literal in their interpretation of statements and idioms, and misunderstand and misuse metaphors and similes (Pence-Turnbull & Justice, 2012). They have difficulty understanding abstract concepts and expressing their wants, needs, thoughts, and feelings even in rudimentary ways, which may result in frustration and behavioral outbursts.

Expressive Language

Expressive language at all ages is difficult for children with specific language impairments. From their earliest days of communicating, they have difficulty expressing their wants and needs, often leaving parents guessing and frustrated. Not only do they have language problems, they frequently have speech problems that make communicating even more difficult.

Articulation and Phonological Problems

Children 3 and 4 years of age who are difficult to understand often have specific language impairments (Leonard, 2000; Reed, 2012). Their reduced speech intelligibility affects their use of expressive language and their interactions with family and peers. As these children enter primary

language comprehension

An active process in which, from instant to instant, a listener infers the meaning of an auditory message based on the context of the information and long-term stored memory of words and general knowledge.

context

The immediate environment of the speaker and listener, including the topic being discussed and past experiences each person brings to the communication encounter.

screening

In speech, any gross measure used to identify individuals who may require further assessment in a specific area (e.g., articulation, language, hearing, fluency, or voice).

mean length of utterance (MLU)

The average length of oral expressions as measured by representative sampling of oral language (e.g., 50–100 spontaneous utterances [Pence & Justice, 2008]); usually calculated by counting the number of morphemes per **utterance** and dividing by the number of utterances; e.g.,

$$\frac{150 \text{ morphemes}}{50 \text{ utterances}} = 3.0 \text{ MLU}.$$

utterance

A unit of vocal expression that is preceded and followed by silence; may be made up of a word or words, phrases, clauses, or sentences.

school they are recognized through **screening** or teacher referral as having articulation problems and are assessed and enrolled in therapy.

Morphological and Syntactic Problems

Morphological and syntactic problems are common in children with SLI. When morphological elements are missing, children's language is grammatically incomplete or incorrect. Children with SLI are late in developing syntactic structures and using them consistently (Owens, 2008; Paul, 2011). These problems usually are evident by 3 to 4 years of age in their **mean length of utterance (MLU)**, morphological markers, and sentence complexity. MLU is considered a valid and reliable indication of general language development (Rice, Redmond, & Hoffman, 2006). Children with morphological and syntactic problems often speak in short, incomplete sentences (e.g., "Milk!") or with simple, active, declarative sentences (e.g., "Me want milk."). As children grow older and have increasingly more complex information to communicate, their numerous morphological and syntactic problems interfere with conveying their messages and listeners become confused or lost. Such morphologic and syntactic problems result in children having difficulty with discourse and pragmatics. The consequences of such difficulty may be frustration and emotional pain for both the children and their parents.

Vocabulary Development and Semantic Problems

Children who have delays in using their first true words and who are slow to develop additional vocabulary (fewer than approximately 20 words by 24 months of age and fewer than approximately 200 words by 36 months of age) are at risk for specific language impairments. Normal children 24 months of age typically are using noun-verb constructions for sentences. Most children have a dramatic increase of new words between 24 and 36 months of age; however, children with SLI often have negligible increases during this time. Children with SLI may be able to name some objects but not be able to use adjectives to describe the objects (e.g., *big, brown,* and *noisy*) or verbs to indicate their actions (e.g., *"Doggy!"* versus *"Doggy bark!"*).

Vocabulary development and concept development are strongly related. Children who have weak vocabulary development typically have poor concept development, which may result in difficulty "making sense" of their world. Many nouns are also concepts; for example, the word *ball* has several concepts that may be related to it. There are many kinds of balls (baseball, basketball, beach ball, etc.), and each kind of ball has numerous concepts that relate to it. A ball is round (shape); it may be big (size) and red (color); it can be rolled, bounced, thrown, hit, or kicked (actions). The noun *ball,* then, can have various parts of speech related to it, such as adjectives, verbs, and prepositions. Children with SLI may not understand or use words that express concepts of shape, size, color, quantity, and quality, or verbs that may relate to an object.

In addition, verb markers (e.g., *-ed* and *-ing*) are particularly difficult for these children (Conti-Ramsden & Windfuhr, 2002). Children with specific language impairments commonly have significant difficulty with literacy skills, that is, learning to read, reading to learn, and writing (see Chapter 7, Literacy Disorders in Children).

Word-finding problems are a characteristic of many children with specific language impairments, that is, they are not able to think of a specific word they want to say (Bayne & Moran, 2005). A study conducted in England found that 23% of children receiving language support services had word-finding problems (Dockrell, Messer, George, & Wilson, 1998). Word-finding problems are commonly characterized by (1) unnatural pauses or *latency* (delays while trying to think of a word), (2) *fillers* (um-um, uh-uh), (3) *nonspecific words* (thing, stuff), (4) *substitutions* of a less desired word for the desired word, (5) the use of *excessive pronouns* that leave the listener uncertain of who or what is being referred to, (7) *repetitions* of a word or phrase until the desired (or an acceptable) word is recalled, (8) *topic avoidance* (avoiding topics for which the child may have difficulty recalling words), (9) **circumlocutions** ("talking around words"), and (10) difficulties with *confrontation naming* (naming objects shown or described to them). These children often say "You know" hoping that listeners can fill in missing words or can guess the meanings of their messages. Because children with SLI cannot provide correct nouns, verbs, and adjectives in conversation, listeners are often confused by their messages.

Asking questions is also difficult for these children and many have problems understanding when to use the "wh"-question words (*who, what, when, where, why, how*). Therefore, they may not get information they need and have difficulty asking for clarification of information for which they are uncertain. They have particular difficulty understanding how to form questions using inverted auxiliaries (e.g., "He is going."— declarative sentence; "Is he going?"—interrogative sentence).

Relating *narratives* (stories with a sequence of events) is one of the most challenging skills for these children. Narratives require (1) recall of the event or events, including the time, place, people, and other important details involved, (2) recall of specific words that could help relate the experience to a listener, (3) formulation of the language structures to communicate the experience as accurately and completely as possible, and (4) pragmatic skills to recognize whether the listener is understanding or even interested in the story. Children with specific language impairments may have breakdowns in all of these skills (Colozzo, Gillam, Wood, et al., 2011).

Metalinguistics

Metalinguistics refers to the ability to think about and eventually talk about language. Metalinguistics goes beyond the ability to understand word meanings and grammar. It is the conscious awareness and use of language as a tool. Metalinguistics encompasses the ability to (1) recognize and interpret multiple meanings in words and sentences, (2) make

circumlocution

The use of a description or "talking around" a word when the specific word cannot be recalled.

metalinguistics

The ability to think about and talk about language.

multiple inferences, (3) interpret figurative language, and (4) plan and organize sentences, paragraphs, and narratives (Nicolosi, Harryman, & Kresheck, 2004). Students with specific language impairments generally have poor metalinguistics skills and are at considerable disadvantage when they reach the middle school years (Cairns, Waltzman, & Schlisselberg, 2007).

In the classroom environment, metalinguistics is often included in **language arts** (i.e., listening, speaking, reading, handwriting, spelling, and written composition). Metalinguistics is a significant linguistic achievement that emerges during primary school and develops through junior and senior high school. It is a skill involved with both spoken and written language and facilitates children's acquisition of independent problem-solving abilities (Cairns, Waltzman, & Schlisselberg, 2004).

As learners of semantics, children must be able to understand and explain word definitions, understand and use similarities and differences, and distinguish between literal and figurative meanings. They must be able to recognize and use various types of sentences (e.g., declarative, interrogative, imperative, and exclamatory, as well as simple, compound, and complex). For children with specific language impairments, metalinguistics is a daunting, increasingly complex task. They are struggling with language basics (comprehension, phonology, morphology, vocabulary, syntax, semantics, discourse, narratives, and pragmatics), and now they need to start thinking about the nebulous concept of language to learn more about language (Botting & Adams, 2005).

Pragmatic Problems

You will recall that pragmatics are the rules governing the use of language in social situations. Many children with specific language impairments have a variety of difficulties with the pragmatic aspects of language, which can significantly interfere with family interactions and friendships (see Figure 6–2). These children have difficulty knowing how to initiate a conversation and when they do initiate a conversation, it may be at the wrong time and in the wrong way, with inappropriate ways of attracting the listener's attention (e.g., shouting or hitting). They tend to have difficulty knowing how to gain access into conversations, so they appear to be interrupting or rude. They have difficulty sustaining topics over several conversational turns, often abruptly trying to change a topic. They usually do not ask for clarification when they misunderstand someone (Pence-Turnbull & Justice, 2012; Reed, 2012).

language arts

Academic activities such as listening, speaking, reading, handwriting, spelling, and written composition.

Multicultural Considerations

About 55% of 3- and 4-year-old children in the non-Latino white population are enrolled in preschool programs, but only 43% of Latino children attend preschool. In addition, 13% more non-poor children 3–5 years of age are enrolled in preschool programs than poor children. The lower the parental education, the younger the mother, the

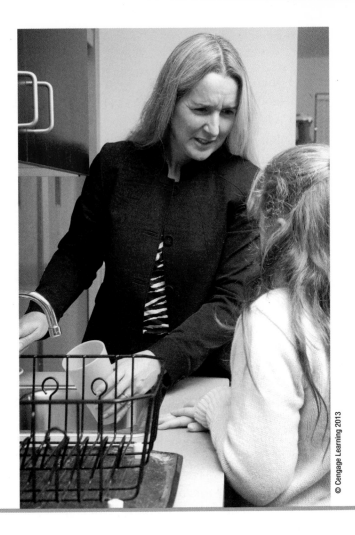

© Cengage Learning 2013

Figure 6-2

Parents sometimes become frustrated with their children who have difficulty communicating.

greater the family's mobility (moving from city to city), the lower the income, and the poorer the English-speaking ability, the less likely children will be enrolled in preschool (U.S. Department of Education, National Center for Education Statistics, 2007).

Bedore & Leonard (2001) found significant grammatical and morphological deficits in Spanish-speaking children with specific language impairments. Without being enrolled in preschool programs, many Latino and poor children do not have the opportunity to be identified and treated for specific language impairments (this is likely true for other non-English-speaking immigrants). Also, because many Latino parents tend to be young and poorly educated, they miss the opportunity to receive information from professionals about things they can do at home to help their children's speech and language development.

LANGUAGE DISORDERS AND LEARNING DISABILITIES

Many children with language disorders also have **learning disabilities (LD)**. Learning disabilities are not diagnosed until a child enters primary school; therefore, preschool children are usually diagnosed as having

learning disability (LD)

A disorder in one or more of the basic psychological processes involved in understanding or using language, spoken or written, that may manifest itself as difficulty listening, speaking, reading, writing, spelling, mathematical calculations, reasoning, and problem solving.

CASE STUDY

Joshua

Joshua was a 4-year-2-month-old boy seen by a speech-language pathologist in a Head Start program. The case history provided by the mother revealed a few of the early "red flags" that indicate a specific language impairment. Joshua did not say his first word until almost 20 months of age and did not combine two words (noun + verb) until 3 years of age. His gestural language was well developed and he often relied on gestures to obtain what he wanted or needed. He had significant difficulty naming objects and using the correct verbs associated with common objects. He did not interact or converse with children his own age.

Joshua's hearing and vision were normal. He had minimal auditory comprehension skills and benefited from gestures that accompanied requests or any communication. The evaluation revealed obvious articulation and phonological problems, some of which interfered with morphological endings (e.g., plurals and past tense). He was inconsistent in his use of various irregular plurals and past-tense forms. His sentences were typically two or three words in length, with occasional four- to six-word sentences; however, the longer his sentences, the more difficult they were to understand.

Joshua had limited receptive and expressive vocabularies, understanding more words than he could use verbally. The *Bracken Basic Concept Scale–Revised* (1998) revealed that he had not yet acquired many of the basic concepts expected for a child his age. His syntax was more like a 2- to 3-year-old child than a 4-year-old child. His sentences were mostly nouns, with some common verbs and occasional adjectives. He tended to avoid discourse and relating stories (narratives), apparently aware that his listener would not likely understand him. He showed some frustration when his parents could not effectively use their "20-question" routine to find out what he wanted or needed. He seemed to avoid frustrating himself by decreasing his verbal interactions. Both mother and father said they were "beside themselves" trying to figure out how to help Joshua communicate.

Therapy was multifaceted, including work on articulation and phonological processes, developing auditory comprehension, vocabulary, concepts, and sentence structure. The parents were encouraged to read simple stories with Joshua and to emphasize the enjoyment of sounds and words and of understanding the sentences and paragraphs in the stories. The parents also were encouraged to require Joshua to use words when he asked for things he wanted or needed rather than allowing him to point or use gestures. Within one year, Joshua was communicating his wants, needs, thoughts, and feelings more completely and accurately, which decreased his frustration significantly. The parents began enjoying their son more and Joshua was interacting more often and appropriately with children his age. ■

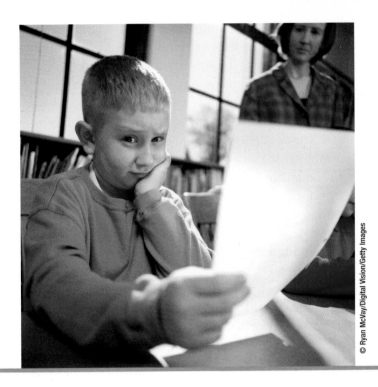

© Ryan McVay/Digital Vision/Getty Images

Figure 6-3

School-age children who have language-learning disorders often show signs of frustration when doing schoolwork.

specific language impairments and this term is often carried over into their school years. After children enter school and struggle academically, an evaluation may reveal that they have a learning disability along with their language impairment. The diagnostic term may be changed to **language-learning disability**, particularly when children are experiencing difficulties with academic achievement in areas associated with language, such as reading, writing, and spelling (Heward, 2008; Pence-Turnbull & Justice, 2012). More than 75% of children with learning disabilities have difficulty understanding and using verbal or graphic language (see Figure 6–3). In many cases a child's learning disability may have as its foundation a language disorder and, therefore, working with an SLP may be essential to helping remediate the child's learning problems (Nelson, 2010; Vinson, 2011).

Children's language problems often manifest themselves differently as they advance through the grades; that is, differences in symptoms and severity levels are reflected in the different communication demands throughout children's education (both auditory–verbal and reading–writing). Because of the increasing demands on children's language abilities as they progress through the grades, various symptoms become apparent that could not be seen in the preschool years. These symptoms often include difficulty (1) understanding increasingly complex verbal information; (2) communicating narrative information in the classroom (e.g., talking during "show and tell time" or making verbal reports on subject matter); (3) learning to read and write (*literacy skills*); and (4) reading to learn (reading for information). When children begin primary school, it becomes clear how their language disorders can impact their academic abilities.

language-learning disability

An impairment of receptive and/or expressive linguistic symbols that affects learning and educational achievement and, consequentially, possible occupational and professional choices and success, in addition to emotional and social development.

Language-learning disabilities tend to run in families. Sixty percent of children with language-learning disabilities have a family member with similar problems, and for 38% it is a parent (Dale, Price, Bishop, & Plomin, 2003). The general prevalence of language-learning disabilities is 12% to 13% for 5-year-old kindergarten children, with approximately 4.5% of children also having speech disorders (Tomblin, Records, Buckwalter, & Zhang, 1996). Most children with language-learning disabilities have the same kinds of problems as younger children diagnosed with specific language impairments; that is, problems with language comprehension, phonology, morphology, syntax, vocabulary development, semantics, discourse or dialogue, narratives, and pragmatics. The severity of these language-learning disabilities may be mild, moderate, severe, or profound, with some areas of language learning being more involved than others.

Many children who receive speech and language therapy also require other special education services, remedial instruction, tutoring, special classroom or special school placement, or a combination of these. The children SLPs work with commonly have more than just speech and language problems, or perhaps their speech and language problems contribute to or exacerbate other academic and social problems. In all cases, however, SLPs are part of a team of professionals doing their best to maximize children's potential.

Motor Skills

Approximately 15% of children with learning disabilities have major difficulty with **gross** and **fine motor skills** and coordination (i.e., **developmental coordination disorder**) (Kurtz, 2007). Fine motor coordination problems also may cause difficulty with articulatory movements, as is seen in *childhood apraxia of speech* (see Chapter 5). Developmental coordination disorders can affect a child's interactions with peers, which complicate the social development of children who already have difficulty with communication.

Adolescents with Language-Learning Disabilities

Some (perhaps many) children who have been diagnosed with specific language impairments or language-learning disabilities have communication problems that persist into secondary school and, probably at some level, throughout life. In addition, their communication problems increasingly affect their educational achievements, choice of vocational and professional careers, potential earning power, and marital and peer relationships. In some cases, language problems may emerge during adolescence because of involvement with drugs. However, many adolescents with language disorders remain unidentified, unserved or underserved, and neglected (Beitchman, Wilson, Douglas, Young, & Adlaf, 2001; Ehren, 2002; Nippold, 2001; Reed, 2012).

gross motor skills

Involvement of the large muscles of the body (e.g., trunk, legs, arms) that require tone, strength, and coordination that enable such functions as standing, lifting, walking, and throwing a ball.

fine motor skills

Movements that require a high degree of dexterity, control, and precision of the small muscles of the body that enable such functions as grasping small objects, drawing shapes, cutting with scissors, fastening clothing, and writing.

developmental coordination disorder

Impairment of groups of gross and fine muscles that prevents smooth and integrated movements, which results in clumsiness during walking, jumping, and athletic movements, and during more refined movements such as using eating utensils and writing; often associated with learning disabilities and complicated by low self-esteem, repeated injuries from accidents, and weight gain as a result of avoiding participating in physical activities.

Receptive Language Problems

Adolescents who had receptive language problems at an earlier age often continue to have significant problems throughout their high school years. In general, they (1) have weak single-word receptive vocabularies, (2) experience problems understanding abstract words and words with multiple meanings, (3) often find figurative language expressions puzzling (including slang and jargon), (4) have difficulty following directions, (5) have difficulty understanding questions, (6) experience problems with semantics, (7) face challenges following rapid speech, (8) have poor listening skills, (9) experience difficulty grasping the essential messages of lectures, and (10) misinterpret facial expressions, body postures, and gestures.

Expressive Language Problems

Expressive language may be even more of a challenge than receptive language for adolescents with language disorders. Because there is a reasonably good chance they do not fully understand a question, message, instructions or directions, their responses or behaviors are likely to be incomplete, inaccurate, and sometimes inappropriate. They have weak vocabularies compared to their normal peers, although they may be able to use teenage figurative language easily (not being able to use more adult vocabulary to express themselves may be an indication of inadequate language development). They often use low-content or no-content words such as *thing* or *stuff.* They use pronouns without clear referents so that listeners are uncertain about who or what is being talked about.

Their syntax tends to be simple and they use fewer compound and complex sentences than other adolescents. Verb tense is often a problem for adolescents with language disorders. They frequently use fragmented sentences that do not clearly convey their messages and leave their listeners confused. They may know what questions they want to ask or what answers they want to give, but do not know how to express them or to do so tactfully. They may have abrasive conversational speech. They violate rules for social distance. They do not know or cannot easily use the necessary concepts and vocabulary needed in community businesses, such as banks, grocery stores, and employment agencies.

Many adolescents with language-learning disabilities who graduate from high school are able to go to college. At the university level, learning disability was the fastest growing category among students with disabilities between 1988 and 2000. In 2000 approximately 40% of university freshmen with disabilities cited a learning disability, compared with only 16% in 1988 (Henderson, 2001).

Overall, preschool children who have specific language disorders may become primary schoolchildren with language-learning disabilities; these schoolchildren may become adolescents with language-learning disabilities, who also may become college students

Application Question

There is a reasonably good chance that a fellow student in the class you are in has a learning disability. Although students with disabilities cannot be pointed out by professors, what could you do to be of assistance to a student with a learning disability?

with language-learning disabilities. Whether or not these adolescents go to college or work, they are likely to enter adulthood with some level of language impairment and they must learn to work and live within their limitations. However, some of these adults become surprisingly and extraordinarily successful despite their language and learning problems.

Multicultural Considerations

In 2006, 11% of people aged 18–24 years were high school dropouts. However, in states where there is a high Hispanic or poor population such as Arizona, New Mexico, Nevada, Texas, Louisiana, Mississippi, and Georgia, the dropout rates are at or above 14% (U.S. Census Bureau, 2008: School Enrollment in the United States, 2006). In some communities within these states the dropout rate is much higher. Teens who drop out of high school are three times more likely to live in poverty than those who complete high school, with the added risk of getting in trouble with the law.

The high dropout rate for Hispanic and poor children may have its roots at the preschool level. Recall that significantly fewer Hispanic and poor children attend preschool and do not have the opportunity to be identified as having or being at risk for communication impairments, including hearing loss. Furthermore, 80% of Hispanic children in the public schools are learning English as a second language. If the 12%–13% of children in the general population having language-learning impairments holds true for the Spanish-speaking population, a significant number of Latinos have language impairments that likely contribute to their educational failures.

ASSESSMENT OF LANGUAGE

As mentioned in Chapter 2, Speech-Language Pathologists and Audiologists, the terms *assessment* and *evaluation* are often used interchangeably; however, *assessment* appears to be the general preference for authors of texts on language disorders in children (e.g., Hegde & Maul, 2006; Owens, 2008; Reed, 2012). Typically the term **diagnosis** is distinguished from *assessment*. Assessment is the work or activity that leads to a clinical decision—the diagnosis. A diagnosis is the determination that there is or is not a disorder, and the label or professional term for the disorder is based on the results of valid and reliable measurements of relevant abilities and skills. However, the intervening part is the **measurement** within the assessment process. Clinicians need to obtain **valid** and **reliable** measures during the assessment to have accurate results from which they can have confidence in their decisions for diagnosis and development of an effective treatment plan. Clinicians need to measure observable behaviors that they, as well as others, can see and hear, and if necessary, **replicate** for research purposes.

---

diagnosis

The determination of the type and possible cause of a hearing, speech, language, cognitive, or swallowing disorder based on the signs and symptoms of a client obtained through case history, interviews, observations, and formal and informal evaluations.

measurement

Procedures that quantify observed behaviors and can be calculated as mathematical results, such as percentages and percentiles.

valid/validity

The extent to which a test measures what it is intended to measure.

reliable/reliability

The dependability of a test or treatment procedure as reflected in the consistency of its scores on repeated measurements of the same group.

replicate

Evaluation or treatment procedures that can be repeated by either the same investigator or other investigators to determine reliability of the data.

Assessment serves numerous purposes:

- It determines whether a child has problems of clinical concern and qualifies for services.
- In some cases, the assessment may help identify the cause or causes of a child's problems.
- It allows the clinician to describe patterns that are both present and absent in a child's language (it is important to observe what the child can and cannot do well).
- Factors that may be associated with the language problems may be noted.
- A diagnosis of the child's communication problems can generally be made.
- A treatment plan should be devised from the assessment, including what further assessment is needed.
- A general prognosis may be made as to the child's improvement.

Adequate evaluation of a child's language is one of the most difficult and demanding tasks faced by speech-language pathologists. The goal is to describe the complex language system of a child. Each child has a unique pattern of language rules and behaviors that need to be revealed and described (Owens, 2008). In order to understand a child's language abilities it is essential to describe the child's strengths and weaknesses. Standard deviation units and other statistical measures (see Chapter 5, Figure 5–5) derived from **standardized tests (norm-referenced tests)** do not fully explain a child's receptive and expressive language abilities. In addition, a serious limitation of standardized tests is that they are often inappropriate for children from ethnically and culturally diverse backgrounds because they have not been standardized on these populations (Dollagham & Horner, 2011; Nelson, 2010; Owens, 2008; Reed, 2010). In many cases, SLPs use **client-specific measurements (clinician devised assessments)** to help "fill in the gaps" that standardized tests might leave in the understanding of a child's communication abilities. Overall, it is the information from the case history and parent interview, interpretations of test scores, analysis of client-specific measurements, and descriptions of the child's language behaviors that provide direction for intervention or, in some cases, further assessment. However, assessment is an ongoing process throughout treatment; that is, we are always collecting data on a child's communication behaviors to make appropriate adjustments in therapy.

Referral and Screening

A child may be referred to a speech-language pathologist soon after birth or during early infancy if there is an identifiable syndrome or physical anomaly, such as a cleft lip or palate (see Chapter 10, Cleft Lip and Palate). Parents and preschool teachers may refer children to an SLP when they are as young as 2 or 3 years of age, but more commonly

---

standardized test (norm-referenced test)

A test that has been administered to a large group of individuals to determine uniform or standard procedures and methods of administration, scoring, and interpretation, and has adequate **normative data** on validity and reliability; tests that are administered to compare one child's performance to others the same age.

normative data (norms)

Data that characterize what is usual in a defined population and that describe rather than explain a particular occurrence; an average of performance of a sample drawn randomly from a population.

client-specific measurements (clinician devised assessments)

Assessments that are not standardized tests that a clinician constructs to make decisions about a specific client's communication abilities.

by 4 or 5 years of age. Parents and teachers also may refer children for a screening at any age while they are in school. Clinicians need to be cautious about the interpretation of screening results when a child uses a dialect such as African American English or is not proficient in English because standardized screening tests do not always contain sufficient numbers of these children for their standardization. We need to remember that there are many individuals from diverse ethnic and linguistic backgrounds who have no problem with language. If an SLP determines there is a problem that needs further investigation, she will recommend the child have a speech, language, and/or hearing evaluation. An interdisciplinary team may become involved in a child's overall evaluation, including an audiologist, a psychologist, special education teacher, physical therapist, occupational therapist, pediatrician, and pediatric neurologist.

Case History and Interview

A complete evaluation of a child includes more than just assessment of language; the process usually includes the following steps:

- Conducting an interview with the parents (the "informants") or other family members (e.g., grandparents) to obtain a detailed case history
- Developing rapport with the child before actual testing begins to help the child "warm up" to the clinician and be willing to participate in the various tasks
- Noting the child's articulation, voice, resonance, and fluency during the rapport-building time
- Evaluating the child's articulation and phonological development
- Examining the orofacial structures and functioning
- Screening hearing
- Evaluating the child's receptive and expressive language, including a language sample
- Meeting with the parents to review the clinician's findings and recommendations

The purposes of a case history and interview are to gather information to help understand the child and his communication problems, to help provide direction of the formal testing, and, ultimately, direction for therapy (Flasher & Fogle, 2012). When possible, one or both parents or other important caregivers of the child are met with in private. The clinician has a list of questions she wants to ask the parents about the child's (1) prenatal and birth history, medical history, speech and language development, (2) hearing ability, (3) the language environment in the home, educational history, (4) possible causes of the communication problem, (5) the child's current communication problems, (6) the child's general behavior, and (7) the parents' feelings about the child's problems.

Developing Rapport and Observing the Child Informally

Before a clinician begins administering tests to a child, she will want to build rapport through relaxed, casual conversation and, when necessary, some play time. Rapport is essential to help a child feel comfortable with the clinician and be willing to participate in the various assessment tasks. The moment the child enters the room, the clinician begins making observations of the child that are important in the overall evaluation. It is during the first several minutes with a child that a clinician often observes many of the strengths and weaknesses of the child's communication abilities. During the initial rapport-building time, the clinician may playfully ask the child to *show me*, *give me*, *hand me*, or *draw me* different objects. This gives the clinician an opportunity to see some of the nouns, verbs, and adjectives the child understands. She may try to "interview" the child, asking about school or play activities, his favorite toys and games, and so on. To the child, what the clinician is doing and asking may appear to make her just a new person in his life who is nice and fun to be with; however, everything the clinician is doing is designed to help understand the child and his communication abilities.

These informal observations can confirm that formal assessment is needed in some additional areas (e.g., a child's voice may be unusually hoarse, his resonance hypernasal, or he may have occasional disfluencies that need to be investigated). Beyond the child's speech and language, the clinician also notes the child's general motor skills and coordination (children with developmental coordination impairments tend to have learning and/or language-learning disabilities [Missiuna, Gaines, Soucie, & McLean, 2006; Webster, Majnemer, Platt, & Shevell, 2005]). During rapport building, screening, and assessment, clinicians must use excellent observational skills. Clinicians become trained listeners and observers—foundational skills for being good speech-language pathologists.

Behavioral Challenges

Not every child is easy to evaluate, usually because of behavioral challenges. As speech-language pathologists we need to learn various methods of behavior modification and techniques to motivate children of all ages to attend to assessment tasks, respond as well as they can, and, ideally, enjoy their time working with the clinician. A positive evaluation session for a child sets him up to be willing to return to the clinician for future therapy.

Evaluating Receptive Language

As discussed earlier, a child with impaired receptive language abilities will often have impaired expressive language abilities. Therefore, a clinician must develop a good impression of a child's receptive language abilities at several levels, including the following:

- Single-word receptive vocabulary and basic concepts
- Morphological structures
- Short sentences
- Longer sentences
- One-, two-, and three-part commands (requests, instructions, and directions)
- Questions
- Conversational speech appropriate for the child's chronological age

A large number of language tests are standardized for different age levels, with some tests targeting specific aspects of receptive language, such as single-word receptive vocabulary. *Comprehensive tests* include evaluations of both receptive and expressive language.

Evaluating Expressive Language

During their education and training SLPs gain experience administering numerous language tests in order to select what they feel are the most appropriate tests to administer to an individual child. SLPs learn to be very flexible and adept in their ability to administer, score, and interpret tests.

Clinicians need to assess many general and specific expressive language abilities, either formally or informally, including the following:

- Spontaneous sounds and words the child uses to communicate
- Morphological units, such as -*ing,* plural -*s,* and past tense -*ed,* used by the child
- Gestures and signs the child often uses to communicate
- Imitation of simple words and phrases
- Vocabulary
- Words, syntax, and semantics the child appears to use easily and others that he appears to have some difficulty using
- Answering of simple questions
- Narrative skills (e.g., describing a picture or telling a story)
- Pragmatic language
- Conversational abilities at an age-appropriate level

Standardized tests are available for assessing each of these areas of expressive language and they are often part of comprehensive language tests. However, as with assessment of receptive language, client-specific measurements are usually needed to fully understand a child's expressive language. A **language sample** is often used as a

language sample

An audio recording of a child's spontaneous conversation or naturalistic verbal interaction with the clinician, family member, or both that is later analyzed.

client-specific measurement. A language sample involves an audio or video recording of a child's spontaneous conversation or verbal interaction with the clinician, family member, or both. However, the interaction is not entirely spontaneous because the clinician designs and guides it to make specific observations. The audio or video recording allows the clinician to later analyze the child's speech and language that was **elicited** during play activities or while having the child describe selected pictures or relate experiences. Open-ended questions (e.g., What did you do last weekend? What is happening in this picture?) allow for more spontaneous elicited language than close-ended questions (e.g., Did you see a movie last weekend? Is the boy throwing the ball?). Clinicians normally attempt to gather 50 to 100 utterances from a child to get an adequate language sample to analyze.

Because context significantly affects the language a child uses, a clinician takes notes on the context of various utterances during the language sample. During the sampling the clinician provides opportunities for the child to demonstrate various pragmatic skills such as greeting, asking questions, *topic initiation* (the skill of introducing new topics for conversation), *topic maintenance* (continuous conversation on the same topic without abrupt interruptions or changing topics), *conversational turn-taking* (talking and listening in an alternating manner), *conversational repair strategies* (verbal behaviors both listeners and speakers use when there are breakdowns in communication), *narrative skills* (telling stories or personal experiences with sufficient details, temporal sequence, characterization, etc.), and *eye contact* (maintenance of mutual eye gaze during conversation) (Hegde & Maul, 2006).

The SLP will transcribe and analyze the language sample in several ways, including phonology, morphology, syntax, semantics, and pragmatics. The clinician will note the frequency of various language skills, including the *comprehension* and *production* (intelligibility) of words, *morphological productions* (e.g., plural -s, past tense -ed, present progressive -ing), *sentence types* (simple, compound, complex, questions), and *conversation skills* (e.g., turn taking, conversational repair). The child's mean length of utterance will be calculated and compared to that of children his **chronological age** (CA). The child's use of vocabulary will be analyzed; for example, naming pictures and objects, objects by category (e.g., foods, clothing), and the use of verbs and adjectives (Hegde & Maul, 2006; Owens, 2008).

Throughout a speech and language evaluation the SLP will attempt to identify possible effective therapy procedures and strategies that will help improve the child's language abilities. Not only is the SLP trying to determine the characteristics of the child's language problems but also what might help remediate them. Any evaluation is a dynamic process where the clinician is always "thinking on her feet," trying to determine from moment to moment what will be the most effective thing to say and do to better understand a child's communication problems and what might be helpful to remediate them.

elicit

Behavior that is drawn out of a person by presenting certain stimuli, e.g., asking a child to name or describe objects to observe his speech and language.

chronological age

The actual age of a person that is derived from date of birth and expressed in days, months, and years.

Diagnosis

It is the responsibility of SLPs to make diagnoses of children's speech and language disorders. This is often not an easy decision and, in reality, a clear diagnosis cannot always be made. All of the information gathered from the case history, parent interviews, and analysis of the assessment results is described, discussed, and included in the clinician's diagnostic report. This information is usually sufficient to provide an understanding of the child's communication strengths and weaknesses, and the clinical decision as to the diagnostic term that best fits the child's communication disorder. Depending on the work setting, certain guidelines may need to be followed when making a diagnosis and qualifying a child for services. For example, public school clinicians may diagnose a language disorder if a child falls below a specified standard deviation below the mean.

SLPs must be able to explain to parents and other family members, as well as to the child himself, what are the child's speech and language strengths and weaknesses. This takes skill in explaining complex speech and language processes in layperson's terms. It also takes considerable tact and good counseling skills when discussing sensitive issues that reveal to parents the type and extent of speech and language problems their child has. Parents can never be objective about their children and parents always have some level of emotional response to hearing the "bad news" (Flasher & Fogle, 2012).

Multicultural Considerations

The challenges of educating children for whom English is their second language are formidable. However, the challenges of learning for these children are formidable as well, including learning to understand, speak, read, and write in English, learning the content of academic subjects, and adjusting to new cultural and linguistic environments. When children have speech and language impairments, in addition to the challenges mentioned here, the tasks are compounded for the teachers, the children, and the speech-language pathologists.

The average percentage of English language learners on school-based speech-language pathologists' caseloads varied from approximately 7% in the Midwest to approximately 20% in the West (Roseberry-McKibbin, Brice, & O'Hanlon, 2005). For example, an estimated 85% of the 1.5 million English language learners enrolled in the California public school system during the 2004–2005 academic year spoke Spanish as their first or home language (California Department of Education, 2006). However, in addition to Spanish, 55 other home languages were reportedly used by families in California schools, including Vietnamese, Hmong, and Cantonese. Nationally, the number of children speaking a language other than English in the United States is increasing rapidly. According to the 2010 U.S. Census, in 2007 62% of people speaking a language other than English in the home reported speaking Spanish. Other languages spoken in American homes include 19% Indo-European (e.g., German, French, Swedish, Italian, Portuguese, Polish, Punjabi); 15% Asian and Pacific Island (e.g., Chinese, Korean, Japanese, Vietnamese, Hmong, Thai, Tagalog), and 4% other languages (e.g., Arabic, Hebrew, languages of Africa).

When bilingual children struggle or fail in their classrooms, SLPs are often involved in assessment teams to determine whether a language disorder or a language difference may be involved. Goldstein (2004) stated that the rapid growth of English language learners has greatly challenged our present system for assessing and treating children who have communication disorders, including such challenges as:

- An inadequate supply of educators and health care providers with knowledge of cultural and linguistic factors that influence communication development
- A paucity of speakers of languages other than English in the provider workforce, along with a lack of trained interpreters and translators
- Health care and early education systems that often are difficult to access for low-income and/or diverse families
- Inadequate assessment tools appropriate for culturally and linguistically diverse children, resulting in over- and underidentification of disabilities
- A mismatch between the cultures of families and those of teachers, with the latter expecting children of these families to fit the dominant culture's expectations

ASHA (1989, p. 93) has provided guidelines for competent clinicians who can provide services in the native language of the child (client):

Speech-language pathologists who present themselves as bilingual for the purposes of providing clinical services must be able to speak their primary language and to speak (or sign) at least one other language with native or near-native proficiency in lexicon (vocabulary), semantics (meaning), phonology (pronunciation), morphology/syntax (grammar), and pragmatics (uses) during clinical management. To provide bilingual assessment and remediation services in the client's language, the bilingual speech-language pathologist or audiologist should possess: (1) the ability to describe the process of normal speech and language acquisition for bilingual and monolingual individuals and how those processes are manifested in oral (or manually coded) and written language; (2) the ability to administer and interpret formal and informal assessment procedures to distinguish between communication differences and communication disorders in oral (or manually coded) and written language; (3) the ability to apply intervention strategies for treatment of communication disorders in the client's language; and (4) the ability to recognize cultural factors that affect the delivery of speech-language pathology and audiology services to the client's language community.

Whenever a test is standardized (the normative sample) there is always risk of biases in the standardization. Wyatt (2002) discusses biases of standardized tests in America. For example, many of the tests that SLPs use are standardized on middle-class individuals from white backgrounds who speak General American English (GAE). The scores of individuals from other socioeconomic, ethnic, cultural, racial, and dialect backgrounds (e.g., African American English) are often grouped with the white, middle-class GAE speakers, which masks group differences.

Kayser (2002) presents three principles concerning the speech and language evaluation of bilingual children:

1. Both languages should always be evaluated, even when the child understands only the home (native) language.

2. If one of the languages is within normal limits, then a language disorder probably does not exist.

3. A concomitant disorder may exist, such as oral–motor disorders, developmental apraxia of speech, phonological impairment, or developmental delay.

THERAPY FOR LANGUAGE DISORDERS

evidence-based treatment (best practices)

The integration of (a) clinical expertise, (b) the current best evidence based on controlled and replicated research, and (c) the client's values, needs, and choices to provide high-quality service.

effective treatment

Treatment with a particular method or approach that has been shown by research to be better than no treatment.

functional treatment

Treatment results that improve communication abilities useful in a person's natural environments (e.g., home, school, community, and job).

attainable treatment

The expectation that an individual can achieve a specific target within a reasonably specified time.

The terms *therapy*, *treatment*, and *intervention* are often used interchangeably by authors, although most SLPs when talking among themselves use the term *therapy* (e.g., "I have some therapy to do."). Therapy methods should be **evidence-based treatment (best practices)**. Treatment methods also should be **effective** (treatment with a particular method or approach has been shown by research to be better than no treatment), **functional** (the treatment results in improved communication abilities useful to the child in natural environments, such as home and school), and reasonably **attainable** (it is expected the child can achieve the specific targeted goals within a reasonably specified time). In all areas of speech-language pathology, including treatment for language disorders in children, more clinically based research is needed. Such research is conducted by clinicians "in the trenches" daily, conducting language therapy with children in the variety of settings in which SLPs work.

By knowing and understanding a child's particular communication problems a clinician can refine general and specific therapy approaches, therapy techniques, individual stimuli, order of presentation of stimuli, and specific types of reinforcement that a child needs. Although the formal assessment may have been completed, therapy is an ongoing assessment process because a clinician is constantly observing, noting, measuring, collecting data (*daily documentation*), analyzing data, and adjusting therapy to the changing needs of each child. Language therapy should be a well-integrated whole in which various aspects of language combine to enhance communication. The purpose of therapy should be to stimulate overall language development and to teach a repertoire of linguistic features that can be used to communicate in all contexts and in all environments (Owens, 2008).

Selecting Goals (Target Behaviors)

A **goal (target behavior)** is any verbal or nonverbal skill a clinician tries to teach a child. The target behaviors clinicians try to "hit" are based on axioms, such as the following:

- The language development of normal children can guide the general selection of therapy targets; that is, there is a hierarchical sequence that helps us know what the child has and needs to acquire. However, for any child, the normative sequence may not be what is "normal" for that child.

- Simple language rules are acquired before complex rules. This is the classic idea that a child needs to learn to walk before he learns to run.

- Certain concepts need to be developed before certain vocabulary can be meaningful. For example, a child who does not have the general notion (concept) of *one* and *more than one* will have difficulty learning plurals.

- Although all verbal skills are important, some are more important than others for a child's developmental and language ages. It is important for clinicians to choose language targets that will be most helpful in a child's family, school, and social environments.

Operationally Defined Goals (Targets)

An **operationally defined goal (target)** means that a specific behavior is observable and measurable. That is, a clinician can observe and measure the accuracy and frequency of a particular language behavior (e.g., *-ing* verbing) before therapy begins, as therapy progresses, and when therapy is terminated. Goals that are operationally defined require several specific points:

- A *specific behavior* that is both observable (can be heard or seen) and measurable (e.g., The child will use *-ing verbing* . . .)
- The *setting* or *environment* in which the target behavior is to be observed (e.g., The child will use *-ing* verbing *in the clinic setting* . . .)
- The *number of times* the particular target behavior is to be observed (e.g., The child will use *-ing* verbing in the clinic setting *10 times* . . .)
- The *percent accuracy* criterion chosen (e.g., The child will use *-ing* verbing in the clinic setting 10 times *with 90% accuracy* . . .)
- The *therapy stimuli* to be used (e.g., The child will use *-ing* verbing in the clinic setting 10 times with 90% accuracy *when shown pictures of actions of people and objects and asked, "What is this person [object] doing?"*)

goal (target behavior)

Any verbal or nonverbal skill a clinician tries to teach a child (client).

operationally defined goal (target)

A specific behavior that is observable (can be heard or seen) and measurable.

In this example, the *long-term goal* is for the child to use -*ing* verbing with 100% accuracy in naturalistic environments (home, school, playground, etc.). In reality, it is impossible for a clinician to observe a child in all natural environments and hear whether -*ing* verbing is used accurately 100% of the time. Therefore, we try to obtain feedback from teachers and parents about how the child is doing with a particular goal in the classroom and home environments.

In most cases, to reach a long-term goal, *short-term goals* are needed. Short-term goals may be thought of as "baby steps" to reach the long-term goal. A short-term goal is operationally defined using language similar to that of the long-term goal; however, the short-term goal usually has a lower percent accuracy rate: for example, "The child will use -*ing* verbing in the clinic setting 10 times with 70% accuracy when shown pictures of actions of people and objects and asked, What is this person [object] doing?" Short-term goals may be written without percentages as well, such as, "The child will use -*ing* verbing without modeling or prompting when shown pictures of actions of people and objects."

Most children with whom SLPs work already have some or even a considerable amount of verbal language; however, there are some children for whom our job is to teach both basic and more advanced language skills. A way to think of *basic* is *functional;* for example, we want young children to learn functional vocabulary words that are important in their home environment and preschool children to learn vocabulary words that are important not only for their home environment but also for their school and community environments (see Figure 6–4). The eventual goal of each is natural, spontaneous conversational speech. As children progress in their language learning, increasing time and emphasis are placed on conversations and narratives.

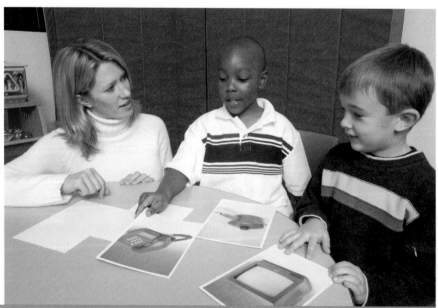

Figure 6–4

A clinician working on functional vocabulary.

© Cengage Learning 2013

There are three primary models that clinicians may choose to follow when working with an individual child who has a communication disorder:

- *Within-discipline model:* The clinician works primarily independently with relatively little interaction with other professionals (classroom teachers, resource teachers, reading specialists, physical therapists, occupational therapists, etc.) who also are working with a child.

- *Interdisciplinary model:* The clinician works with other disciplines and participates in regular (usually weekly) meetings with other professionals to share information about a child's progress in the various intervention programs.

- *Transdisciplinary model:* The various professionals working with a child learn the therapy programs a child is involved in and incorporate information and procedures from all programs into each therapeutic discipline.

Clinicians also may choose combinations of the three. The model or models selected depend on the needs of the individual child. The transdisciplinary model is particularly helpful when working with children who have multiple impairments, such as a child with cerebral palsy who has physical impairments, speech and language problems, and learning disabilities (see Figure 6–5).

Organization and Structure of Therapy Sessions

A few general principles help clinicians determine the organization and structure of individual therapy sessions. In general, young children and children just beginning therapy benefit from well-organized and tightly structured therapy sessions. Tightly structured sessions are more efficient when establishing target behaviors, especially at the morpheme, word, phrase, short-sentence, and simple-question levels. Also, children who have moderate to severe language impairments and behavioral challenges from various neurological causes (e.g., attention deficit disorders, developmental delays, autism spectrum disorders, or traumatic brain injury) benefit from well-organized and highly structured therapy.

A *well-organized therapy session* means that the clinician has carefully preplanned the structure and sequence of therapy tasks and the materials that will be used. She has materials readily available so there are no unnecessary and distracting delays moving from one task to another. She has carefully chosen *tangible reinforcers* (stickers, stamps, bubbles, etc.) that are easily accessible but usually out of sight so that the child is not constantly distracted by them while trying to focus on therapy tasks. The clinician knows how she is going to start the session, what will likely be the middle parts, and how she wants to end the session.

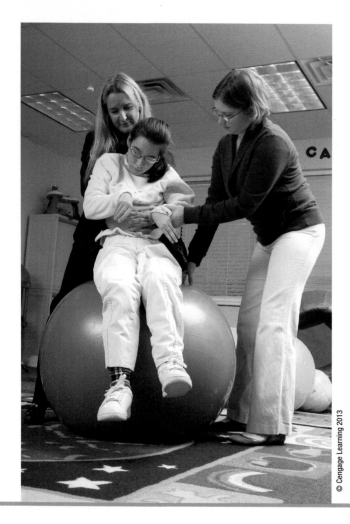

Figure 6-5

A child with cerebral palsy working with a transdisciplinary team.

© Cengage Learning 2013

Nevertheless, the clinician remains flexible throughout the session to accommodate the child's needs, unpredictable behaviors, inability to perform that day as had been expected, internal distractions of the child (e.g., being upset for having gotten in trouble at home or school before coming to therapy), and so on. A clinician's flexibility allows her to make the most of what may otherwise turn out to be a minimally productive session. Clinician flexibility is a hallmark of a good speech-language pathologist at all levels of training and throughout a professional career.

A General Therapy Session Model

It is helpful for clinicians to have in mind a general therapy session model that will likely be functional when working with most children. Within the general therapy session model, there is considerable flexibility that allows clinicians to adapt to the ever-changing and sometimes unpredictable needs of a child. A general therapy session model that works well for many clinicians is the following:

1. *Start the session with a minute or two of general conversation,* asking, for example, how the day is going, how the child did on a recent test, or anything that the clinician can think of that is applicable or

pertinent to the child. This moment or two may provide considerable information that is valuable to the clinician. The clinician will likely receive an answer to the question that was asked; however, she also may hear how the child is producing particular sounds or using certain morphemes, vocabulary, syntactic structures, or pragmatic skills they have been working on. That is, she may be able to see and hear how well the child is generalizing the targeted speech and language skills into connected, spontaneous speech.

Beyond those benefits, the clinician also may get a sense of how the child is feeling about school, classmates and playmates, and other important areas of the child's life. Special bonds are often developed between a child and his "speech teacher," and sometimes a child may share important information with a clinician that is appropriately and necessarily (sometimes mandated) shared with a supervisor, parent, teacher, or other professional (see Flasher & Fogle, 2012, for a discussion of confidentiality as it relates to children).

2. *Review what the child has worked on that he is generally successful with.* This helps reinforce and strengthen what he has been accomplishing, but it also helps him feel that he already has a good start with his speech therapy session for that day. This review time may take just a few minutes, with the child receiving reinforcements for his successes.

3. *Work on new or more difficult therapy targets that need structured teaching and careful monitoring by both the clinician and the child.* This is the hard work of the session that needs intense focus, and the child deserves frequent rewards for his hard work even before he is having correct responses.

4. *Do a quick review of another speech or language skill to give the child a break from the intense focus of the previous task.* The child should be able to respond rapidly and accurately to each stimulus and earn reinforcements for his successes. If time does not allow further work, this is a good way to end the session, with the child feeling he has demonstrated what he has learned, and learned (or started to learn) some new skills.

5. *Work on another challenging task to keep the child working hard and learning new language skills.* At this time, reinforcement is more for hard work than accuracy with such challenging tasks.

6. *End the session on a high note.* A moment of review or going over some skill the child will have high success with helps the child feel that no matter how hard some of the therapy tasks were, he did a great job at the end. This is always appreciated by children.

Eliciting Large Numbers of Responses

For a child to make gains in speech and language abilities, it is important for the clinician to elicit large numbers of responses. As discussed in

Chapter 3, "Anatomy and Physiology of Speech and Language," all therapy involves working with the brain, literally down to the neuron and synapse levels. For a child to learn new vocabulary, morphemes, syntax, semantics, and pragmatics, information (stimuli) must get into the brain and the brain must use or process the information in various locations within the cortex, integrate the information with other language concepts, and be able to retrieve and use the information appropriately when needed. For example, a child may learn some new vocabulary words quickly, such as *male* and *female* for *man* and *woman;* however, the understanding of the appropriate times to use the synonyms may take a considerable amount of additional learning.

Form, content, and use of language a child has not learned automatically through his environment may take a considerable amount of time, effort, and "brain work" in therapy. The concept of making a footpath through grass may clarify this. When you walk across some grass once, the grass quickly springs back up and in a short time there is no trace that you had even walked across it. However, if you walk across the grass many times, you eventually develop a pathway. That is similar to what happens inside the brain; we need to present numerous stimuli and receive numerous responses to develop strong neural pathways.

Multicultural Considerations

In 1998, ASHA adopted the following position statement on the role of speech-language pathologists in providing services to individuals learning English as a second language (ESL):

> It is the position of the American Speech-Language-Hearing Association that speech-language pathologists who possess the required knowledge and skills to provide English as a second language (ESL) instruction in school settings may provide direct ESL instruction. ESL instruction may require specialized academic preparation and competencies in areas such as second-language acquisition (SLA), comparative linguistics, and English as a second language (ESL) methodologies, assessment and practicum. Speech-language pathologists who do not possess the requisite skills should not provide direct instruction in ESL but should collaborate with ESL instructors in providing preassessment, assessment, and/or intervention with English as second-language speakers in school settings.

Battle (2011) offers several points that clinicians need to consider when providing services to individuals with cultural and linguistic differences, some of which are as follows:

- When providing clinical services to all individuals, it is important to consider one's own personal cultural beliefs, attitudes, and values and to be aware that they contribute to and are a major factor in the multicultural, cross-cultural clinical encounter.

- Do not use generic terms as substitutes or synonyms for more descriptive racial or ethnic terms. For example, avoid using *minority* to refer to African Americans, *bilingual* to refer to Hispanics, or *culturally diverse* or *multicultural* to refer to individuals. Note: *African American* does not apply to all black individuals in North America. For example, individuals from Haiti or the Caribbean often want to be referred to based on their home country (Haitian, Bahamian, etc.). Likewise, *Hispanic* does not apply to all individuals from Latin backgrounds. For example, individuals from Puerto Rico or Cuba often want to be referred to based on their home country (Puerto Rican, Cuban, etc.) (Kanzki-Veloso, 2006).

- Be aware that some terms have questionable or negative racial, ethnic, or socioeconomic connotations, such as *culturally deprived* and *culturally disadvantaged.*

EMOTIONAL AND SOCIAL EFFECTS OF LANGUAGE DISORDERS

Language disorders in children can affect them both emotionally and socially throughout their education and possibly into adulthood. The research on psychosocial problems on children dates back to the 1980s. For example:

- Of approximately 300 consecutive intakes of children to a community-based speech and language clinic, 95% of the children with expressive language problems had some form of psychosocial difficulties according to 1980 criteria used by the American Psychiatric Association (Baker & Cantwell, 1982).

- Of 40 consecutive admissions to a child psychiatric unit, 50% of the children had language problems (Gualtieri, Koriath, Van Bourgondien, & Saleeby, 1983).

- Of the children consecutively admitted because of behavioral or emotional problems to an inpatient facility, 67% failed a speech and language screening (Prizant, Audet, Burke, et al., 1990).

As clinicians we need to assess and treat all manner of communication disorders in children, but we also need to recognize that not all children we work with are emotionally stable and may have psychological problems concurrent with their communication disorders. As SLPs, we do not work with the psychological problems of children or other clients, but try to work with individuals in ways that their psychological problems do not interfere with our therapy (Flasher & Fogle, 2012). SLPs need to refer clients to the proper mental health professionals when we feel there are psychological or emotional concerns outside of our scope of practice.

The communication disorders of children often result in parents being in a quandary about what is different about their children, what they might have done to cause or contribute to their children's problems (a considerable amount of soul-searching is done by parents), and what they can do to help their children (parent support groups are often helpful in these areas). Parents naturally want to boast to family and friends about their children's academic achievements; however, parents of children who have communication and learning problems may find it difficult to talk about the school struggles of their children.

The effects of language disorders on the education of children at all ages can be devastating. Good receptive and expressive language skills are essential for learning, and anything less than good skills can affect a child's academic performance and potential success in life. Being undereducated and underemployed are common results of adults having language disorders that were unidentified or undertreated in school. It also has been recognized for years that there is a relationship between juvenile delinquency and adolescent language disorders, and now there is increasing awareness of communication disorders in the adult prison population (Castrogiovanni, 2002; U.S. Department of Education, 2005).

Addendum

As speech-language pathologists, we seldom know the long-term (lifelong) benefits of the work we do with children. After many years of work, we may occasionally come across adults whom we had in therapy as children, and they may remember us. Often we are gratified with how well they are doing. Although we do not try to take credit for their successes in their education, work, and life, we may feel that we were a small part of all of the help they needed to get them where they are.

> For the want of a horseshoe nail the shoe was lost; for want of a shoe the horse was lost; for want of a horse the rider was lost; for want of a rider the battle was lost; for want of the battle, the war was lost—all for the want of a horseshoe nail.
> Sometimes we might be the nail—and that makes all the difference.

CHAPTER SUMMARY

Speech-language pathologists work with children who have both receptive and expressive language delays and disorders that may involve the form, content, and function of language. Specific language impairments (SLI) refer to significant receptive and/or expressive language impairments that cannot be attributed to any general or specific cause or condition.

SLI may include problems with receptive language, morphology, vocabulary, syntax, semantics, discourse, narratives, and pragmatics. When children enter primary school and their SLI begins to interfere with their educational achievement they will likely be diagnosed as having a language-learning disability (language disorder). Clinicians need to obtain valid and reliable measures during their assessments of children to have accurate results from which they can have confidence in their decisions about diagnosis and development of an effective treatment plan. Treatment methods should be effective, functional, and reasonably attainable. Multicultural issues need to be taken into consideration with many of the children identified and treated. As clinicians, we need to be aware of and concerned about possible emotional and social effects of language disorders on children.

STUDY QUESTIONS

Knowledge and Comprehension

1. What is ASHA's definition of a language disorder?
2. Define *specific language impairment.*
3. Define *language-learning disability.*
4. What are three purposes of an assessment of language?
5. What elements need to be included in an operationally defined goal (target)?

Application

1. How does ASHA's definition of language disorder help clinicians understand their professional scope of practice?
2. What are some of the "red flags" parents should note during an infant's first year of life that may indicate the infant is at risk for developing a language disorder?
3. How could understanding a preschool child's specific language impairments help you understand his current language-learning disability?
4. What are some strengths and weaknesses of a child's language that you might observe during the rapport-building time?
5. Outline an organized, structured general therapy session model.

Analysis/Synthesis

1. How can you apply the information about specific language impairments to children with language-learning disabilities?
2. How could language impairments affect children throughout primary and secondary education?

3. How could a high school student's language-learning disability influence decisions about further education and choice of occupations and professions?

4. What are the differences between an assessment and a diagnosis?

5. Discuss the importance of eliciting large numbers of responses during therapy.

REFERENCES

ASHA. (1989). Bilingual speech-language pathologists and audiologists. *ASHA, 31*, 93.

ASHA's Ad Hoc Committee on Service Delivery in the Schools. (1993). Definitions of communication education disorders and variations. *ASHA, 35*(Supplement 10), 40–41.

Baker, L., & Cantwell, D. P. (1982). Psychiatric disorders in children with different types of communication disorders. *Journal of Communication Disorders, 15*, 113–126.

Battle, D. (2011). *Communication disorders in multicultural populations* (4th ed.). Boston, MA: Butterworth-Heinemann.

Bayne, G., & Moran, C. (2005). The effect of single word semantic-phonological intervention on developmental word finding difficulties at single word and discourse levels. *New Zealand Journal of Speech-Language Therapy, 60*, 31–44.

Bedore, L. M., & Leonard, L. B. (2001). Grammatical morphological deficits in Spanish-speaking children with specific language impairments. *Journal of Speech, Language, and Hearing Research, 44*, 905–924.

Beitchman, J., Wilson, B., Douglas, L., Young, A., & Adlaf, E. (2001). Substance abuse disorders in young adults with and without LD: Predictive and concurrent relationships. *Journal of Learning Disabilities, 34*, 317–332.

Bishop, D. V. (2006). What causes specific language impairment in children? *Association for Psychological Science, 15*(5), 217–221.

Botting, N., & Adams, C. (2005). Semantics and inferencing abilities in children with communication disorders. *International Journal of Language and Communication Disorders, 40*(1), 49–66.

Cairns, H. S., Waltzman, D., & Schlisselberg, G. (2004). Detecting the ambiguity of sentences: Relationship to early reading skills. *Communication Disorders Quarterly, 25*, 68–78.

Cairns, H. S., Waltzman, D., & Schlisselberg, G. (2007). Development of a metalinguistics skill: Judging the grammaticality of sentences. *Communication Disorders Quarterly, 27*, 213–220.

California Department of Education. (2006). *Dataquest* (online). Available at http://www.cde.ca.gov/ds/sd/cb/dataquest.asp.

Castrogiovanni, A. (2002). *Special populations: Prison populations - 2002 edition*. Rockville, MD: ASHA.

Choudhury, N., & Benasich, A. (2003). A family aggregation study: The influence of family history and other risk factors on language development. *Journal of Speech, Language, and Hearing Research, 46,* 261–272.

Conti-Ramsden, G., & Windfuhr, K. (2002). Productivity with word order and morphology: A comparative look at children with SLI and children with normal language abilities. *International Journal of Language and Communication Disorders, 37*(1), 17–30.

Colozzo, P., Gillam, R. B., Wood, M., Schnell, R. D., Johnston, J. R. (2011). *Journal of Speech, Language, and Hearing Research, 54,* 1609–1627.

Dale, P. S., Price, T. S., Bishop, D., & Plomin, R. (2003). Outcomes of early language delay, I: Predicting persistent and transient language difficulties at 3 and 4 years. *Journal of Speech, Language, and Hearing Research, 46,* 544–560.

Delange, F. (2000). The role of iodine in brain development. *Proceedings of the Nutrition Society, 59*(1), 75–79.

Dockrell, J., Messer, D., George, R., & Wilson, G. (1998). Children with word-finding difficulties: Prevalence, presentation, and naming problems. *International Journal of Language and Communication Disorders, 33,* 445–454.

Dollagham, C. A., & Horner, E. A. (2011). Bilingual language assessment: A meta-analysis of diagnostic accuracy. *Journal of Speech, Language, and Hearing Research, 54,* 1077–1088.

Ehren, B. J. (2002). Speech-language pathologists contributing significantly to the academic success of high school students: A vision for professional growth. *Topics in Language Disorders, 10,* 192–203.

Erwin, M. (2001). Specific language impairments: What we know and why it matters. *ASHA Leader, 6,* 4.

Flasher, L. V., & Fogle, P. T. (2012). *Counseling skills for speech-language pathologists and audiologists* (2nd ed.). Clifton Park, NY: Delmar Cengage Learning.

Gualtieri, L., Koriath, U., Van Bourgondien, M., & Saleeby, N. (1983). Language disorders in children referred for psychiatric service. *Journal of the American Academy of Child Psychiatry, 22,* 165–171.

Goldstein, B. A. (2004). *Bilingual language development and disorders.* Baltimore, MD: Paul H. Brookes.

Hegde, M. N., & Maul, C. A. (2006). *Language disorders in children: An evidence-based approach to assessment and treatment.* Boston, MA: Pearson Allyn and Bacon.

Henderson, C. (2001). *College freshmen with disabilities: A biennial statistical profile.* Washington, DC: American Council of Education.

Heward, W. L. (2008). *Exceptional children: An introduction to special education* (9th ed.). Upper Saddle River, NJ: Merrill Prentice Hall.

Johnson, C., Beitchman, J., Young, A., Escobar, M., Atkinson, L., & Wilson, B. (1999). Fourteen-year follow-up of children with and without speech/language impairments: Speech-language stability and outcomes. *Journal of Speech and Hearing Research, 42*(3), 744–760.

Kanzki-Veloso, E. (2006). *Counseling skills for difficult conversations with supervisees, staff, clients, and families.* ASHA Convention Workshop.

Kayser, H. R. (2002). Bilingual language development and language disorders. In D. E. Battle (Ed.), *Communication disorders in multicultural populations* (3rd ed.). Boston, MA: Butterworth-Heinemann.

Kurtz, L. A. (2007). *Understanding motor skills in children with dyspraxia, ADHD, autism, and other learning disabilities: A guide to improving coordination.* Philadelphia, PA: Jessica Kingsley Publishers.

Leonard, L. B. (2000). *Children with specific language impairment.* Cambridge, MA: MIT Press.

Missiuna, C., Gaines, R., Soucie, H., & McLean, J. (2006). Parental questions about developmental coordination disorder: A synopsis of current evidence. *Pediatric Child Health, 11*(8), 507–512.

Nelson, N. W. (2010). *Language and literacy disorders: Infancy through adolescence.* Boston, MA: Pearson Allyn and Bacon.

Nicolosi, L., Harryman, E., & Kresheck, J. (2004). *Terminology of communication disorders: Speech-language-hearing* (5th ed.). Philadelphia, PA: Lippincott Williams & Wilkins.

Nippold, M. A. (2001). Adolescents with language disorders: An underserved population. *New Zealand Journal of Speech-Language Therapy, 55,* 27–32.

Owens, R. E. (2008). *Language disorders: A functional approach to assessment and intervention* (5th ed.). Boston, MA: Pearson Allyn and Bacon.

Paradis, J. (2005). Grammatical morphology in children learning English as a second language: Implications of similarities with specific language impairment. *Language, Speech, and Hearing Services in the Schools, 36,* 172–187.

Paul, R. (2011). *Language disorders from infancy through adolescence: Assessment and intervention* (4th ed.). St. Louis, MO: Mosby.

Pence-Turnbull, K. L., & Justice, L. M. (2012). *Language development from theory to practice.* Upper Saddle River, NJ: Pearson Prentice Hall.

Prizant, B., Audet, L., Burke, G., Hummel, L., Maher, S., & Theadore, G. (1990). Communication disorders and emotional and behavioral disorders in children and adolescents. *Journal of Speech and Hearing Disorders, 55,* 179–192.

Reed, V. A. (Ed.). (2012). *An introduction to children with language disorders* (4th ed.). Boston, MA: Pearson Allyn and Bacon.

Rice, M. L., Redmond, S. M., & Hoffman, L. (2006). Mean length of utterance in children with specific language impairment and in young control children shows concurrent validity and stable and parallel growth trajectories. *Journal of Speech, Language, and Hearing Research, 49*, 793–808.

Roseberry-McKibbin, C. (2001). *The source for bilingual students with language disorders*. East Moline, IL: LinguiSystems.

Roseberry-McKibbin, C., Brice, A., & O'Hanlon, L. (2005). Serving English language learners in public school settings: A national survey. *Language, Speech, and Hearing Services in the Schools, 36*, 48–61.

Tomblin, J. B., Records, N. L., Buckwalter, P., & Zhang, X. (1996). Prevalence of specific language impairment in kindergarten children. *Journal of Speech, Language, and Hearing Research, 40*, 1245–1260.

Tomblin, J. B., Zhang, X., Buckwalter, O., & O'Brian, M. (2003). The stability of primary language disorder: Four years after kindergarten diagnosis. *Journal of Speech, Language, and Hearing Research, 46*, 1283–1296.

U.S. Census Bureau. (2010). *Language use in the United States: 2007*. Available at http://www.census.gov/prod/2010pubs/acs-12.pdf.

U.S. Census Bureau. (2008). *School enrollment in the United States: 2006*. Washington, DC: U.S. Census Bureau.

U.S. Department of Education. (2008). *Twenty-eighth annual report to Congress on the implementation of the Individuals with Disabilities Education Act (IDEA), 2006, Vol. 1*. Washington, DC: U.S. Department of Education.

U.S. Department of Education, National Center for Education Statistics. (2007). *The condition of education: 2005*. Washington, DC: U.S. Department of Education.

Vinson, B. P. (2011). *Language disorders across the lifespan* (3rd ed.). Clifton Park, NY: Delmar Cengage Learning.

Webster, R. I., Majnemer, A., Platt, R. W., & Shevell, M. I. (2005). Motor function at school age in children with a preschool diagnosis of developmental language impairment. *Journal of Pediatrics, 146*, 80–85.

Wyatt, T. A. (2002). Assessing the communicative abilities of children from diverse cultural and language backgrounds. In D. E. Battle (Ed.), *Communication disorders in multicultural populations* (3rd ed.). Boston, MA: Butterworth-Heinemann.

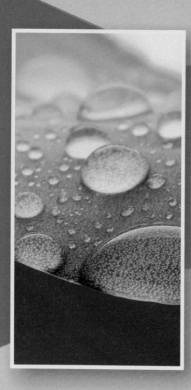

CHAPTER 7
Literacy Disorders in Children

LEARNING OBJECTIVES

After studying this chapter, you will:

- Be familiar with the ASHA guidelines for the roles and responsibilities of speech-language pathologists with respect to literacy for children and adolescents.

- Understand the justification for speech-language pathologists' involvement in literacy.

- Be aware of possible contributions of the English language to reading difficulties.

- Be able to discuss common problems of children with reading and writing disabilities.

- Recognize the multicultural considerations related to literacy problems.

KEY TERMS

alphabetic principle

conventional literacy

dysgraphia

emergent literacy (preliteracy) skills

literacy (reading, writing)

literacy disorder (disability)

orthography

phonics method

phonological awareness

reading disability (dyslexia, developmental dyslexia)

scaffolding

CHAPTER OUTLINE

INTRODUCTION

Students beginning their studies of speech-language pathology and audiology are usually familiar with only the basics of what these professions study and work with clinically—that is, speech, language, and hearing. They are always surprised to find out how much these three areas of study involve. When students learn that speech-language pathologists work with cognition and cognitive disorders, there is an increased realization of the scope and depth of practice of the profession. However, when students learn that speech-language pathology includes learning about **literacy (reading, writing)** and literacy problems (*dyslexia*), they sometimes think these areas are tangential or unrelated to what the profession works with or perhaps *should* work with.

Literacy development is within the scope of practice of speech-language pathologists (ASHA, 2001). When we consider that speech-language pathologists are communication specialists (both normal and impaired communication) and that reading and writing are essential components of communication, it becomes clear that we must learn about and work with literacy and disorders of literacy (Manzo, Manzo, & Thomas, 2009; Nelson, 2010). Kamhi and Catts (2012) and Goldsworthy (2003; Goldsworthy & Lambert, 2010) emphasize that reading and writing are extensions of a child's auditory perception, receptive language, and verbal expressive language skills. In the past, it was assumed that reading disorders were primarily caused by visual perceptual deficits. However, no other factor better justifies speech-language pathologists' involvement in literacy than the research-supported view that reading and writing are *language-based* activities; therefore, language delays, disorders, or both can contribute to or cause literacy problems (Hegde & Maul, 2006).

literacy (reading, writing)

The ability to communicate through written language, both reading and writing.

THE DIFFERENCES BETWEEN LEARNING TO UNDERSTAND SPEECH AND LEARNING TO READ

Kamhi and Catts (2012) discuss three main differences between learning to understand speech and learning to read.

- The human auditory perceptual system is biologically adapted to process spoken words (Lieberman, 1973). In contrast, the human visual system is not biologically adapted to process written words. Learning to read requires specific knowledge of the phonological system of the language; that is, a reader must first know the sounds (phonemes) that correspond with the letters *(graphemes)* in the alphabet (remember, however, that there are many more sounds in the English language than there are letters in the alphabet, which complicates the pronunciation of written words).

- Reading is a comparatively new human ability for which there is no specific biological adaptation. That is, learning to talk is *caught,* but learning to read must be *taught.*

- The nature of the reading system children develop depends on the relative proficiency of all aspects of language, not just phonology.

Geffner (2005), a dual certified speech-language pathologist and audiologist, emphasizes the interrelationship among hearing, phonological processing, reading, and dyslexia. The brain's auditory system and visual system are interconnected by complex pathways of nerve fibers *(sensory-neural integration).* Because of these interconnections, children who have problems in one mode of communication often have problems in another mode. Longitudinal studies have consistently shown that 50% or more of children with language impairments in preschool or kindergarten go on to have reading disabilities in primary or secondary grades and that another 20% of these children are classified as poor readers (Catts, Fey, Tomblin, & Zhang, 2002).

EMERGENT LITERACY/PRELITERACY PERIOD (BIRTH–KINDERGARTEN)

Emergent literacy skills or **preliteracy skills** are terms that have been applied to the skills developed during the preschool years that prepare children for learning to read and write. During the early years, children lack the knowledge of the phoneme–grapheme (sound–letter) correspondence that they later learn. The path to proficient reading and writing skills begins well before children have formal reading and writing instruction in classrooms (Snow, Scarborough, & Burns, 1999).

Before babies can even talk or walk, they may be turning pages of books and spending considerable time looking at pictures in books. Parents often make a big deal about which book they think their child wants to have read, talking animatedly about each book. Children learn that books must be interesting things because there is so much talk about them and parents become excited about reading them. Through *shared book reading,* over time, children begin to learn the names of letters, their shapes, and the sounds they make. For some preschoolers these can lead to the discovery of the underlying **alphabetic principle**—that words consist of discrete sounds represented by letters in print. This principle becomes the foundation of reading.

The National Early Literacy Panel (2004) analyzed several hundred research studies on emergent literacy to identify skills that consistently

emergent literacy (preliteracy) skills

Early skills developed in the preschool years that precede or are presumed prerequisites for later-developing reading and writing skills.

alphabetic principle

Letters and combinations of letters represent speech sounds; speech can be turned into print; and print can be turned into speech.

Application Question

If you are a parent, can you recall when you first started to read to your baby? Can you recall some of the things you did to try to make the experience fun and interesting? If you are not a parent, can you imagine some benefits of reading to a baby at an early age?

and most strongly related to literacy achievement. It found the following to be the strongest skills:

- *Phonological awareness*—Sensitivity to the sound structure of spoken language
- *Oral language*—Grammatical, lexical, and narrative abilities
- *Alphabet knowledge*—Receptive and expressive knowledge of the individual letters of the alphabet
- *Concepts about print*—Knowledge of the rules governing how print is used and organized across various genres, including books and general print in the home and community environments (e.g., labels on boxes, newspapers, and billboards)
- *Name writing*—Representation of one's own name in print

Adult involvement (**scaffolding**) during the emergent literacy and early literacy periods is essential for children to develop these skills in a timely manner (Justice, 2006). Scaffolding involves adults providing whatever supports are needed for children to achieve competence in an activity (such as reading and writing). Gradually, these supports are removed until the child is able to perform independently. Quality emergent literacy assistance involves scaffolding children's achievements in language development, phonological awareness, print knowledge, and writing.

Phonological Awareness

Phonological awareness has an important role in the development of reading skills (Gillon, 2004; Hogan, Catts, & Little, 2005). Phonological awareness is not a simple concept to define. It involves recognizing and understanding (1) sound–letter associations; (2) that individual sounds can be combined to form words; (3) that a single-syllable word (e.g., *dog*) is heard as one word but can be segmented into its beginning, middle, and ending sounds; and (4) that longer words have more "middle" sounds (Foy & Mann, 2003).

The single best predictor of reading success is phonological awareness and the ability to accurately process sounds and words auditorily. Children need to be aware of sounds in speech to acquire sound–letter correspondence knowledge and use this knowledge to *decode* (understand) the printed word. Because phonemes are the fundamental elements of the language system, they are the essential building blocks of all spoken and written words.

Before words can be identified, understood, stored in memory, or retrieved from it, they must be broken into phonemes. When first learning a word, the individual phonemes are processed by the brain's language system. Readers need to convert the letters of words on a page into their corresponding sounds and appreciate that words are composed of smaller segments or phonemes. Children learning to read must rely on hearing sounds to make letter-sound associations to "sound out the word" (the basis of the **phonics method** of reading) and identify the

---

scaffolding

Support that adults provide to children for them to achieve competence in an activity (e.g., reading and writing), with the support gradually removed until the child is able to perform independently.

---

phonological awareness

Recognition and understanding of sound–letter associations; that individual sounds can be combined to form words; that a single-syllable word is heard as one word but can be segmented into its beginning, middle, and ending sounds; and that longer words have more "middle" sounds.

---

phonics method

The method of teaching reading and pronunciation by learning the sounds of letters and groups of letters ("sounding out words"); the association of the sounds (phonemes) of a language with the equivalent written forms (graphemes).

first, middle, and last sounds in words. Phonics is heavily influenced by phonological awareness. Children who learn the phonics approach develop *word-attack skills* that allow them to take complex words and sound out each letter and syllable (*letter–sound association*) and to hear themselves say the word. When they can blend the sounds and syllables together, they can often pronounce a word that they have never seen in print or perhaps even heard before. Children who are unable to make such associations are at risk for reading disabilities (Culatta & Hall, 2006; Ehri et al., 2001).

Proficient Word Recognition

When confronted with a new word while reading, we typically try to sound it out in order to say it. However, when it becomes part of our lexicon we visually recognize the word rather than sound out the letters and syllables. For example, we see and read the word *computer;* however, when reading it silently we are not likely to hear ourselves say *c-ah-m-p-ew-t-r,* or even *com-put-er.* Accurate, effortless word recognition requires the ability to use a direct visual route without phonological mediation to access semantic memory and word meaning. It is not surprising that it is unclear how children become automatic, fluent readers.

Emergent Writing: Preschool

Scribbling is likely the beginning of early writing. From about their first birthday, children achieve the fine motor control required to handle a crayon. Most children make horizontal lines before they make vertical lines, and later circular motions are added. Children appear to get considerable pleasure from watching the lines or the colors appear on paper. Then, from about their second birthday, controlled scribbling starts. Children produce patterns of simple shapes: rough circles, crosses, and starbursts. They also begin to arrange shapes and patterns on paper. Learning to hold a crayon and make purposeful lines may be considered the beginnings of **orthography**—learning how to write (print).

LEARNING TO READ AND READING TO LEARN

Although children are expected to understand the spoken language and be able to proficiently verbally express their basic wants, needs, thoughts, knowledge, and feelings well before they enter elementary school, they are not expected to be able to read and write. Not all children attend preschool or are provided the benefit of emergent literacy skills. Schools, therefore, are expected to provide the training and education for children to learn to read and write and later read to learn and write to communicate. To eventually become a proficient reader, a

---

Application Question

Can you recall the way you were taught to read? Did it include learning how to "sound out words"? What do you think are the benefits and difficulties of learning how to sound out words?

---

orthography

The part of language study concerned with letters and spelling; the representation of the sounds of a language by written or printed symbols.

child must be able to visually recognize words accurately and with little effort, which requires knowledge of letter sequences and orthographic patterns (Kamhi and Catts, 2012). Although phonological skills are essential in learning to read and in sounding out new words, mature, fluent readers rely more on their visual systems. That is, during rapid silent reading people do not "sound out" words through the auditory system (*subvocalize*—hear themselves say the words in their heads), but visually process words as units.

Good Raedres Can Raed Tihs

I culod not blveiee taht I cluod aulaclty uesdnatnrd waht I was rdanieg. The phaonmeanl pweor of the hamun bairn to raed no mttaer in waht oredr the ltteers in a wrod are. Wahts iprmoatnt tohguh is taht the frist and lsat ltteer be in the rghit pclae. The rset can be a taotl mses and you can sitll raed it wouthit a rael porbelm. Tihs is bcuseae the biarn deos not raed ervey lteter by istlef, but the wrod as a wlohe. And I awlyas tghuhot slpelnig was ipmorantt!

---

conventional literacy

Reading and writing according to the rule-governed system of the alphabetic principle and being able to read to learn.

literacy disorder (disability)

Reading and writing impairments in a heterogeneous population of children.

reading disability (dyslexia, developmental dyslexia)

An inability or difficulty reading that is of neurological origin.

dysgraphia

A developmental motor and/ or literacy disorder that affects a child's or adult's ability to write, characterized by messy or illegible handwriting, misspellings, and difficulty with grammar and organizing sentences; note: *agraphia* is a loss of ability to write resulting from injury to the brain.

Children reach **conventional literacy** when they can read and write according to the rule-governed system using the alphabetic principle and are able to read to learn. For most children, this occurs around 8 years of age or the third grade. By this age, they have a considerable sight vocabulary, as well as sophisticated word-attack skills. When children are able to automatically read many words they encounter or can easily sound out and figure out a new word through word-attack skills, they are able to shift important cognitive processes from a focus on decoding and word recognition to the act of reading for understanding and acquiring new knowledge (Feifer & De Fina, 2000). When children's cognitive processes are occupied with basic reading tasks and each word must be individually processed, there may not be sufficient cognitive reserve to fully appreciate the meaning of a sentence, paragraph, or story.

LITERACY DISORDERS IN CHILDREN

In the definition of **literacy disorder (disability)** used by speech-language pathologists, both reading and writing disabilities are included. However, the International Dyslexia Association (IDA) definition of **reading disabilities (dyslexia, developmental dyslexia)** does not include writing disabilities or disorders (**dysgraphia**). Dyslexia is defined by the IDA (Lyon, Shaywitz, & Shaywitz, 2003) in the following manner:

> Dyslexia is a specific learning disability that is neurological in origin. It is characterized by difficulties with accurate and/or fluent recognition and by poor spelling and decoding abilities. These difficulties typically result from a deficit in the phonological components of language that is often unexpected in relation to other cognitive abilities and the provision of effective classroom instruction. A few of the secondary consequences may include problems in reading comprehension and reduced reading experience that can impede growth of vocabulary and background knowledge.

Dyslexia is the most common learning disability in both children and adults, and 75%–85% of all children with learning disabilities have reading impairments (Nelson, 2010; Reed, 2012). To be diagnosed as having dyslexia, hearing and vision acuity problems must be excluded (this includes with amplification such as hearing aids, corrected vision with eyeglasses or contact lenses, or both). The problem is more prevalent in males, with a ratio of about four boys to every one girl with the disability. The cause or causes of a reading impairment for any one child usually cannot be determined. However, reading disabilities have long been recognized as tending to run in families and are often seen in siblings, parents, and grandparents (Stevenson, Graham, Fredman, & McLoughlin, 1987).

Considerable evidence suggests a strong and reciprocal link between language development and emergent literacy development in preschool children (Goldsworthy, 2003; Justice, Invernizzi, & Meier, 2002). Kamhi & Catts (2012) and Hesketh (2004) maintain that reading disabilities are best characterized as developmental language disorders. That is, reading is a language activity that relies on a person's knowledge of the phonological, morphological, syntactic, semantic, and pragmatic aspects of language. Therefore, impairment in one or more of these aspects of auditory or verbal language, could lead to significant disruptions in the ability to read and communicate effectively in writing (see Figure 7–1).

ASHA (2001) published guidelines for the roles and responsibilities of speech-language pathologists with respect to reading and writing (literacy) for children and adolescents. Our roles and responsibilities include designing and implementing programs to do the following:

1. Prevent reading and writing language problems by fostering language acquisition and emergent literacy.

2. Identify children at risk for reading and writing problems.

3. Assess reading and writing.

4. Provide intervention and document outcomes for reading and writing intervention programs.

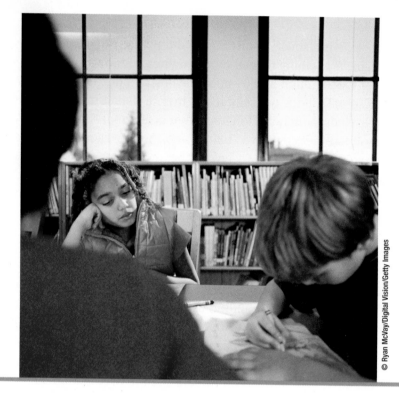

© Ryan McVay/Digital Vision/Getty Images

Figure 7-1

Some children find letters, printed words, and reading incomprehensible.

5. Provide assistance to general education teachers, parents, and students.

6. Advocate effective literacy practices and advance the knowledge base.

Insufficient opportunities for children during their first 5 years of life to be exposed to the printed word have become an important issue in speech-language pathology (Justice, 2006; Snow, 2006).

POSSIBLE CONTRIBUTIONS OF THE ENGLISH LANGUAGE TO READING DIFFICULTIES

The causes of children's literacy problems may be the same as those that cause speech and language delays and disorders, including heredity (Snowling, Gallagher, & Firth, 2003) (see Chapter 5). However, for children with speech and language delays and disorders, learning to read and write can be even more challenging, especially because of the numerous inconsistencies in pronunciation of words based on the context, inconsistencies in letter–sound correspondence, and even in shapes of letters (consider the number of type fonts a child has to become accustomed to).

Inconsistencies in Pronunciation of Words Based on the Context

Understanding of the intended meaning of a written statement can be affected by pronunciation of words depending on the context. For example, we can use two different pronunciations of the same word in a single sentence: "He couldn't read what she read" (i.e., *read* is pronounced "reed" and "red"). Likewise, the stress on words changes the meaning: "*Maybe* he *may be* willing to do it." and "It is *apparent* he is a *parent*." In the phrases "He is going to *be wilder*" and "He is going to *bewilder*," the change in the pronunciation of the vowel "i" in the last word significantly changes the meaning. Even adult readers sometimes have to reread a sentence to place the proper pronunciation and stress on some words in order to understand the intended meaning.

Inconsistencies in Letter–Sound Correspondence

English is challenging to read due to frequent inconsistencies of the letters in a word and the sounds that correspond to them. This lack of one-to-one letter-to-sound correspondence makes spelling even more difficult for children (and adults). Some classic examples are our use of *ph* to represent the sound *f* (e.g., *phone*) and the many silent consonants and vowels we use in printed words, such as *talk*, *write*, and *though*. Children's misspellings often reflect the spelling of words as they hear them. Irregularities of English spelling present another obstacle. There are 251 spellings for the 42 phonemes in English (Horn, 1926). There are, for example, 7 spellings for the sound /i/: *e, ie, ei, i, y, ea,* and *ee*. Likewise, the consonant /f/ has 4 spellings: *f, ff, gh,* and *ph*.

Inconsistencies in Shapes and Styles of Letters

Children learning to read usually start with large print that is *sans-serif* (in typography, letters that do not have *serifs*—terminal strokes at the top and bottom of main strokes. The large, plain letters of sans-serif are easier for young children to read. However, usually by second or third grade children are able to read both sans-serif and serif print. Most all casual reading (newspapers, magazines, novels) and formal reading (textbooks) are in serif; however, telephone text messages and computer e-mails are typically in sans-serif. Children must eventually be able to easily shift back and forth from sans-serif to serif while reading different material. Students and other writers have scores of *font* choices on their computers. Publishers of children's books and textbooks for all educational levels make critical choices as to what will be the primary font to use for a book and its *point size* (the size of the letters), as well as which fonts will be selected to highlight or emphasize certain information or illustrations.

COMMON PROBLEMS OF CHILDREN WITH LITERACY DISABILITIES

The International Dyslexia Association's definition of dyslexia provided earlier in this chapter highlights several general and specific areas commonly seen in children with reading disabilities. Any one area may have an interacting and compounding effect on the other areas.

Deficits in Phonological Processing

The IDA definition of dyslexia states that difficulties in word recognition and spelling are typically the result of a deficit in the phonological component of language. As discussed earlier, phonological processing deficits are considered the foundation of dyslexia (Culatta & Hall, 2006; Geffner, 2005; Goldsworthy, 2003). Research has shown that phonological processing deficits are inheritable; however, a common cause of phonological problems (auditory processing disorders) is middle ear infections (Musiek & Chermak, 2007; Olson & Bryne, 2005).

Leitao and Fletcher (2004) stated that phonological processing disorders may be detected before children are challenged to learn to read. This has some important educational and therapeutic implications for early identification of risk factors. That is, if children can be recognized and diagnosed with an auditory processing disorder and can receive appropriate intervention for the disorder, it may help prevent them from developing reading problems. This is a proactive approach rather than a reactive approach; the child receives help to prevent likely problems that would need help anyway (Kamhi & Catts, 2012).

Problems in Word Recognition and Spelling

Historically, the word *dyslexia* has been associated with visual processing deficits that resulted in disturbances such as letter reversals (e.g., *b–d* and *p–q*), letter confusion (e.g., *m–n, s–z,* and *O–Q*), sequencing errors (e.g., *was–saw*), and "misreading" (e.g., *house–horse* and *boy–toy*) that had been seen in children with reading problems. Children with reading problems have significant difficulty decoding printed words, which results in problems recognizing and figuring out new words and building good *sight vocabularies* (words that can be automatically recognized without needing to sound them out). With sufficient help, many children with dyslexia can improve their word-reading accuracy (particularly by developing *word-attack skills*); however, most do not become *fluent readers* (i.e., reading effortlessly).

Children with reading problems typically have difficulty with spelling, which may be a lifelong struggle. Problems with spelling may be the result of several interacting factors, such as phonological problems with sound–letter correspondence, inconsistencies in letter–sound correspondence, and the need to memorize the spelling of words with silent letters.

Underachievement Unrelated to Other Factors

Children with reading disabilities often do not achieve the academic levels that may be expected based on their general intellectual abilities.

However, the use of IQ is controversial when diagnosing or trying to relate intelligence to reading abilities. IQ tests do not directly measure potential for reading achievement; rather, they assess current cognitive abilities, some of which overlap with abilities important for reading. In addition, poor readers generally read fewer books and other materials than good readers and, therefore, acquire less of the knowledge measured by verbal IQ tests, resulting in lower IQs for the poor readers (Siegel, 1989).

Secondary Consequences

Children with reading disabilities face numerous secondary consequences. Secondary consequences include academic difficulties, possible influences on occupation and career choices (with resulting effects on future income), difficulty using reading as a leisure-time activity, and possible effects on interpersonal relationships (Justice, 2006; Stothard, Snowling, Bishop, Chipchase, & Kaplan, 1998).

Reading Comprehension and Academics

Children who have difficulty learning to read also have difficulty reading to learn; that is, reading comprehension and, likely, memory for what they have read may be seriously impaired because the information has not been coded well. As children progress through school, increasing amounts of learning come from independent reading. Thus, children with reading problems learn less, and what they do learn may be partly, largely, or totally in error. These children may argue that what they are saying is what they understood (or misunderstood) from their readings. They wonder why they receive poor grades on tests because they are certain they had written what their textbook said. Their reading and writing problems become more evident in each new grade as learning and grading increasingly depend on these skills.

Reading to learn, among other things, requires the ability to find the main ideas in a passage or story. Finding the main ideas is a complex task involving a child's knowledge of language and text conventions on many levels. A child who cannot determine the main ideas in material he reads has difficulty answering the questions, "What is this story about?" and "What are the important points?"

Reading disabilities affect all areas of academic learning. Consequently, these children have poor academic performance even though they may put out extreme effort to do well. Many of these children become disheartened and eventually develop an "I don't care" attitude as a self-defense for their failures. Their self-esteem and self-confidence deteriorates, and they may create problems in the classroom, interfering with other children's learning. Reading disabilities commonly determine how much children enjoy school and how far they go in school (Institute of Community Integration, 2000).

Application Question

Imagine that you had a reading disability. How would that have affected your education? Your choice of profession? Your life?

Writing Problems

Throughout children's educations, reading and writing are inextricably connected. First and second graders are asked to read aloud the short stories they write. However, by third grade and throughout the rest of their education, students read to find out what to write and write to demonstrate that they understood what they read.

Different types of writing call on different cognitive abilities, use different vocabulary, and employ different sentence forms. For example, writing a narrative story about a personal experience is quite different from writing a cogent argument about a point of view for a controversial topic, and both of these forms of writing are different from writing text material for a book. Children of all ages who have reading and writing problems write shorter compositions than do other children. This is a consistently good predictor of quality of writing; that is, shorter compositions usually do not have well-developed compound or complex sentence structure and often have missing components needed to make a good composition (see Figure 7–2). Overall, writing is a formidable mental process for individuals of all ages (Feifer & De Fina, 2000; Sun & Nippold, 2012). Compared to speaking, writing requires a higher level of abstraction, elaboration, conscious reflection, and self-regulation (we may speak without careful thought, but we seldom write without it).

Common writing problems seen in children (and adults) include inadequate or incorrect reference to the subject (i.e., the reader cannot easily determine who or what is being written about); inconsistent or inaccurate noun–pronoun agreement; inconsistent or inaccurate gender words; shifting inappropriately between first and third person; and inaccurate subject–verb agreement. Punctuation problems are common for individuals with writing disorders, particularly inconsistent or inaccurate use of periods and commas and lack of capitalization.

Figure 7–2

Writing complete sentences seems a nearly impossible task to some children.

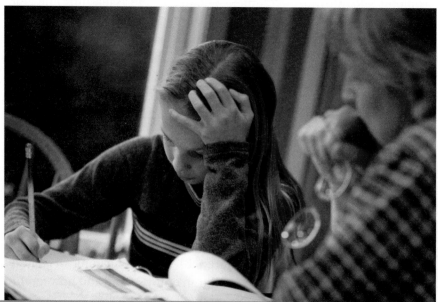

© Keith Brofsky/Photodisc/Getty Images

These problems result in sentences that are fragmented and unclear. In addition, spelling errors are abundant.

ASSESSMENT OF READING AND WRITING SKILLS

We need to keep in mind that not all children come from home environments that foster emergent literacy by having books and other reading material readily available, nor are there drawing and writing utensils easily available, such as crayons, markers, pencils and paper. Although SLPs may gently inquire about such things during parent interviews or even make an occasional home visit, other than encouraging parents to provide a literacy enriched environment, little can be done to change the home milieu.

Assessing Pre-reading and Reading Skills

Preschool children are referred to SLPs for evaluations of speech and language rather than for literacy problems. Therefore, before assessing reading and writing skills, SLPs should assess a child's receptive and expressive language skills. The initial investigation of a child's literacy skills may be more of a screening than an actual assessment, with more in-depth assessment carried out after the child is enrolled in therapy for language problems.

When children enter primary school and are screened for speech, language, and hearing problems, a clinician may detect possible literacy problems as well. These children should be referred to a *reading specialist* (a specially trained teacher who works with students experiencing reading difficulties) for a complete evaluation. However, because there is an important relationship between phonological awareness and reading, phonological awareness needs to be probed by the SLP (Hogan, Catts, & Little, 2005). At the emergent level, children as young as age 3 should be able to detect and produce rhyming words and recognize alliteration, which can be screened in the context of verbal play, nursery rhymes, songs, and books (Schuele, Skibbe, & Rao, 2007). At the kindergarten and early primary levels, children should be able to isolate a phoneme within a word (e.g., the first sound of *dog*); recognize the same sound in different words (e.g., *cat, car, can*); segment phonemes (e.g., *d-, o-, g-* for *dog*); delete sounds (e.g., saying the word *phone* without the /f/ sound); and substitute sounds (e.g., "Say '*can.*' Now say it again but change the /c/ to /m/.") (Hegde & Maul, 2006).

At the kindergarten and early primary levels, children can be assessed for their ability to name letters (*letter identification* or *alphabet knowledge*) (Schatschneider et al., 2002). *Sound–letter (alphabetic principle) association* also can be assessed; for example, asking what sound different letters make and asking children to "sound out" three-letter printed words and then to say the sounds fast and tell what the word is or means (e.g., *man* [*m-a-n*]). Some children become fluent readers although their comprehension of words, sentences, and paragraphs is weak. Comprehension of words, sentences, and short paragraphs can be assessed by having children read both aloud and silently, and then asking them to explain what they have read. Alternatively, clinicians can ask them specific questions about the material they read to see if they understood it.

Assessing Writing Skills

A clinician may ask children to print individual letters or the letters that correspond with certain sounds presented by the clinician. Children may be asked to write (print) short words. If they cannot do this independently, the clinician may ask them to copy letters and words, and if this is too difficult, clinicians can ask them to trace a letter outlined either with dots or dashes. It is important for children to be able to write basic identification information, such as their name, age, telephone number, address, and names of parents or primary caregivers. For more advanced writing skills, the SLP may assess children's legibility of individual letters and words, spelling, word usage, grammar, and punctuation. Content of sentences and paragraphs may be evaluated for cohesiveness, logical sequences, and ability to communicate information. When an SLP obtains information about children's reading and writing abilities, the information should be shared with the children's teachers and reading specialists.

INTERVENTION FOR READING AND WRITING PROBLEMS

Speech-language pathologists' academic training relating to early language and literacy development help prepare them to be an important member of the team that works with children who have reading and writing problems. Other members of the team include the child, classroom teacher, and parents, and, when available, a reading specialist and resource teacher. The ASHA National Outcomes Measurement (NOMS) (2009) data indicate that more than 70% of teachers who responded to a survey believed that students who received speech-language pathology services demonstrated improved pre-reading, reading, or reading comprehension skills. A majority of teachers also cited improvements in the students' listening, written language skills, and ability to communicate in socially appropriate ways (pragmatics). We need to keep in mind that most of our training is in the area of speech and language disorders rather than reading disorders; reading specialists (when available) are specifically trained to work with children who have literacy problems. Some SLPs, however, take additional course work and training in literacy assessment and treatment and provide direct services to children and consultation to other clinicians and teachers.

Teaching Reading Skills in the Context of Speech and Language Therapy

As discussed previously, because reading and writing are language-based activities and auditory processing is an important factor in developing reading skills, speech-language pathologists are appropriate professionals to help children develop their literacy skills. We can be part of the team that involves the child, parents, classroom teacher, and reading specialist. Because literacy is directly linked to speech and language, intervention provided for phonologic, morphologic, syntactic, and semantic aspects of language may improve literacy. Integrating reading and writing skills training can be accomplished within the context of traditional speech and language therapy, although oral communication skills should remain the priority for most speech-language pathologists (ASHA, 2001; Goldsworthy, 2003; Goldsworthy & Lambert, 2010; Hegde & Maul, 2006; Nelson, 2010).

SLPs can pair written material with pictured and modeled verbal stimuli at every level of therapy—from isolated speech sounds paired with printed letters to verbal stimuli of words, phrases, and sentences paired with those words in print. Specifically selected storybooks can be used in conjunction with both speech and language therapy. For older children, *guided reading* (having a child read aloud while providing direct feedback) can simultaneously work on articulation, syntax, semantics, and pragmatics (Hegde & Maul, 2006; National Reading Panel, 2000, 2001; Nelson, 2010). We need to encourage parents to be actively involved with their children's literacy opportunities such as reading to their children (*shared book reading*), patiently listening to their children read aloud, and reading their children's school writing assignments and providing appropriate feedback (Senechal & Cornell, 1993).

Teaching Writing Skills in the Context of Speech and Language Therapy

Young children learning how to write (print) can be asked to write the letter representing a speech sound they are working on. This may initially require helping guide their hands, tracing individual letters, or using "dot-to-dot" outlines. At the word level, children can be asked to write the words they are practicing saying. For older children, writing phrases and sentences can work on spelling, syntax, semantics, and pragmatics. This writing practice can reinforce their work on articulation and language. Consultation with teachers and parents is helpful to devise lists of words and syntactical structures that are important to classroom work and communication at home.

MULTICULTURAL CONSIDERATIONS

Children from culturally and linguistically diverse backgrounds have a greater likelihood than most other groups of children beginning school inadequately prepared to learn to read and to become successful readers (Culatta, Aslet, Fife, & Setzer, 2004; Justice, Chow, Capellini, Flanigan, & Colton, 2003; Thomas-Tate, Washington, & Edwards, 2004). In 2005, the National Assessment for Educational Progress (NAEP) reported that by fourth grade, 59% of African American children and 56% of Latino or Hispanic children read below basic levels, compared with 25% of majority-culture children. The 2005 NAEP report also stated that 54% of children living in poverty demonstrated reading proficiency below basic reading levels.

For preschoolers who are known to be at risk for language and literacy problems, it is essential to provide appropriate interventions so that they may enter kindergarten on par with other children (Rosin, 2006). This should include providing emergent literacy opportunities that respect and build on children's home culture while simultaneously preparing them to succeed in the majority culture.

Ample evidence supports early proactive interventions that focus intensively on promoting emergent literacy and language skills in minority cultures, as well as in children living in poverty. In addition, early intervention for children with language difficulties, rather than focusing exclusively on language acquisition, should include reciprocal and similarly intensive focus on emergent literacy development (Justice et al., 2002; Washington, 2006).

Several differences in narrative writing of children from culturally and linguistically diverse backgrounds are reported by Fiestas and Pena (2004), including story length, level of description, content, sequence and structure of the story, and prominent verb forms used (e.g., past tense versus present progressive). Support may be provided along a continuum for helping these children develop their narrative skills, from labeling pictures with a single word, to telling and retelling stories based on shared book reading, to personal accounts and language–experience activities in which a child's experiences are used as the foundation of the written narrative (e.g., a trip to the zoo), to development of imagined stories.

EMOTIONAL AND SOCIAL EFFECTS OF LITERACY DISORDERS

Although it is a real issue, little is written about the emotional and social effects of literacy disorders on children and adults. Most early elementary school children who are learning to read are aware of the ease or difficulty they are experiencing with this new skill. They fairly easily recognize what reading "group" they are in and take pride in being known as a good reader or feel embarrassment and sometimes rejection in being a poor reader. They soon realize the effects of their reading and writing difficulties when studying various subject matter and writing stories and answering questions on tests. They are confronted with their reading and writing problems on a daily basis at school and often at home. For these children, reading and writing difficulties are a daily frustration that can take a toll on their self-confidence, self-image, and self-esteem throughout their education and determine how much and how good of an education they receive. Their reading and writing impairments can affect the kinds of occupations and professions they pursue and even their social lives. (I am aware of one woman [a speech-language pathologist] who chose to end a relationship because the gentleman was a "non-reader.") The quality of life of people who have literacy problems can be significantly affected because they miss the enjoyment of reading recreational material and struggle with reading daily (Alexander-Passe, 2010).

CHAPTER SUMMARY

Reading disabilities are the most common learning disability in both children and adults. Reading disabilities are best characterized as developmental language disorders. Emergent literacy is the reading and writing behaviors of young children before they become readers and writers in the conventional sense. Adult involvement (scaffolding) during the emergent literacy and early literacy periods is essential for children to develop these skills in a timely manner. Speech-language pathologists need to take a proactive role in preventing reading difficulties among children with whom they work, as well as in the more general population of at-risk children for whom emergent literacy intervention may be the most powerful mechanism for improving the likelihood that they will become lifelong readers.

For many children, English is a challenging language to learn to read, especially because of the numerous inconsistencies in pronunciation of words based on the context, in letter–sound correspondence, and even in shapes of letters. There are numerous secondary consequences for children with reading disabilities, including academic difficulties, possible influences on occupation and career choices (with resulting effects on future income), difficulty using reading as a leisure-time activity, and possible effects on self-esteem and interpersonal relationships. An SLP can be an important member of the team to help children with literacy problems, including providing assessment and remediation.

Children from culturally and linguistically diverse backgrounds have a greater likelihood than most other groups of children of beginning school inadequately prepared to learn to read. For those preschoolers who are known to be at risk for language and literacy problems, it is essential to provide appropriate interventions so that they may enter kindergarten on par with other children.

STUDY QUESTIONS

Knowledge and Comprehension

1. Define *literacy disorder.*

2. What must be excluded for a child to be diagnosed as having a literacy disorder or dyslexia?

3. What is emergent literacy?

4. Explain *scaffolding*.

5. What are some secondary consequences of reading disabilities?

Application

1. What does ASHA say are the roles of speech-language pathologists in regard to working with children who have reading disabilities?

2. How could speech-language pathologists incorporate storybook reading into their work with children who have language disorders?

3. In what areas might scaffolding be used other than reading development?

4. Why is it important to encourage parents to read to their children?

5. What are two methods speech-language pathologists could use to integrate literacy skills while working on speech and language?

Analysis/Synthesis

1. Why are reading disabilities best characterized as developmental language disorders?

2. Discuss ways in which the English language may contribute to reading difficulties.

3. How can children's automatic recognition of many words and development of word-attack skills help them in their learning the content of written material?

4. How could reading problems set up children for academic problems and other problems throughout their lives?

5. Why would children with reading problems be likely to have problems with writing, particularly expository and narrative compositions?

REFERENCES

Alexander-Passe, N, (2010). *Dyslexia and depression: The hidden sorrow.* London South Bank University: London.

ASHA. (2001). *Roles and responsibilities of speech-language pathologists with respect to reading and writing for children and adolescents: Practice guidelines.* Rockville, MD: ASHA.

ASHA. (2009). *National Outcomes Measurement System Fact Sheet: Do SLP services have an impact on students' classroom performance? What teachers think.* Rockville, MD: ASHA.

Catts, H. W., Fey, M. E., Tomblin, J. B., & Zhang, X. (2002). A longitudinal investigation of reading outcomes in children with language impairments. *Journal of Speech, Language, and Hearing Research, 45*, 1142–1157.

Culatta, B., Aslet, R., Fife, M., & Setzer, L. A. (2004). Project SEEL: Part I. Systemic and engaging early literacy instruction. *Communication Disorders Quarterly, 25*, 79–88.

Culatta, B., & Hall, K. A. (2006). Phonological awareness instruction in early childhood settings. In L. M. Justice (Ed.). *Clinical approaches to emergent literacy intervention.* San Diego, CA: Plural Publishing.

Ehri, L., Nunes, S., Willows, D., Schuster, B., Uagoub-Zadeh, K., & Shanahan, T. (2001). Phonic awareness instruction helps children learn to read: Evidence from the National Reading Panel's meta-analysis. *Reading Quarterly, 36*(3), 250–287.

Feifer, S. G., & De Fina, P. A. (2000). *The neuropsychology of reading disorders: Diagnosis and intervention.* Washington, DC: National Association of School Psychologists.

Fiestas, C., & Pena, E. (2004). Narrative discourse in bilingual children: Language and task effects. *Language, Speech, and Hearing Services in Schools, 35*, 155–168.

Foy, J., & Mann, V. (2003). Home literacy environment and phonological awareness in preschool children: Differential effects for rhyme and phoneme awareness. *Applied Psycholinguistics, 24*, 59–88.

Geffner, D. (2005). What is the role of audition in literacy? *The ASHA Leader, 10*(13), 8–9, 33.

Gillon, G. (2004). *Phonological awareness: From research to practice.* New York, NY: Guilford Press.

Goldsworthy, C. (2003). *Developmental reading disabilities: A language-based treatment approach* (2nd ed.). Clifton Park, NY: Delmar Cengage Learning.

Goldsworthy, C., & Lambert, K. (2010). *Linking the strands of language and literacy: A resource manual.* San Diego, CA: Plural Publishing.

Hegde, M. N., & Maul, C. A. (2006). *Language disorders in children: An evidence-based approach to assessment and treatment.* Boston, MA: Allyn and Bacon.

Hesketh, A. (2004). Early literacy achievement of children with a history of speech problems. *International Journal of Language and Communication Disorders, 39*(4), 453–468.

Hogan, T. P., Catts, H. W., & Little, T. D. (2005). The relationship between phonological awareness and reading. *Language, Speech, and Hearing Services in Schools, 36*, 285–293.

Horn, E. (1926). *A basic writing vocabulary.* University of Iowa Monographs in Education, No. 4. Iowa City, IA: University of Iowa Press.

Institute of Community Integration. (2000). *Impact: Feature issue on postsecondary education supports for students with disabilities.* Minneapolis, MN: University of Minnesota Press.

Justice, L. M. (2006). *Clinical approaches to emergent literacy intervention*. San Diego, CA: Plural Publishing.

Justice, L. M., Chow, S., Capellini, C., Flanigan, K., & Colton, S. (2003). Emergent literacy intervention for vulnerable preschoolers: Relative effects of two approaches. *American Journal of Speech-Language Pathology, 12*, 320–332.

Justice, L. M., Invernizzi, M., & Meier, J. (2002). Designing and implementing an early literacy screening protocol: Suggestions for speech-language pathologists. *Language, Speech, and Hearing Services in Schools, 33*(2), 84–101.

Kamhi, A. G., & Catts, H. W. (2012). *Language and reading disabilities* (3rd ed.). San Antonio, TX: Pearson/Allyn & Bacon.

Leitao, S., & Fletcher, J. (2004). Literacy outcomes for students with speech impairments: Long-term follow-up. *International Journal of Language and Communication Disorders, 39*(2), 245–256.

Lieberman, P. (1973). On the evolution of language: A unified view. *Cognition, 2*, 59–94.

Lyon, G., Shaywitz, S., & Shaywitz, B. (2003). A definition of dyslexia. *Annals of Dyslexia, 53*, 1–14.

Manzo, U. C., Manzo, A. V., & Thomas, M. M. (2009). *Content area literacy: Strategic teaching for strategic learning* (5th ed.). New York, NY: Wiley.

Musiek, F. E., & Chermak, G. D. (2007). *Handbook of (central) auditory processing disorders: Vol. 1, Auditory neuroscience and diagnosis*. San Diego, CA: Plural Publishing.

National Assessment for Educational Progress. (2005). *The nations report card* [online]. Available at http://nces.ed.gov.nationsreportcard/reading/.

National Early Literacy Panel. (2004). *The National Early Literacy Panel: A research synthesis on early literacy development*. Paper presented at the National Association of Early Childhood Specialists Conference, Anaheim, CA.

National Reading Panel. (2000). *Teaching children to read: An evidence-based assessment of the scientific research literature on reading and its implications for reading instruction* (NIH Pub. No. 00–4769). Washington, DC: National Institutes of Child Health and Human Development.

National Reading Panel. (2001). *Put reading first: The research building blocks for teaching children to read*. Washington, DC: U.S. Department of Education.

Nelson, N. W. (2010). *Language and literacy disorders: Infancy through adolescence*. Boston, MA: Allyn and Bacon.

Olson, D., & Bryne, B. (2005). Heredity of word reading and phonological skills. In H. W. Catts, T. P. Hogan, & S. M. Adolf (Eds.). *Connections between language and reading disabilities*. Mahwah, NJ: Erlbaum.

Reed, V. A. (2010). *An introduction to children with language disorders* (4th ed.). Boston, MA: Pearson Allyn and Bacon.

Rosin, P. (2006). Literacy intervention in culturally and linguistically diverse worlds: The Linking Language and Literacy Project. In L. M. Justice (Ed.), *Clinical approaches to emergent literacy intervention*. San Diego, CA: Plural Publishing.

Schatschneider, C., Carlson, C. D., Francis, D. J., Floorman, R., & Fletcher, J. M. (2002). Relationship between rapid automatized naming and phonological awareness in early reading development: Implications for the double-deficit hypothesis. *Journal of Learning Disabilities, 35*(3), 245–257.

Schuele, C. M., Skibbe, L. E., & Rao, P. K. S. (2007). Assessing phonological awareness. In K. L. Pence (Ed.). *Assessment in emergent literacy*. San Diego, CA: Plural Publishing.

Senechal, M., & Cornell, E. H. (1993). Vocabulary acquisition through shared reading experiences. *Reading Research Quarterly, 28,* 360–375.

Siegel, L. S. (1989). IQ is irrelevant to the definition of learning disabilities. *Journal of Learning Disabilities, 22,* 469–478.

Snow, C. E., Scarborough, H. S., & Burns, M. S. (1999). What speech-language pathologists need to know about early reading. *Topics in Language Disorders, 20*(1), 48–58.

Snow, K. L. (2006). Measuring school readiness: Conceptual and practical considerations. *Early Education Development, 17,* 7–14.

Snowling, M. J., Gallagher, A., & Firth, U. (2003). Family risk of dyslexia is continuous: Individual differences in precursors of reading skills. *Child Development, 74,* 358–373.

Stevenson, J., Graham, P., Fredman, G., & McLoughlin, V. (1987). A twin study of genetic influences on reading and spelling ability and disability. *Journal of Child Psychology and Psychiatry, 28,* 229–247.

Stothard, S., Snowling, M., Bishop, D., Chipchase, B., & Kaplan, C. (1998). Language-impaired preschoolers: A follow-up into adolescence. *Journal of Speech, Language, and Hearing Research, 41,* 407–418.

Sun, L., & Nippold, M. A. (2012). *Narrative writing in children and adolescents: Examining the literate lexicon.* Language, Speech, and Hearing Services in Schools, *43,* 2–13.

Thomas-Tate, S., Washington, J., & Edwards, J. (2004). Standardized assessment of phonological awareness skills in low income African American first graders. *American Journal of Speech-Language Pathology, 13,* 182–190.

Washington, J. (2006). *Emergent literacy in high-risk communities: Research considerations.* Presentation at the Department of Communicative Disorders, University of Wisconsin-Madison, Madison, WI.

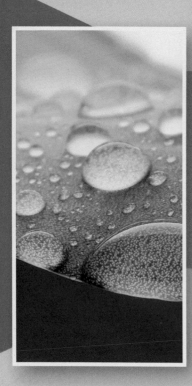

CHAPTER 8
Fluency Disorders

LEARNING OBJECTIVES

After studying this chapter, you will:

- Be able to define stuttering.
- Understand normal disfluency.
- Know some of the audible and visible overt behaviors of stutterers.
- Be familiar with general information about stuttering.
- Be familiar with the general theories of stuttering.
- Understand some multicultural considerations regarding stuttering.
- Be able to discuss the evaluation and treatment of children and adults who stutter.
- Appreciate the emotional and social effects of stuttering.

KEY TERMS

affect/affective

biofeedback

cluttering

cognitive behavioral therapy

congruent/congruence

external motivation

family systems therapy

fluency shaping (modification)

internal motivation

normal disfluency

secondary/overt/concomitant stuttering behaviors

stuttering (disfluency)

stuttering modification

CHAPTER OUTLINE

INTRODUCTION

Stuttering (disfluency) is probably the most common problem people think of when they think of a speech disorder. The problem has been discussed since the earliest days of recorded history with Chinese writings from 4000 B.C.E., Egyptian hieroglyphs from 3500 B.C.E., and early Biblical references (Bobrick, 1995). The earliest work in speech pathology focused on the causes and treatments of stuttering (Travis, 1931). Even then, theorists and therapists "projected their observations with a definiteness that suggests that they believe the problem to be solved" (West, 1942). The same may be said today.

Stuttering is perhaps the most researched of all speech disorders. In addition to SLPs, professionals such as psychologists, psychiatrists, pediatricians, neurologists, and others have investigated and written about this fascinating problem. It is no wonder there are so many views of what stuttering is, what causes it, what maintains it, and what can be done to help children and adults who do it.

---

stuttering (disfluency)

A disturbance in the normal flow and time patterning of speech characterized by one or more of the following: audible or silent blocks; sound, syllable, or word repetitions; sound prolongations; interjections; broken words; circumlocutions; or sounds and words produced with excessive tension.

Most speech-language pathologists refer to the disorder as either *stuttering* or *disfluency*—a disorder of fluency (note: most authors use the Latin prefix *dis* whereas some use the Greek prefix *dys*). The term *stammering* is now rarely used in the United States but is often used in Europe, Great Britain, and other countries. Even among those who have the disorder, there is disagreement about what to call people who stutter. Many people who stutter say "I am a stutterer," and others are adamant that they only be referred to as a "person who stutters" (i.e., a person-first reference—the person is not the disorder but is a person *with* a disorder). Some people want to say they are *disfluent* rather than say they stutter. For some clinicians and individuals who stutter, perhaps the word *stutter* sounds too harsh and has too many automatic negative connotations or mental images. Although ASHA emphasizes *person-first* when referring to individuals with any disorder, speech-language pathologists who stutter and are considered experts in the area of stuttering and author articles and texts on this disorder commonly use the term *stutterer* (Bloodstein & Berstein Ratner, 2008; Gregory, 2003; Conture, 2001; Guitar, 2006; Van Riper, 1982). This chapter follows the convention of well-known SLPs who are themselves stutterers and author texts on stuttering.

NORMAL DISFLUENCY

normal disfluency

The repeating, pausing, incomplete phrasing, revising, interjecting, and prolonging of sounds that are typical in the speech of young children.

All children and adults are disfluent to some degree. Essentially all verbally disfluent behaviors that clinicians attribute to individuals who stutter may be heard in normal-speaking children and adults but not necessarily with the same frequency or degree (Ward, 2006). As children are simultaneously developing speech, language, and fluency, their rates of development can be significantly different (Zebrowski & Kelly, 2002). **Normal disfluencies** include occasional repetitions of syllables or words once or twice, li-li-like this. Disfluencies also may include hesitations and the use of fillers such as "uh," "er," and "um." Such disfluencies occur most often between 1½ and 5 years of age and they tend to come and go. They are usually signs that a child is learning to use language in new ways. Sometimes disfluencies will disappear for several weeks and then return, which means the child may be going through another stage of learning (Gregory, 2003; Guitar, 2006; Manning, 2010). Children do not begin to stutter on their first attempts to speak. Children who go on to stutter do not seem to have difficulty with the earliest speech sounds such as cooing and babbling. Most children develop a considerable vocabulary and grammatical base before exhibiting abnormal disfluency (Ramig & Dodge, 2010; Yairi & Ambrose, 2005).

Some children and adults are remarkably fluent and articulate, and we may envy their communication abilities. Other children and adults may be particularly disfluent much of the time and have moderate to severe difficulty communicating with ease. However, a person can have significant disfluencies and still may not be considered a stutterer. The question for parents and SLPs is whether a child's disfluencies are normal or abnormal. It is not always easy to say.

DEFINING STUTTERING

One of the historical and ongoing problems of stuttering is how to define the disorder. Van Riper (1982, p. 15) provided a definition that continues to be appreciated by many clinicians: "Stuttering occurs when the forward flow of speech is interrupted by a motorically disrupted sound, syllable, or word, or by the speaker's reactions thereto." Guitar (2006) defines stuttering as an abnormal high frequency or duration of stoppages in the forward flow of speech affecting its continuity, rhythm, rate, and effortfulness. In 1977 the World Health Organization (WHO) provided a definition of stuttering that states stuttering includes "disorders in the rhythm of speech in which the individual knows precisely what he wishes to say, but at the time is unable to say it because of an involuntary repetitive prolongation or cessation of a sound" (p. 202). This definition uses the word "disorders" to imply that the symptoms of stuttering can take many forms and have more than one etiology (Manning, 2010).

Gregory (2003) says that stuttering is a problem related to the fluency of a person's speech or the way in which the sounds, syllables, and words of speech flow together in a forward-moving temporal sequence, and that a definition should consider both *overt behaviors* (audible and visible characteristics) and *covert reactions* (thoughts and feelings). The overt behaviors and covert reactions are essential elements to describing, understanding, and treating stuttering. We cannot change the cause of a child's stuttering, but we can work with the child who stutters and, when appropriate and possible, the parents or other caregivers important in a child's life.

Secondary/Overt/Concomitant Stuttering Behaviors

The **secondary, overt, or concomitant (accompanying) behaviors** of stuttering refer to the quantitative and qualitative audible and visible characteristics of the disorder. They are what most people think of when they think of stuttering. However, the difficulty is deciding what constitutes stuttering based on *which behaviors occur* (qualitative) and *how often these behaviors occur* (quantitative).

Audible Overt Behaviors

Audible refers to what is heard. Stutterers have "core behaviors" (Guitar, 2006; Van Riper, 1982) that are the basic speech behaviors of

secondary/overt/ concomitant stuttering behaviors

Extraneous sounds and facial and body movements a person who stutters uses during moments of stuttering; e.g., repetitions of "uh" or "um," eye blinks, and unusual head, hand, or other body part movements.

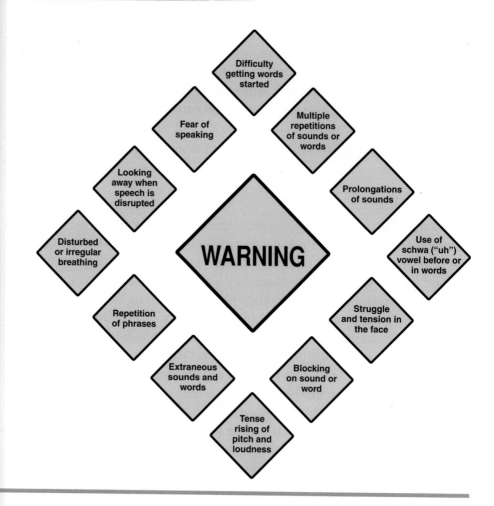

Figure 8–1

Warning signs of stuttering.

© Cengage Learning 2013.

stuttering: repetitions of sounds, prolongations of sounds, and "silent blocks." Repetitions of a sound, syllable, or single-syllable word are the core behaviors observed most frequently among children who are just beginning to stutter. Prolongations of voiced or voiceless sounds for as brief as a half second to a minute or more (with pauses for breaths) usually appear somewhat later in the speech of children who are beginning to stutter. Silent blocks are the inappropriate stopping of the flow of air or voice and often movements of the articulators that may last an instant to several minutes. (I once had a 19-year-old male client have a 10-minute silent block on the word "I.") Blocks may occur at each level of the speech production mechanism—respiratory, phonatory, or articulatory. Blocks are usually the last core behavior to appear in children as they are developing stuttering. As stuttering persists, blocks often become longer and more tense and tremors may be noticed in the lips or mandible (Guitar, 2006). (See Figure 8–1.)

The following audible overt behaviors indicate stuttering and are described by Bloodstein & Berstein Ratner, 2008; Conture, 2001; Gregory, 2003; Guitar, 2006; Manning, 2010; Ramig & Dodge, 2010; Reardon-Reeves & Yaruss, 2004; Ward, 2006; Zebrowski & Kelly, 2002. All of these audible overt behaviors may be repeated once, twice, or numerous times, and accompanied by visible signs of tension.

- *Part-word repetitions*—Sound or syllable repetitions that are involuntary and occur at the beginning of words (e.g., "M-m-m-mommy's home to make d-d-dinner!")
- *Whole-word repetitions*—Repetitions of an entire word (e.g., "Mommy-mommy-mommy's home to make dinner!")
- *Phrase repetitions*—Repetitions of units consisting of two or more words (e.g., "Mommy's home-mommy's home to make dinner.")
- *Interjections of sounds, syllables, words, and phrases*—Sounds or words that occur between words in a sentence that do not have a linguistic purpose in messages, such as "uh" (schwa [ə] vowel), "um," "well," and "you know" (e.g., "Mommy's-uh-uh-home to make-um-um-um-dinner! I'm well you know really hungry.")
- *Revisions of phrases and sentences*—A change in the content or the intended message, grammatical form, or pronunciation of a word (e.g., "Mommy's home to make lunch-dinner," "Mommy's home to have-make dinner," and "Mommy's home to take-make dinner!")
- *Prolongations of sounds and syllables*—Inappropriate lengthening of sounds and syllables, which may be accompanied by pitch change (often a tense rising pitch) (e.g., "Mmmmommy's home to mmmake dinner!")
- *Blocks*—Inappropriate timing in the initiation of a sound that is often accompanied by tension (a tense pause that may be just an instant to many seconds—or longer) (e.g., ". . . . . Mommy's home to make dinner!")
- *Dysrhythmic phonations*—Disturbances in the normal rhythm of speech that may include a variety of behaviors, such as a break between syllables ("Mom—my"), unusual timing (rapid "Mommy's home to" slow "make dinner!"), or any abnormal rhythm in speech that draws attention to how the person is speaking rather than what is being said.

Curlee (2007, p. 3) gives the following advice to parents to help them recognize whether their child is stuttering:

First, children who stutter often have problems getting words started, and many of these disruptions occur at the beginning of sentences. When they stutter, they tend to repeat parts of words, for example, sounds or syllables, rather than whole words or phrases. In addition, they frequently repeat portions of words two or more times before they are able to say what they want. Sometimes a child may exaggerate or prolong a sound in a word. The child may seem to be stuck with no sound or word coming out, perhaps working hard at speaking, or look away just as his speech is disrupted.

Visible Overt Behaviors

Stuttering is not just about verbal disfluencies; it is also about what the person is doing literally from head to toe that is associated with stuttering behaviors. Some people are verbally fluent by using countless extraneous and often subtle body movements. The overt or secondary stuttering behaviors are often the true handicap of stuttering because listeners (observers) are usually more distracted by what they see a stutterer doing than by what they hear the stutterer saying (Sheehan, 1970). Overt stuttering behaviors may include losing eye contact at the moment of stuttering, blinking the eyes rapidly, furrowing the forehead, tensing facial muscles, jerking the head, tensing or raising the shoulders, swinging an arm, jerking the arm or hand, clenching the fist, pressing the thumb and a finger together, tensing the chest muscles (which affects breathing), moving the upper or lower part of a leg, pulling the foot up toward the shin, tapping a foot, tensing the toes, and countless other almost imperceptible "tricks and crutches to be fluent" (Bloodstein & Berstein Ratner, 2008; Gregory, 2003; Guitar, 2006; Manning, 2010; Ramig & Dodge, 2010; Sheehan, 1970; Ward, 2006). As Williams (1979, 2004) pointed out, trying not to stutter usually involves some form of physical struggle or interference with talking.

Covert Reactions

Covert (i.e., emotional and cognitive) reactions to stuttering include feelings and thoughts such as frustration, anxiety, anger, guilt, hostility, shame, and expectations of difficulty talking, which leads to inhibitory and avoidance behaviors (Conture, 2001; Gregory, 2003; Guitar, 2006; Iverach, Menzies, O'Brian, Packman, & Onslow, 2011; Ramig & Dodge, 2010). Gregory (2003) said that as the overt behaviors of stuttering increase, the covert reactions grow stronger. Furthermore, increased negative emotions associated with speaking lead to more tension and stuttering, and more stuttering results in more negative emotions. However, it is difficult to know which comes first: the stuttering or the emotional effects of stuttering (see Figure 8–2). The covert reactions of individuals who stutter can be some of the most serious challenges they face while in therapy.

Figure 8–2

It is difficult to know which comes first: the stuttering or the emotional effects of stuttering.

© Cengage Learning 2013.

Which Comes First?

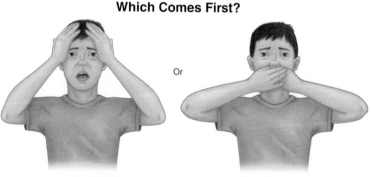

Or

Anxiety about Stuttering

Stuttering Causes Anxiety

GENERAL INFORMATION ABOUT STUTTERING

Much information about stuttering has been obtained over the decades. Areas of general concern include such things as the incidence of stuttering, the male–female ratio, family history of stuttering, physiological characteristics of stutterers, and psychological characteristics of stutterers.

- **Incidence:** The general incidence of stuttering is 1% in the population (Bloodstein & Berstein Ratner, 2008; Yairi & Ambrose, 2006).

- **Age of Onset:** Ninety percent of disfluent children begin to stutter between 2 to 6 years of age, and only 10% begin to stutter after 6 years of age (Ramig & Dodge, 2010).

- **Male–Female Ratio:** In cultures around the world, slightly more boys than girls begin to stutter, but girls are more likely to recover so that by school age and beyond, there are 3 or 4 males to every 1 female who stutter (Goldman, 1967; Yairi & Ambrose, 2005).

- **Family History of Stuttering:** Stuttering tends to run in families and stuttering appears to have a genetic basis in many individuals, although genes must interact with environmental factors for stuttering to appear (Buck, Lees, & Cook, 2002; Guitar, 2006; Yairi & Ambrose, 2005).

- **Stuttering and Other Speech and Language Disorders:** Many children who stutter have concurrent communication disorders, including articulation, phonology, and language disorders (Blood, Ridenour, Qualls, & Hammer, 2004; Ntourou, Conture, & Lipsey, 2011; Paden, 2005).

- **Physiological Characteristics:** Bloodstein & Berstein Ratner (2008) reviewed the literature on physiological characteristics of stutterers (e.g., respiration, cardiovascular, biochemical) and found that, in general, there are no significant differences between stutterers and nonstutterers other than just preceding and during the moment of stuttering (e.g., respiratory and pulse rates increase). That is, on average, stutterers are normal physiologically other than when they stutter. As these authors state, the "necessary and sufficient [physiological] conditions for stuttering" have not yet been found (p. 190).

- **Brain Function and Stuttering:** The general themes of the available research are that (1) the neural systems of individuals when stuttering can be distinguished from those when they are not stuttering; (2) areas known to be associated with motor speech and language production are found to show differences in levels of activity among individuals who stutter compared to individuals who do not stutter; (3) stuttering is not necessarily related to one structure or neural pathway; and (4) stuttering is particularly associated with hemispheric asymmetry, including increased activity in motor centers in the nondominant (typically the right) hemisphere (DeNil, 2004; Manning, 2010; Ward, 2006). However, whether the differences that have been observed represent the underlying problem that leads to stuttering or reflect the speakers' attempts to compensate for the deficit is unclear (Bloodstein & Berstein Ratner, 2008).

- **Cognitive and Personality Characteristics:** The general cognitive abilities of children who stutter are similar to those of their non-stuttering peers (Yairi & Ambrose, 2005). Sufficient research over the decades that has compared stutterers to nonstutterers has shown that people who stutter are generally adequately adjusted and that there are no specific character and personality traits of stutterers; that is, stuttering is not the symptom of a basic personality disorder (Bloodstein & Berstein Ratner, 2008).

Stutterers Are in Good Company

Many successful and famous people have stuttered at some time in their lives (De Keyser, 1973; Silverman, 2004; Tillis & Wager, 1984; see also www.stutteringhelp.org):

- *Actors and TV personalities*—Jane Seymour, Julia Roberts, Marilyn Monroe, Mike Rowe (*Dirty Jobs*), Anthony Quinn, Bruce Willis, Harvey Keitel, James Earl Jones (voice of Darth Vader), Nicholas Brendon, Jimmy Stewart, Peggy Lipton, Samuel L. Jackson, Emily Blunt, John Stossel (broadcast journalist)

- *Authors*—Aesop (*Aesop's Fables*), Andrew Lloyd Weber (playwright—*Phantom of the Opera, Cats*), Lewis Carroll (*Alice in Wonderland*), Jim Davis (cartoonist—*Garfield*), John Updike, Washington Irving, Somerset Maugham

- *Politicians*— President George Washington, President Thomas Jefferson, President Theodore Roosevelt, Joseph Biden (U.S. Vice President), Prince Albert of Monaco, King George VI of England (1895–1952 [film—"The King's Speech"]), Napoleon the 1st, Winston Churchill, Demosthenes (ancient Greek statesman)

- *Scientists*—Charles Darwin, Isaac Newton, Steven Hawking, Alan Rabinowitz

- *Singers*—Marc Anthony, Carly Simon, Mel Tillis, Nat King Cole, B. B. King

- *Sports figures*— Tiger Woods (world-champion golfer), Bill Walton (professional basketball player), Bo Jackson (football and baseball), Bob Love (basketball), Horace Grant (basketball), Johnny Damon (baseball), Ken Venturi (champion golfer), Herschel Walker (football Heisman Trophy winner), Sophie Gustafson (champion golfer), Kenyon Martin (basketball), Lester Hayes (football), Darren Sproles (football), Gordie Lane (hockey), Michael Spinks (heavyweight boxing champion), Ron Harper (basketball), Rubin "Hurricane" Carter (professional boxer), Ty Cobb (baseball)

- *Other prominent figures*—Alan Turning (founder of computer science), Annie Glenn (wife of U.S. Senator and astronaut John Glenn), Aristotle (ancient Greek orator), Arthur Blank (cofounder of Home Depot and owner of the NFL's Atlanta Falcons), Clara Barton (American founder of the Red Cross), Henry Luce (founder of *Time* magazine and *Sports Illustrated*), Jack Welch (former head of General Electric), John Scully (executive at Apple Computers), Moses (biblical Hebrew prophet)

THEORIES OF THE ETIOLOGY OF STUTTERING

Numerous theories of the etiology of stuttering and what occurs at the moment of disfluency have been proposed and there have been strong disagreements among authorities on the factors involved. The number of proposed etiologies by different authorities suggests that there is no certainty about the cause or the moment of stuttering, and no one theory fully explains these for all individuals.

Many factors, including characteristics of the child and characteristics of the environment, come into play when considering the etiology of stuttering. For example, characteristics of the child include genetic, gender, physiological, neurological, psychological, and linguistic. Characteristics of the environment include parental attitudes and behaviors such as expectations of the child's speech and other behaviors. Essentially all major theorists believe that environmental factors are important in the development and maintenance of stuttering (Bloodstein & Berstein Ratner, 2008; Conture, 2001; Gregory, 2003; Guitar, 2006).

Theories of the etiology and moment of stuttering are divided into *breakdown theories*, *repressed need theories*, and *anticipatory struggle behavior theories* (Bloodstein & Berstein Ratner, 2008; Silverman, 2004). Within each theory, more specific hypotheses help explain the cause of stuttering and, ideally, lead to some direction for its treatment. However, rather than focusing on possible individual etiologies of stuttering, it may be more productive to consider stuttering as having *multifactorial* causes for many children; that is, two or more potential causes may need to come into play for any one child to develop stuttering.

The *breakdown theories* of the onset of stuttering attribute the disorder to the effects of early environmental stress and usually assign an important role to neurological predisposition factors. Increasing evidence supports the theory of a neurological predisposition to stutter (Biermann-Ruben, Salmelin, & Schnitzler, 2005; DeNil, 2004; Ingham, 2001). That is, if a child had a stressful environment but did not have the predisposition to stutter, he would not likely stutter; likewise, if he had a predisposition to stutter but did not have a stressful environment, he would not likely stutter (Ramig & Dodge, 2010). (See Figure 8–3.)

Repressed need theories of the etiology of stuttering tend to merge with theories of the etiology of neurotic behavior. That is, a stutterer has an emotional need that has not been met, and the stuttering behaviors are a symbolic expression or symptom of that repressed need (Bloodstein & Berstein Ratner, 2008).

Anticipatory struggle behavior theories attribute stuttering to parental penalties for normal disfluency or to pressures extending to other speech failures. That is, stuttering is a learned behavior somehow precipitated by the child anticipating and fearing it, and the struggle is to avoid it, with the struggle itself becoming the stuttering (Silverman, 2004).

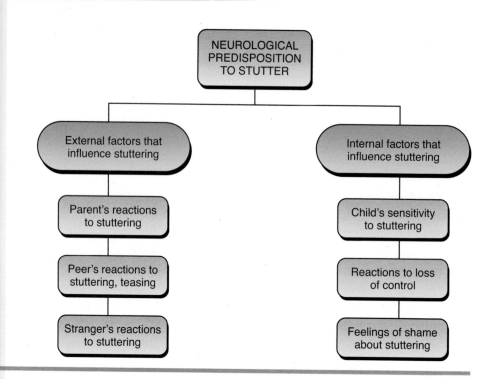

Figure 8-3

External and internal factors that influence a child's neurological predisposition to stutter.

Source: Ramig & Dodge, 2010/
© Cengage Learning 2013.

Guitar (2006) integrates these theories with a two-stage model. The first stage is primary stuttering, which involves repetitions and prolongations that are frequently the first signs of stuttering. These signs are thought to be the result of constitutional factors: a "dyssynchrony" at some level of the speech and language production process. The second stage is secondary stuttering, which involves the tension, struggle, escape, and avoidance behaviors that are often present in persistent stuttering. These behaviors may be the result of a separate constitutional factor: a reactive temperament that triggers a defense response that makes the individual more emotionally conditioned than the average speaker (see Figure 8–4).

Conditions That Increase Stuttering

Two of the most challenging words for stutterers to say are their own name and the word *I*. Many (most) stutterers will avoid saying their name at all costs, including simply not identifying themselves. Having to take a turn reading aloud to a class or having to wait to speak (particularly having to wait to introduce himself when in a group) creates increased anxiety and pressure for stutterers, which increases their likelihood of stuttering. Speaking to authority figures (the disciplinary parent, the bully in the classroom, or a teacher, principal, supervisor, or boss) is particularly difficult for stutterers. Speaking on the telephone can be terrifying to many stutterers, and they will sometimes try to convince other

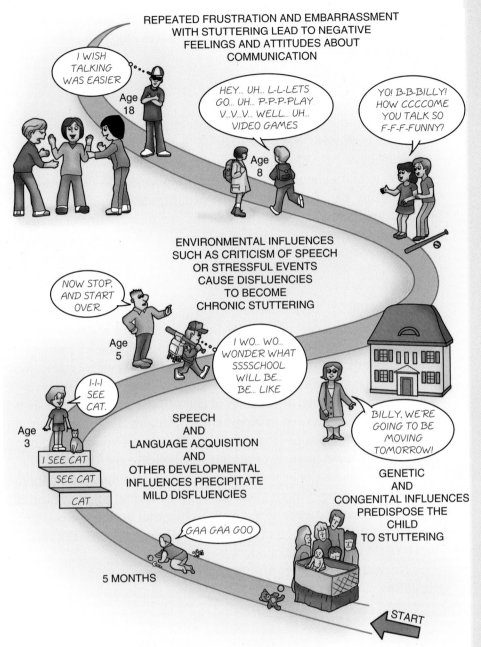

Figure 8-4

A developmental pathway
to stuttering.

Source: Figure 1–1, p. 6 In Guitar, B. (2006).
*Stuttering: An integrated approach to its nature
and treatment.* Baltimore, MD: Lippincott Williams
& Wilkins. Copyright © 2006 by Lippincott Williams
& Wilkins. Adapted with permission. http://lww.com.

people to make calls for them to avoid confronting one of their worst
fears (Gregory, 2003; Ramig & Dodge, 2010).

CLUTTERING

Cluttering is a speech and language disorder that shares some of the
characteristics of stuttering but differs in many important ways (Ward,
2006). Although stuttering has been well researched, cluttering has
not. Like stuttering, however, cluttering is difficult to define because of

cluttering

A fluency disorder characterized
by a speech rate that is
abnormally fast or irregular that
may be affected by (1) failure
to maintain normally expected
sound, syllable, phrase and pause
patterns, and (2) evidence of
greater than expected incidences
of disfluency, the majority of
which are unlike those typical
of people who stutter.

differences in opinions as to which behaviors are associated with the disorder. St. Louis, Raphael, Myers, and Bakker (2003) describe cluttering as follows:

> A syndrome characterized by a speech delivery which is either abnormally fast, irregular, or both. In cluttered speech the person's speech is affected by one or more of the following: (1) failure to maintain normally expected sound, syllable, phrase and pausing patterns, and (2) evidence of greater than expected incidents of disfluency, the majority of which are unlike those typical of people who stutter.

Daly (1992, p. 107), however, emphasizes the language difficulties of clutterers when he describes cluttering as a "disorder of speech and language processing resulting in rapid, dysrhythmic, sporadic, unorganized and frequently unintelligible speech. Accelerated speech is not always present, but an impairment in formulating language almost always is."

As with stuttering, the etiology of cluttering is uncertain. The speech of clutterers is considered to be primarily disorganized (motorically, linguistically, or both) rather than disfluent. Daly and Cantrelle (2006) presented 10 common features of cluttering, which are shown in Figure 8–5.

Cluttering results in reduced speech intelligibility and incoherent sentences because of incomplete phrases, abnormal prosody, and disorganized discourse. Listeners are left feeling that the person had something to say, but the person said it so fast and in such a confusing manner that it could not be understood.

Note: The emphasis of this chapter is on stuttering rather than cluttering.

Figure 8–5

Ten common features of cluttering.

Adapted from Daly & Cantrelle, 2006.

1. Telescoping or condensing of words (e.g., omission of sounds)
2. Lack of effective self-monitoring of speech
3. Lack of pauses
4. Lack of awareness of speech difficulties
5. Imprecise consonants (e.g., distortion of sounds)
6. Irregular rate of speech; speaking in spurts (staccato-like speech)
7. Use of numerous interjections, revisions, and filler words
8. Compulsive talking, verbosity, and circumlocutions (i.e., talking around words rather than using a specific word)
9. Disorganized language with confused wording
10. Apparent verbalization before adequate thought formulation

WORKING WITH CHILDREN WHO STUTTER

Before clinicians can provide intervention (therapy) for a child who stutters, they need to interview the parents and evaluate the child's general speech and language development. In a way, the initial parent interview, which always involves answering their questions about stuttering and their child's speech, is the beginning of therapy. A clinician's first meeting with the parents and child often establishes the future working relationship with the family. Throughout the working relationship with a family, the **family systems therapy, family-centered service delivery**, and **cognitive behavioral therapy** models are helpful (Gregory, 2003; Guitar, 2006; Maul, 2011; Yu & Kashinath, 2011; Zebrowski, 2002). Family systems therapy emphasizes collaboration with all family members who have significant involvement with the child. The child is the person who is brought into therapy but other family members are essential in the overall treatment of the child's fluency problem. Cognitive behavioral therapy emphasizes that there are numerous perspectives or interpretations of any given event or behavior. Furthermore, the way in which people think about events and behaviors (their perceptions) determine how they feel about themselves, others, and the future. The essential purpose of cognitive therapy is to help individuals recognize and examine tightly held but problematic beliefs and replace them with more adaptive and flexible ways of thinking (Flasher & Fogle, 2012).

Evaluation of a Child

Depending on the environment in which a clinician works, the setting for an evaluation may differ significantly. In a university clinic, the evaluation usually takes place in a relatively small, often somewhat "sterile" clinic room with the child and at least one parent present. In the schools, the speech therapy room is used and the clinician and child are likely surrounded by many colorful posters and therapy materials, although a parent is not likely present to give information and be asked questions. In hospital settings, one or both parents usually bring the child and the evaluation may be done in an office environment or therapy room. In private practice, the evaluation may be done in an office setting, a therapy room, or the family home (with all of the variables you can imagine) with one or both parents present. In all settings, excellent interviewing and counseling skills are essential when questioning and talking to parents and children about such sensitive issues as a child's fluency. Some parents and children become emotional and clinicians need to know how to handle such emotions professionally and gracefully (Flasher & Fogle, 2012).

During the evaluation of a child, the clinician will observe the types and frequency of his disfluencies under different conditions, such as interacting with his parents and interacting with the clinician during play, conversation, direct questioning, reading (if he is a reader), and

family systems therapy/ family-centered service delivery

Models of counseling and service delivery that focus on variables regarding the family unit as a whole; i.e., each family member is part of a system (the family), each member affects the others, and the system is interdependent; that is, within the system there are sub-systems: e.g., mother–father, mother–son, father–son, grandparent–grandchild.

cognitive behavioral therapy

A model of counseling designed to help individuals recognize and examine problematic beliefs and replace them with more adaptive and flexible ways of thinking.

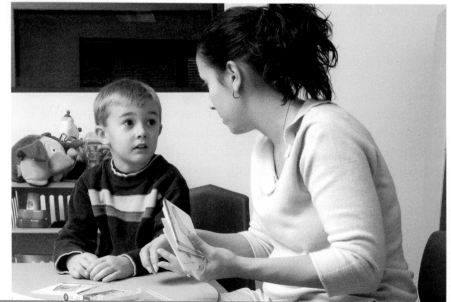

Figure 8-6

A clinician evaluating a preschool child who stutters. (Notice that the child is sitting to the side of the clinician rather than across the table so there is not a physical or psychological barrier between them.)

© Cengage Learning 2013

even talking on a telephone. Audio- or video-recording is important for a later analysis. Requesting the parents to bring an audio- or video-recording of the child talking in various situations at home is very helpful in getting a more true-to-life example of the child's speech.

Beyond the interview and fluency evaluation, the clinician will want to evaluate the speech systems (respiratory, phonatory, resonatory, and articulatory) and may choose to administer standardized articulation and language assessments. Upon completion of the evaluation of the child, the clinician should be able to diagnose whether stuttering is occurring and its severity level. Impressions also need to be made about the child's covert reactions to his stuttering, such as frustration, anger, shame, and inhibitory and avoidance behaviors (see Figure 8–6).

Analysis of the child's disfluencies may include the *percent disfluency rate* (e.g., 54 disfluent words divided by 318 words in a speech sample, equals 17% disfluency rate). The actual percent disfluency may not be as clinically significant as what the child is doing at the moment of disfluency; that is, what he tries to do to prevent being disfluent (e.g., avoiding talking or long pauses); what he does during the disfluency (e.g., rapid repetitions or prolongations of a sound, blinking his eyes and looking away); and what he does to end the disfluency (e.g., jerks his head and finishes the word in a high-pitched, tense voice). The clinician should take notes on all of the "core stuttering" and verbal and secondary stuttering behaviors that she observes to include in her analysis and evaluation report.

The first major decision the clinician needs to make is whether the child's speech has normal disfluencies. Guitar (2006) uses the following criteria for determining normal disfluencies: (a) the child has fewer than 10 disfluencies per 100 words; (b) the disfluencies consist mostly of multisyllabic word and phrase repetitions, revisions, and interjections;

(c) when disfluencies are repetitions, they have two or less repeated units per repetition that are slow and regular in tempo; (d) the ratio of stuttering-like disfluencies to total disfluencies is less than 50%; (e) all disfluencies will be relatively relaxed and the child will seem to be hardly aware of them and is not upset when he is aware.

Severity Levels

When a child is diagnosed as having abnormal disfluencies (i.e., stuttering), it is important to determine the severity level to help guide the direction of therapy. Guitar (2006) says children may be considered to have *borderline stuttering* if they have more than 10 disfluencies per 100 words, but the disfluencies are loose and relaxed. The disfluencies may be part-word repetitions, single-syllable word repetitions, prolongations, and/or repetitions with two repeated units (sounds, syllables, words, or phrases) per instance.

Key features of *beginning stuttering* include rapid, abrupt repetitions; pitch rises during repetitions and prolongations; difficulty with airflow or phonation; and tension while talking. Beginning stutterers appear to be aware of their difficulty talking and may be frustrated by it. They may use escape behaviors such as head nods or eye blinks to try to end stuttering blocks. They may begin avoiding words by substituting more easily spoken words for words they have difficulty with (e.g., using "me" for "I").

Children at the *intermediate stuttering* level have most of the characteristics of children who are at the beginning level, but repetitions and prolongations of sounds and syllables are more common. In addition, they may use a variety of starters (e.g., "uh uh uh," "um um," "You know") to begin sentences and look away (lose eye contact) or appear embarrassed about their difficulty talking. They may have "silent blocks." They appear to anticipate stuttering and use *avoidance behaviors*, that is, extraneous behaviors such as eye blinking before saying *feared words* (words they expect to stutter on). Children may use *escape behaviors* to terminate blocks, such as head jerking or forcing the word out using excessive tension, as though the word explodes from the mouth. They anticipate feared people (people with whom they expect to do considerable stuttering), places (e.g., talking in front of the class), and situations (e.g., having to answer questions or large family gatherings).

Advanced stuttering includes longer and more tense blocks, often with tremors of the lips, tongue, or jaw. Numerous repetitions and prolongations of sounds and syllables occur. Complex patterns of avoidance and escape behaviors may be so well habituated that stutterers are unaware they are doing them. Stuttering behaviors may be suppressed in some individuals through extensive avoidance behaviors, making them appear more fluent than they really are. Emotions, fears, embarrassment, and shame are very strong in advanced stuttering. Stutterers usually have negative feelings about themselves as competent speakers and these feelings may be pervasive in their self-concept.

Personal Story — Jonathan

I received a call from a mother who sounded intense and somewhat desperate. She had been referred to me by the mother of another child who stuttered whom I had worked with the previous year. The mother explained that Jonathan was 4 years old, a sweet and bright little boy who was stuttering. The father was a fairly new police officer and the mother was a librarian with a degree in English. I scheduled an appointment to see the family in their home.

When first meeting the parents, I had the impression of meeting Ken and Barbie in person. Both parents looked perfect in every way, with manners that seemed to have come from a manual on etiquette. The house was neat and clean (spotless), and there was a nicely circumscribed area in the family room for Jonathan's play area. Jonathan was polite and well mannered. He shook my hand as though he had been well trained. After visiting with the parents for a few minutes, the parents asked Jonathan to show me his room. A nice room it was; neat and orderly. When Jonathan finished playing with one toy, he put it back in its place and took out another. Jonathan was definitely exhibiting some signs of disfluency.

Over the next 2½ months, I met with the family once or twice a week in the family home. Both parents were always present and if one could not make the scheduled appointment, they rescheduled. I worked with Jonathan for a while in his room during each visit, with the parents just outside the door to listen. The parents and I then sat around the formal dining room table to discuss stuttering in general, their child's stuttering in particular, and specific things the parents could do during the week that could help Jonathan's speech. Never had parental perfectionism been so helpful. They did every assignment perfectly and began to see that the little changes they needed to make in their daily family lives could have big benefits for Jonathan. The parents began to accept Jonathan's occasional disfluencies and not react to them; his imperfect, but normal for his age, articulation of sounds and words; and his normal 4-year-old playfulness and other behaviors of a child his age. The parents eventually became less perfect (i.e., "lightened up"), and Jonathan's speech became more fluent. This story helps illustrate the importance of working with the parents of children who stutter. ■

Treatment of Children Who Stutter

When a child is at risk for stuttering but is not yet stuttering, a speech-language pathologist can focus on prevention strategies, rather than providing direct therapy. ASHA (1988) published a position statement on applying prevention strategies, stating that speech-language pathologists should play a significant role in the development and application of prevention strategies in all areas of communication disorders. Hill (2003) describes primary prevention strategies for children at risk for stuttering.

Primary prevention refers to SLPs being involved in eliminating or inhibiting the onset and development of stuttering by changing the susceptibility of children or modifying exposure conditions that may lead to the development of the disorder (ASHA, 1988; Nelson, 1999). The goal of primary prevention is educating parents so they can support the development of communication skills in their children by understanding normal speech, language, and fluency development; providing appropriate language stimulation; identifying signs of speech, language, and fluency concerns; and seeking advice from knowledgeable resources—such as speech-language pathologists. Of particular help to parents of children at risk for stuttering are publications from the Stuttering Foundation of America (www.stutteringhelp.org [Spanish: www.tartamudez.org]), especially *Stuttering and Your Child: Questions and Answers* (2002a), *Stuttering and the Preschool Child: Help for Families* (2002b), *Stuttering: Straight Talk for Teachers* (2002c), and *Fundación Americana de la Tartanudez* (2002d) (information in Spanish).

Although parents may not be the cause of the stuttering problem, they can be an important part of the solution. Some helpful points for parents include (Stuttering Foundation of America, 2002a–c):

- Speak with your child in an unhurried manner, pausing frequently. Wait a few seconds after your child finishes speaking before you begin to speak so that the child does not feel the conversation is being rushed.
- Refrain from making remarks such as "Slow down," "Take a breath," "Relax," or "Think before you talk." Such advice can feel demeaning to a child and it is not helpful.
- Refrain from finishing his sentences or filling in words when your child is having trouble talking.
- Maintain natural eye contact and try not to look embarrassed when he is disfluent. Just wait patiently and naturally until your child is finished.
- Let your child know by your manner and actions that you are listening to *what* he is saying, not *how* he is saying it.
- Reduce the number of questions you ask your child. Instead of asking questions, simply comment on what your child has said.
- Set aside a few minutes at a regular time each day when you can give your undivided attention to your child.
- Help all members of the family learn to take turns talking and listening.
- Accept your child and find ways to show your child that you love and value him and that you enjoy your time together.

Ramig and Dodge (2010) have several major emphases in their stuttering program for children and adolescents, including (a) counseling and helping parents learn about stuttering; (b) assessment of the

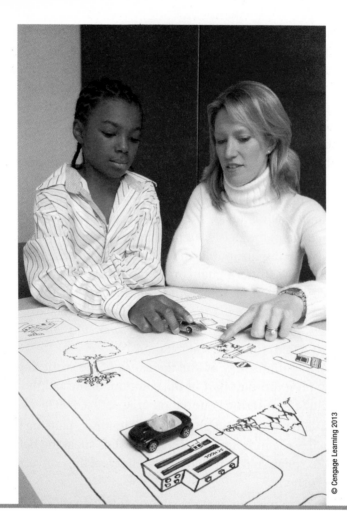

Figure 8–7

A speech-language pathologist playing "On the Road" with a child who stutters.

© Cengage Learning 2013

child's disfluencies; (c) working with teachers so they will understand stuttering and how to be supportive of a child who stutters; (d) direct therapy approaches with children, such as fluency shaping and stuttering modification; and (e) transference and maintenance. Ramig and Dodge emphasize a cooperative model of stuttering treatment that includes the child, the parents or caregivers, and the speech-language pathologist.

Zebrowski and Kelly (2002, pp. 75–76) provide a creative way of helping children identify and then learn to change their stuttering behaviors. The authors call it "On the Road" (illustrated in Figure 8–7). The clinician draws or sets up objects to form a roadway that has smooth stretches and various obstacles, including railroad tracks, a mud slick or oil spill, a drawbridge, and a closed roadway with a detour. For every obstacle, there should be an alternative path or way to move through the obstacle. The child and clinician use their vehicles to go "on the road." Each obstacle represents a type of disfluency; for example, bumpy speech for railroad tracks, mud slick or oil spill for sound prolongations, drawbridge for broken words, and closed roadway for silent "blocks." Using the child's own terms for the various types of disfluencies, the clinician shows the child how to take the smooth detour around or through all obstacles by using easy speech techniques.

Therapy for children who stutter requires a sound base of knowledge and understanding of the problem based on the best available literature, insight into both children and adults (parents), and creativity. To become confident and successful when working with children who stutter, you will need to take a genuine interest in the problem and seek every opportunity to expand your education and training in this complex area. The rewards for the children and families you help, and for you, can be enormous.

Direct Therapy

Stuttering therapy is a dynamic process, meaning that the goals and procedures used are determined by the child's behaviors and needs and the specific goals are likely to change during the process. A clinician typically fine-tunes the overall therapy plan as she becomes familiar with the child's abilities, attitudes, and concerns during the early stages of treatment. The work with the parents is likewise fine-tuned as trust is developed and the parents further understand stuttering in general and their child's in particular (Zebrowski & Kelly, 2002).

The relationship we develop with the child is important in our ability to help him. We work to develop an open child–clinician relationship as an important component for building trust, confidence, and understanding (Ramig & Dodge, 2010; Reardon-Reeves & Yaruss, 2004). Our general approach is to be understanding and accepting so that the child views us as someone who is genuinely interested in him and accepting of whatever he says and however he says it. By having a good child–clinician relationship, our social reinforcement will be more important to the child. It is important for the therapist to model for the parents what will be helpful to the child's speech. Our calm, warm, and accepting manner along with our relaxed, easygoing way of talking with the child may be quite different from how the parents normally interact and communicate with their child.

Building the child's self-confidence is important throughout therapy (Chmela & Reardon, 2005). Providing the child with successful speaking activities and opportunities, such as single-word and phrase-level tasks, can be helpful. Therapy activities may be built around child-level conversations and games. Games are not therapy; rather, therapy lies in the speech and communication that occurs while games are being played. Blocks, memory-matching card games (e.g., Go Fish), toy trains, and action figures can be used in creative ways. The goal of a game is not to see who wins but for the clinician to model easy speech and for the child to have numerous opportunities for successful, easy, and relaxed speech attempts.

Some clinicians choose to use published fluency therapy packages. Some of these programs provide speech modification games, drill activities, role-playing scenarios, and counseling activities that can

Personal Story Shot in the Heart

Jared was 7 years old when he was referred to me by a public school speech therapist. Jared was a severe stutterer and had been in therapy for more than a year with only minimal progress. The therapist was going to continue, but then something drastic happened. On a Saturday morning, Jared was playing in the front yard of his house when a teenager who lived across the street fired a BB gun through his screen door and hit Jared. The BB went through Jared's T-shirt, passed through his skin and chest muscles between two ribs, and entered his heart. Jared did not fall but quickly grabbed his chest. His mother saw that something was wrong and ran to him. She saw the hole in his T-shirt and some blood. She immediately called 911, and within minutes the fire department ambulance was at the home.

Jared was rushed to the hospital. In the emergency room, the doctor tried to extract the BB from Jared's heart, but he could not find it. From Jared's chest X-rays, the doctor discovered the BB lodged in his right shoulder. Apparently, the BB had entered Jared's heart directly into the left ventricle and was pumped out through the aorta and then traveled to the right subclavian artery that carried it to his right shoulder, where it lodged in a smaller artery. The doctor removed the BB from Jared's shoulder and "patched him up."

After the shooting incident, Jared was seen by a psychologist who was helpful with him "working through" the incident. However, after Jared returned to school, his speech therapist thought he needed a different approach to help his stuttering, as well as someone who could work with the parents. Working with the parents was essential, and I spent many hours in Jared's home talking with them about stuttering in general and Jared's stuttering in particular. Because Jared was aware of his stuttering and motivated to work on it, a direct approach was used. Although Jared made significant improvements in his fluency, he continues even now to have some difficulty with stuttering. It is important for clinicians to appreciate that even when we provide our best therapy, not all outcomes are what we or the clients and their families hope for. ■

be adapted to or integrated with other approaches. General therapy approaches have been used with preschool and school-age children who stutter to teach a slow, smooth, relaxed pattern of speech through clinician and parent modeling. The usual practice is to progress systematically from one- or two-word utterances to longer and more complex sentences (Conture, 2001; Gregory, 2003; Guitar, 2006; Ramig & Dodge, 2010; Reardon-Reeves & Yaruss, 2004).

Fluency Shaping (Modification)

With both children and adults, **fluency shaping (modification)** therapy attempts to directly train stutterers to speak with relaxed respiration, relaxed vocal folds, and relaxed articulation muscles. The goal is to teach stutterers how to talk fluently. Fluency shaping therapy tends to be highly structured behavior modification that works directly on the physical aspects of speech and fluency, that is, respiratory, phonatory, and articulatory movements. Fluency controlling techniques are used through a series of exercises that are usually implemented within a slow-speech framework, which fundamentally changes the way that respiration, phonation, and articulation are coordinated for speech (Ward, 2006). Essentially, the stutterer is taught to do the opposite of what he does when he stutters. That is, rather than speaking with (a) tense, shallow intake of breaths, he learns to take relaxed full breaths; (b) tense and tight vocal mechanism, he learns to relax the vocal folds and laryngeal muscles; (c) tense articulatory system, he learns to relax the articulators; and (d) rapid and tense rate of speech, he learns to speak with a slower and more relaxed rate.

Fluency shaping uses various direct modifications of the speech act. The speech act starts with an intake of air followed by controlled exhalation, and a smooth continuous airflow is needed to produce fluent speech. The clinician teaches the child to have a *smooth airflow* by using diaphragmatic breathing to help him learn to fill his lungs so that he does not run out of breath while talking. This can be demonstrated by placing the hand on the upper abdomen and feeling the abdomen rise during inhalation and lower during exhalation. The child also learns to exhale a small amount of air a second or two before he starts to speak, which initiates a smooth exhalation that helps produce smooth phonation.

A *soft glottal onset* or *gentle initiation of sound* builds on the smooth airflow technique. The soft glottal onset helps decrease tension of the vocal folds and other muscles of the larynx. The soft glottal onset is used primarily with vowels and glides (semivowels) as an attempt to make the smooth airflow technique carry over into a gentle initiation of vocal fold vibration so that the sound emerges rather than being abruptly produced. Initially this may sound as though an /h/ has been placed before the initial vowel of a word, for example, *am* may sound like *hhaam*; however, with further development of the technique the /h/ is less noticeable and the person acquires a steady yet inaudible airflow while speaking.

Soft consonant contacts are taught to reduce the force of the contact between articulators and reduce tension in the articulatory system. The initial consonants of words are produced by bringing the two articulators lightly together. Clients can practice by attempting a soft contact consonant and contrasting that with the production of a hard contact, for example, on the word *big*. However, the client must simultaneously use a smooth air flow and soft glottal onset so that all three systems are working smoothly and effortlessly. The fluency shaping approach tends

fluency shaping (modification)

A therapy approach for children and adult stutterers that attempts to directly train individuals to speak with relaxed respiration, relaxed vocal folds, and relaxed articulation muscles; the approach attempts to teach stutterers how to talk fluently.

to slow the stutterer's speech rate, although the clinician also may work with the stutterer to intentionally slow his speech rate by prolonging syllables in words. Later, as the stutterer increases and habituates his fluency a more natural speech rate may be used.

Stuttering Modification

The **stuttering modification** therapy approach was first developed by Charles Van Riper in his early writings (Van Riper, 1939; 1971) and has continued to be the foundation of many fluency experts since that time (Gregory, 2003; Ramig, 1997; Sheehan, 1970; Williams, 2004). A primary premise of this approach is the stutterer recognizing and confronting his fears, avoidances, and struggles to escape his stuttering, and, therefore, a primary focus of therapy is the reduction and management of his fears, avoidances, and struggle behaviors. The acronym "MIDVAS" (Van Riper, 1971, 1982) outlines the principle components of stuttering modification therapy:

- *Motivation* of the stutterer is the most important underlying factor throughout the therapy process, and the stutterer must be an active participant in the therapy. The stutterer is changed by what he does, not by what he thinks about.

- *Identification* of the stuttering behaviors, both verbal and secondary, is essential before they can be changed or eliminated. The stutterer needs to identify, analyze, and confront his specific patterns of stuttering (most stutterers have never looked at themselves in a mirror to see what they do when they stutter). Beyond looking at his behaviors he also needs to confront his anxieties and fears associated with his stuttering.

- *Desensitization* is partly achieved by a stutterer's willingness to examine what he has always avoided—his stuttering behaviors. The stutterer is expected to talk openly to family and friends about his stuttering problem. Negative practice (stuttering voluntarily but in a new and easier way) further helps desensitize the feelings of frustration, guilt, and shame.

- *Variation* provides the individual alternative stuttering behaviors to increase speaking control. The stutterer goes from his old, reflexive, and automatic pattern of stuttering to small but important changes that he intentionally uses to vary his stuttering behaviors.

- *Approximation* of increasingly "normal" fluency includes using specific techniques such as "cancellations" (after finishing a stuttered word, saying the word again but in an easier, less tense manner) and "pull-outs" (changing the stuttering behavior as it is occurring).

- *Stabilization* is the transference of the speaker's new perceptions and skills to situations outside of the therapy setting. From the earliest therapy sessions the client is asked to do assignments in his home, community, school, and work place. The goal is for the speaker to become resilient in responding to the variety of communicative pressures encountered in daily speaking situations.

---

stuttering modification

A therapy approach for children and adult stutterers that requires the speaker to recognize and confront his fears, avoidances, and struggles to escape his stuttering, and the speaker reducing and managing those fears, avoidances, and struggles.

Multicultural Considerations when Working with Children

Stuttering exists in all known cultures, with some having a higher or lower incidence than others (Bloodstein & Berstein Ratner, 2008; Botterill & Fry, 2005; Ezrati-Vinacour & Amir, 2005; Kenjo, 2005; Limongi, 2005; Lundstrom & Garsten, 2005; Robinson & Crowe, 2002; Subramanian & Prabhu, 2005; Yang, 2005). Proctor, Yairi, Duff, & Zhang (2008) in their study on the prevalence of stuttering in African American preschoolers (2,223 African American children compared with 941 European American children) found no statistically significant difference in the incidence of stuttering between the two groups.

Watson and Kayser (1994) discussed several fluency issues in bilingual and bicultural children that should be considered when evaluating and treating children who stutter:

- Bilingual children may exhibit pauses, repetitions, revisions, or a combination of these related to second-language acquisition.

- Distinguish true stuttering from disfluencies associated with second-language acquisition.

- Disfluencies observed only in a second language that are not accompanied by secondary behaviors are most likely not stuttering behaviors.

- Monolingual clinicians should be able to identify tension and secondary characteristics in a bilingual child even if they do not understand the child's language.

WORKING WITH ADOLESCENTS AND ADULTS WHO STUTTER

Adolescents and adults who stutter come to a speech-language pathologist because they want help (**internal motivation**) or because someone else, such as a parent, spouse, or employer, wants the person to receive help (**external motivation**). Internal motivation is essential; however, some external motivation can be helpful to keep the person in therapy. Treatment of adolescents and adults who stutter is sometimes the result of earlier (preschool or school-age) therapy that was not successful. Therapy's success relies on numerous variables, including the readiness of the person to receive help, motivation and maturity, and having the right therapist with the right therapy at the right time.

Adult stutterers come for help at all ages (I have worked with some adults in their 60s who decided that they wanted to "conquer" their stuttering before they die); however, many adults appear to seek therapy when they recognize that their stuttering problem is interfering with or holding them back in their occupations and professions. Sometimes when a stutterer is promoted to a job with more speaking responsibilities (e.g., a managerial position) and increased pressure to communicate fluently, the person recognizes that the stuttering problem is going

internal motivation

Motivation that is self-generated or intrinsic in which a person decides what is important and needed.

external motivation

Motivation that is provided by the encouragement of someone else, often family or an employer.

to become obvious to others and that something needs to be done—even starting therapy.

Evaluation of Adolescents and Adults

The evaluation of adolescents and adults is considerably different from that of preschool and school-age children. (Note: Because of the wide range of maturity levels from early adolescence to late adolescence, evaluation and therapy techniques may overlap from the childhood-adolescence group and the adolescence-adult group.) When evaluating adolescents, the parents may play a role in providing some history of the adolescent's stuttering and some family background information; however, the emphasis is on the stutterer and her problem and her perceptions of the problem. With adults, however, there is typically no parental involvement, with the only information about the parents and family history being provided by the client.

congruent/congruence

The agreement among a person's thoughts, feelings, words, tone of voice, and body language; communication in which a person sends the same message on both verbal and nonverbal levels.

The interview and evaluation of both adolescents and adults are direct. As mentioned previously, interviewing is an essential skill for clinicians to develop, and all interviewing involves counseling skills. Interviewing and therapy require clinicians to be **congruent**; that is, our thoughts, feelings, words, tone of voice, and body language all need to be in agreement. Our clients are probably going to "read" us better than we can read ourselves. They can tell if we are faking knowledge, understanding, and confidence. People most readily trust us when we are congruent (Flasher & Fogle, 2012). In a university clinic setting, clients realize that their student clinicians are "learning on them," and they tacitly accept that students probably do not really know what they are doing, but hope that the supervisor behind the mirror does know and is giving the student good direction.

affective/affect

Relating to, arising from, or influencing feelings or emotions; *affect* is revealed by facial expressions, body posture and gestures, tone of voice, and choice of words.

Knowledge about stuttering is not sufficient to be a good or excellent clinician; it also takes the ability to enter into the person's world and develop a strong therapeutic relationship. The relationship has dynamics that are inevitably affected by what the client and clinician bring to it. Variables contributing to the therapeutic relationship are illustrated in Figure 8–8. The client–clinician relationship emphasizes the **affective**

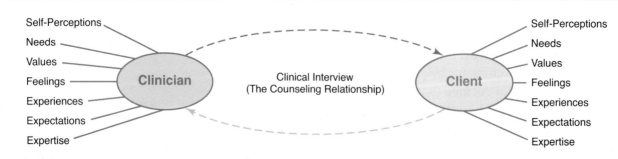

Figure 8–8

Variables contributing to the therapeutic relationship.

Adapted from Brammer & McDonald, 1999.

Too Good at Hiding

Personal Story

Two of my recent adult male clients who stuttered had both "successfully" hidden their stuttering from their wives and employers for years. One stutterer had been a forklift driver for several years (he chose the job because he did not need to talk much), and the other was a police officer who liked working in the toughest areas of a well-known high-crime city. However, both men said that their stuttering was "eating them up inside." Even though to other people they appeared fluent and generally normal speakers, they both knew they were "faking" having fluent speech. One of the early assignments both men were given was to talk to their wives about their stuttering. Although both men found this a very challenging assignment, they were extremely relieved for their wives to learn about their problems and to find out how accepting their wives were and how supportive they were of therapy. ■

mode because, like any relationship, there is an emotional quality to the interaction. The client and clinician influence each other as their relationship evolves. How clients behave toward us is invariably linked to how we think, feel, and behave toward them. The relationship can change subtly or even significantly from session to session and sometimes from moment to moment. However, mutual respect and trust help the client and clinician through the "rocky" times of their therapeutic relationship.

During the interview, the clinician takes notes about stuttering behaviors she sees and hears. Often, as the interview progresses, the clinician can begin to recognize stuttering patterns. For example: *When she stutters she tends to repeat the first sound of the word three times, then stops, then looks away (usually up and to her right), then clenches her left hand, then clears her throat, then tries to say the word again as she is looking around the room, and then says the word.* Clinicians develop astute behavioral observation skills.

Some stutterers will be remarkably fluent—too fluent—during the evaluation. The clinician may wonder where the stuttering is. The client has found such subtle tricks for concealing her stuttering from others (even family members) that she can be as fluent—or more fluent—than nonstutterers. However, the stutterer knows she stutters, and her hiding and dishonesty with herself can be tormenting. It is unlikely that an adult would come for stuttering therapy if she did not stutter. If there is not a legitimate problem, therapy is too time and emotionally consuming and financially expensive to pursue. Therefore, when a fluent adult enters therapy, believe her when she says she stutters.

When adolescents and adults talk about their stuttering, be aware of the emotions that may be released (having a box of tissues handy is helpful).

Application Question

How important do you think having a strong background in counseling would be to becoming an excellent clinician?

Application Question

What do you like friends to do when you are crying? What would you want someone you did not know well to do if you are crying?

You may be the first person they have ever been open with about their problem, and that may open the floodgates. Most people are not comfortable with the tears of people they do not know well, and even experienced clinicians are not always certain just what to say or do. Flasher and Fogle (2012) provide suggestions on managing such delicate times.

A stuttering evaluation with an adult usually lasts an hour. During that time the clinician should have enough information to decide on the direction of therapy. Most adults are not particularly keen on long, protracted evaluations of every nuance of their stuttering (much less their receptive and expressive language abilities) before starting to work on their problem. Still, in a sense, all therapy involves continual evaluation of the client—and the therapy itself.

Treatment of Adolescents and Adults

Adolescents and adults do not enter therapy with a clean slate. That is, they have some preconceived notions about what will help and what will not. They (especially adults) have beliefs and often strong opinions about therapy based on their past experiences with it or what they have imagined. It is helpful to learn about their beliefs and opinions. Your therapy may reinforce what they think might help, or it may run counter to what they had imagined. The one certainty is that they will be asked to do things that they are uncomfortable doing and may resist doing. It is important for clinicians to appreciate that behind resistance is fear; often the fear of change.

If therapy is to be successful, change is required. People change in essentially three ways (Flasher & Fogle, 2012):

1. *Evolution*—A person slowly, sometimes almost imperceptibly, changes over time (e.g., normal maturation and growth, education, and rehabilitation).

2. *Revolution*—A significant event in a person's life changes the way she thinks, believes, or behaves (e.g., marriage, parenthood, loss of a loved one, or a stroke).

3. *Resolution*—A person decides that it is now time to change (e.g., going back to school, stopping drinking or taking drugs, or starting therapy or taking responsibility for improvements in therapy).

As clinicians, we know that the person's stuttering evolved over time and is, in a way, still evolving as the person develops new tricks and crutches to replace (or add to) the old ones that no longer help her be fluent. We also know that therapy is an *evolutionary* process and that it will take time for the stutterer to change old beliefs and attitudes and behaviors. We are aware that most stutterers are impatient with therapy. They want a *revolutionary* change: "I want to take care of this problem I've had all of my life in the next couple of months." As clinicians, we know that for the stutterer to improve she needs to have *resolve* (a *resolution*); she needs to stay with therapy even when she most wants to quit.

Brian

Brian was a fluent stutterer who had "successfully" hidden his stuttering from everyone, including his wife and employer. Brian was also a veteran police officer who preferred to work the night shift in the roughest, high-crime areas of a large city. He had done plenty of "take downs" and had "taken men out." During one therapy session, he told me about an experience he had just the night before. He was in hot pursuit on foot of an armed robber. He knew the robber could turn at any moment and shoot at him. Brian admitted that his greatest fear was not whether he might be shot by the man he was chasing but whether he would stutter badly at the moment he caught him. ■

Gregory (2003) describes four areas of emphasis in therapy for adolescents and adults who stutter. There is a sequence to therapy, but fairly soon the client will be working on the stuttering in all four areas during each therapy session.

1. *Developing insight into attitudes, thoughts, and feelings about stuttering.* Stutterers have strong feelings about their stuttering, and they have conjured and imagined how other people must think about stuttering and stutterers, although they most likely have never asked people what they think about stuttering. Part of therapy may involve a "reality check" in which the stutterer asks family, friends, and others their opinions about stuttering and stutterers. Most clients find that people do not think nearly as much or as negatively about stuttering and stutterers as what clients have imagined. In therapy, speech changes accompany attitude changes.

2. *Increasing awareness of muscular tension through the use of relaxation exercises.* Stutterers are aware that they have muscular tension, but for many of them the tension is so chronic that it becomes their "norm" and they hardly notice the tension in their face, throat, shoulders, chest, and back. Some stutterers who have been placed on **biofeedback** instruments have been able to see graphically displayed the sometimes extraordinary tension in some muscles. Stutterers often need to become aware of muscle tension in the large muscle groups before they can become aware of and modify the tension in their speech and facial muscles. Many stutterers do not know what normal muscle tension feels like, and it comforts them to begin their first perceptions of normalcy.

3. *Analyzing and modifying speech.* Early in therapy, audio and videotaping may be used to help the client hear and see what she does when she stutters. Stutterers often initially deny that certain

biofeedback

The process of becoming aware of various physiological functions of the body using instruments that provide information on the activity of muscles or systems being monitored, with the goal of being able to control or manipulate those muscles or systems voluntarily.

behaviors (tricks and crutches to help them be fluent) are part of their stuttering: "It's just the way I talk." These tricks and crutches are "avoidance" behaviors. But when they try to talk without using some of these behaviors, they discover that they become more disfluent. What the clinician knows, the stutterer has to learn. As therapy progresses, clients learn to modify their stuttering and overall speech production.

A speech modification technique that has been used by many clinicians is referred to as "voluntary stuttering" or "voluntary disfluency," in which the person is asked to do the very thing she does not want to do—stutter. The difference is that the person learns that she has a choice as to *when* she stutters, *how* she stutters, and *how long* she stutters—voluntarily (Gregory, 2003; Guitar, 2006; Sheehan, 1970; Van Riper, 1982). By using voluntary stuttering, the client is performing an "approach" behavior, which will decrease fear and tension. Stutterers learn that *monitoring* (paying attention to their speech) and *modifying* are continuous processes. Stuttering modifications need to be carried from the clinic room to the real world if they are going to be used in daily conversations.

4. *Building new speech skills.* Therapy does not focus only on stuttering but includes communication in general. We work with stutterers head to toe and even sometimes with their articulation and use of language. The more confidence stutterers can develop that they are good communicators, despite some disfluencies, the better they feel about themselves. Stutterers learn that they can say what they want and not resort to saying whatever is easiest at the moment (stutterers have eaten countless meals in restaurants that they did not want; stutterers often order what they can say easily rather than what they really want).

Clinicians need to have a clear organization in their therapy so that they know where they have come from, where they are, and where they are going with therapy. However, therapy is unscripted; it is not, "If she says that, I'll say this." Therapy requires moment-to-moment decision making about what is the best thing to say, when to say it, and how to say it. The ability to integrate all of your perceptions of the client at the moment and your knowledge and understanding of stuttering and the ability to "think on your feet" are essential in stuttering therapy.

Stuttering therapy is a marathon, not a sprint. To be most successful, stuttering therapy needs to be long-term. After a foundational period of therapy (usually 3 to 6 months), a follow-through program of 12 to 18 months is most beneficial. People who stutter need to realize that they will continue to experience challenging situations that will require time to process. Many concepts not well understood during therapy are clarified with further experience. Stutterers develop new insights into their feelings and behaviors, and therapy techniques they resisted earlier are used more effectively and more willingly.

A $40,000 Phone Call

Personal Story

A private client of mine who was in his late 20s was already success-ful farming orchard crops. John had avoided the telephone all of his life; he even had his wife make the initial phone call to set up the first appointment with me. After several weeks of therapy, John was increasingly working on overcoming his feared situations, especially those involving the telephone. At the beginning of one appointment, he smiled, shook my hand, and thanked me for helping him make $40,000 that week. He told me that for the first time he made a phone call to talk directly to one of his buyers and from that conversation landed an additional $40,000 contract that he had never expected to obtain. Beyond all of the emotional and psychological "costs" of stuttering, for many people their fears and avoidances can be finan-cially costly. ■

Success of Therapy

How successful therapy will be for a stutterer depends on many variables. If the therapy approach is well researched and understood, appropriate, and well presented by the clinician, the variables that determine suc-cess mostly depend on the individual stutterer. Many stutterers do not stay with therapy for the entire time that it takes to fully understand and integrate the principles and techniques they learn from their clinician. Many drift away or in and out of therapy, perhaps because they develop some level of comfort. For those who stay with therapy, are reasonably diligent in following the principles and techniques they learn, and do the exercises, there is a good chance they will have long-lasting benefits. Gregory, in his Adult Stuttering Program at Northwestern University and in his private practice, has found that approximately 8 out of 10 clients are pleased with the results of therapy and consider it successful. Success is defined as gaining sufficient confidence to be comfortable about communication, being able to speak easily in most situations, and having a program for continuing to work on speech goals.

EMOTIONAL AND SOCIAL EFFECTS OF STUTTERING

Clinicians who have considerable experience working with children and adults who stutter recognize that stuttering is a communication disorder that is fraught with emotional and social distress (which are different from emotional and social disorders) (Gregory, 2003; Guitar, 2006; Zebrowski, 2002). As a group, children and adults who stutter have a more sensitive temperament, which may be associated with more physical tension in laryngeal muscles (Guitar, 2006). Children and adults have anxiety about their stuttering, and stuttering causes anxiety (Iverach et al., 2011). They tend to have low self-esteem and excessive needs for social approval. Individuals who stutter often feel punished by their disfluency and avoid certain speaking situations (e.g., speaking up in class or speaking in meetings) and talking to certain people (particularly people they perceive as "authority figures"). One of the indications of strong emotional reactions to stuttering is habitual avoidance of speaking (Bloodstein & Berstein Ratner, 2008). Most stutterers have spent most of their lives trying to hide their stuttering from others and even from themselves—denying that it is a problem. Many people who stutter choose their daily social interactions based on how fluent they feel they will be when they start their day.

People who stutter may choose their occupations or professions based on their fluency, preferring jobs in which speaking is a minimal part of their work. Parents often wonder whether they may have caused or contributed to their child's stuttering problem, and frequently feel some guilt and embarrassment about their child's stuttering (Flasher & Fogle, 2012; Guitar, 2006; Zebrowski, 2002). However, in spite of the emotional toll their stuttering takes, many people who have been and are stutterers have had remarkably happy and successful lives.

CHARLES VAN RIPER (1905–1994)

Perhaps no single person has had a greater effect on the profession of speech-language pathology, and stuttering therapy in particular, than Charles Van Riper. In speech-language pathology, he was a legend in his own time. The first quarter-century of his life was plagued by profoundly severe stuttering (perhaps the most profoundly severe stuttering of any person known to the profession). His stuttering led him to become a pioneering founder of this new profession and widely recognized world authority on stuttering. Dr. Van Riper was a prodigious author, with more than 200 publications spanning seven decades. His *The Nature of Stuttering* (1982) and *The Treatment of Stuttering* (1973) are classics in the specialty.

Beyond his professional writing, he also was a poet. While an undergraduate at Northern Michigan College in an honors class with the resident poet, Robert Frost, the renowned Frost awarded Van Riper first prize for his poetry, which was later published. Van Riper earned his master's degree at the University of Michigan with a specialty in Old English literature and Elizabethan ballads. He earned his doctoral degree in clinical psychology at the University of Iowa. During his years at Iowa, he worked with Lee Edward Travis and others to help his stuttering, and it was there that he developed his theories of and therapy for stuttering. After leaving Iowa, he taught at Western Michigan University in Kalamazoo and remained there most of his professional career. As Van Riper once wrote, "The potential in any living thing is immense, but to release that potential someone has to intervene. . . . After a bum beginning, I've had a very rewarding life—love to see the human flowers bloom, and take no credit except for the weeding and fertilizing."

A Sun

For reasons that I do not know,
I am a sun, a small, small sun
Whose warmth helps others grow,
Bear fruit and seed
So other human suns
May glow.

—Charles Van Riper

CHAPTER SUMMARY

Stuttering typically comprises both verbal overt behaviors and visible overt behaviors. The covert, emotional, and social reactions of individuals who stutter can be some of the most serious challenges they face in therapy. The incidence of stuttering is generally considered to be 1% of the childhood population. The gender ratio is three or four males to one female stutterer. Stuttering tends to run in families. Physiologically, the only difference between stutterers and nonstutterers occurs just before and at the moment of stuttering. Stutterers are within the norms for intelligence. There do not appear to be any particular personality traits that are typical of individuals who stutter.

Throughout the working relationship with a family, the family systems model coupled with a cognitive therapy counseling model is helpful. Not all children who are disfluent need direct therapy, particularly those who are at risk for stuttering but are not yet stuttering. The function of the speech-language pathologist with such children is in the area of prevention. In direct therapy with children and adolescents, our general approach is to be understanding and accepting so that the child views us as someone who is genuinely interested in him and accepting of whatever he says and however he says it. Providing children with successful speaking activities and opportunities can be helpful. Fluency shaping and stuttering modification approaches are used with both children and adults.

Four areas of emphasis in therapy for adolescents and adults who stutter may include developing insight into attitudes, thoughts, and feelings about stuttering; increasing awareness of muscular tension through the use of relaxation exercises; analyzing and modifying speech; and building new speech skills. To be most successful, stuttering therapy needs to be long-term. Success is defined as gaining sufficient confidence to be comfortable about communication, being able to speak easily in most situations, and having a program for continuing to work on speech goals.

STUDY QUESTIONS

Knowledge and Comprehension

1. What are normal disfluencies?
2. What is family systems therapy and what does it emphasize?

3. Discuss what a clinician should be able to do after completion of a fluency evaluation.

4. What is primary prevention?

5. What might be a reasonable definition of success in therapy for adults who stutter?

Application

1. How could covert reactions contribute to a person's disfluency?

2. Explain why stuttering therapy is a dynamic process.

3. What are some helpful points for how parents should react when their child is disfluent?

4. Discuss the importance of the relationship a clinician develops with a child who is disfluent.

5. Why is interviewing an essential skill for clinicians to develop?

Analysis/Synthesis

1. Why are visible overt behaviors considered part of stuttering?

2. Why would no one theory fully explain the cause of stuttering in all children?

3. What are the similarities and differences between fluency shaping and stuttering modification approaches?

4. Why is the *affective* mode so important in understanding the variables that contribute to the therapeutic relationship?

5. Discuss the three essential ways people change and how these may be applied to stuttering therapy.

REFERENCES

American Speech-Language-Hearing Association. (1988, March). *Position statement: Prevention of communication disorders.* Washington, DC: ASHA.

Biermann-Ruben, K., Salmelin, R., & Schnitzler, A. (2005). Right rolandic activation during speech perception in stutterers: A MEG study. *NeuroImage, 25,* 793–801.

Blood, G. W., Ridenour, C., Qualls, C. D., & Hammer, C. S. (2004). Co-occurring disorders in children who stutter. *Journal of Communication Disorders, 36,* 427–488.

Bloodstein, O., & Berstein Ratner, N. (2008). *Handbook on stuttering* (6th ed.). Clifton Park, NY: Delmar Cengage Learning.

Bobrick, B. (1995). *Knotted tongues: Stuttering in history and the quest for a cure.* New York, NY: Kodansha International.

Botterill, W., & Fry, J. (2005). Stuttering research and treatment around the world: United Kingdom. *ASHA Leader, 9*, 41.

Buck, S. M., Lees, R., & Cook, F. (2002). The influence of family history of stuttering on the onset of stuttering in young children. *Folia Phoniatrica, 54*, 117–124.

Chmela, K. A., & Reardon, N. (2005). *The school-age child who stutters: Working effectively with attitudes and emotions: A workbook.* Memphis, TN: Stuttering Foundation of America.

Conture, E. G. (2001). *Stuttering: Its nature, diagnosis, and treatment.* Boston, MA: Allyn and Bacon.

Curlee, R. F. (2007). Does my child stutter? In *Stuttering and your child: Questions and answers,* Publication no. 0022. Memphis, TN: Stuttering Foundation of America.

Daly, D. A. (1992). Helping the clutterer: Therapy considerations. In F. L. Meyers & K. O. St. Louis (Eds.), *Cluttering: A clinical perspective.* Kibworth, England: Far Communications.

Daly, D. A., & Cantrelle, R. P. (2006). *Cluttering: Characteristics identified as diagnostically significant by 60 fluency experts.* Paper presented at the 5th International Fluency Association World Congress on Disorders of Fluency, Dublin, Ireland.

De Keyser, J. (1973). The stuttering of Lewis Carroll. In Y. Lebrun & T. Hoops (Eds.), *Neurolinguistic approaches to stuttering.* The Hague: Mouton.

DeNil, L. (2004). Recent developments in brain imaging research in stuttering. In B. Maassen, R. D. Kent, H. F. Petters, P. H. van Lieshout, & W. Hulstijn (Eds.), *Speech motor control in normal and disordered speech.* Oxford: Oxford University Press.

Ezrati-Vinacour, R., & Amir, O. (2005). Stuttering research and treatment around the world: Israel. *ASHA Leader, 9*, 8–9.

Flasher, L. V., & Fogle, P. T. (2012). *Counseling skills for speech-language pathologists and audiologists* (2nd ed.). Clifton Park, NY: Delmar Cengage Learning.

Goldman, R. (1967). Cultural influences on the sex ratio in the incidence of stuttering. *American Anthropologist, 69*, 78–81.

Gregory, H. H. (2003). *Stuttering therapy: Rationale and procedures.* Boston, MA: Allyn and Bacon.

Guitar, B. (2006). *Stuttering: An integrated approach to its nature and treatment* Baltimore, MD: Lippincott Williams & Wilkins.

Hill, D. G. (2003). Differential treatment of stuttering in the early stages of development. In H. H. Gregory, *Stuttering therapy: Rationale and procedures.* Boston, MA: Allyn and Bacon.

Ingham, R. (2001). Brain imaging and studies of developmental stuttering. *Journal of Communication Disorders, 34*, 493–516.

Iverach, L., Menzies, R. G., O'Brian, S., Packman, A., & Onslow, M. (2011). Anxiety and stuttering: Continuing to explore a complex relationship. *American Journal of Speech-Language Pathology, 20*, 221–232.

Kenjo, M. (2005). Stuttering research and treatment around the world: Japan. *ASHA Leader, 9,* 36.

Limongi, F. P. (2005). Stuttering research and treatment around the world: Brazil. *ASHA Leader, 9,* 6.

Lundstrom, C., & Garsten, M. (2005). Stuttering research and treatment around the world: Sweden. *ASHA Leader, 9,* 36–37.

Manning, W. H. (2010). *Clinical decision making in fluency disorders* (3rd ed.). Clifton Park, NY: Delmar Cengage Learning.

Maul, C. A. (2011). *Family-centered service delivery: Is there an evidence base?* CSHA Magazine, 41(1), 8–9.

Nelson, L. A. (1999). How does our home life influence his stuttering? In *Stuttering and your child: Questions and answers.* Memphis, TN: Stuttering Foundation of America.

Ntourou, K., Conture, E. G., & Lipsey, M. W. (2011). Language abilities of children who stutter: A meta-analytical review. *American Journal of Speech-Language Pathology, 20,* 163–179.

Paden, E. (2005). Development of phonological ability. In E. Yairi & N. Ambrose (Eds.). *Early childhood stuttering: For clinicians by clinicians.* Austin, TX: Pro-Ed.

Proctor, A., Yairi, E., Duff, M. C., & Zhang, J. (2008). Prevalence of stuttering in African American preschoolers. *Journal of Speech, Language, and Hearing Research, 51*(6), 1465–1479.

Ramig, P. R. (1997). Various paths to long-term recovery from stuttering. Paper presented at 2nd World Congress on Fluency Disorders, San Francisco, CA.

Ramig, P. R., & Dodge, D. M. (2010). *The child and adolescent stuttering treatment and activity resource guide* (2nd ed.). Clifton Park, NY: Delmar Cengage Learning.

Reardon-Reeves, N. A., & Yaruss, J. S. (2004). *The source for stuttering: Ages 7-18.* East Moline, IL: LinguiSystems.

Robinson, T. L., & Crowe, T. A. (2002). Fluency disorders. In D. E. Battle (Ed.), *Communication disorders in multicultural populations* (3rd ed.). Boston, MA: Butterworth-Heinemann.

Sheehan, J. G. (1970). *Stuttering: Research and therapy.* New York, NY: Harper & Row.

Silverman, F. H. (2004). *Stuttering and other fluency disorders.* Long Grove, IL: Waveland Press.

St. Louis, K. O., Raphael, L. J., Myers, F. L., & Bakker, K. (2003). Cluttering updated. *ASHA Leader, 18,* 4–5, 20–21.

Stuttering Foundation of America. (2002a) *Stuttering and your child: Questions and answers.* Memphis, TN: Stuttering Foundation of America.

Stuttering Foundation of America. (2002b). *Stuttering and the preschool child: Help for families.* Memphis, TX: Stuttering Foundation of America.

Stuttering Foundation of America. (2002c). *Stuttering: Straight talk to teachers.* Memphis, TN: Stuttering Foundation of America.

Stuttering Foundation of America. (2002d). *Foudacion Americana de la tartanudez.* Memphis, TN: Stuttering Foundation of America.

Subramanian, U., & Prabhu, B. (2005). Stuttering research and treatment around the world: India. *ASHA Leader, 9,* 7–8.

Tillis, M., & Wager, W. (1984). *Stutterin' boy.* New York, NY: Rawson Associates.

Travis, L. E. (1931). Diagnosis and treatment of stuttering cases. *Proceedings of the American Speech Correction Association, 1,* 121–127.

Van Riper, C. (1939). *Speech correction, principles and methods.* New York, NY: Prentice-Hall.

Van Riper, C. (1971). *The nature of stuttering.* Englewood Cliffs, NJ: Prentice Hall.

Van Riper, C. (1982). *The nature of stuttering* (2nd ed.). Englewood Cliffs, NJ: Prentice Hall.

Ward, D. (2006). *Stuttering and cluttering: Framework for understanding and treatment.* East Sussex, England: Psychology Press.

Watson, J., & Kayser, H. (1994). Assessment of bilingual/bicultural children and adults who stutter. *Seminars in Speech and Language, 15,* 149–164.

West, R. (1942). The pathology of stuttering. *The Nervous Child, 2*(2), 96–106.

Williams, D. E. (1979). A perspective on approaches to stuttering therapy. In H. Gregory (Ed.), *Controversies about stuttering therapy.* Baltimore, MD: University Park Press.

Williams, D. E. (2004). *The genius of Dean Williams* (compiled by the Stuttering Foundation of America). Memphis, TN: Stuttering Foundation of America.

World Health Organization. (1977). *Manual of the international statistical classification of diseases, injuries, and causes of death* (Vol. 1). Geneva: World Health Organization.

Yairi, E., & Ambrose, N. (2005). *Early Childhood Stuttering.* Austin, TX: Pro-Ed.

Yang, E. (2005). Stuttering research and treatment around the world: Taiwan. *ASHA Leader, 9,* 37–38.

Yu, B., & Kashinath, S. (2011). *Family-centered care and other labors of love: Culturally competent service delivery for young children and their families.* CSHA Magazine, 41(1), 12–13.

Zebrowski, P. M. (2002). Counseling: An approach for speech-language pathologists. *Contemporary Issues in Communication Sciences and Disorders, 29,* 91–100.

Zebrowski, P. M., & Kelly, E. M. (2002). *Manual of stuttering intervention.* Clifton Park, NY: Delmar Cengage Learning.

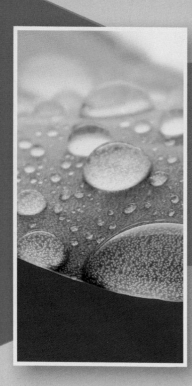

CHAPTER 9
Voice Disorders in Children and Adults

LEARNING OBJECTIVES

After studying this chapter, you will:

- Be able to describe the major voice disorders.
- Be able to discuss the evaluation of voice disorders by the otolaryngologist and speech-language pathologist.
- Be familiar with two of the foundational voice therapy approaches.
- Be able to discuss voice therapy for patients who have had laryngectomy surgery.
- Be aware of the emotional and social effects of voice disorders on clients.

KEY TERMS

acute

acute laryngitis/
  traumatic laryngitis

breathiness

cancer (carcinoma)

chronic

chronic laryngitis

contact ulcer

conversion reaction
  (disorder)

diplophonia

direct laryngoscopy

dystonia

edema

electrolarynx/
  artificial larynx

endoscopy

esophageal speech

facilitating techniques

functional aphonia

functional
  dysphonia

hard glottal attack

harshness

hoarseness

holistic

hyperadduction

hyperfunction

hypoadduction

hypofunction

indirect
  laryngoscopy

intubation

laryngectomy

laryngitis

laryngopharyngeal
  reflux (LPR)

lesion

malignant

muscle tension
  dysphonia (MTD)

mutational falsetto
  (puberphonia)

otolaryngologist/
  otorhino-
  laryngologist
  (ear, nose, and
  throat [ENT]
  doctor)

KEY TERMS continued

papilloma
(papillomatosis)

phonotrauma

polypoid thickening
(degeneration)

referred pain

spasmodic
dysphonia (SD)

stoma

tracheoesophageal
prosthesis
(TEP)

vocal abuse

vocal fold paralysis

vocal hygiene

vocal misuse

vocal nodule

vocal polyp

voice disorder
(dysphonia)

CHAPTER OUTLINE

Introduction

Classification of Voice Disorders

Voice Disorders Related to Functional Etiologies
and Faulty Usage
Laryngitis
Vocal Nodules
Vocal Polyps
Contact Ulcer
Functional Dysphonia
Functional Aphonia
Mutational Falsetto/Puberphonia

Voice Disorders Related to Organic Etiologies
Papillomas
Blunt, Penetrating, and Inhalation Traumas
Cancer/Carcinoma

Voice Disorders Related to Neurological Etiologies
Hypoadduction Vocal Fold Problems
Hyperadduction Vocal Fold Problems

Multicultural Considerations

Assessment of the Voice
The Otolaryngologist's Examination
The Speech-Language Pathologist's Assessment

Voice Therapy
Voice Therapy Approaches
Laryngectomy

Emotional and Social Effects of Voice Disorders
Young Children
Adolescents
Adults

Chapter Summary

Study Questions

References

voice disorder (dysphonia)

Any deviation of loudness, pitch, or quality that is outside the normal range of a person's age, gender, or geographic or cultural background that interferes with communication, draws unfavorable attention to itself, or adversely affects the speaker or listener.

INTRODUCTION

Voice disorders (dysphonias) have been recognized for more than 3,500 years. The Edwin Smith Papyrus from an ancient Egyptian burial tomb, dated about 1600 B.C., described in some detail a crushing injury to the neck, which caused the loss of speech. The Egyptian writings contained a hieroglyph portraying the lungs and trachea, although the larynx was not pictured because no organ for voice had yet been identified (Fink, 1975). To treat recognized voice disorders, different cultures used treatments such as gargles derived from fruit juices, cabbage, garlic, the juice of crabs, centipedes, owl's brain, and the urine of sacred cows. Other remedies included wearing beads of various kinds or a black silk cord around the throat (Stevenson & Guthrie, 1949; Wright, 1941). In more modern times, before speech-language pathologists began working with voice disorders, singing teachers, phoneticians (recall Henry Higgins [Rex Harrison] working with Eliza Doolittle [Audrey Hepburn] in the movie *My Fair Lady*), and voice and diction teachers worked with trained and untrained singers and other individuals with voice problems (Curry, 1940). Since that time, speech-language pathologists have become the professionals who work with disorders of the speaking voice.

The voice has long been considered a mirror of the person—the inner self. The voice is a reflection of an individual's personality and is a sensitive indicator of emotions, attitudes, and the roles we play. People can recognize the typical voice of intense, hard-driving people and the nasal, singsong voice of the constant whiner. We detect a depressed or withdrawn person's monotone, deenergized voice and we know the voice of the outgoing, charismatic, happy person. A soft, soothing voice tends to calm an agitated person, and a tense, strident voice tends to be discomforting (Andrews, 2006; Boone, McFarlane, & Von Berg, 2009; Colton, Casper, & Leonard, 2011).

The loudness, pitch, and quality of voice are influenced by multiple factors involving the anatomy and physiology of the respiratory system, the vocal folds, and the *supraglottal vocal tract's* (above the vocal folds) tuning characteristics (Scherer, 2006; Stemple, Glaze, & Klaben, 2009; Titze, 2000). A variety of terms are used to subjectively describe the quality of dysphonia, such as *hoarse, breathy, harsh, husky, raucous, grating, strident, thin, strained, tense, weak, tremulous,* and *monotone.* The subjective term *hoarse* is the most commonly used by professionals who work with voice disorders.

TABLE 9-1	Voice Disorders Speech-Language Pathologists Work With	

FUNCTIONAL	NEUROLOGICAL	ORGANIC
Diplophonia	Ataxic dysarthria	Cancer
Falsetto	Essential tremor	Congenital abnormalities
Functional aphonia	Guillain-Barré syndrome	Contact ulcers
Functional dysphonia	Hyperkinetic (spasmodic dysphonia, essential tremor)	Endocrine changes
Muscle tension dysphonia	Hypokinetic (Parkinson's disease)	Granuloma
Nodules	Lower motor neuron (LMN)	Hemangioma
Phonation breaks	Mixed (amyotrophic lateral sclerosis, TBI, multiple sclerosis)	Hyperkeratosis
Pitch breaks	Myasthenia gravis	Infectious laryngitis
Polyps	Resonance disturbance	Laryngectomy
Reinke's edema	Spasmodic dysphonia	Leukoplakia
Traumatic laryngitis	Spastic dysarthria	Papilloma
Ventricular dysphonia	Sulcus vocalis	Pubertal changes
Vocal cord thickening	Unilateral dysarthria	Reflux
Vocal fold paralysis	Upper motor neuron (UMN)	Webbing

Adapted from Boone, McFarlane, and Von Berg, 2009.

CLASSIFICATION OF VOICE DISORDERS

Boone, McFarlane, and Von Berg (2009) use a three-way classification of voice disorders: functional, neurological, and organic (see Table 9–1). *Functional voice disorders* usually are considered to be caused by faulty use of a normal vocal mechanism. *Neurological voice disorders* are related to muscle tone and control of the muscles used for respiration and phonation. *Organic voice disorders* are related to some physical abnormality in the larynx. However, many voice disorders also include an emotional or psychological component. Two other important classifications are vocal **hyperfunction** and vocal **hypofunction**. Hyperfunction describes a pervasive pattern of excessive effort and tension that affects many different structures and muscles in the phonatory system, as well in some cases in the respiratory, resonatory, and articulatory systems (Andrews, 2006). Signs of hyperfunction include a tense sounding voice and **hard glottal attacks**. Hypofunction describes inadequate muscle

hyperfunction

A pervasive pattern of excessive effort and tension that affects many different structures and muscles in the phonatory system and, in some cases, the respiratory, resonatory, and articulatory systems; signs of hyperfunction include a tense sounding voice and hard glottal attacks.

hypofunction

Inadequate muscle tone in the laryngeal mechanism and associated structures, including the muscles of respiration; signs of hypofunction include breathiness because of inadequate closure of the vocal folds, weak vocal power that can affect speech intelligibility, and reduced vocal endurance.

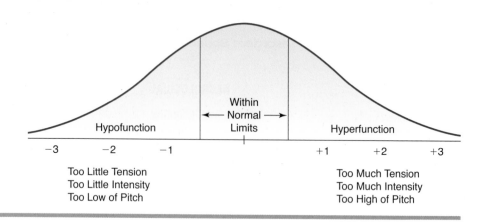

Figure 9–1

Bell-shaped curve with examples of hyperfunctional and hypofunctional voice problems.

© Cengage Learning 2013.

---

hard glottal attack

Forceful *approximation* (closing) of the vocal folds during the initiation of phonation.

vocal nodule

A *benign* (nonmalignant or not cancerous) vocal fold growth that tends to be *bilateral* (both sides, i.e., both vocal folds) and occurs at the same location as vocal polyps (i.e., juncture of the anterior 1/3 and middle 1/3 of the vocal folds), caused by continuous vocal fold hyperfunction (abuse and misuse).

phonotrauma

Deleterious acute or chronic vocal behaviors, such as excessive yelling, screaming, cheering, coughing, throat clearing, inappropriate pitch or loudness, singing beyond the range of the vocal mechanism, hard glottal attacks, inadequate respiratory support, talking loudly over noise, poor hydration, and smoking that are damaging to the vocal folds and the laryngeal and pharyngeal muscles and tissues.

---

tone in the laryngeal mechanism and associated structures, including the muscles of respiration. Signs of hypofunction include breathiness because of inadequate closure of the vocal folds, weak vocal power that can affect speech intelligibility, and reduced vocal endurance (Andrews, 2006). Some voice disorders (e.g., **vocal nodules**) may be caused by hyperfunctional vocal activity (e.g., **phonotrauma**) and result in a hypofunctional (e.g., breathy, weak) voice.

It may be helpful to visualize a bell-shaped curve, where hyperfunction refers to excess tension or forcing in the laryngeal region (i.e., +1, +2, or +3) and hypofunction refers to decreased or inadequate tension or reduced vocal capacity (i.e., –1, –2, or –3) (see Figure 9–1). The two concepts can be extended to hyperfunction referring to too much intensity, too high of a pitch, too much talking, too much **vocal abuse** and **misuse**, and so on. Hypofunction can refer to too low of intensity, too low of a pitch, too little vocal fold vibration, and so on. For a person diagnosed with a hyperfunctional voice disorder, the general therapeutic goal is to teach and train the person to use more hypofunctional behaviors to bring the voice closer to normal limits. When someone has a hypofunctional voice disorder, the goal is to teach and train the person to use more hyperfunctional behaviors to bring the voice closer to normal limits.

Many cases of voice disorders have both functional and organic components that may be causing and maintaining the disorder. For example, individuals with vocal nodules may have originally caused the voice problem (e.g., **hoarseness**) from either **acute** or **chronic** phonotrauma (also referred to by some authorities as *vocal abuse* and *misuse* [Boone et al., 2009; Colton et al., 2011]), such as excessive yelling, screaming, cheering, coughing, throat clearing, chronic loudness, use of the wrong pitch, and hard glottal attacks. Smoking is also considered to cause phonotrauma. These could be considered "functional" behaviors that may lead to an "organic" disorder—the vocal nodules (Andrews, 2006; Boone et al., 2009; Colton et al., 2011). Individuals with neurologically based voice disorders also may have organic and functional components to their voice problems.

VOICE DISORDERS RELATED TO FUNCTIONAL ETIOLOGIES AND FAULTY USAGE

The concepts of hyperfunction and hypofunction, as discussed previously, are important to understanding the various voice disorders that are related to functional etiologies and faulty usage. Many of these disorders have a hyperfunctional component (e.g., tension) that can include a hypofunctional component (e.g., breathiness).

Laryngitis

Laryngitis is a general term that refers to an acute or chronic voice disorder that may have a variety of etiologies, such as phonotrauma or bacterial or viral infections of the larynx. The term *laryngitis* is used to describe an inflammation of the vocal fold mucosa that causes mild to severe dysphonia with lowered pitch and *intermittent phonation breaks* (the voice cuts in and out randomly). Laryngitis is one of the most common hyperfunctional laryngeal problems that results in a voice disorder. The vocal quality that is typically heard in laryngitis is hoarseness, that is, a combination of **harshness** and **breathiness** (Stemple et al., 2009; Swigert, 2005).

Acute Laryngitis/Traumatic Laryngitis

Acute laryngitis (traumatic laryngitis) is often caused by yelling, screaming, and cheering (e.g., at sports events). When in large, noisy crowds, people try to talk over the noise and cheer loud enough so others can hear them (drinking alcohol also decreases inhibitions and awareness of irritation and pain). Many people, after they start to lose their voice, will try to yell or cheer harder to make up for their decreased loudness and vocal control, thereby traumatizing their vocal folds even more and causing **edema** (see Figure 9–2; compare to Figures 3–5 and 3–6). Acute laryngitis also may be caused by bacterial or viral infections that result in *membranous laryngitis*.

Chronic Laryngitis

Chronic laryngitis is laryngitis that lasts more than 10 days and may be caused by a variety of behaviors; for example, (1) acute laryngitis where the vocal folds were not allowed to return to their normal healthy condition because of continued vocal abuses and misuse behaviors; (2) allergies and chemical irritants (including **laryngopharyngeal reflux [LPR]**) that may result in irritation and chronic coughing (Boone et al., 2009; Rees & Belafsky, 2008); (3) singing excessively at damaging intensity levels and in vocal registers outside of a singer's normal range (rock singers sometimes have severely dysphonic voices that become part of their singing style); and (4) smoking, which has numerous effects on the larynx and lungs, such as drying and irritating the vocal folds and irritation of the lungs, both of which can cause chronic coughing and

vocal misuse

Deleterious chronic vocal behaviors that may have a cumulative effects on the structure and functioning of the laryngeal mechanism, such as chronic inappropriate loudness or pitch, singing beyond the range of the vocal mechanism, frequent hard glottal attacks, and speaking with inadequate respiratory support.

hoarseness

A common dysphonia that is a combination of breathiness and harshness that may affect loudness (usually decreased loudness or a monoloudness), pitch (usually a low pitch with reduced pitch range), and quality (usually decreased "pleasantness" of the sound of the voice).

acute

Intense and of short duration, usually referring to a disease or injury.

chronic

Of long duration with slow progress, usually in reference to a disease or disorder.

laryngitis

An acute or chronic inflammation of the mucous membranes of the larynx that often results in hoarseness or loss of voice.

harshness

A "rough" sounding vocal quality resulting from a combination of hard glottal attacks, low pitch, and high intensity caused by *overadduction* (hyperfunction) of the vocal folds.

breathiness

Incomplete closure of the vocal folds during phonation that results in excessive unvibrated air escaping.

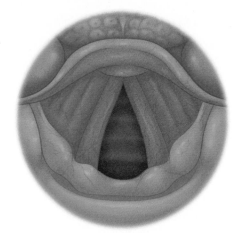

Acute Laryngitis

Figure 9–2

Acute traumatic laryngitis; compare to Figures 3–5 and 3–6.

© Cengage Learning 2013.

acute laryngitis/ traumatic laryngitis

An abrupt, intense, and usually relatively brief inflammation of the mucous membrane lining in the larynx, accompanied by edema of the vocal folds with hoarseness and loss of voice that is often caused by severe vocal abuse.

edema

Accumulation of excessive fluid in tissue that is associated with inflammatory conditions and results in swelling of the tissue.

chronic laryngitis

A persistent laryngitis lasting more than 10 days with inflammation of the mucous membrane lining in the larynx, accompanied by edema of the vocal folds with hoarseness and loss of voice that is often caused by heavy smoking, coughing, allergies and chemical irritants, and ongoing vocal abuse and misuse.

vocal fold trauma (not to mention the potential for laryngeal cancer, lung cancer, or both). It is standard practice that anyone with chronic dysphonia in the absence of a throat infection or *upper respiratory infection* (common cold) needs to undergo a laryngeal examination by an **otolaryngologist** to determine the possible cause or causes of the problem and to rule out serious laryngeal disease (e.g., cancer).

Vocal Nodules

Vocal nodules are the most common benign **lesions** of the vocal folds in both children and adults (Sataloff, 2005). They have been referred to as "cheerleaders' nodes," "screamers' nodes," and "singers' nodes" in reference to the individuals who sometimes develop them. They are a vocal hyperfunction problem caused by continuous abuse and misuse of the voice. Common causes of vocal nodules are yelling and screaming, hard glottal attacks, singing in an abusive manner, frequent speaking in noisy environments, coughing, and excessive throat clearing. Nodules are usually bilateral, but may be *unilateral* (one side).

In the early stage of development, nodular masses are soft and pliable; however, with continuous abuse and misuse of the vocal mechanism, the masses may become larger, harder, and more fibrous. Upon direct visual examination of the vocal folds, nodules generally look like whitish *protuberances* (bumps) on the edges of the vocal folds, typically at the juncture of the anterior one-third and middle one-third of the folds (Boone et al., 2009) (see Figure 9–3). Nodules occur at this location because this is the point on the vocal folds where there is the greatest impact during phonation. As miniscule as the difference may be in terms of pressure on that point compared to any other location on the vocal folds during vibration, if we consider the average number of times the vocal folds vibrate per second (in adult males approximately 120 Hz and in females approximately 225 Hz), we can see that over time the vocal folds may adduct millions of times over months and years.

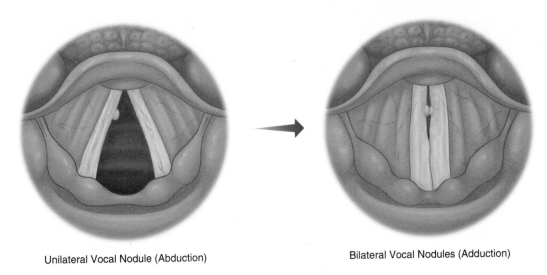

Unilateral Vocal Nodule (Abduction)   Bilateral Vocal Nodules (Adduction)

Figure 9–3

Vocal nodules.

© Cengage Learning 2013.

Individuals with vocal nodules have a hoarse voice quality caused by the nodules preventing the vocal folds from completely adducting. The nodules allow excessive air to escape during phonation, resulting in a breathy quality. The harshness is the result of the extra mass on the vocal folds causing *aperiodicity* (irregular vocal fold vibration). The added mass of tissue (as minute as it is) also can cause the pitch to lower slightly compared to what is optimal for a person (Andrews, 2006; Swigert, 2005).

Evaluation of individuals with vocal nodules involves a detailed case history; perceptual judgments of the loudness, pitch, and quality of the voice; and instrumental evaluations. Voice therapy for vocal nodules is a behavioral, symptomatic approach, often following a four-step program: (1) identifying abuses and misuses of the voice; (2) reducing the occurrence of the abuses and misuses; (3) searching with the patient for various voice therapy facilitating approaches that seem to produce an easy, optimal vocal production; and (4) using the **facilitating techniques** that work best as a practice method (Boone et al., 2009; Stemple et al., 2009). Voice therapy with an SLP is usually needed for at least 6 to 8 weeks. For many children and adults, there is a need for strong psychological and counseling support by the SLP (Andrews, 2006). With appropriate symptomatic behavioral therapy and counseling, surgical removal of vocal nodules is generally not needed.

Vocal Polyps

Vocal polyps are benign vocal fold lesions that tend to be unilateral and typically occur at the same location as vocal nodules; that is, the juncture of the anterior one-third and middle one-third of the vocal folds.

laryngopharyngeal reflux (LPR)

Gastric reflux (stomach acids causing heartburn) that flows through the esophagus, past the upper esophageal valve, and into the larynx or pharynx; reflux may spill over onto the vocal folds and irritate them, causing coughing and inflammation.

otolaryngologist/ otorhinolaryngologist (ear, nose, and throat [ENT] doctor)

A medical doctor who specializes in diseases of the ears, nose, and throat; often referred to as an "ear, nose, and throat" (ENT) doctor.

lesion

A wound, injury, or area of pathological change in tissue.

facilitating techniques

The selected therapy exercises that help to achieve a "target" or a more optimal vocal response by the patient.

Personal Story | Beverly

Beverly was a 45-year-old woman who was referred to me by an otolaryngologist for voice therapy to help with her vocal nodules. Beverly had been an elementary school teacher for 20 years. She loved teaching and loved the children. She was a single mother struggling financially to support 14- and 17-year-old daughters. She was active in her church and sang in the choir. She was, in many ways, typical of many adults with vocal nodules: she had a job that required excessive use of her voice, sometimes with vocal abuses such as yelling to children on the playground; she had a variety of stresses in her life, from financial pressures to trying to raise teenage children; and she tried to reach the extremes of her vocal range during choir practice, choir performances, and singing around the house. She had little time to take care of herself and relax and she felt guilty when she tried to do something for herself. She was both intense and tense.

Besides symptomatic voice therapy and **vocal hygiene** education, I used considerable counseling skills to help Beverly learn to take better care of herself. She eventually began to appreciate that if she "used herself up and burned herself out" she would not be able to continue teaching or singing and she may have difficulty using her voice when trying to talk with her family and friends and on the job. As she learned to balance her life better and manage her stresses better, some of her generalized tension—as well as the tension in her larynx—began to diminish. Voice therapy helped prevent Beverly from requiring surgery to remove the vocal nodules. ■

vocal hygiene

Behaviors that are helpful to achieve and maintain a healthy vocal mechanism and prevent or decrease vocal pathologies, such as eliminating phonotrauma, speaking in an appropriate pitch, turning the television or radio down while talking, using amplification when speaking to an audience in a large room, and singing within the optimal pitch range.

vocal polyp

A benign vocal fold growth that may take various forms and is caused by vocal abuse and misuse and results in vocal hoarseness.

polypoid thickening (degeneration)

A condition in which a vocal fold becomes edematous, flabby, and almost jelly-like as the result of vocal hyperfunction, making the voice chronically low pitched and hoarse.

Polyps may take various forms and are caused by vocal hyperfunction (abuse and misuse). For otolaryngologists, the observable distinctions and *histological* (microscopic study of tissue) differences are not always clear between vocal nodules and vocal polyps, and occasionally one may be mistaken for the other (Colton et al., 2011; Sataloff, 2005).

Polyps may be *pedunculated* (attached to the vocal fold only by a slim stalk of tissue), *sessile* (a broad-based mass adhering to the mucosa of the vocal fold) (see Figure 9–4), or *hemorrhagic* (appearance of a blood blister). Vocal polyps are often precipitated by a single hyperfunctional vocal episode, much like what causes acute laryngitis. The hyperfunctional vocal episode may cause a small capillary to hemorrhage (*intracordal hemorrhage*) in the membranous covering of a vocal fold. A polyp may form out of the hemorrhagic irritation by adding mass that is filled with blood. Further vocal abuse or misuse will cause increased irritation that results in the formation of **polypoid thickening (degeneration)**. If the growth is diffuse, it may cover half to two-thirds of the length of a

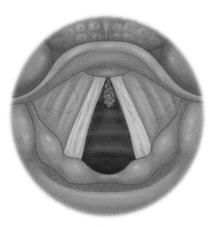

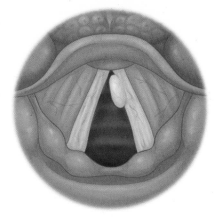

Pedunculated Polyp   Sessile Polyp
at Anterior Commissure

Figure 9–4

Pedunculated and sessile
vocal polyps.
© Cengage Learning 2013.

vocal fold (Case, 2002). The polyp, like a vocal nodule, interferes with vocal fold vibration, causing breathiness and harshness and results in a severe hoarse voice quality (Zhang & Jiang, 2004).

The evaluation and therapy for vocal polyps is much the same as it is for vocal nodules. To avoid surgery as the initial management of a vocal polyp, the "sandwich approach" may be used by some otolaryngologists. That is, voice therapy from an SLP to eliminate the kinds of vocal behaviors that cause a vocal polyp, and then surgery only if necessary. If surgery is still needed to remove the vocal polyp, the patient will likely benefit from follow-up voice therapy to reinforce the vocal hygiene techniques that were taught before the surgery (Andrews, 2006; Colton et al., 2011; Stemple et al., 2009).

Contact Ulcer

A **contact ulcer** is a small ulceration that develops in the posterior region on the *medial surface* of a vocal fold (i.e., the edge of one vocal fold that makes contact with the edge of the other vocal fold) (see Figure 9–5). They are usually caused by hyperfunctional use of the voice with persistent and excessive slamming together of the arytenoid cartilages during production of a chronic low-pitched voice in conjunction with hard glottal attacks and other vocal fold abuses and misuses. Contact ulcers tend to occur in hard-driving males who frequently experience gastroesophageal reflux (GERD) that spills over onto the vocal folds causing irritation, coughing, and frequent throat clearing. They may have pain in the laryngeal region that radiates out to one ear (**referred pain**) (Andrews, 2006; Colton et al., 2011; Rubin & Sataloff, 2006).

Surgical removal of contact ulcers is usually not needed; however, medical management of the gastric reflux is essential. These individuals often respond well to voice therapy, where elimination of vocal

contact ulcer

A benign vocal fold ulceration at the juncture of the middle one-third and posterior one-third of a fold that is caused by persistent and excessive vocal hyperfunction that is most commonly seen in adult males.

referred pain

Pain felt at a site different from that of an injured or diseased organ or part of the body, e.g., *angina*, the pain of coronary artery insufficiency, may be felt in the left shoulder, arm, or mandible.

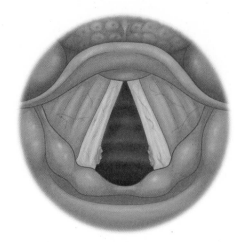

Contact Ulcers

Figure 9–5

Contact ulcers.

© Cengage Learning 2013.

functional dysphonia

A voice disorder that may be either hyperfunctional or hypofunctional and has no organic, physical, or neurological cause but is heard in patients with extreme tension in both the laryngeal and the supralaryngeal regions; the voice may have hypofunctional qualities such as low-pitch and breathy or hyperfunctional qualities such as high-pitch, strident, or hoarse.

abuses and misuses (including using an abnormally low-pitched voice) and learning how to initiate the voice gently without hard glottal attacks. Teaching voice conservation techniques is also essential (Ferrand, 2012).

Functional Dysphonia

Functional dysphonia may be the diagnosis when an otolaryngologist has determined that there is no organic, physical, or neurological cause for a voice disorder. Patients with functional dysphonia may have severely disturbed voices with a range of vocal symptoms, from hypofunctional vocal folds that produce a low-pitched, breathy voice to hyperfunctional vocal folds that produce a high-pitched, tense, strident, harsh, or hoarse vocal quality. Functional dysphonia is the result of extreme tension in both the laryngeal and the *supralaryngeal* (vocal tract above the larynx) regions. There is no medical or surgical treatment for functional dysphonia. The voice therapist (SLP) works on dimensions that directly help improve the sound of the voice, including appropriate vocal intensity for the speaking environment (e.g., a quiet conversational environment), helping establish the patient's best pitch, and improving the quality of the voice. Considerable counseling, similar to individuals with vocal nodules, is often needed. The person's motivation and commitment to improving the voice are key factors in the success of therapy (Andrews, 2006; Boone et al., 2009; Ferrand, 2012; Rubin & Sataloff, 2006).

Individuals with functional dysphonia often benefit from psychological support from the clinician. Although few individuals need referral for specialized professional counseling from a psychologist or psychiatrist, speech-language pathologists need to take into consideration the psychological correlates of functional dysphonia (Andrews, 2006; Boone et al., 2009; Colton et al., 2011; Mirza, Ruiz, Baum, & Staub, 2003).

Margaret

Margaret was a successful attorney and prominent person in the community. Her husband had held a high political office in the state and together they made a dynamic team. Margaret also had functional dysphonia and was referred to me by an otolaryngologist for voice therapy. After the evaluation and several therapy sessions in the client's home, she asked to have a session in her office so that I could see the environment she worked in.

The office was large and imposing with a massive desk. When she sat behind her desk and I sat where her clients normally would, I noticed that she automatically raised the loudness of her voice. I also noticed a noisy heater and air conditioner vent directly over her desk, which may have contributed to her automatically raising her voice loudness. Margaret agreed to try talking with clients in a small conference room adjacent to her office where it was quieter and she did not have to raise her loudness level to be easily heard. Often when therapists are working with clients with functional dysphonia, clients can make many small changes in their vocal behaviors that, together, make significant improvements in their voices. ■

Muscle Tension Dysphonia

In a type of functional dysphonia called **muscle tension dysphonia (MTD)** the voice is adversely affected by excessive muscle tension that ranges from mild to severe (Boone et al., 2009; Andrews, 2006). MTD is a hyperfunctional voice disorder. Various subtypes of MTD have been discussed in the literature but are beyond the scope of this text. In general, individuals who demonstrate MTD tend to have weak voices with a lack of intensity range and variation. A rough, hoarse, or thin vocal quality that lacks resonance and carrying power, along with a voice that fatigues easily are common. Differential diagnosis depends on clear evidence that the dysphonia does not have an organic etiology. MTD is generally responsive to voice therapy from an SLP who specializes in voice disorders (Andrews, 2006).

muscle tension dysphonia (MTD)

A hyperfunctional voice disorder in which the voice is adversely affected by excessive muscle tension that ranges from mild to severe; characteristics include a weak voice that lacks intensity, range and variation, a rough, hoarse, or thin vocal quality that lacks resonance, and a voice that fatigues easily.

Functional Aphonia

Functional aphonia is a hyperfunctional voice disorder, although it first may appear to be hypofunctional because patients speak with a whisper (i.e., the vocal folds are held in an abducted position during phonation). As with all voice disorders, an otolaryngologist needs to evaluate these patients to determine whether there are structural or neurological causes of the voice problem. Functional aphonia may have a variety of causes, most of which have some psychological foundation.

functional aphonia

A hyperfunctional voice disorder in which a person speaks mostly with a whisper although is able to use a normal voice when laughing, coughing, clearing the throat, and humming; often associated with psychological stressors or conflicts.

CASE STUDY

Irene

Irene had suffered with intermittent functional aphonia for several years, and the aphonia was becoming more persistent. When her lack of voice began to threaten her job security, she sought help from a speech-language pathologist who specialized in voice disorders. The therapist saw Irene for one session, and she was able to achieve some phonation during various nonspeech tasks. However, before proceeding further, the therapist requested that Irene be seen by an otolaryngologist. She scheduled an appointment with an otolaryngologist at a time the voice therapist could be present. The physician, therapist, and client were all able to view her vocal folds clearly with *videostroboscopy* (to be discussed later). There were no apparent organic or neurological causes for her aphonia. Within two more therapy sessions, Irene was able to achieve and sustain good phonation but with intermittent phonation breaks when talking about certain job stresses. The therapist recognized that she needed to work with another professional to help her manage some personal stresses in her life and that by having a functional and generally reliable voice she would be able to better communicate with a professional counselor. Sometimes as voice therapists we can help prepare clients to work with other professionals who can work on areas outside of our scope of practice (Flasher & Fogle, 2012). It is difficult for mental health professionals to provide "talk" therapy when an individual does not have a voice for communicating. Speech-language pathologists can help clients achieve voice so that they can more fully benefit from the help of other professionals. ■

conversion reaction (disorder)

An ego defense mechanism in which *intrapsychic conflict* (mental struggle of opposing impulses or wishes within oneself) is expressed symbolically through physical symptoms that may manifest as actual illness or delusions of illness or incapacity (including voice disorders); causal factors may include a conscious or unconscious desire to escape from or avoid some unpleasant situation or responsibility, or to obtain sympathy or some other secondary gain.

The disorder has been referred to as a **conversion reaction (disorder)** because of its association with psychological stressors or emotional conflicts that produce such emotional pain that a physical symptom such as aphonia is more tolerable to the individual than dealing with the emotional pain directly (Rubin & Sataloff, 2006). Individuals with aphonia may receive reinforcing gains from their loss of voice by not having the ability to use their voice to assume personal responsibilities for life problems (Andrews, 2006; Baker, 2003; Case, 2002).

When patients with functional aphonia are able to produce some sound, it is usually high pitched, strident, weak, and breathy. Paradoxically, patients are able to use a normal voice during nonspeech vocalizations such as laughing, coughing, clearing the throat, and even humming, as though they do not associate these voice uses with the same voice needed for talking. That is, individuals with functional aphonia often do not recognize that these sound productions reveal that the vocal folds are physiologically capable of vibrating to produce sound. Therapeutically, these nonspeech sounds can be used to help patients "merge" into vocalization for speech. Most patients with functional aphonia respond well to voice therapy, often achieving a normal functioning voice in either the first therapy session or within the first few sessions (Andrews, 2006; Case, 2002; Stemple et al., 2009).

Mutational Falsetto/Puberphonia

Mutational falsetto (puberphonia) is a high-pitched, breathy voice produced by the vibration of the anterior one-third of the vocal folds, with the posterior two-thirds held tightly in a slightly open position or else so tightly adducted that little or no posterior vibration occurs (Colton et al., 2011; Seikel et al., 2010). Falsetto is the voice quality produced at the upper end of the normal range and represents the highest register of the voice (e.g., some songs sung by James Blunt, Aaron Neville, Robin Thicke, and Greg Pritchard are in falsetto, also the Bee Gees singing group used their falsetto voices for many of their songs in *Saturday Night Fever* with John Travolta).

Falsetto voice occurs in adolescent males where psychological factors may lead to inhibition of the transitional events that produce a lower-pitched, more masculine voice (Andrews, 2006). A falsetto voice in a male projects a female vocal quality. These males may have occasional downward pitch breaks, although they quickly resume their more habituated high-pitched falsetto voice. The social penalties for this kind of voice can be significant.

Voice therapy focuses on helping these patients lower their pitch to produce a more natural male voice. *Digital manipulation* (using the fingertips to lower the larynx while the person is phonating or using light finger pressure on the thyroid cartilage) can often bring the vocal pitch down so the patient can hear and feel the more natural and appropriate pitch. Another therapy approach is to use *masking* (a *white noise* [sound that contains energy at all frequencies in the audible spectrum] that is fed through headphones) while the person is reading aloud. Typically, the person will quickly and automatically begin to use a more normal adult male's voice. Once the more appropriate male pitch is established (often in the first or at least the first few sessions), the patient has little or no difficulty maintaining it.

VOICE DISORDERS RELATED TO ORGANIC ETIOLOGIES

There are a variety of voice disorders related to organic etiologies and in most cases medical management, including surgery, is needed. However, as a member of the team who specializes in helping children and adults with voice disorders, a speech-language pathologist is often involved in the rehabilitation of the voice.

Papillomas

Papillomas (papillomatosis) are wartlike growths on the vocal folds. They have a viral origin and occur mostly in young children 4 to 6 years

mutational falsetto (puberphonia)

A high-pitched, breathy voice produced by the vibration of the anterior one-third of the vocal folds, with the posterior two-thirds held tightly in a slightly open position or else so tightly adducted that little or no posterior vibration occurs.

papilloma (papillomatosis)

Soft, wartlike, benign growths on the vocal folds of children that have a viral origin and may grow to a size that can obstruct the airway.

Personal Story   Jason

Jason was a 17-year-old adolescent referred to me by an otolaryngologist. He had the highest-pitched voice of any adolescent male I had ever heard (almost 290 Hz), plus being tense and strained. He was cooperative and said he wanted to achieve a normal-sounding male voice. After interviewing Jason and evaluating his voice, I decided to ask him to do something that I believed he did not expect. Rather than asking him to try to lower his voice pitch, I asked him to try to raise his pitch "just a little." With some effort, he was able to raise his pitch noticeably. I then had him lower back to his "normal" voice, which he did easily. I had him practice raising his pitch a little higher several times and then back down to his accustomed (*habitual*) pitch level. When he had developed some control of his pitch, I asked him to lower it just a little below his normal pitch, which he was able to. After numerous successful attempts at raising his pitch quite a lot and then lowering it just a little, he was able to start lowering it significantly. By the third session, his voice was at a comfortable (optimal) 120–130 Hz. We discussed his new "voice image" and how he was going to manage when his friends made comments about his new voice.

Often in therapy we use several well-researched techniques to establish which technique evokes the desired response from the client. This information then is helpful in designing approaches for stabilizing the individual client's new voice behaviors. Sometimes we may try a new technique that we have not seen in the literature. If the new technique or approach is beneficial, it may be added to our therapy repertoire, and perhaps eventually be included in our professional literature. ■

of age but may occur up to the age of puberty (much like warts that occur on the hands of children and tend to end by puberty because by that age children have developed a natural immunity to the virus that causes both warts and papillomas). Although papillomas can cause severe voice disorders because the masses produce breathiness and harshness that results in chronic severe hoarseness, the major threat is to the child's airway (see Figure 9–6). The glottis is very small in children, and it takes only small masses to potentially occlude it, which can be life threatening. Because of the potential of papillomas for airway obstruction, children who are hoarse for more than 10 days, independent of a cold or allergy, should have a laryngeal examination by an otolaryngologist to rule out papillomas (Lindman, Gibbons, Morleir, & Wiatrak, 2004).

When papillomas are identified, they need to be removed surgically or through other medical procedures. Beyond the removal of the

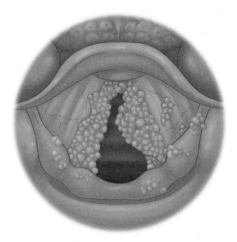

Juvenile Papillomatosis

Figure 9–6
Juvenile papillomas.
© Cengage Learning 2013.

tissue mass, the goal is to prevent damage to the vocal folds that can cause more permanent voice problems. SLPs are often needed to help the children develop their best voices and to teach vocal hygiene techniques. On a more long-term basis, it is helpful to monitor children's voices for early detection of hoarseness caused by recurrence of papilloma growths (Swigert, 2005).

Blunt, Penetrating, and Inhalation Traumas

A variety of traumatic injuries may affect the larynx, including the larynx being compressed or crushed by the steering wheel of a car (this tends to occur when individuals are in accidents while not wearing seat belts), attempted strangulation, and penetrating neck wounds such as from bullets or other projectiles that occur in war (Kleinsasser, Priemer, Schulze, & Kleinsasser, 2000). The trauma can immediately compromise the airway and needs emergency medical or surgical treatment. Later, voice therapy is needed to help patients achieve their most functional voice within the limits of their altered larynges.

Inhalation injuries may occur from inhalation of gases, steam, and smoke (all of which may occur during a house fire). The reflexive closure of the vocal folds is brief and then a person will gasp for air, causing the chemicals and heat to penetrate the larynx, trachea, and lungs. Likewise, *thermal injuries* from hot smoke or steam (sometimes seen in children with severe scald injuries) can damage the larynx and entire respiratory system. Within moments of inhaling hot fumes, the laryngeal and supraglottal structures usually have extensive edema, which can occlude the airway (Belanger, Scott, Scholten, Curtiss, & Vanderploeg, 2005; Casper, Clark, Kelley, & Colton, 2002). Severe edema of the respiratory tract may appear immediately or may develop within hours, and it can quickly lead to bronchial obstruction and death. Emergency *tracheotomy* and **intubation** are needed for survival. Voice therapy can be a concern

intubation

The passage of a breathing tube through the mouth, through the nose, or directly into the trachea through a *tracheotomy* (endotracheal intubation) to ensure a *patent* (open; pronounced "pAtent") airway for delivery of oxygen.

only after treatment of the bodily and organ injuries. However, speech-language pathologists can be helpful to the patient, family, and medical staff during the early stages of medical management by providing a functional and efficient means for the burn victim to communicate through *augmentative* or *alternative systems* (see Chapter 13).

Fires

During my years working as an EMT in ambulances in Southern California and my tour of duty as a combat medic in Vietnam in 1969, I saw many cases of burn (thermal) injuries. In those days, my first concern was pulling people out of the fires and to safety, making certain their airways were open, and treating the burns as best I could before moving them to the hospital or *medevac* (medical evacuation [usually by helicopter]) for further treatment. I remember breathing in the hot, smoky, noxious air and fumes and how drying and irritating they were to my throat, sometimes causing severe coughing spasms afterward. When I began studying voice disorders as a student of speech-language pathology, I began to more fully understand the effects of smoke, heat, and fumes on my larynx and lungs and those of the people I was trying to rescue and help. The study of speech-language pathology provides us information that helps us understand experiences in our own lives well beyond what we do in our professional work.

---

cancer (carcinoma)

A malignant *neoplasm* (new growth) characterized by uncontrolled growth of cells that tend to invade surrounding tissue and *metastasize* (spread) to distant body sites.

malignant

A neoplasm with uncontrollable growth and dissemination that invades and destroys neighboring tissue.

hypoadduction

Difficulty making the vocal folds close strongly enough or long enough for normal phonation that results in a weak, breathy voice that often deteriorates with increasing amounts of vocal use throughout the day.

hyperadduction

Difficulty with the vocal folds closing too tightly or for too long that results in a voice that sounds tense and strained and tends to fatigue with use as a result of hypertonicity.

Cancer/Carcinoma

Cancer or **carcinoma** in the vocal tract is a life-threatening disease that requires medical and surgical management. If a **malignant** lesion affects one or both vocal folds, the vocal symptom will be hoarseness (Colton et al., 2011) (see Figure 9–7). For this reason, all voice cases speech-language pathologists work with must be evaluated by an otolaryngologist to determine whether there is a malignant mass on the vocal folds causing the voice problem. As is well known, cigarette smoking is a major cause of cancers of the lungs, larynx, and oral cavity (Stewart & Semmler, 2002; Zhang, Morgenstern, & Spitz, 2000). However, cancer may be caused by other agents, including environmental irritants, chemicals and other contaminants, metabolic disorders, and unknown causes.

VOICE DISORDERS RELATED TO NEUROLOGICAL ETIOLOGIES

As mentioned earlier, neurological voice disorders are related to muscle control and innervation of nerves into the muscles of respiration and phonation. Many neurological voice disorders are associated with dysarthrias, with either **hypoadduction** or **hyperadduction** of the vocal folds (Colton et al., 2011; Stemple et al., 2009).

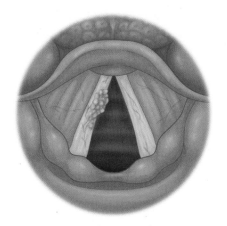 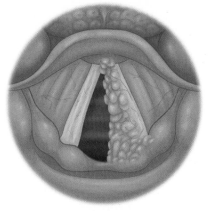

| Early Carcinoma of Right Vocal Fold | Extensive Carcinoma of Left Vocal Fold Involving Arytenoid Region |

Figure 9-7

Laryngeal cancer.

© Cengage Learning 2013.

Hypoadduction Vocal Fold Problems

Individuals with hypoadduction voice problems have difficulty making the vocal folds close strongly enough or long enough (Shrivastav & Sapienza, 2003). Their voices are often weak and breathy and deteriorate with increasing amounts of vocal use throughout the day. Their voices are often stronger in the morning than in the afternoon, making jobs that require extensive voice use (e.g., teaching) more difficult (Rubin & Sataloff, 2006). Various neurological disorders have hypoadduction problems, including muscular dystrophy and Parkinsonism (these disorders are discussed in more detail in Chapter 11).

Vocal Fold Paresis and Paralysis

One or both vocal folds may be paretic or paralyzed. Vocal fold paresis or paralysis may be caused by damage to one or more areas of the central and peripheral nervous systems, such as the motor strip in the cerebral cortex, the pyramidal tract, cerebellum, brainstem, vagus nerves, and recurrent laryngeal nerves (Loughran, Alves, & MacGregor, 2002; Marchant, Supiot, Choufani, & Hassid, 2003; Segas, Stravroulakis, Monolopoulos, Yiotakis, & Adamopoulus, 2001). Patients with unilateral **vocal fold paralysis** present with varied vocal symptoms, ranging from mild to severe dysphonias, depending on the *resting position* (the position of the folds during quiet breathing) of the paralyzed vocal fold. When a unilateral paralyzed vocal fold is positioned in the midline, voice quality is less impaired than when it is further from the midline because the healthy vocal fold comes closer to approximating the paralyzed fold. Typically, the voice is characterized by breathiness, low intensity, and **diplophonia**.

Bilateral vocal fold paralysis is often the result of damage to the brainstem, such as strokes, tumors, carcinoma, or trauma. If both vocal

vocal fold paralysis

Unilateral or bilateral loss of laryngeal movements (including vocal fold opening or closing) that may be caused by damage to the brainstem, vagus (X cranial) nerves, recurrent laryngeal nerves, or the neuromuscular junctions (where the nerve fibers connect with the muscle tissue), resulting in a weak, breathy voice, or possible difficulty breathing if the vocal folds are paralyzed in the closed position.

diplophonia

Two distinct pitches perceived simultaneously during phonation that is caused by the two vocal folds vibrating under different degrees of tension (as in unilateral vocal fold paralysis) or vibration of the ventricular folds concurrently with the true vocal folds.

folds become paralyzed in the midline position, the immediate medical concern is respiratory survival; that is, the closed vocal folds prevent normal respiration. If the vocal folds are paralyzed in the abducted position, there is increased risk of aspiration of food or liquid because the vocal folds are not adequately closed during swallowing (see Chapter 12, Swallowing Disorders/Dysphagia for a discussion of vocal fold closure during swallowing).

Hyperadduction Vocal Fold Problems

Patients with hyperadduction problems have difficulty with the vocal folds closing too tightly or for too long. Their voices are often tense and strained and tend to fatigue with use as a result of hypertonicity. Individuals with spastic dysarthria are good examples of hyperadduction problems (see Chapter 11, Neurological Disorders in Adults). However, the most striking cases with hyperadduction disorders are those with spasmodic dysphonia.

Spasmodic Dysphonia

spasmodic dysphonia (SD)

A relatively rare voice disorder that may have either or both neurological and psychological etiologies; characterized by a strained, strangled, harsh voice quality, or an absence of voice because of tight abduction of the vocal folds; clients typically do not respond well to voice therapy.

dystonia

A general neurological term for a variety of problems characterized by excessive contraction of muscles with associated abnormal movements and postures.

Spasmodic dysphonia (SD) is relatively rare. Individuals with this voice disorder exhibit a strained, strangled, harsh voice quality with observable effort to push air through the vocal folds to obtain useable voice. The vocal folds are typically held closed with such extreme tension while trying to phonate that normal vibration is prevented. In many cases, the false vocal folds also are adducted tightly. In some cases, however, the vocal folds may be held rigidly in an open position during efforts to phonate, resulting in an absence of vibration of the vocal folds and a tense, breathy sounding "voice." The voice disorder is usually insidious in onset and progresses over months or years. Schweinfurth, Billante, and Courey (2002), in a study of 168 patients with spasmodic dysphonia, found that 79% of the patients were female and 21% were male, with an average age of 45 years. Thirty percent of patients directly associated the onset of spasmodic dysphonia symptoms with an upper respiratory tract infection, and 21% to a major life stress. However, the general consensus in the medical and voice disorder literature, as well as the National Spasmodic Dysphonia Association (NSDA; www.dysphonia.org) is that spasmodic dysphonia is a central nervous system disorder and a form of **dystonia** (Haslinger, Erhard, Dresel, et al., 2005; Simonyan, & Ludlow, 2010; Sulica, 2004).

Regretfully, most individuals with spasmodic dysphonia do not respond well to voice therapy approaches alone. Most success for the voices of these individuals occurs when medical-surgical approaches are used, such as injection of *botulinum toxin* (botox) into one vocal fold to create weakness of the fold that temporarily (usually months) decreases vocal fold tension, or the severing of the recurrent laryngeal nerve that innervates one vocal fold to permanently decrease vocal fold tension. Voice therapy from an SLP is needed to maximize the benefits of the medical-surgical techniques (Andrews, 2006; Boone et al., 2009; Stemple et al., 2009).

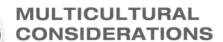

MULTICULTURAL CONSIDERATIONS

There is little literature investigating multicultural considerations and voice disorders. Haller and Thompson (1975), in their study of 1,000 African American children in Harlem, New York, found that 22% of the children exhibited dysphonia marked by hoarseness (compared to Ramig and Verdolini's 1998 estimated 3%–6% of school-age children with dysphonia). However, Duff, Proctor, and Yairi (2004), in their study of the prevalence of voice disorders in 2,445 African American and European American young children (1,246 males and 1,199 females, 2 to 6 years of age), hoarseness was identified in 3.9% of the total sample, with no statistically significant differences among those children in age, gender, or race. Holland and DeJarnette (2002) did an extensive review of the literature on voice-related pathologies in minority groups in the United States, health issues related to voice dysfunction, ethnographic and racial factors related to voice, and the role of the speech-language pathologist in prevention, assessment, and intervention. Their review of the literature on *epidemiology* (the study of the determinants of disease in different populations) of voice-related pathologies in minority groups revealed the need for increased research on the incidence and prevalence of causal factors and types of disorders among minority populations. However, the available literature suggests that health risk factors include occupational and daily living exposure to *teratogens* (any substance that interferes with normal prenatal development, causing developmental abnormalities in a fetus) in pregnant women, substance abuse, and possible predisposition to certain disease processes that are the combined effect of biological inheritance and environmental conditions. Holland and DeJarnette (2002, p. 329) state, "Developing culturally sensitive, client centered, and relevant approaches to voice service delivery permits speech-language pathologists to fulfill their roles and responsibilities as preventionists, diagnosticians, and interventionists in working with multicultural groups."

ASSESSMENT OF THE VOICE

An otolaryngologist (ENT) is essential in the diagnosis of a person with a voice disorder and often in the treatment. However, the speech-language pathologist (with clients who have voice disorders, we are often referred to as *voice therapists*) frequently needs to be on the team who evaluates and treats voice disorders. The ENT may refer a patient to an SLP after her initial evaluation and diagnosis of a patient. However, in other cases a person with a voice disorder may first contact an SLP for help and the therapist may conduct an evaluation and initiate therapy; however, therapy cannot continue until an ENT has evaluated the patient and referred the patient back to the voice therapist. In the schools an SLP can screen, evaluate, and initiate therapy with a child who has a voice disorder, but therapy cannot continue unless the child also is evaluated by an ENT.

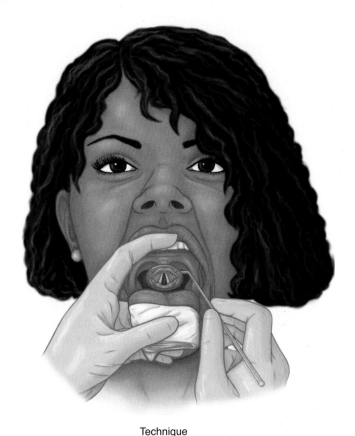

Figure 9-8

Indirect laryngoscopy with a laryngeal mirror.
© Cengage Learning 2013.

Technique

---

indirect laryngoscopy

A method of examining the larynx and vocal folds by placing a *laryngeal mirror* (a small round mirror attached to a long handle) into the back of the mouth and directing a reflected light source onto the mirror to shine on the vocal folds.

direct laryngoscopy

Examination by an ENT physician of the interior of the larynx by direct vision with the aid of a **laryngoscope**, usually while the patient is anesthetized.

laryngoscope

A hollow tube used by an ENT physician that is inserted into the larynx through the mouth for examining or operating on the interior of the larynx.

The Otolaryngologist's Examination

Otolaryngologists use three primary procedures to view the vocal folds (*laryngoscopy*): **indirect laryngoscopy, endoscopy,** and **direct laryngoscopy.** The indirect laryngoscopy examination is usually the first method the ENT specialist uses to view the vocal folds. During this procedure, the physician attempts to view the larynx and vocal folds using a laryngeal mirror (see Figure 9-8). Indirect laryngoscopy is considered a fairly noninvasive procedure because it does not require anesthesia or cause any pain or trauma to the patient (Colton et al., 2011). The ENT physician also may choose to evaluate the laryngeal mechanism by using endoscopy with a rigid scope that is passed through the oral cavity with the tip of the scope reaching near the posterior pharyngeal wall, and the physician viewing the vocal folds and laryngeal region on a monitor (see Figure 9-9). A video recording (*videoendoscopy*) or video recording with strobe lighting (*videostroboscopy*) may be chosen for later study of the images. The physician also may choose to use a *flexible fiberoptic scope* that is passed *transnasally* (through the nose and down to the level of the epiglottis) to view the vocal folds and laryngeal area (Woo, 2006) (see Figures 9-10 and 9-11). *Direct laryngoscopy* is less commonly used by ENT physicians and is the most invasive of the laryngeal examination procedures. It is usually performed in a hospital with

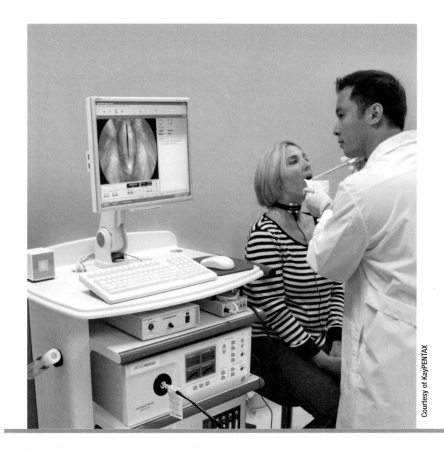

Courtesy of KayPENTAX

Figure 9–9

Videoendoscopy using a rigid scope through the oral cavity (note the microphone pressed against the neck to record the patient's voice simultaneously while the vocal folds are being viewed).

a patient under general anesthesia. Direct laryngoscopy allows an ENT physician to examine the laryngeal structures in more detail and, when necessary, obtain a biopsy of a lesion (Colton et al., 2011).

The Speech-Language Pathologist's Assessment

A complete voice evaluation includes numerous components, and the entire evaluation may not be completed on the first *visit* (appointment) with a client. The SLP must do a thorough evaluation of the person's respiratory and phonatory systems to determine the best course of therapy. However, the voice evaluation and voice therapy cannot be separated. Effective voice therapy is an ongoing, continuous evaluation process (Boone et al., 2009; Shipley & McAfee, 2009). This is necessary to be continually listening to subtle changes in the client's voice, as well as to incorporate increased understanding of the person as the client reveals more information about what may have contributed to the voice problem and what is maintaining it.

Case History

If the client already has been examined by an ENT physician, then the speech-language pathologist should read the medical report before seeing the client the first time. The first meeting between the client and

endoscopy

Methods of viewing the velopharyngeal mechanism, vocal tract, or both that use a rigid endoscope introduced *intraorally* (through the mouth) or flexible fiberoptic endoscope *transnasally* (through the nose) with a camera lens and fiber-optic light source at the tip of the scope that can illuminate the nasopharynx, oropharynx, and larynx; the structures may be videotaped (*videoendoscopy*), and the light source can be put in *strobe mode* (rapid flashing) so that the vibrating vocal folds appear to move in slow motion for more detailed viewing (*videostroboscopy*); (note: SLPs may be trained to perform endoscopic evaluations and in most states are allowed to perform them).

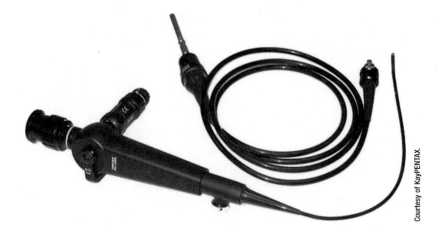

Courtesy of KayPENTAX.

Figure 9–10

Flexible fiberoptic endoscope that can be passed transnasally to view the velopharyngeal mechanism, vocal folds, and laryngeal region.

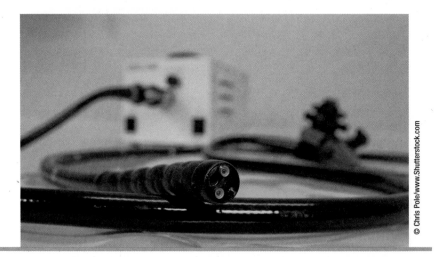

© Chris Pole/www.Shutterstock.com

Figure 9–11

Tip of a flexible fiberoptic endoscope showing the very small light source and camera lens.

the clinician is important because rapport must be established for open and honest sharing of information. The interview with a client who has a voice disorder requires some of the most sensitive skills we use during any interaction with clients (Flasher & Fogle, 2012). An individual's voice is a personal expression of the individual, and most people feel that it represents them as individuals. The kinds of questions we ask and the way we ask them can significantly influence the responses we receive.

During the interview, we want the client to describe the problem, what she feels may have caused it, and what is contributing to its continuation. We want to learn when the voice is at its best and worst; for example, during various times of the day, in different environments (home, work, etc.), with different people, and when talking about different topics. We want information about any vocal abuses and misuses. We also need to know about medications the client takes (some may have effects on the voice) and any smoking and drinking habits. As you can imagine, considerable tact is needed to investigate certain areas.

Throughout the interview, we also are listening to and observing the client's vocal behaviors. For example, we are noting the loudness, pitch, and quality of the voice; vocal abuses such as frequent throat clearing or coughing; and tension in the voice, face, and body. During the interview we are using some of our most astute observational and listening skills to understand the person and the voice problem. It is the *observational skills* (auditory, visual, and sometimes even tactile) that help clinicians recognize nuances of attitudes, feelings, and behaviors that indicate relaxation and tension in a person's body and throat. Keen listening skills help the clinician hear the subtleties in the voice that indicate positive or negative changes, or no changes.

Quantification of the Voice

A clinician may choose from several voice rating scales that are commercially available to help quantify the various characteristics of the voice. Most published voice rating scales quantify several key areas of voice based on the evaluator's perceptual judgments. During a voice evaluation, the clinician is trying to investigate the *perceptual*, *acoustic*, and *physiologic* correlates. The perceptual correlates refer to what we hear, such as loudness, pitch, and quality. The *acoustic* correlates refer to the biomechanical characteristics of the vocal folds, such as *habitual pitch* (what the person typically uses), *pitch range* (highest pitch and lowest pitch), *optimal pitch* (the most comfortable and appropriate pitch for the person's vocal mechanism), and *maximum phonation time* in seconds (how long a person can hold a sound). To measure the acoustic correlates, sophisticated computerized instruments such as the Visi-Pitch™ or the Computerized Speech Lab™ (CSL) by KayPentax may be used. The physiologic correlates of the vocal folds refer to *aerodynamic features* and *vibratory behavior*, such as *airflow rates* (volume of air passing between the vibrating vocal folds in a fixed period of time), *airflow pressures* (force of the air passing between the vocal folds), *abnormal movements* of the vocal folds during vibration, and *masses on the vocal folds* (ASHA, 2004a). Sophisticated computerized instruments may be used to measure the physiologic correlates.

Resonance of the voice, from the posterior pharyngeal wall through the nasal passages, influences the quality of the voice. Individuals who use their articulators in a constricted manner (e.g., speaking with their mandible nearly closed or with their teeth clenched) affect their ability to project their voice because they are not using the "megaphone effect" of their mouth, which results in the need for increased laryngeal tension to achieve adequate loudness to be easily heard. A hearing screening should always be a part of a complete assessment.

During the assessment, in addition to the interview and formal voice evaluation, it is important to try various voice therapy stimulability techniques to hear how they may affect the voice. In a way, the voice evaluation and voice therapy merge into one another when we say to a client, "I want you to try . . . to see what happens." When we have tried a few therapy techniques that give a positive change to the client's voice, we have a better idea of the direction of therapy.

Application Question

How would you rate the loudness, pitch, and quality of your voice compared to that of your friends of the same age and gender?

VOICE THERAPY

Voice therapy usually involves a multifaceted approach that integrates several areas of knowledge, training, skills, and understanding. Voice clinicians rely on several strong foundations: (1) a thorough understanding of the anatomy and physiology of all speech systems, but especially the respiratory and phonatory systems; (2) knowledge of the many voice disorders; (3) a thorough evaluation of the client or patient; (4) knowledge and understanding of the various voice therapy approaches and techniques; (5) training in both auditory and visual perceptual discrimination; and (6) good listening skills and a "good ear" to help recognize nuances of voice. Technical expertise is essential in our work with individuals who have voice disorders (or any disorder); however, it is not sufficient for being a good or excellent clinician. A good background in psychology and counseling is essential when working with individuals (Flasher & Fogle, 2012). Almost all skills of a well-trained speech-language pathologist come into play when working with people who have voice disorders. In voice therapy, we are confronted with the job of trying to disentangle the organic, psychological, and social factors that are intertwined in the person with a voice disorder (Andrews, 2006; Boone et al., 2009; Case, 2002; Colton et al., 2011; Rubin & Sataloff, 2006; Stemple et al., 2009) (see Figure 9–12).

Voice Therapy Approaches

A number of factors influence the design of voice therapy programs, including the age of the person, the type and severity of the disorder, the patient's personality and understanding of the problem, and the person's commitment to change. Clinician variables also are important. Some clinician variables include education and training in voice disorders, previous experience working with a variety of individuals and types of voice disorders, interest in voice disorders, and personality. Some voice

Figure 9-12

A speech-language pathologist helping a client with a voice disorder understand how the vocal folds work.

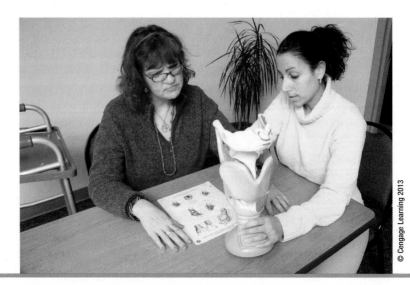

© Cengage Learning 2013

Using Metaphors in Therapy — Personal Story

Beth was a 43-year-old woman who was diagnosed by an ENT physician as having functional dysphonia and was referred to me for an evaluation and therapy. I noticed that Beth tended to talk rapidly and to change subjects often, as well as to be unusually animated, all in a somewhat tense manner. She also liked to describe herself using metaphors, such as "I feel like a turtle in mud" (i.e., she felt she could never talk fast enough or say everything she wanted). I realized that Beth would relate well to metaphors and used them to illustrate various concepts about voice and her voice problem. For example, I told her that the conversation reminded me of a race-horse rider who kept changing horses in the middle of a race; each horse rode a little differently, but she never stayed on one horse long enough to get a real "feel" for it—to finish a topic. Beth liked that metaphor and thought about it often in her conversations outside of therapy. As therapy progressed, she recognized that she was "staying on one horse longer" in a conversation and eventually "rode one horse all the way to the finish" (the end of a topic of conversation). Over time, and with the use of various therapy approaches, she decreased her overall tension and had a more relaxed-sounding voice. This example illustrates how, as clinicians, we always need to be "thinking on our feet" and finding novel ways to help our clients understand subtle (and not so subtle) concepts that help them make attitudinal and behavioral changes to improve their voices. ■

clinicians are more physiological and instrumentation oriented and their therapy tends to have more emphasis in those directions. Other clinicians are more psychosocially oriented and their therapy may have more emphasis on the psychological and emotional aspects of the voice disorder. Most clinicians, however, are probably somewhat balanced in their orientation to therapy and draw on a combination of approaches (Andrews, 2006; Stemple et al., 2009). Although various approaches may be used, voice therapy has been demonstrated to be an effective treatment for dysphonia (MacKenzie, Millar, Wilson, Sellars, & Deary, 2001). Three of the foundational voice therapy approaches are *physiologic voice therapy*, *hygienic voice therapy,* and *symptomatic voice therapy.*

Physiologic Voice Therapy

Physiologic voice therapy attempts to directly alter or modify the physiology of the vocal mechanism. Normal voice production relies on normal functioning and balance of the respiratory, phonatory, and resonatory systems; that is, their anatomy and physiology. A disturbance in the physiologic balance of these systems may lead to a voice disorder. The causes of the disorders may be mechanical, neurological, or psychological. In physiologic voice therapy, addressing the cause of the voice problem is not the focus of therapy. Modification of the inappropriate physiologic activity through exercises and manipulation of the respiratory, phonatory, and resonatory systems is the focus. This approach uses objective data obtained through physiologic measurements of laryngeal functioning to guide the direction of therapy for altering the function of the laryngeal musculature and the respiratory support of voice production (Andrews, 2006; Stemple, Glaze, & Klaben, 2009).

Hygienic Voice Therapy

Hygienic voice therapy (i.e., vocal hygiene education) is often the first step in many voice programs. For many individuals, poor vocal hygiene may contribute to their voice disorder. Some examples of poor vocal hygiene include shouting, screaming, yelling, coughing, frequent throat clearing, talking loudly over noise, and poor hydration. These behaviors are often considered *vocal abuses*. Other damaging behaviors include frequently speaking too loudly or for prolonged periods, speaking or singing with a pitch outside of the person's best pitch range, poor phonatory habits such as hard glottal attacks, making playful animal sounds or sounds of motors, and speaking with inadequate respiratory support. These behaviors are often referred to as *vocal misuses*.

Vocal hygiene therapy strives to instill healthy vocal behaviors in the person's habitual speech patterns. *Internal hydration* (i.e., drinking plenty of fluids) is often a key component of vocal hygiene therapy. Therapy is usually behaviorally oriented; that is, determining what vocal abuses, misuses, or both a person has; helping the person become aware of the damaging behaviors; and helping the person eliminate the inappropriate or damaging vocal behaviors.

Symptomatic Voice Therapy

Symptomatic voice therapy is based on the premise that most voice disorders are caused by the functional misuse or abuse of the respiratory, phonatory, or resonatory systems, as well as inappropriate loudness, vocal pitch, and rate of speaking. When identified through the evaluation process, the abuses and misuses are reduced or eliminated through various voice therapy facilitating techniques. The focus of symptomatic voice therapy is on the modification of a person's vocal symptoms, finding the person's "best" voice in the presence of the disorder, and facilitating techniques to stabilize the improved voice production. A few of the facilitating techniques used by voice clinicians include the following (Boone et al., 2009):

- Auditory feedback: Used to enhance a client's listening of her voice with *real-time amplification* (client uses an amplifier, microphone, and headset to hear her own voice as she phonates), or

Mathew and Mark

Mathew and Mark were both 8-year-old boys attending a private school who were referred to me by an ENT doctor for voice therapy because of their chronic laryngitis and vocal nodules. They were in the same class, lived near each other, and did most everything together, including, as their mothers said, "yelling their voices away." Initially I saw them individually in their homes for the evaluations and the first several therapy sessions. One of the fathers was on the school board and made arrangements for me to see the boys together twice a week for half-hour sessions at the school. They needed to learn what they were doing that caused them to lose their voices, develop vocal nodules, and then make the slow behavioral changes so that they could regain and maintain their voices and eliminate the nodules. With the support of their teacher and parents, the boys began remembering some voice therapy techniques that helped them have successful outcomes. Voice therapy is a team approach, and for children it is helpful to have both teachers and parents who are supportive and willing to help the children monitor their vocal abuses. ▪

loop feedback (client uses a device that provides immediate feedback by replaying a tape or digital recording of her voice).

- Counseling: Explanation of the voice problem is essential for the client to understand her voice disorder, but explanations must be made in ways a client can understand them and in ways that will not make a client defensive (Flasher & Fogle, 2012).

- Elimination of abuses (phonotrauma): Therapy cannot be successful for many clients until contributory vocal abuses and misuses are significantly reduced, which first requires identifying the abuses and misuses and then consciously attempting to decrease and then eliminate them.

Laryngectomy

There are various medical and surgical approaches to treating laryngeal cancer, including radiation, chemotherapy, and partial or total **laryngectomy** (Back & Sood, 2005; Zeitels, Jarboe, & Franco, 2001). (Note: A person who has had a laryngectomy surgery is commonly referred to as a *laryngectomee* and does not always follow the person-first rule.) There are a variety of types of laryngeal cancer and some respond better to one mode of treatment than another, but all have consequences for the voice. The effect of voice production capability will depend on the extent and nature of the surgery performed. For example,

laryngectomy

Surgical removal of the larynx because of cancer and includes the trachea being brought forward and sutured to the skin in the lower midline of the neck to create a permanent stoma; the pharynx is closed as a separate tract for swallowing.

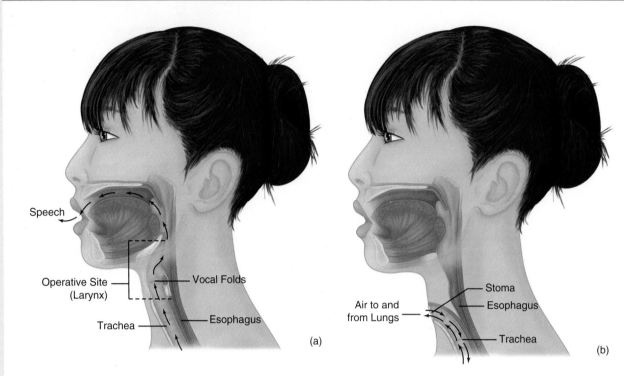

Figure 9-13

(a) Larynx before laryngectomy and (b) after laryngectomy.

© Cengage Learning 2013.

stoma

An opening about the diameter of a finger or thumb made surgically into the neck that allows a person to breathe directly through the trachea.

tracheoesophageal prosthesis (TEP)

A surgical procedure (*tracheoesophageal puncture*) in which an incision through the trachea and esophageal walls is created to fit a one-way plastic valve (*prosthesis*) that directs air from the trachea into the esophagus where it can reach the oral cavity and be articulated for speech.

some patients may be able to have just a small cancerous growth *excised* (cut out), others may have a *partial laryngectomy* with part of the larynx removed or a *hemilaryngectomy* with half of the larynx removed, and still others may need to have the entire larynx removed—a *total* or *complete laryngectomy*. In a total laryngectomy surgery a **stoma** is created in the neck just above the *sternum* (breastbone). A stoma is an opening about the diameter of a finger or thumb that connects to the trachea through which the patient will breathe for the rest of her life (see Figure 9-13).

Speech-language pathologists have important roles both before and after laryngectomy surgery. Before surgery, it is helpful for the SLP to meet with the patient and family to discuss the clinician's role in vocal rehabilitation and the various choices the patient has for eventual voice production. It is also important for both the patient and the family to understand that after the surgery the patient will not be able to make *any* vocal sound, not even crying or whispering (patients do not always realize that). Establishing some form of communication, such as writing or a communication board will assist the patient in communicating important medical and personal needs. Providing the patient and family members with information about the *International Association of Laryngectomees* (IAL) and its website (http://www.theial.com) can help them feel that they are not alone and will have a means to communicate with other laryngectomees both locally and around the world. The three general postlaryngectomy alaryngeal speech options (listed in the order most commonly used) are: **tracheoesophageal prosthesis (TEP)**, esophageal speech, and electrolarynx (Brown, Hilgers, Irish, & Balm, 2003).

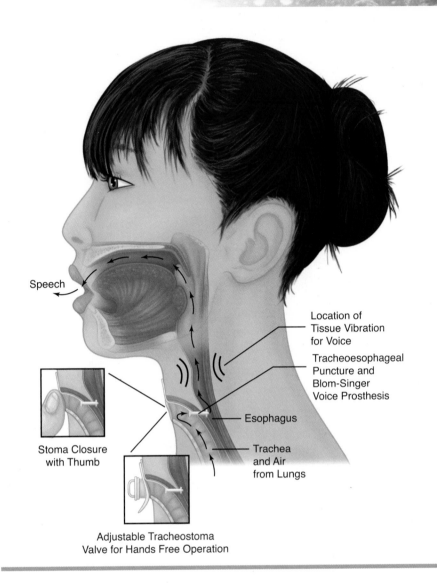

Speech

Location of
Tissue Vibration
for Voice

Tracheoesophageal
Puncture and
Blom-Singer
Voice Prosthesis

Esophagus

Trachea
and Air
from Lungs

Stoma Closure
with Thumb

Adjustable Tracheostoma
Valve for Hands Free Operation

Figure 9-14

Representation of speech
being produced using
a tracheoesophageal
puncture (TEP) shunt,
and examples of various
prostheses.

© Cengage Learning 2013.

Tracheoesophageal Prosthesis (TEP)

Many laryngectomees today are candidates for the tracheoesophageal prosthesis and many have the tracheosphageal (TE) puncture
performed at the time of the laryngectomy surgery (ASHA, 2004b). In
the TE puncture procedure, the surgeon makes an incision (puncture)
through the tracheal and esophageal walls, creating a *fistula* (passageway). A one-way plastic valve (*prosthesis*) is inserted into the fistula that
allows the laryngectomee to cover the stoma with his fingers or thumb.
With the stoma covered, air coming up the trachea is directed into the
prosthesis that sends the air into the esophagus. From there, it travels
up to the pharynx and into the mouth, where it is articulated for speech
(see Figure 9–14).

Esophageal Speech

When a patient uses **esophageal speech**, she must be trained to take
air into the esophagus by compressing the air within the *oropharynx*

esophageal speech

The compression of air within
the oropharynx and injection of it
into the esophagus, followed by
the rapid expelling of the air out
of the esophagus that causes it
to vibrate the upper esophageal
valve, which produces a low-
pitched, monotone "voice" that
is shaped by the articulators to
produce "burp" speech.

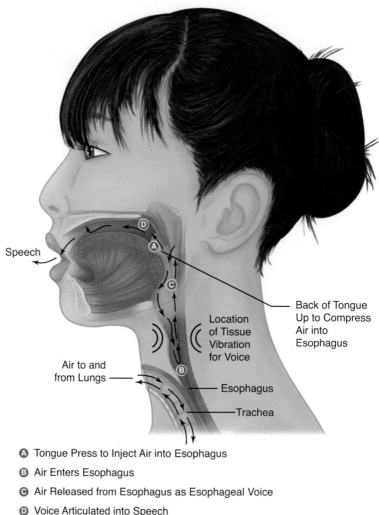

Speech

D

A

C

B

Back of Tongue
Up to Compress
Air into
Esophagus

Location
of Tissue
Vibration
for Voice

Air to and
from Lungs

Esophagus

Trachea

Ⓐ Tongue Press to Inject Air into Esophagus

Ⓑ Air Enters Esophagus

Ⓒ Air Released from Esophagus as Esophageal Voice

Ⓓ Voice Articulated into Speech

Figure 9-15

Representation of speech being produced using esophageal speech.

© Cengage Learning 2013.

(back of mouth and top of pharynx), injecting it into the esophagus (but not down into the stomach), and then expelling the air out of the esophagus. This causes the air to vibrate the *pharyngoesophageal segment/upper esophageal valve* (top of the esophagus), which produces a low-pitched, monotone "voice." The patient then learns how to shape the sound by using the articulators to produce "burp" speech (see Figure 9-15).

Two methods for teaching esophageal speech are commonly used: the *injection method* and the *inhalation method*. Both methods compress air within the oropharynx and inject the compressed air into the space of the esophagus. Once the compressed air flows into the esophagus, the greater pressure from the elasticity of the esophageal walls forces the air back up the esophagus, through the pharyngoesophageal segment, and into the oral cavity where the air can be articulated. As an analogy, consider blowing up a balloon (compressed air from the lungs flowing into the balloon), holding the neck of the

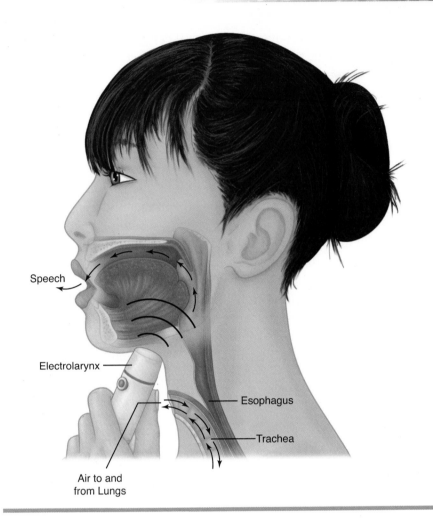

Speech

Electrolarynx

Esophagus

Trachea

Air to and
from Lungs

Figure 9-16

Representation of speech
being produced with a
neck-type electrolarynx.

© Cengage Learning 2013.

balloon closed for a second, and then releasing the hold slightly. The
walls of the balloon (esophagus) force the air out of the balloon and
through the mouth of the balloon (PE segment), producing a rather
raucous sound. The sound that the PE segment produces in the laryngectomee is then modified and resonated by the oropharyngeal and
oral cavities for speech. (A detailed discussion of the specifics of the
injection and inhalation methods of teaching esophageal speech is
beyond the scope of this text.)

Electrolarynx/Artificial Larynx

The use of an **electrolarynx (artificial larynx)** during the first few
days following surgery can provide patients a voice while healing, and
some individuals choose to continue using the device as their main
source of oral communication. There are a variety of brands and types
of artificial larynges and usually one or more will work well for a patient.
Most are neck-type devices with a vibrating source within the electrolarynx that produces the sound. The head of the device is placed against a
spot on the neck (sometimes called the "sweet spot") where the sound
is transferred into the pharyngeal region (see Figure 9–16). The sound in

**electrolarynx/artificial
larynx**

An electronic (battery powered)
device used by laryngectomees
that produces a vibrated
mechanical sound that is held
against the neck, with the sound
entering the pharynx and oral cavity
where it is articulated for speech.

the pharyngeal region moves into the oral cavity where it is articulated in a normal manner. When an electrolarynx is used, all sounds (vowels, voiced and unvoiced consonants) are voiced because of the continuous vibration of the electrolarynx; however, listeners fairly easily become accustomed to this continuous voicing, and most laryngectomees are at least moderately intelligible using an electrolarynx (Liu, Wan, Wang, & Niu, 2004; Watterson, Cox, & McFarlane, 1998).

Regardless of the method of speech a person eventually uses, all individuals with a laryngectomy benefit from counseling support provided by a speech-language pathologist. Patients undergo adjustment difficulties with acceptance of themselves as being cancer survivors, permanently losing their normal way of producing voice, their way of communicating with family and friends, social obstacles, and possible loss of employment they may have had for decades. These individuals benefit from meeting other individuals who have successfully adjusted to their laryngectomy and can encourage the new laryngectomee. Successful voice and speech rehabilitation includes the person's overall life adjustment, coping skills, and general well-being (Schuster et al., 2003).

EMOTIONAL AND SOCIAL EFFECTS OF VOICE DISORDERS

Our normal voices can reflect our emotions from moment to moment and our reactions to our voice disorders can cause us emotional distress. A person's facial expressions and voice are the two most important ways of communicating emotions. Because we know that our voices can reveal our feelings, we learn how to suppress emotionally charged cues. We want to communicate our thoughts but we do not always want to communicate all of the feelings behind our thoughts (Andrews, 2006; Rammage et al., 2001).

Young Children

Most preschool children with hyperfunctional voice disorders appear unaware of or unconcerned about the problems that clinicians hear. Voice therapy for young children is often deferred until they are in kindergarten or first grade; however, the parents may be counseled about how they can encourage their children to be less abusive to their voices when talking and playing. Even when children are in the early elementary grades they typically have little concern about the quality of their voices; to them, a hoarse voice is as acceptable as a clear voice. It is SLPs and perhaps ENT doctors and parents who have to try to instill in children enough emotional concern about their voice problems to motivate them to participate in therapy. As children get older they usually become increasingly aware of their voices and are better candidates for voice therapy (Andrews, 2006; Boone et al., 2009).

To change their behaviors, people of all ages need to be sufficiently emotionally concerned and engaged to carry out the often long-term tasks to accomplish the changes. This takes a level of emotional maturity, the cognitive abilities to understand the need for the changes, the memory to carry out the tasks, and the ability to accept delayed gratification ("If I do what I need to now, then later on I will have the rewards.").

Adolescents

It is usually during adolescence when children begin focusing on their every little imperfection that they begin to be concerned about their voices. Adolescent boys and girls may "yell their voices away" while cheering at football, soccer, or rugby games. In a way, the acute laryngitis they develop is a badge of honor—they had cheered their team on. It is only when adolescents develop chronic voice problems that interfere with verbal communication that they may be sufficiently motivated to follow a voice therapy regimen. However, adolescents are able to do much of their communicating now without their voices, using instant messages (IMs) on their computers and text messages on their mobile phones, which may have a secondary benefit of providing some voice rest.

Adolescent boys with falsetto voices may have serious emotional reactions to their voice disorders (most individuals with falsetto voices have sought help by early adulthood). The social penalties can be significant for adolescent boys and men who sound effeminate or child-like. They typically feel rejected and isolated, and are ridiculed by their peers. Because of the social penalties most individuals with falsetto voices are highly motivated and have good prognoses for change (Andrews, 2006; Boone et al., 2009; Peppard, 2000).

Adults

It is normal for the voice to change in some ways as a person grows older; however, normal voice changes should not be in the direction of a pathology (Stathopoulos, Huber, & Sessman, 2011). According to Boone (1997), approximately 25% of adults in the United States are displeased with the sound of their voices and believe that their social lives and/or careers have been affected. However, the incidence of voice disorders in the United States is estimated to be 3% to 9% of the adult population (Ramig & Verdolini, 1998). It is unknown whether some adults may attribute lack of social and/or career success to their voices, over which they may feel they have little control.

Many adults with hyperfunctional voice disorders have considerable stress in both their home and work place, and stressors in either location can contribute to a voice disorder. The voice is often a mirror of a person's reactions to what is going on in the person's life. As clinicians, our understanding of the voice's reflection of the person and of the human condition in general allows us to help many people regain their voices and then maintain them by better coping with life's vicissitudes.

holistic

A philosophic concept in which an entity (e.g., person) is seen as more than the sum of its parts; a prominent approach to psychology, biology, nursing, medicine, and other scientific, sociologic, and educational fields of study and practice (including speech-language pathology and audiology).

Application Question

If you ever had a voice disorder, what emotional effects do you recall it having on you?

By considering our clients and patients **holistically**, we can better address both the physical and emotional causes of their voice disorders and their reactions to their disorders (Merrill, Anderson, & Sloan, 2011).

CHAPTER SUMMARY

A voice disorder (dysphonia) occurs when the loudness, pitch, or quality is outside the normal range for voice use for a person's age, gender, or both. The quality of voice relies on multiple factors involving the anatomy and physiology of the respiratory system, the vocal folds, and the supra-glottal vocal tract resonating characteristics. Functional voice disorders usually are considered to be caused by faulty use of a normal vocal mechanism. Neurological voice disorders are related to the muscle control and innervation of the muscles of respiration and phonation. Organic voice disorders are related to some physical abnormality. With many cases of voice disorders, both functional and organic factors may be causing and maintaining the disorder. Hyperfunctional voice disorders refer to too much tension, intensity, breathiness, talking, vocal abuse and misuse, and too high of a pitch. Hypofunctional voice disorders refer to too low of intensity or pitch and too little vocal fold vibration. Some individuals have laryngectomy surgery to remove laryngeal cancer and must learn an alternative method of producing a functional voice. Our normal voices can reflect our emotions from moment to moment and our reactions to our voice disorders can cause us emotional distress.

STUDY QUESTIONS

Knowledge and Comprehension

1. Define voice disorder.
2. Explain hoarseness.
3. What is an otolaryngologist?
4. Why might the interview of a client with a voice disorder be sensitive?
5. What is acute (traumatic) laryngitis, and what are some common causes?

Application

1. Discuss why many voice disorders have both functional and organic components or factors that may be causing and maintaining the disorders.
2. What are some of the observations a clinician would want to make during an interview with a client who has a voice disorder?
3. Explain the use of the bell-shaped curve in understanding voice disorders.

4. Why is effective voice therapy an "ongoing, continuous evaluation process"?

5. Why are preschool children and many early elementary school children not good candidates for voice therapy?

Analysis/Synthesis

1. Discuss the similarities and differences between vocal abuse and vocal misuse.

2. Compare and contrast hyperfunction and hypofunction.

3. Discuss the similarities and differences between vocal nodules and contact ulcers.

4. What is meant by *perceptual, acoustic,* and *physiologic correlates* of the vocal folds?

5. Explain mutational falsetto (puberphonia) voice and why adolescents and young adults with falsetto voices may have serious emotional reactions to their voice disorders?

REFERENCES

Andrews, M. L. (2006). Manual of voice treatment: Pediatrics through geriatrics (3rd ed.). Clifton Park, NY: Delmar Cengage Learning.

ASHA. (2004a). Knowledge and skills for speech-language pathologists with respect to vocal tract visualization and imaging. *ASHA (Supplement 24),* 184–192.

ASHA. (2004b). Evaluation and treatment for tracheoesophageal puncture and prosthesis: Technical report. *ASHA (Supplement 24),* 135–139.

Back, G., & Sood, S. (2005). The management of early laryngeal cancer: Options for patients and therapists. *Current Opinions in Otolaryngology and Head and Neck Surgery, 13,* 85–91.

Baker, J. (2003). Psychogenic voice disorders and traumatic stress experience: A discussion paper with two case reports. *Journal of Voice, 17*(3), 308–313.

Belanger, H., Scott, S., Scholten, J., Curtiss, G., & Vanderploeg, R. (2005). Utility of mechanism-of-injury-based assessment and treatment: Blast injury program case illustration. *Journal of Rehabilitation Research and Development, 42*(4), 403–412.

Boone, D. R. (1997). *Is your voice telling on you* (2nd ed.). Clifton Park, NY: Delmar Cengage Learning.

Boone, D. R., McFarlane, S. C., & Von Berg, S. L. (2009). *The voice and voice therapy* (8th ed.). Boston, MA: Pearson Allyn and Bacon.

Brown, D. H., Hilgers, F., Irish, J., & Balm, A. (2003). Postlaryngectomy voice rehabilitation: State of the art at the millennium. *World Journal of Surgery, 27*(7), 824–831.

Case, J. L. (2002). *Clinical management of voice disorders* (4th ed.). Austin, TX: Pro-Ed.

Casper, J., Clark, W., Kelley, R., & Colton, R. (2002). Laryngeal and phonatory status after burn/inhalation injury: A long-term follow-up study. *Journal of Burn Care and Rehabilitation, 23*(4), 235–243.

Colton, R. H., Casper, J. K., & Leonard, R. (2011). *Understanding voice problems: A physiological perspective for diagnosis and treatment* (4th ed.). Philadelphia, PA: Lippincott Williams & Wilkins.

Curry, R. (1940). *The mechanism of the human voice.* New York, NY: Longmans, Green & Co.

Duff, M. C., Proctor, A., & Yairi, E. (2004). Prevalence of voice disorders in African American and European American preschoolers. *Journal of Voice, 18*(3), 348–353.

Ferrand, C. T. (2012). *Voice disorders: Scope of theory and practice.* San Antonio, Tx: Pearson/Allyn & Bacon.

Fink, R. (1975). *The human larynx: A functional study.* New York, NY: Raven Press.

Flasher, L. V., & Fogle, P. T. (2012). *Counseling skills for speech-language pathologists and audiologists* (2nd ed.). Clifton Park, NY: Delmar Cengage Learning.

Haller, R. M., & Thompson, E. A. (1975). Prevalence of speech, language, and hearing disorders among Harlem children. *Journal of the National Medical Association, 4*, 299–306.

Haslinger, B., Erhard, P., Dresel, C., Castrop, F., Roettinger, M., & Ceballos-Baumann, A. (2005). Silent event-related fMRI reveals reduced sensorimotor activation in laryngeal dystonia. *Otolaryngology—Head and Neck Surgery, 133*(5), 654–656.

Holland, R. W., & DeJarnette, G. (2002). Voice and voice disorders. In D. Battle (Ed.). *Communication Disorders in Multicultural Populations* (3rd ed.). Boston, MA: Butterworth-Heinemann.

Kleinsasser, N., Priemer, F., Schulze, W., & Kleinsasser, O. (2000). External trauma to the larynx: Classification, diagnosis, therapy. *European Archives of Oto-Rhino-Laryngology, 257*(8), 439–444.

Lindman, J., Gibbons, M., Morleir, R., & Wiatrak, B. (2004). Voice quality of prepubescent children with quiescent recurrent respiratory papillomatosis. *International Journal of Pediatric Otorhinolaryngology, 68*(5), 529–536.

Liu, H., Wan, M., Wang, S., & Niu, H. (2004). Aerodynamic characteristics of laryngectomee breathing quality and speaking with the electrolarynx. *Journal of Voice, 18*(4), 567–577.

Loughran, S., Alves, C., & MacGregor, F. B. (2002). Current etiology of unilateral vocal fold paralysis in a teaching hospital in the West of Scotland. *Journal of Laryngology and Otology, 116*(11), 907–910.

MacKenzie, K., Millar, A., Wilson, J., Sellars, C., & Deary, I. (2001). Is voice therapy an effective treatment for dysphonia? A randomized controlled trial. *British Medical Journal, 323*, 658–663.

Marchant, H., Supiot, F., Choufani, G., & Hassid, S. (2003). Bilateral vocal fold palsy caused by chronic axonal neuropathy. *Journal of Laryngology and Otology, 117*(5), 414–416.

Merrill, R. M., Anderson, A. E., & Sloan, A. (2011). Quality of life indicators according to voice disorders and voice-related conditions. *Laryngoscope, 121*(9), 2004–2010.

Mirza, N., Ruiz, C., Baum, E. D., & Staub, J. P. (2003). The prevalence of major psychiatric pathologies in patients with voice disorders. *Ear, Nose, and Throat Journal, 82*(10), 808–814.

Peppard, R. C. (2000). Functional falsetto. In J. C. Stemple (Ed.), *Voice Therapy: Clinical Studies*. Clifton Park, NY: Delmar Cengage Learning.

Ramig, L. O., & Verdolini, K. (1998). Treatment efficacy: Voice disorders. *Journal of Speech-Language-Hearing Research, 41*, 101–116.

Rammage, L., Morrison, M., & Nichol, H. (2001). *Management of the voice and its disorders* (2nd ed.). Clifton Park, NY: Delmar Cengage Learning.

Rees, C. J., & Belafsky, P. C. (2008). Laryngopharyngeal reflux. In R. Leonard & K. Kendall (Eds.), *Dysphagia assessment and treatment: A team approach*. San Diego, CA: Plural Publishing.

Rubin, J. S., & Sataloff, R. T. (2006). *Diagnosis and treatment of voice disorders* (3rd ed.). San Diego, CA: Plural Publishing.

Sataloff, R. T. (Ed.). (2005). *Professional voice: The science and art of clinical care* (3rd ed.). Clifton Park, NY: Delmar Cengage Learning.

Scherer, R. C. (2006). Laryngeal function during phonation. In J. S. Rubin & R. T. Sataloff (Eds.), *Diagnosis and treatment of voice disorders* (3rd ed.). San Diego, CA: Plural Publishing.

Schuster, M., Lohscheller, J., Kummer, P., Hoppe, U., Eysholdt, U., & Rosanowski, F. (2003). Quality of life in laryngectomees after prosthetic voice restoration. *Folia Phoniatrica, 55*(5), 211–219.

Schweinfurth, J. M., Billante, M., & Courey, M. S. (2002). Risk factors and demographics in patients with spasmodic dysphonia. *Laryngoscope, 112*(2), 220–223.

Segas, J., Stravroulakis, P., Monolopoulos, L., Yiotakis, J., & Adamopoulus, G. (2001). Management of bilateral vocal fold paralysis: Experience at the University of Athens. *Otolaryngology—Head and Neck Surgery, 124*, 68–71.

Seikel, J. A., King, D. W., & Drumright, D. G. (2010). *Anatomy & physiology for speech, language, and hearing* (4th ed.). Clifton Park, NY: Delmar Cengage Learning.

Shipley, K. G., & McAfee, J. G. (2009). *Assessment in speech-language pathology: A resource manual* (4th ed.). Clifton Park, NY: Delmar Cengage Learning.

Shrivastav, R., & Sapienza, C. (2003). Objective measures of breathy voice quality obtained during an auditory model. *Journal of Acoustical Society of America, 114*(4), 2217–2224.

Simonyan, K., & Ludlow, C. L. (2010). Abnormal activation of the primary somatosensory cortex in spasmodic dysphonia: An fMRI study. *Cerebral Cortex 20*(11), 2749–2759.

Stathopoulos, E. T., Huber, J. E., & Sessman, J. E. (2011). Changes in acoustic characteristics of the voice across the life span: Measures from individuals 4–92 years of age. *Journal of Speech, Language, and Hearing Research, 54,* 1011–1021.

Stemple, J., Glaze, L., & Klaben, B. (2009). *Clinical voice pathology* (4th ed.). San Diego, CA: Plural Publishing.

Stevenson, S., & Guthrie, G. (1949). *A history of otolaryngology.* Edinburgh, Scotland: E. & S. Livingston.

Stewart, B. W., & Semmler, P. C. (2002). Establishing causation of laryngeal cancer by environmental tobacco smoke. *Medical Journal of Australia, 176,* 113–116.

Sulica, L. (2004). Contemporary management of spasmodic dysphonia. *Current Opinion in Otolaryngology & Head and Neck Surgery, 12*(6), 543–548.

Swigert, N. B. (2005). *The source for children's voice disorders.* East Moline, IL: Lingui Systems.

Titze, I. R. (2000). *Principles of voice production* (2nd ed.). Iowa City, IA: National Center for Voice and Speech.

Watterson, T. L., Cox, T., & McFarlane, S. C. (1998). Speech intelligibility using four different electric-neck larynges. *Phonoscope, 1,* 21–26.

Woo, P. (2006). *Stroboscopy.* San Diego, CA: Plural Publishing.

Wright, J. (1941). *A history of laryngology and rhinology* (2nd ed.). Philadelphia, PA: Lea and Febiger.

Zeitels, S. M., Jarboe, J., & Franco, R. A. (2001). Phonosurgical reconstruction of early glottic cancer. *The Laryngoscope, 111*(10), 1862–1865.

Zhang, Z. F., & Jiang, J. J. (2004). Chaotic vibration of a vocal fold model with a unilateral polyp. *The Journal of the Acoustical Society of America, 115*(3), 1266–1269.

Zhang, Z. F., Morgenstern, H., & Spitz, M. R. (2000). Environmental tobacco smoke, mutant sensitivity and head and neck squamous cell carcinoma. *Cancer Epidemiology Biomarkers Prevention, 9,* 1043–1049.

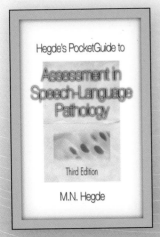
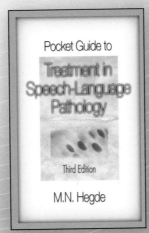
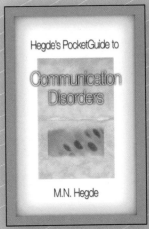
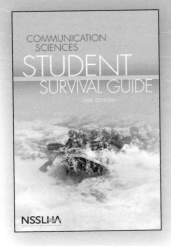

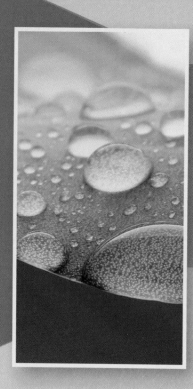

CHAPTER 10
Cleft Lip and Palate

LEARNING OBJECTIVES

After studying this chapter, you will:

- Know how to describe the various types of clefts of the lip and palates.

- Be able to discuss the anomalies and disorders associated with clefts.

- Understand the need for a team approach to help the child and family.

- Be aware of the complexity of cleft lip and palate repair.

- Understand the involvement of the speech-language pathologist from the formation of the team into, in some cases, the patient's adulthood.

- Describe common speech-language pathology evaluation techniques.

- Be familiar with general therapy techniques for children with structurally competent velopharyngeal mechanisms to help them use more normal oral resonance.

- Understand some of the emotional and social effects of a child's cleft lip or palate on the parents and the child.

KEY TERMS

anesthesia

atrophy

cul-de-sac resonance

denasal/denasality

Eustachian (auditory) tube

glottal stops

hypernasal/hypernasality

hyponasal/hyponasality

interdisciplinary team

intraoral breath pressure

nasal air emission/nasal escape

nasometer

nasopharyngoscopy

palatal fistula

palatal lift

palatal obturator

palatoplasty

pharyngeal fricatives

pharyngoplasty

pressure-airflow technique

prosthetic device (prosthesis)

rule of 10s

social worker

speech bulb obturator

submucous cleft

teratogen

velopharyngeal incompetence (inadequacy, insufficiency, dysfunction)

CHAPTER OUTLINE

Introduction

Etiologies of Cleft Lip and Palate

Clefts of the Lip and Alveolar Ridge

Clefts of the Hard and Soft Palates

    Submucous Clefts

Multicultural Considerations

Associated Problems with Cleft Lip and Palate

    Feeding

    Hearing

    Dental Anomalies

    Resonance Disorders

    Articulation and Phonological Disorders

    Language Delays and Differences

Surgical Management of Cleft Lip and Palate

    Cleft Lip and Nose Repair

    Primary Surgery for Cleft Palate Repair

Speech and Resonance Evaluation

    Noninstrumental Tests

    Instrumental Procedures

Speech Therapy

    The First Years

    Preschool Through School Age

Speech Appliances (Prosthetic Devices, Prostheses)

Multicultural Considerations

Emotional and Social Effects of Cleft Lip and Palate

    Parents' Initial Shock and Adjustment

    Children's Preschool and Early Elementary School Years

    School-Age Years

    Adolescents

    Adults

Chapter Summary

Study Questions

References

INTRODUCTION

Hippocrates (400 B.C.) mentioned cleft lip but not cleft palate in his writings. For centuries clefts were considered to be caused by syphilis, and it was not until 1556 that Pierre Franco recognized that clefts of the lip and palate were congenital disorders. Cleft lip is sometimes referred to as "harelip," a term now considered inaccurate and insensitive. The term originated in the 16th century when a French doctor referred to a patient with a cleft as having the "lip of a hare [rabbit]," which was later shortened in English to "harelip." During the dark ages of history and into the 17th century, there was superstition that children born with cleft lips were born to women who, when pregnant, were frightened by the devil, who had assumed the shape of a hare. A woman who gave birth to an infant with a cleft lip was assumed to have had relations with the devil, and both she and the infant were put to death.

A variety of clefts can occur. Some clefts affect just the lip, either unilaterally or bilaterally; others affect the hard palate; and still others affect just the soft palate. The most severe clefts occur when all three structures are involved. One other form of cleft may occur when the mucosal tissue covering the hard palate is intact but there is a small hole (*fistula*) in the hard palate. A cleft of any type is not painful to the infant because the cleft is not a wound but a malformation; therefore, the tissue around the cleft is not tender or sore to touch.

The latest worldwide data (30 countries) from the WHO reveals that the overall prevalence of cleft lip and/or cleft palate is approximately 1 in 1,000 births (9.92 per 10,000) (International Perinatal Database of Typical Oral Clefts, 2011).

Hippocrates

Hippocrates (460–377 B.C.) was a Greek physician. He is called the "father of medicine" because he introduced a scientific approach to healing by seeking physical causes of disease rather than magic, superstition, possession of evil spirits, or disfavor of the gods. He also compiled case records of illnesses, including results of treatments administered, and developed the art of ethical bedside care. He believed that the body must be treated as a whole and not just a series of parts (the beginning of *holistic* [wholistic] medicine, a philosophic approach that considers a person is more than the sum of his parts). He believed in the natural healing process of rest, good diet, fresh air, and cleanliness. He was also the first physician to hold the belief that thoughts, ideas, and feelings come from the brain and not the heart (Asimov, 1982).

The "Hippocratic oath" is attributed to Hippocrates and serves as an ethical guide for all medical professions, including speech-language pathology and audiology. The oath reads, in part, as follows (Collier, 1910):

To consider dear to me as my parents him who taught me this art . . . I will prescribe regimen for the good of my patients according to my ability and my judgment and never do harm to anyone. . . . In every house where I come I will enter only for the good of my patients, keeping myself far from all intentional ill-doing. . . . All that may come to my knowledge in the exercise of my profession or outside of my profession or in daily commerce with men, which ought not to be spread abroad, I will keep secret and will never reveal. If I keep this oath faithfully, may I enjoy my life and practice my art, respected by all men and in all times, but if I depart from it or violate it, may the contrary be my lot.

Note: The basis of the ASHA Code of Ethics is the Hippocratic Oath.

ETIOLOGIES OF CLEFT LIP AND PALATE

No single cause or etiological model can explain the occurrence of cleft lip, cleft palate, or both. Clefts may be caused by single genes, chromosomal disorders, or intrauterine environmental factors. A cleft is a feature in more than 300 genetic syndromes (e.g., Apert syndrome, Crouzon syndrome, Pfeiffer syndrome, Pierre Robin sequence, Rett syndrome, Stickler syndrome, Treacher Collins syndrome, and velocardiofacial syndrome). When a child has a cleft lip, cleft palate, or both, it is reasonable to consider the possibility that a syndrome is involved. Likewise, when a child has a syndrome, it is wise to look closely for any type of clefting. People without syndromes may have clefts and their clefts may be the result of a single *mutant* (abnormal) gene (Sekhon, Ethunandan, Markus, Krishnan, & Rao, 2011; Mitchell & Risch, 1992).

Most human traits, however, are *multifactorial;* that is, there are probably several genes, possibly combined with environmental factors (e.g., maternal nutrition), that determine the expression of traits such as height, hair color, and eye color, as well as intelligence and other cognitive traits. The multifactorial model suggests that there is a "threshold" at which sufficient predisposing factors (genetic and environmental) cause an abnormality to occur, whether it is a cleft or some other abnormality. The multifactorial model is widely accepted as an explanation of clefts without accompanying syndromes (Peterson-Falzone, Hardin-Jones, & Karnell, 2010; Rahimov, Jugessur, & Murray, 2012).

During the first trimester of pregnancy, the embryo is particularly vulnerable to the influences of harmful agents or **teratogens**, including cigarettes, alcohol, drugs, and some medications (e.g., antiseizure medications) (Diehl & Erickson, 1997; Ericson, Kallen, & Westeholm, 1979; Khoury, Gomez-Farias, & Mulinare, 1989; Koren, Pastuszak, & Ito, 1998; Sampson, 2000). Peterson-Falzone et al. (2010) state that the influence of various illegal drugs on the incidence of birth defects has been under investigation for years. Many babies with structural (e.g., clefts) and neurological deficits have parents who abuse multiple substances

teratogen

Any substance, agent, or process that interferes with prenatal development, causing the formation of one or more developmental abnormalities in a fetus.

(tobacco, alcohol, marijuana, cocaine, heroin, etc.). For this reason, it is nearly impossible to segregate the effects of these various substances. Maternal nutritional deficiencies have been implicated in causing clefts and other malformations. In particular, inadequate folic acid in the maternal diet may affect embryonic and fetal development (Rosenblatt, 1995).

CLEFTS OF THE LIP AND ALVEOLAR RIDGE

Recall that the central (*median*) and side (*lateral*) portions of the upper lip have fused by eight weeks gestation and have formed the three segments of the lip: left side, middle (philtrum), and right side (the small philtril ridges are the fusion lines). There are various types of cleft lip and different degrees of severity. An *incomplete cleft lip* can be as minor as a small notch in the lip tissue with no involvement of the alveolar ridge (see Figure 10–1a). In more severe cases, the cleft may extend on one side through what would have been the philtral ridge up to the floor of the nostril (*unilateral complete cleft lip*) (Figure 10–1b and 10–1c). More severe yet is when there are clefts through both sides of the lip that extend to the floor of the nostrils (*bilateral complete cleft lip*) (Figure 10–1d). The more severe the cleft of the lip, the more likely the alveolar ridge will be involved as well as the hard and soft palates. When a bilateral cleft lip extends through the alveolar ridge, the tissue that would have formed the philtrum and alveolus is often a mass that protrudes and may cover the nostrils. In these cases, the nose is often involved and is wide, flat, and malformed.

In a cleft lip, the orbicularis oris muscle that forms the upper lip is divided and misaligned as it curves upward with the cleft. A cleft lip that extends through the alveolar ridge results in disunity of the orbicularis oris muscle in unilateral, and more severely in bilateral, clefts. Clefting can affect an infant's ability to suck and nurse. If a cleft lip is not repaired in infancy (as is the case in many countries around the world), articulation can be affected where the child is not able to develop normal **intraoral breath pressure** to produce pressure consonant sounds such as plosives (e.g., /p/, /b/), fricatives (e.g., /f/, /th/, /z/, /sh/), and affricates (e.g., /ch/). Numerous complicated dental anomalies, including missing teeth, rotated teeth, and misaligned teeth, require the services of dentists and orthodontists (see Figure 10–1e).

intraoral breath pressure

A buildup of air pressure in the oral cavity that provides the force for the production of oral consonants, particularly plosives, fricatives, and affricates.

CLEFTS OF THE HARD AND SOFT PALATES

Between the 8 and 12 weeks of gestation, the roof of the mouth is formed and fused together with the fusion occurring in an anterior to posterior direction (see Chapter 3, Figure 3–8). This direction of fusion allows for normal development of the anterior portions of the hard and soft palates

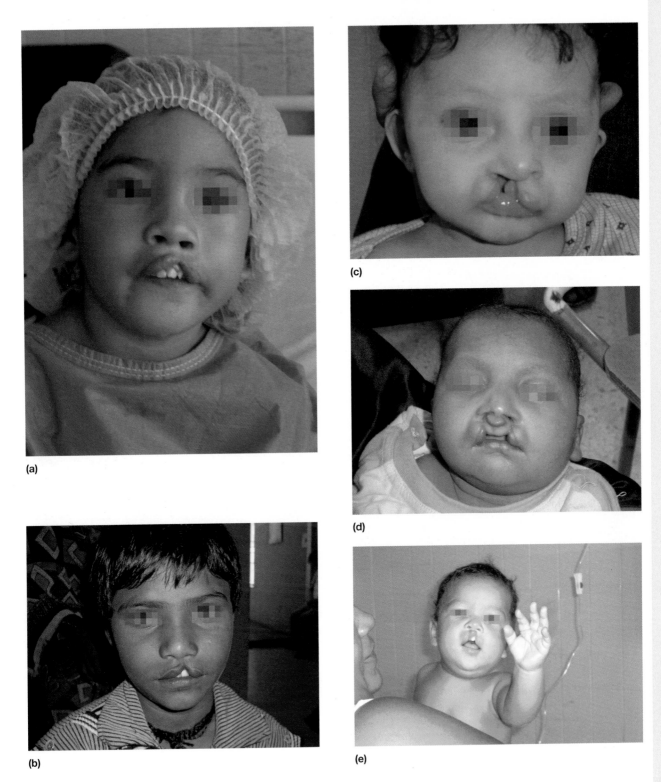

Figure 10-1

(a) Mild incomplete unilateral cleft left. (b) Unilateral complete cleft lip. (c) Unilateral complete cleft of the lip and alveolar ridge. (d) Bilateral complete cleft lip. (e) Dental anomalies are common with cleft lips and palates.

Source: All images courtesy of Paul Fogle, Ph.D., Rotaplast (Rotary) International Cleft Palate Missions, Cumaná, Venezuela, 2008, Sohag, Egypt, 2010, Nagamangala, India, 2011.

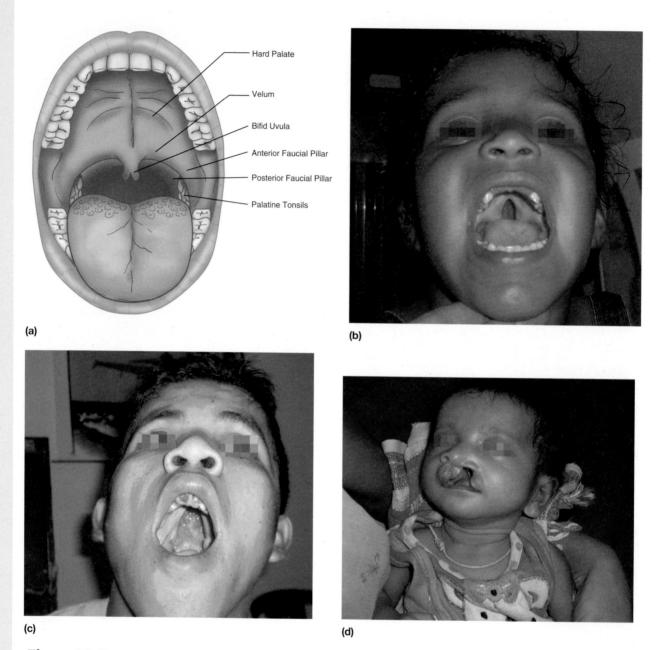

Figure 10–2

(a) A bifid uvula. (b) Cleft of the soft palate. (c) Clefts of the hard and soft palates—*complete cleft palate*.
(d) Clefts of the lip, alveolar ridge, and hard and soft palates.

Source: Image (a) © Cengage Learning 2013; Images (b) through (d) courtesy of Paul Fogle, Ph.D., Rotaplast (Rotary) International Cleft Palate Missions, Cumaná, Venezuela, 2008, Sohag, Egypt, 2010, Nagamangala, India, 2011.

and only a minor defect of the uvula, resulting in a *bifid uvula* (divided uvula) (see Figure 10–2a). Clefts of the soft palate may occur (Figure 10–2b), of the hard and soft palates (referred to as a *complete cleft palate*) (Figure 10–2c), of the alveolar ridge and hard and soft palates, or of the lip, alveolar ridge and hard and soft palates (Figure 10–2d).

A cleft of the soft palate results in *velopharyngeal inadequacy/insufficiency* (i.e., the palate does not have adequate or sufficient tissue to make contact with the posterior pharyngeal wall), which results in **velopharyngeal incompetence (VPI)** and is heard as hypernasal speech. In the literature on cleft palate and velopharyngeal closure, the terms velopharyngeal "incompetence," "inadequacy," "insufficiency," and "dysfunction" are often used interchangeably (Peterson-Falzone et al., 2010).

Submucous Clefts

A **submucous cleft** (sometimes referred to as *occult submucous cleft*) is a defect in the hard palate in the absence of an actual opening into the nasal cavity; that is, the mucosal tissue of the palate covers the defect. A defect in the muscles of the soft palate that cannot be seen through the mucosal tissue also may be considered a submucous cleft (Peterson-Falzone et al., 2010). Indications that a submucous cleft may be present are a bifid uvula and a bluish tint in the midline of the soft palate. Although the hard and soft palates may appear intact, there may be some disunity of the muscles of the soft palate that results in velopharyngeal incompetence and hypernasality. However, some individuals do not have any noticeable speech problems and the submucous cleft may go undetected throughout life.

Famous People with Repaired Clefts

There are several contemporary famous people with repaired cleft lips, cleft palates, or both, including Blaise Winter (football player); Jesse Jackson (reverend and politician); Cheech Marin (actor and comedian, in comic duo Cheech and Chong); Gale Gordon (actor); Nikki Payne (comedian from Canada); Jason Robards (actor); Lee Raymond (CEO of Exxon); Mary Crosby (actress, daughter of Bing Crosby); Nick Palmer (British Member of Parliament); Rita McNeil (country-western singer); Joaquin Phoenix (actor); Stacy Keach (actor who always wore a heavy mustache); Tom Brokaw (TV news anchor); and Tom Burke (British actor).

MULTICULTURAL CONSIDERATIONS

Vanderas (1987) examined the literature on *epidemiological* (study of the determinants of diseases or disorders in populations) studies of cleft lip, cleft palate, and cleft lip and cleft palate in African Americans, American Indians, Chinese, and Japanese using both U.S. and international studies. Clefts vary in different racial groups, but in general there are twice as many clefts in Asians than in Caucasians and twice as many clefts in Caucasians than in blacks (Chung & Kau, 1985; Vanderas, 1987; Peterson-Falzone et al., 2010). The causes of the variations of incidence of cleft lip and palate among various racial groups have not been clearly determined.

Application Question

If you were a new mother or father and your newborn infant with a bilateral cleft lip was presented to you for the first time, what do you think your reaction would be?

velopharyngeal incompetence (inadequacy, insufficiency, dysfunction)

A term generally used to describe abnormal velopharyngeal function, regardless of the cause (i.e., an anatomical or structural defect [e.g., a cleft] or a neuromotor or physiological disorder [e.g., weakness of the soft palate caused by a CVA or TBI]) that typically results in hypernasality and/or nasal emission; various authors use different terms, such as *incompetence*, *inadequacy*, *insufficiency*, and *dysfunction*.

submucous cleft

A defect in the hard palate in the absence of an actual opening into the nasal cavity or a defect in the muscles of the soft palate that cannot be seen through the mucosal tissue but may cause disunity of the velar muscles, resulting in velopharyngeal incompetence and hypernasality.

Personal Story

Working with Philanthropic Organizations

I have been involved with philanthropic organizations that provide cleft lip and palate care to infants, children, adolescents, and adults in countries around the world. These organizations send complete teams to hospitals, including plastic surgeons, anesthesiologists, surgical and recovery room nurses (my wife Carol, a recovery nurse, was on a mission to Sohag, Egypt in 2010), pediatricians, dentists, a speech-language pathologist, and nonmedical volunteers such as instrument sterilizers, logisticians, team directors, and others. The working conditions are always less than ideal, including no air conditioning (except for surgical suites), unsterile work areas, ventilation provided by open windows that allow dust, dirt, and insects into work areas, and long hours—usually 12- to 14-hour days for a typical two-week "mission" (see Figure 10–3). In this setting, team members from different countries quickly build a sense of camaraderie and pride for providing assistance to those who would never have surgical and speech management of their clefts without their help.

If the SLP does not speak the language of the country, a translator works with the SLP during all interactions with patients and family members. Most countries have speech-language pathologists who also act as translators. The SLP's roles typically include evaluating and helping determine the best candidates (*triage*) for surgery, working with family members prior to and after the patient's surgery, instructing families about feeding techniques post-surgery to help prevent damaging the sutured areas, providing parents information about speech and language development, and helping the surgeons evaluate the success of the surgical repairs of the palates.

Figure 10–3

Dr. Fogle with mother, child, and "Mohammed" in Sohag, Egypt, 2010.

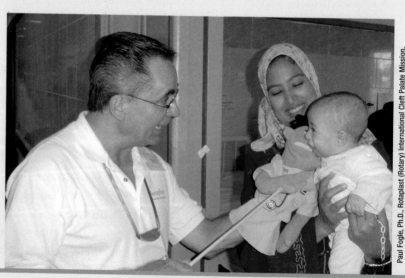

Paul Fogle, Ph.D., Rotaplast (Rotary) International Cleft Palate Mission, Sohag, Egypt, 2010

Teaching and training resident SLPs and providing inservices and workshops for SLPs and medical staff is often a part of missions. SLPs who want to be members of international teams need considerable expertise and experience working with individuals who have cleft lips and palates. Several philanthropic organizations provide cleft lip and palate and oral–facial anomaly surgery in many parts of the world. Examples include Operation Smile (www.operationsmile.org); Rotaplast International Cleft Palate Team (www.rotaplast.org); and Smile Train (www.smiletrain.org).

Culture and country of origin must be considered when developing a complete profile of people with clefts. In many cases, these factors influence families' attitudes toward treatment and even the availability of treatment (Middleton & Pannbacker, 1997). In some developing countries, treatment for cleft lip and palate may be a relatively low priority because of economics, availability of treatment, and other factors. In addition, social, cultural, and religious attitudes about birth defects affect both societal willingness to provide medical treatment to individuals with all types of disabilities and individual willingness to seek treatment (Strauss, 1985).

Because of individual, family, cultural, and socioeconomic differences, it is important for the cleft palate team to be sensitive to the family's culture and values and to listen carefully to the parents' perceptions about the cause of the cleft, preferred treatments, and expectations for improvement (Mollar & Glaze, 2009; Strauss, 1991). However, it is important to avoid stereotyping individuals' attitudes based on their cultural identity. Not all individuals adhere to traditional values and beliefs, and these values and beliefs may be influenced by, among other things, a person's or a family's level of education and acculturation into a society. It is, therefore, important not only to understand the beliefs of a cultural group but also to understand how closely the family identifies with and subscribes to these beliefs (Salas-Provance, 2012).

ASSOCIATED PROBLEMS WITH CLEFT LIP AND PALATE

Feeding difficulties, middle ear infections, and dental anomalies are some of the myriad problems associated with cleft lip and palate. Resonance disorders caused by velopharyngeal incompetence are the hallmarks of cleft palate. Speech and language problems are common for children with clefts, particularly when associated with syndromes (e.g., Treacher Collins syndrome and Pierre-Robin sequence). Even after surgical management of a cleft palate, many children are left with some velopharyngeal dysfunction that can significantly affect speech intelligibility.

Feeding

Difficulty or inability to feed efficiently is an immediate problem for infants born with cleft lip, cleft palate, or both. Severe clefts present significant oral feeding problems, resulting in low volumes of oral intake, decreased nutrition, and poor weight gain (Kummer, 2008; Redford-Badwal, Mabry, & Frassinelli, 2003). Adequate nutrition and weight gain are necessary before lip and palatal surgery can be performed. Infants born with clefts resulting in feeding problems may have other pediatric feeding and swallowing problems that can complicate the already-challenging task of acquiring adequate nutrition for growth and weight gain. Such problems include gastroesophageal and gastrointestinal tract disorders, respiratory disorders, central and peripheral nervous system damage, and cardiac defects, particularly when syndromes are involved (see Chapter 12, "Normal Swallow Function and Dysphagia," for more information).

Feeding problems for these infants typically include poor oral suction, poor intake that causes inadequate nutrition, lengthy feeding times, excessive energy expenditure, *nasal regurgitation* (reflux of milk or other material into the nasopharynx and nasal cavity during feeding), gagging, choking, excessive air intake, discomfort with feeding, and stressful feeding interactions between the infant and the caregivers (Carlisle, 1998; Kummer, 2008).

New mothers have to learn specialized feeding techniques for the infant to receive sufficient nutrition for growth and health. No single feeding method is successful for infants with clefts. A variety of special bottles and nipples are commercially available to help with feeding problems. Feeding specialists (including speech-language pathologists trained and specialized in this area) can help mothers find the best method of providing nutrition to their infants.

Hearing

Children with various craniofacial anomalies may have ear deformities, particularly when syndromes are involved. The *auricle* (outer ear) as well as the middle ear and *ossicles* (3 small bones in the middle ear) may be abnormally formed. Conductive hearing losses are common. The maxilla and mandible also may be severely deformed, typically on one side. The facial nerve may be damaged unilaterally, resulting in weak or flaccid muscles on one side of the face.

Middle Ear Infections

Infants and children with cleft palates are considered to be at high risk for *otitis media* (*middle ear infections*) and associated conductive hearing loss (Kwan, Abdullah, Liu, van Hasselt, & Tong, 2011; Antonelli, Jorge, Feniman, et al., 2011). (Hearing loss is discussed in detail in Chapter 14.)

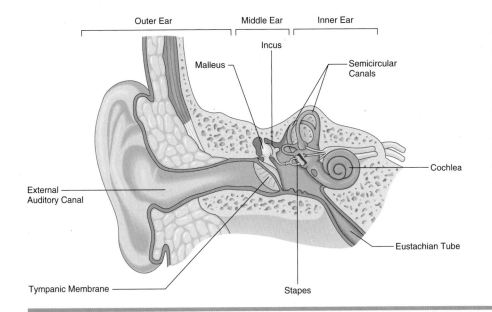

Figure 10-4

Eustachian (auditory) tube and the ear.

© Cengage Learning 2013.

The otitis media is the result of malfunction of the **Eustachian (auditory) tubes** that connect the nasopharynx to the middle ear (see Figure 10–4).

Dental Anomalies

Cleft lip and palate can contribute to dental anomalies (Kummer, 2008; Al Jamal, Hazza, & Rawashdeh, 2010). One of the most common problems is missing teeth. One or more teeth are often absent from clefts in the alveolar ridge; however, when teeth are present, they may be smaller than normal, misshapen, or malformed. Children with clefts have various problems with their bite as a result of maxillary and mandibular misalignment. *Pedodontists* (dentists who specialize in children) and *orthodontists* are essential professionals on the cleft palate team (see Figure 10–5).

Resonance Disorders

Resonance is the quality of the voice that results from the vibration of sound in the pharynx, oral cavity, and nasal cavity. Resonance disorders are commonly seen in children with clefts of the hard and soft palates. Functional hard and soft palates are necessary for normal oral–nasal resonance balance. Velopharyngeal incompetence can affect speech and resonance in a variety of ways, but in particular it can cause hypernasality and nasal air emission. The speech intelligibility of many individuals with cleft palate is severely affected by velopharyngeal incompetence. The term *"cleft palate speech"* is often used to describe the typical consonant productions, abnormal nasal resonance, abnormal nasal airflow, altered laryngeal voice quality, and nasal or facial grimaces of children with clefts of the hard and/or soft palates.

Eustachian (auditory) tube

A tube lined with mucous membrane that joins the nasopharynx and the middle ear cavity; normally closed but opens during yawning, chewing, and swallowing to allow equalization of air pressure in the middle ear with atmospheric pressure (named after Bartolomeo Eustachio, an Italian anatomist, 1524–1574).

DENTAL CLASSIFICATION	EXAMPLE	SKELETAL CLASSIFICATION	EXAMPLE
Class I Occlusion The mesiobuccal cusp of the upper molar occludes in the buccal groove of the lower molar. The remaining teeth are arranged upon a smoothly curving line.	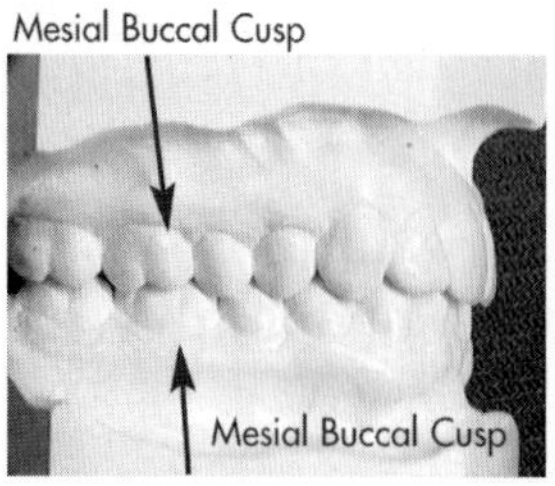 *Mesial Buccal Cusp* *Mesial Buccal Cusp*	**Class I–Normal**	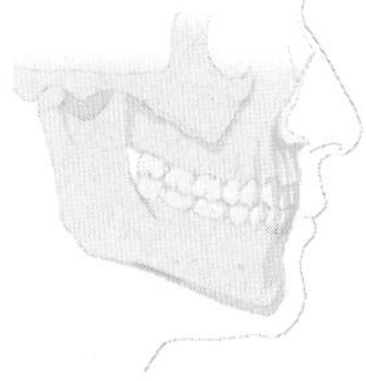
Class I Malocclusion Normal relationship of the molars, but line of occlusion is incorrect because of malpositioned teeth, rotations, or other causes.	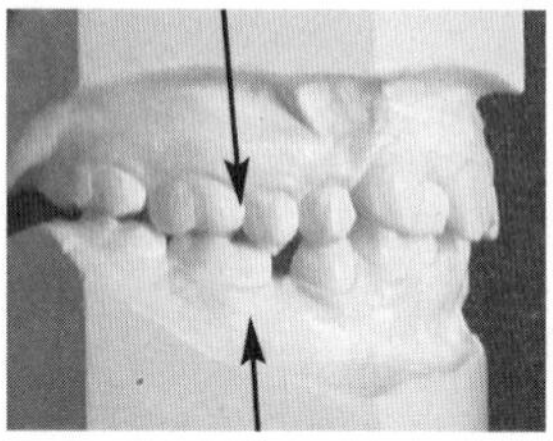	**Class I–Normal**	
Class II Malocclusion Lower molar distally positioned relative to upper molar; line of occlusion is not specified.	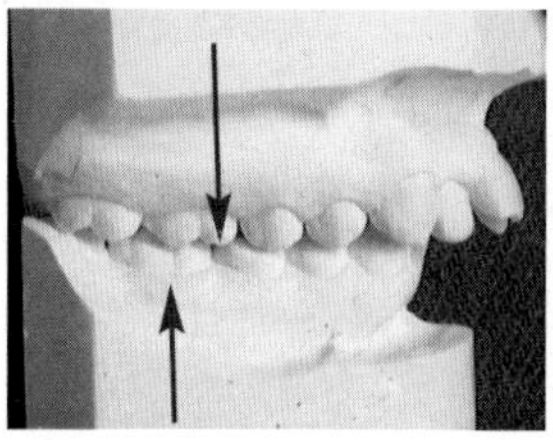	**Class II–Mandibular Retrusion and/or Maxillary Protrusion**	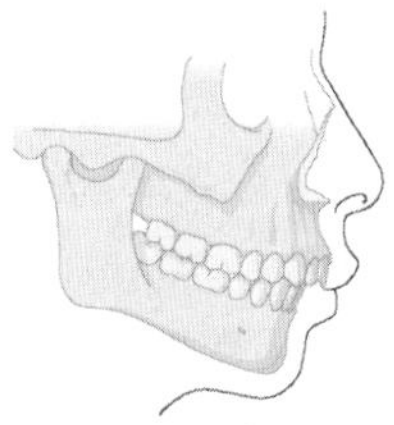
Class III Malocclusion Lower molar mesially positioned relative to upper molar; line of occlusion is not specified.	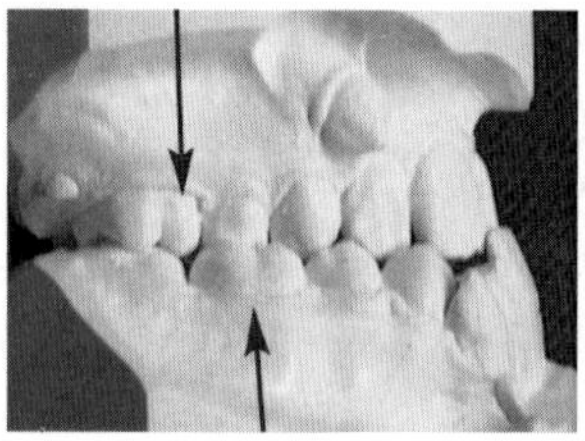	**Class III–Mandibular Protrusion and/or Maxillary Retrusion**	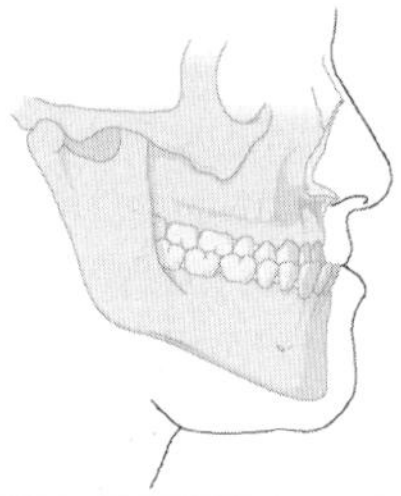

Figure 10-5

Angle's classification of occlusion and skeletal relationships.

Adapted from Kummer, 2008. © Cengage Learning 2013.

Hypernasality

Hypernasality refers to an excessive and undesirable amount of perceived nasal cavity resonance during speech. Hypernasality occurs when there is abnormal coupling of the oral and nasal cavities, resulting in distorted or nasal-sounding vowels and oral consonants. In general, consonants that require more intraoral breath pressure will force more air into the nasal cavity and increase the perception of hypernasality (e.g., voiced plosives /b/, /d/, /g/; fricatives /z/, /v/; and affricates /tʃ/ [ch]). The voiced plosives often sound as if they are substituted with their nasal cognates (/m/ for /b/, /n/ for /d/, and /n/ for /g/). Hypernasality is easiest to perceive in connected speech; it often increases during faster rates of speech (Ha & Kuehn, 2011).

Nasal Air Emission/Nasal Escape

Nasal air emission refers to the inappropriate release of air pressure through the nose during speech, causing distortion of speech. Nasal air emission occurs primarily on voiceless consonants (e.g., plosives /p/, /t/, /k/ and fricatives /s/, /f/) because voiceless consonants require more intraoral breath pressure than voiced consonants. (This can be tested by placing your hand in front of your mouth and producing the /p/ sound and then the /b/ sound. On which sound do you feel more air pressure on your hand?) Velopharyngeal incompetence affects consonants by causing decreased intra oral air pressure, nasal emission, or both. The combination of hypernasality, decreased intraoral air pressure, and nasal air emission on the phonemes of any single word can seriously affect a word's intelligibility Baylis, Munson, & Moller (2011).

Hyponasality/Denasality

Hyponasality (**denasality**) refers to a reduction in nasal resonance during speech that is caused by partial blockage (*occlusion*) in the nasopharynx or the posterior entrance to the nasal passages, as might occur when the *adenoids* (masses of lymphoid tissue on the posterior pharyngeal wall of the nasopharynx) are enlarged. Hyponasality particularly affects the nasal consonants (/m/, /n/, and /ŋ/ [ng]), often distorting them.

Cul-de-sac Resonance

Cul-de-sac resonance is a variation of hyponasality. It differs in the place of obstruction and in the way the speech sounds. The nasal sounds are trapped in a blocked passage with only one outlet: back the direction it came and then out through the mouth. The speech has a muffled characteristic, which you can hear in your own speech if you repeat the consonant–vowel (CV) combination "me, me, me" and then, continuing to produce the sounds, pinch your nostrils together tightly. You will hear and feel the air stream necessary for the nasal sounds as it enters the open posterior nasal passage, but you will trap it by the tight anterior constriction. The resonating cavity, which is normally an open tube, becomes a cul-de-sac with the consequent changes in nasal resonance.

Articulation and Phonological Disorders

The various associated problems with cleft lip and palate can have cascading effects on speech. For example, the middle ear problems and infections can negatively affect the development of speech sounds and the phonetic repertoire that are the building blocks for words, sentences, and language. Clefts can severely affect the development of many sounds. Studies have revealed that during speech development young children with clefts have a smaller phonetic repertoire and use

nasal air emission/ nasal escape

The inappropriate release of air pressure through the nose during speech, causing distortion of speech.

denasal/denasality

The perceived sounds when there is complete blockage of the entrance to the nasal passages and the /m/, /n/, and /ŋ/ (ng) sounds are eliminated; when this occurs, the nasal consonants sound more like /b/, /d/, and /g/.

cul-de-sac resonance

A variation of hyponasality that differs in the place of obstruction (anterior, compared to posterior in hyponasality or denasality), resulting in distortion (a muffled quality) of the nasal consonants /m/, /n/, and /ng/.

restricted syllables and structures in the formation of their early words, although there is considerable variation among children (Chapman & Hardin, 1992; Salas-Provance, Kuehn, & Marsh, 2003). Severe dental anomalies can negatively affect sound productions (Peterson-Falzone et al., 2010).

Compensatory Articulation Errors

In individuals with cleft palate, some articulation errors appear to develop to compensate for velopharyngeal incompetence. **Glottal stops** are the most common compensatory articulations produced by individuals with cleft palate (Peterson-Falzone, 1989; Sulprizio, 2010). Glottal stops are compensatory articulation productions primarily for plosive sounds (e.g., /p/, /b/, /t/, /d/). Individuals with velopharyngeal incompetence are unable to build the necessary intraoral air pressure to produce stop sounds because the air escapes into the nasal passages, resulting in hypernasality and nasal emission. Glottal stops are characterized by the forceful adduction of the vocal folds and the buildup and release of air pressure under the glottis, resulting in a grunt-type sound (Kummer, 2008). **Pharyngeal fricatives** also are used as compensatory articulation patterns. Pharyngeal fricatives are produced when the tongue is retracted so that the base of the tongue approximates, but does not touch, the pharyngeal wall, which causes a friction sound as air pressure passes through the narrow opening during production of fricatives and affricates (e.g., /f/, /v/, /s/, /z/, /ʃ/ [sh], and /ʧ/ [ch]).

glottal stops

Compensatory articulation productions primarily for plosive sounds (e.g., /p/, /b/, /t/, /d/) used by individuals with velopharyngeal incompetence; characterized by the forceful adduction of the vocal folds and the buildup and release of air pressure under the glottis, resulting in a grunt-type sound.

pharyngeal fricatives

Compensatory articulation productions primarily for fricatives and affricates (e.g., /f/, /v/, /s/, /z/, /ʃ/ [sh], and /ʧ/ [ch]) used by individuals with velopharyngeal incompetence; characterized by tongue retraction so that the base of the tongue approximates, but does not touch, the pharyngeal wall, which causes a friction sound as air pressure passes through the narrow opening.

CASE STUDY

Daddy Wanted to Hear "Daddy"

I was conducting a research study on the speech-sound development of 11-month-old babies with cleft palate. One of the babies produced many glottal stops. The parents were proud of their daughter because she produced this sound to communicate in an expressive manner. It sounded like "uh uh uh." She was a "daddy's girl," and Daddy was happy with the glottal stops but was hurt because the baby had only one recognizable word, "mamma." No matter how hard the father worked with her, she would never say "daddy." When I explained to him that it was physically impossible at this time for her to make a /d/ sound, he was so relieved he just squeezed his little girl and said, "You do love daddy, I knew you did!" In addition, I took the opportunity to tell the parents not to reinforce the glottal stop sounds and taught them how to help their daughter make other speech sounds with her lips and tongue. ■

Source: Marlene Salas-Provance, Ph.D.

Language Delays and Differences

Children with cleft palates are at risk for various language delays and disorders compared with children without clefts, particularly when clefts are associated with syndromes or other disorders. Children with clefts tend to have poor receptive and expressive language skills, shorter mean length of utterance, reduced structural complexity, smaller vocabularies, and poor reading skills (Broen, Devers, Doyle, Prouty, & Moller, 1998; Chapman, 2011; Scherer & D'Antonio, 1997). In general, the poorer the speech intelligibility, the poorer the expressive language (Pannbacker, 1975).

SURGICAL MANAGEMENT OF CLEFT LIP AND PALATE

Management of children with cleft lip and palate, as well as other craniofacial anomalies, requires an **interdisciplinary team** approach in which the team members collaborate and coordinate the care of the patient and family (Hodgkinson et al., 2005; Moller & Glaze, 2009; Taub & Lampert, 2011). The parents are always essential members of the team. Various other team members are involved at different stages of the care of the infant and child. Team members who may be involved at various times include an audiologist, geneticist, neurosurgeon, nurse, nutritionist, ophthalmologist, oral surgeon, orthodontist, otolaryngologist, pediatrician, pedodontist, plastic or craniofacial surgeon (Gk. *plastikos,* to mold or form), prosthodontist, psychologist, radiologist, social worker, and a speech-language pathologist (see Figure 10–6). The American Cleft

interdisciplinary team

A group of professionals from various disciplines who work together to coordinate the care of a patient through collaboration, interaction, communication, and cooperation.

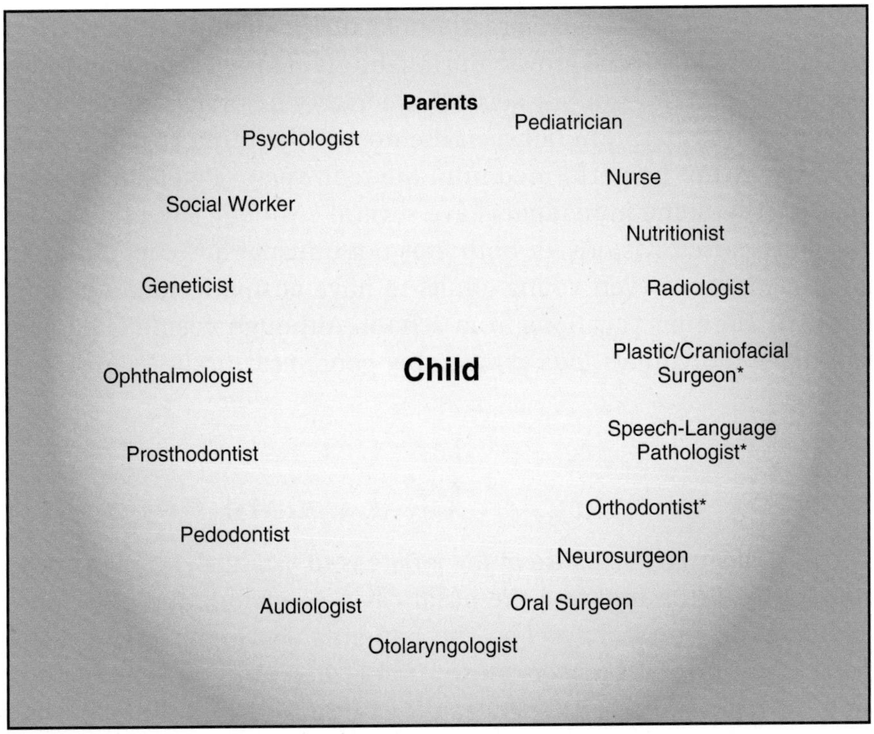

Figure 10–6

Potential members of a cleft palate–craniofacial anomalies team (* indicates essential team members).

© Cengage Learning 2013.

rule of 10s

A guideline for the appropriate time for a cleft lip repair, which says that the infant must be at least 10 weeks of age, weigh 10 pounds, and have a hemoglobin count of 10 grams before the lip repair.

anesthesia

The administration of a topical, local, regional, or general drug or agent capable of producing a partial or complete loss of sensation or consciousness.

palatoplasty

The surgical repair of a cleft palate.

pharyngoplasty

A surgical procedure of the pharynx that is designed to correct velopharyngeal dysfunction.

Palate–Craniofacial Association has established basic standards for what constitutes a professional cleft palate or craniofacial team. The minimum core professionals must include a surgeon, speech-language pathologist, and orthodontist who are qualified by virtue of their education, experience, and credentials to provide craniofacial and cleft care (American Cleft Palate-Craniofacial Association, 1996).

Cleft Lip and Nose Repair

Many plastic surgeons follow the **rule of 10s** guidelines to determine an infant's readiness for lip repair. This rule says that the infant should be at least 10 weeks of age, weigh 10 pounds, and have a hemoglobin count of 10 grams. By doing the initial cleft lip surgery sometime between the 2nd and 3rd month of life, physicians have more time to investigate other potential problems the infant may have, such as syndromes or medical complications. The infant also will have established a feeding technique that allows weight gain. However, the most important reason is for the surgery team to be assured that the infant will survive the long period (usually 1 to 2 hours) under general **anesthesia**. The goals of cleft lip surgery are to achieve unity of the orbicularis oris muscle and normal lip configuration with a cupid's bow. The size of the cleft (incomplete vs. complete) and whether the cleft is unilateral or bilateral determine the complexity of the surgery (Lazarus et al., 1998; Kuehn & Henne, 2003) (see Figure 10–7).

Most children with cleft lips undergo some *secondary surgery* (revisions) in early childhood to reduce scar tissue on the lip, improve the symmetry of the lip, and improve the symmetry and appearance of the nose. Other secondary surgeries may not be performed until there is more complete facial growth during the elementary school and adolescent years. For example, secondary surgery to straighten the *nasal septum* (fleshy partition between the nostrils) and improve the nasal airway may not be performed until the teen years (Peterson-Falzone et al., 2010). Some individuals have several cosmetic surgeries for lip revisions, nose revisions, or both. It is not unusual for older children, adolescents, and even young adults to have cosmetic surgeries during their summer vacations from school. Although cosmetic surgery can make individuals look remarkably good, scar tissue may still be noticeable.

Primary Surgery for Cleft Palate Repair

The goal of surgical closure of the palate is to establish an intact division between the oral and the nasal cavities, including a fully functional velopharyngeal system. The patient's age for the cleft palate repair (**palatoplasty**, **pharyngoplasty**) depends on whether the surgeon follows the early (between 6 months and 15 months) or late (between 15 months and 24 months) surgery philosophy (Kuehn &

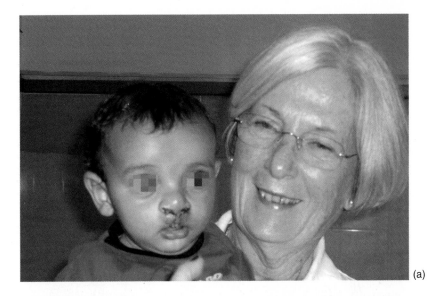

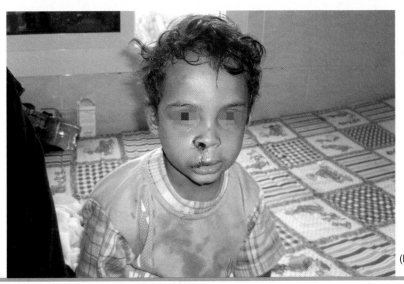

Figure 10–7

(a) Post-cleft-lip-repair patient with operating room nurse. (b) Post cleft lip repair.

Source: Paul Fogle, Ph.D., Rotaplast (Rotary) International Cleft Palate Missions, Cumaná, Venezuela, 2008, Sohag, Egypt, 2010.

Henne, 2003). Primary palatal surgery performed before 12 months of age is more likely to prevent compensatory articulation behavior, such as the production of glottal stops (Murthy, Sendhilnathan, & Hussain, 2010). Achieving a good result with palatal surgery is often more difficult than achieving a good result with lip surgery. Palatal surgery is technically more challenging with potentially more complications. In addition to closing the hard and soft palates so that they form a barrier between the mouth and the nasal passages, the surgeon needs to repair the soft palate so that it functions dynamically (i.e., is able to move) for normal speech. Surgeons may choose from various types of repairs, such as a *Von Langenbeck* repair or a *Wardill-Kilner* repair (see Figure 10–8 and Figure 10–9).

When the primary palatal repair does not provide adequate velopharyngeal closure, or when closure appears adequate for speech in

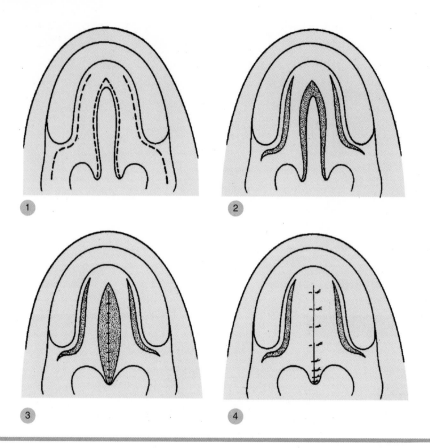

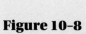

Figure 10-8

The Von Langenbeck surgical technique of palatal repair. Note the markings on the palate where incisions will be made and the illustrations of how the tissue will be moved to close the cleft.

From *Plastic Surgery*, by Joseph McCarthy, 1990, Vol. 4, Fig. 54–12. Orlando, FL: W.B. Saunders Company. Reprinted with permission.

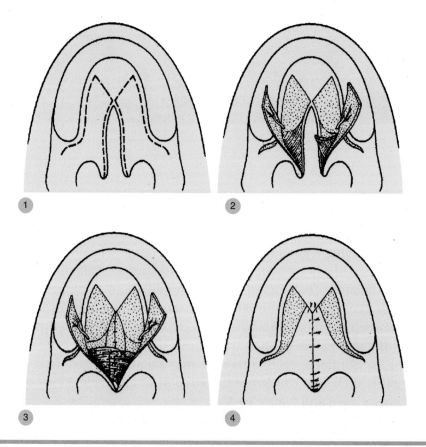

Figure 10-9

The Wardill-Kilner surgical type of palatal repair. Note the markings on the palate where incisions will be made and the illustrations of how the tissue will be moved to close the cleft.

From *Plastic Surgery*, by Joseph McCarthy, 1990, Vol. 4, Fig. 54–11. Orlando, FL: W.B. Saunders Company. Reprinted with permission.

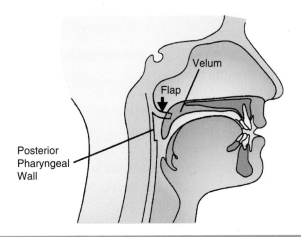

Velum

Flap

Posterior
Pharyngeal
Wall

Figure 10–10

A lateral view of a
pharyngeal flap.
© Cengage Learning 2013.

early childhood but then changes to inadequate closure as a result of natural growth of the craniofacial bones or **atrophy** of the adenoids, the craniofacial team needs to consider how to best reestablish good velopharyngeal function (Peterson-Falzone et al., 2010). Surgical approaches include creation of a *pharyngeal flap;* that is, sewing a flap of tissue from the back of the throat (posterior pharyngeal wall) into the soft palate, leaving an opening (*port*) on either side for breathing and nasal drainage (see Figure 10–10). A few surgical options are available to alter the position and function of the pharyngeal muscles (Liedman-Boshki, Lohmander, Persson, Lith, & Elander, 2005).

atrophy

A shrinking in size or wasting away that is usually caused by injury, disease, lack of use (e.g., muscles), or natural reduction in size over time (e.g., adenoids and tonsils).

SPEECH AND RESONANCE EVALUATION

The speech-language pathologist is always in an evaluation process of an infant, child, adolescent, and even adult who has had a cleft palate. The emphasis changes as the child matures. The first concern is feeding for nutrition and growth, followed by language development, and then speech development and intelligibility. Ongoing counseling with the parents and later with the child is part of the evaluation process (Flasher & Fogle, 2012).

Noninstrumental Tests

Speech-language pathologists have several simple noninstrumental, low-tech techniques to evaluate children for velopharyngeal incompetence and nasal emission (Kuehn & Henne, 2003; Kummer, 2008; Peterson-Falzone et al., 2010). These techniques include the mirror test, nostril pinching, and air paddle. During the *mirror test,* the clinician places a small mirror, such as a dental mirror, under the child's nostrils and asks the child to produce nonnasal voiceless and voiced consonants (e.g., /p/, /t/, /k/, /b/, /d/, /g/, /s/, /z/) and several words loaded with these consonants (e.g., *badges, boat, cookie, cupcake, dishes, foot, juices, kitty, pipe, safety, shoes, tooth,* and *top*). Sentences also may be used, such as "Take the dog to the park" and "I like Coca Cola." The clinician watches for fogging (condensation) of the mirror from either nostril. If fogging occurs, it indicates that the velopharyngeal port is not closing properly.

Nostril pinching (occluding) is another technique to evaluate for velopharyngeal incompetence. While lightly pinching the nostrils closed, the clinician has the child produce nonnasal words (see earlier examples). The clinician listens for a change in perceived nasality compared to the sound with the nostrils unoccluded. If there is increased oral resonance and decreased nasal resonance, it indicates that the velopharyngeal port is not working properly.

Nasal emission can be detected by using an *air paddle.* An air paddle can be cut from a piece of paper and placed underneath each nostril individually while the child is rapidly producing pressure-sensitive voiceless consonants (e.g., "pa pa pa, ta ta ta, ka ka ka"). If the paddle moves during the production of these sounds, it indicates that there is nasal air emission.

Instrumental Procedures

If hypernasality or nasal emission is detected, further assessment of velopharyngeal function is indicated. **Nasopharyngoscopy** is a minimally invasive procedure that is commonly used by SLPs that allows visual observation and analysis of the velopharyngeal mechanism (Garrett & Deal, 2002; Kummer, 2008). See Figure 10–11. Nasopharyngoscopy uses the same flexible fiberoptic endoscopic equipment as is used for laryngoscopy (see Figure 9–10 and Figure 9–11). However, the purpose of nasopharyngoscopy is to view the nasal surface of the velum and all of the structures of the velopharyngeal valve during speech.

nasopharyngoscopy

A minimally invasive procedure commonly used by SLPs for evaluation of velopharyngeal dysfunction that allows visual observation and analysis of the velopharyngeal mechanism during speech; equipment includes a flexible fiberoptic endoscope, the same that is used in laryngoscopy.

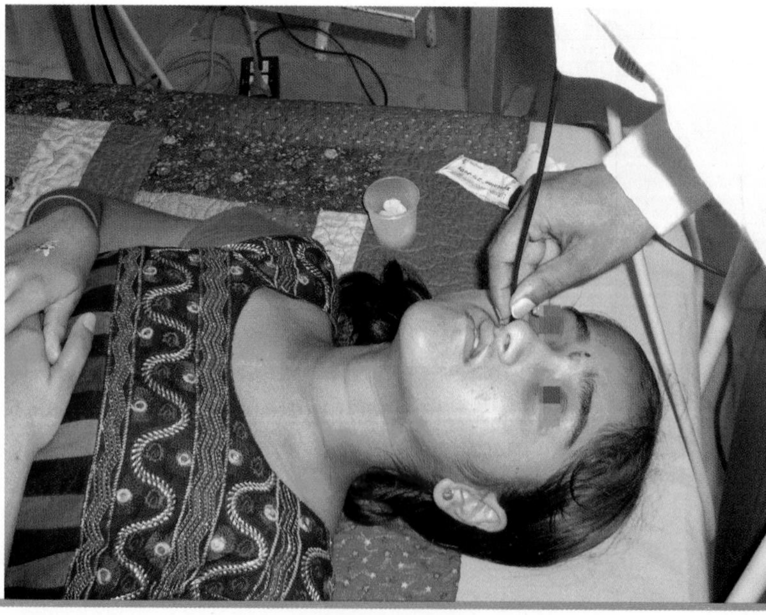

Figure 10–11

Nasopharyngoscopy being performed by an ENT on a 13-year-old girl to determine feasibility of pharyngeal flap surgery.

Paul Fogle, Ph.D., Rotaplast (Rotary) International Cleft Palate Team Mission, Nagamangala, India, 2011

Other instrumental evaluations (e.g., *nasometry*) may be conducted before recommendations for further surgery designed to improve speech (Peterson-Falzone et al., 2010). A **nasometer** is a computer-based instrument that measures the relative amount of nasal acoustic energy in an individual's speech, resulting in a *nasalance* score. **Pressure-airflow techniques** may detect various pressures in the oral and nasal cavities.

SPEECH THERAPY

Most children with cleft palates will need the services of a speech-language pathologist at some time in their lives. Speech therapy can improve their articulation or phonological development, general expressive language abilities, or a combination of these. For many of these children, the course of speech and language therapy will be complex. Clinicians must determine when it is appropriate to initiate therapy, when it is appropriate to refer for physical management, and when it is prudent to defer management of all kinds. The initial assessment will not always provide the information needed to develop a long-term course of management. The therapy process itself often must provide the information needed to arrive at a diagnosis and ongoing modifications in clinical management (Peterson-Falzone et al., 2010).

The First Years

During the first year, the primary speech pathology concerns are feeding and the development of the prerequisites for verbal communication (Kummer, 2008; Moller & Glaze, 2009; Sulprozio, 2010). Nursing staff and speech-language pathologists help train the parents on feeding techniques of the baby; however, if feeding continues to be a problem, the speech-language pathologist needs to evaluate the infant's swallowing abilities so that the problem can be resolved quickly (see Chapter 12, Dysphagia/Swallowing Disorders).

The speech-language pathologist does considerable teaching, explaining, and training with the parents on methods of speech and language stimulation. During the first 3 years, language development is the primary focus, rather than good intelligible speech; that is, during the early years, the quantity of speech is more important than the quality of speech. During these years, the clinician will likely meet with the parents periodically (at least annually) to assess the child's language development, provide further information to the parents, and answer their questions. Most clinicians are able to spend only 1 to 2 hours per week working directly with a patient and family (there are 168 hours in a week, leaving 166 without direct clinician involvement); therefore, extensive parent participation is essential to successful speech and language development—not only for children with clefts, but other communication disorders (Pamplona & Ysunza, 1999; Pamplona, Ysunza, & Uriostegui, 1996; Scherer & D'Antonio, 1997).

Infants and young children with cleft palates should be given normal language stimulation. Parents should talk to their children frequently

nasometer

A computer-based instrument that measures the relative amount of nasal acoustic energy in a person's speech.

pressure-airflow technique

A procedure using *aerodynamic instrumentation* to evaluate the dynamics of the velopharyngeal mechanism during speech; also used to evaluate nasal respiration and to quantify upper airway obstruction through measurements of nasal airway resistance.

and listen to them. Parents should avoid using nonsense words and should speak clearly, using correctly formed words and short phrases. Infants with cleft palates should be allowed to babble freely and naturally. Children should be encouraged to communicate using speech. Even though the speech sounds of children born with cleft palates will be nasally produced before primary palatal surgery, these sounds are preferred over glottal stops. Orally produced sounds, or attempts at orally produced sounds, should be reinforced even though they are produced nasally. Glottal stops should be ignored and not reinforced. Once glottal stops become habitual, they may be difficult to change with therapy as the child grows older (Golding-Kushner, 2001; Kuehn & Henne, 2003; Kuehn & Moller, 2000).

About age 3, the child should receive a comprehensive evaluation of speech and language. Parents' reports of their child's speech and language progress are good indications of the child's communication development. Resonance and velopharyngeal function can be assessed in the child's connected speech through perceptual (i.e., listening) evaluations described above.

Preschool Through School Age

Most children with clefts require intervention to improve their articulation, phonological development, or expressive language development (Blakely & Brockman, 1995; Chapman, 1993; Peterson-Falzone et al., 2010; Sulprizio, 2010). The speech therapy techniques used with articulation disorders related to resonance disorders (compensatory productions) are similar to those used in basic articulation and phonology therapy (see Chapter 5, Articulation and Phonological Disorders). Kummer (2008) provides several general therapy techniques that may be helpful to encourage children with structurally competent velopharyngeal mechanisms to use more normal oral resonance:

- Auditory discrimination training to hear the difference between normal oral speech and hypernasal speech
- Visual feedback using instruments (e.g., nasometer or pressure-flow instrumentation) that allow a child to see increases in oral resonance
- Tactile-kinesthetic training to allow the child to increase awareness and sensation of soft palate movement
- Tactile feedback using the child's fingers on the side of her nose to feel for vibration during the production of oral and nasal phonemes
- Increasing oral activity and using an open-mouth approach when talking to reduce intraoral resistance and increase oral resonance

Chapman, Hardin-Jones, and Halter (2003) made the following additional recommendations for speech and language therapy for children with clefts:

- When evaluating, be sure to include whether or not the sound inventories contain stops and other true consonants.

- These sounds should be targeted in early treatment because the ability to produce them early can affect later speech development.
- Therapy goals should focus not only on acquisition of new words but also on acquisition of new sounds.

Overall, the goal for children who have had successful cleft palate repairs and have achieved functional velopharyngeal mechanisms is normal speech. The team approach is essential in the successful management of children with clefts. Speech and language therapy should continue as long as a child is making progress (Blakely & Brockman, 1995; Hardin-Jones, Chapman, & Scherer, 2006; Sulprizio, 2010).

SPEECH APPLIANCES (PROSTHETIC DEVICES, PROSTHESES)

When surgical correction of velopharyngeal dysfunction is not an option or when surgical management and speech therapy have not been able to sufficiently improve oral-nasal resonance balance, prosthetic management may be used (Kummer, 2008; Peterson-Falzone et al., 2010). **Prosthetic devices (prostheses)** can be fabricated out of acrylic (plastic) and metal to close the palate or the velopharyngeal port for speech. Various types of speech appliances may be used to lift the soft palate to hold it in place close to or against the posterior pharyngeal wall (**palatal lift**), to cover an open defect in the hard palate (**palatal obturator**), or occlude the velopharyngeal port during speech (**speech bulb obturator**) (see Figure 10–12).

prosthetic device (prosthesis)

An artificial device to replace or augment a missing or impaired part of the body.

palatal lift

A prosthetic appliance that can be used to raise the velum for speech if the velum is long enough to achieve velopharyngeal closure but does not move well, often because of central or peripheral neurological impairment.

palatal obturator

A prosthetic appliance that can be used to cover an open palatal defect, such as an unrepaired cleft palate or a **palatal fistula**; it can be used to improve an infant's ability to achieve compression of the nipple for suction or can be used to close a palatal defect for speech.

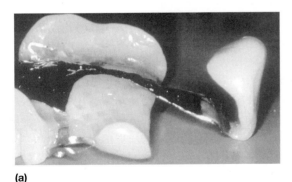

(a)

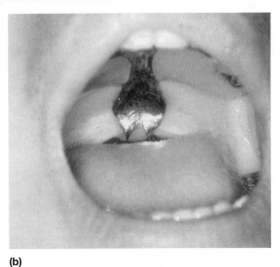

(b)

Figure 10–12

(a) A speech bulb obturator, and (b) the speech bulb obturator in place. The bulb sits in the nasopharynx to occlude the velopharyngeal port during speech. This improves speech and can improve swallowing because it eliminates nasal regurgitation.

Source: Kummer, 2008.

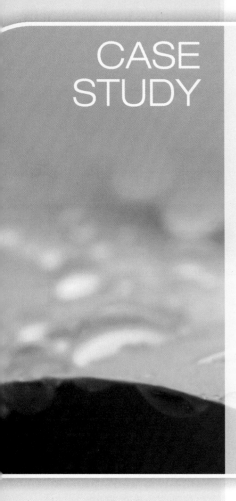

CASE STUDY

Marty

Marty was a 4-year-old boy referred to a speech-language pathologist in private practice. He was born with a bilateral cleft lip and complete cleft of the hard and soft palates. He had undergone repair of the lip and palates but likely would need more than one lip revision. He met the guideline for being a candidate for speech therapy. He was seen twice weekly for 1-hour sessions in his home, primarily to help him use the velopharyngeal structures that were functioning adequately and to learn appropriate articulatory placement and oral airflow. The parents were concerned about Marty developing good speech before entering kindergarten. The parents were obviously proud of Marty and had a series of framed portraits of him on the wall, both before his initial lip surgery and about every 6 months after to show his growth.

Marty had become accustomed to getting his way in his home and tried to avoid working in therapy, even when play therapy and a variety of motivators and reinforcers were incorporated. The therapist had to make numerous adjustments in the therapy approach, always keeping in mind the goals and targets of therapy. Marty made significant gains over time in use of his velopharyngeal mechanism and articulatory placement and airflow despite himself. Although "drill" is an essential component of much of therapy, the clinician's creativity in making the drill "palatable" is an important skill that needs to be developed. ■

speech bulb obturator

A prosthetic device that may be considered when the velum is too short to close completely against the posterior pharyngeal wall; it consists of a retaining appliance and a bulb (usually made of acrylic) that fills in the pharyngeal space for speech.

palatal fistula

Usually a small opening or passage between the oral cavity and the nasal cavity that allows air or sound to escape from the oral cavity into the nasal cavity, causing some hypernasality.

EMOTIONAL AND SOCIAL EFFECTS OF CLEFT LIP AND PALATE

A baby born with a serious facial disfigurement sets in motion an array of emotions in everyone related to or involved with the newborn. The delivery team's first concern is the physical well-being of both the infant and the mother, but the team also knows there will be emotionally trying times for the family who will be taking home a less than perfect baby (Fallowfield & Jenkins, 2004). This section is about the parents who must adjust to their disappointments and fears and about the children who develop increasing awareness that they look and sound different from everyone in their family and, likely, all of their playmates.

Parents' Initial Shock and Adjustment

Probably all soon-to-be-parents have said, "I don't care if it's a boy or girl; I just want my baby to be healthy." In some cases, because of increasingly refined ultrasound techniques, a cleft lip or other craniofacial anomaly may be detected in utero. Learning about their baby's cleft at this stage of development is emotionally shocking for the parents, and from that point on they need to receive information and counseling from the obstetrician and pediatrician (Despars, Peters, Borghini, et al., 2011). The early knowledge that the unborn child is not perfect—that it has a cleft—allows the parents time to learn about the problem and perhaps develop some adjustment to the reality of the birth.

Most parents, however, have no advanced warning and opportunity to prepare for the birth of a child with a cleft; the baby is born, and the parents' first awareness of the facial anomaly is when they are shown their new baby (Strauss et al., 1995). Many parents of babies with clefts have never heard of or seen pictures of clefts ("harelip" is usually the term adults have heard) before their child's birth.

Parental reactions to first seeing their baby's birth defect include disbelief, shock, anger, guilt, depression, feelings of inadequacy, resentment, grief, frustration, anxiety, fear, and protectiveness—all common reactions to any serious physical defect of a newborn (Bradbury & Hewison, 1994; Dolger-Hafner, Bartsch, Trimbach, Zobel, & Witt, 1997; Van Staden & Gerhardt, 1995). These emotions are not just fleeting feelings. Because a cleft is a "chronic" problem, the parental reactions may become chronic too, sometimes being externalized (e.g., frustration and anger) to the spouse or team of professionals involved in trying to help the child and family. Realizing that this might occur, it is wise not to take the parents' frustration and anger personally but to appreciate that it is the entire situation and all of the stressors around it that are frustrating and anger-producing for the parents. While the SLP plays an important role in assisting a child with a cleft to develop speech and language properly, another team member, such as a **social worker** or psychologist, would be better equipped to deal with the parents' feelings about having a child with a disability.

We do not want to forget that the newborn may have older brothers and sisters who also will be reacting to the baby's appearance. The grieving behavior of a child will often be similar to that of the same-gender parent. For example, a son may try to be stoic and "strong," much as he sees his father trying to be (Flasher & Fogle, 2012; Sanders, 1998). Likewise, grandparents have their own reactions but do the best they can to be supportive of the new parents and the other grandchildren. A *family systems counseling model* is usually the most helpful in these cases (see Chapter 8).

A major cause of stress for many parents is the cost of a cleft palate team, surgery, and the care needed for these children. A family's health insurance, Health Maintenance Organization (HMO), or various other third-party payers may cover the cost of certain aspects of an infant's and child's care. However, parents need to be advocates for their child and themselves when insurance companies and HMOs deny claims because they are considered "cosmetic" surgeries, dental problems rather than medical problems, "preexisting" conditions, or because the claims agent feels that an entire cleft palate team is not necessary. In addition, beyond what might be covered by third-party payers, there are always numerous expenses that come out of the pockets of the family.

Many parents have had little experience with hospitals before the birth of their baby, and now they must learn to navigate the complexities

social worker

A professional who helps families coordinate appointments, deal with insurance and other funding sources, and manage their stress and emotional reactions to the many problems associated with a patient's treatment.

Application Question

How do you think you might react if your baby was born with a serious physical defect? What can you do to try to develop some empathy for the new parents of a baby born with a cleft or other serious physical defect?

of the medical system, as well as insurance companies. A knowledgeable and compassionate social worker can be most helpful to the parents at this time. As the first surgery time (usually closing the lip) approaches, the stress and anxiety of the parents and family increase.

Parent–infant attachment and bonding have been a concern for years (Koepp-Baker & Harkins, 1936). The more severe the cleft, the more likely the following behaviors will occur: parents perceive their infants as irritable and having less pleasing personality characteristics; mothers delay in touching their babies; and mothers are less interactive (less playful, less responsive, and less facially expressive) with their babies (Coy, Speltz, & Jones, 2002; Slade, Emerson, & Freedlander, 1999).

Children's Preschool and Early Elementary School Years

During the preschool years, children's self-images and feelings about themselves are influenced primarily by the attitudes and behaviors of their parents. The relationship between parents' attitudes and a child's self-concept is crucial during the preschool years. As children's interactions with the community expand in the school years, the effects on self-image, socialization, school adjustment, and academic achievement become more complex (Collett & Speltz, 2006; Endriga, Jordan, & Speltz, 2003). How children look and sound when entering elementary school affects how they perceive themselves and their social interactions. A child's facial appearance is strongly correlated with attractiveness and social acceptance (Krueckeberg, Kapp-Simon, & Ribordy, 1993; Turner, Rumsey, & Sandy, 1998).

A number of studies have looked at how early elementary school children with craniofacial anomalies perceive themselves. In general, the children felt more alienated, sadder, and more scared, angry, and upset than the normal-appearing control groups (Elder, 1995; Slifer et al., 2006). Parents and teachers often need help to realize that many children with clefts feel rejected and are rejected by their peers and that children with clefts may need special training and experiences in ways to positively handle teasing and ridiculing and to develop good social skills. Parents may want to discuss with their children how to handle negative social situations related to their clefts. A child who is entering school should learn the proper (and age-appropriate) terms related to the cleft. The ability to confidently explain the condition to others may limit feelings of awkwardness and embarrassment and reduce negative social experiences.

School-Age Years

Self-perceptions and self-concepts of children during the elementary school years become increasingly complex, with many factors influencing how they feel about themselves almost moment to moment. Children with clefts generally have a significantly lower self-concept than their noncleft peers. They generally perceive themselves as less socially adept and more often sad and angry than children without clefts. They report significantly greater dissatisfaction with their appearance, less success in school, and greater general unhappiness and anxiety than do other children (Millard & Richman, 2001; Warschausky, Kay, Buchman, Halberg, & Berger, 2002). Richman and Millard (1997) found that girls with clefts tend to be more socially inhibited than boys. Pillemer and Cook (1989) found that for school-age children with a history of cleft, better physical attractiveness correlated with better overall adjustment.

Overall, clinicians need to be aware of the potential for children and adolescents with repaired or unrepaired clefts to have self-concept and self-esteem issues and need to be willing to listen when they want to talk about how they feel about themselves. Being empathic is more helpful to these children than being sympathetic, and working on social skills (particularly on handling teasing) as part of pragmatic language development can be helpful.

Adolescents

The adolescent years are a tremendous challenge—even for individuals with no apparent physical or other abnormality. Adolescents view appearance as the most important characteristic, above intelligence and humor (Prokhorov, Perry, Kelder, & Klepp, 1993). Physical appearance concerns are consistently higher in adolescents with a history of clefts, particularly in girls (Berger, Hons, & Dalton, 2011).

Adolescents with repaired clefts have the same challenges as other adolescents, plus the likely addition of some that are related to residual surgical scars, facial features, and speech patterns associated with cleft lips and palates. Adolescents are susceptible to comments and ridicule because they cannot hide their facial differences from their peers. Males often deal with their concerns about their facial appearance by internalizing and developing anxiety and depression. They often externalize by withdrawing from others, becoming aggressive, or both. Females also often develop problems relating to self-image with anxiety and depression, and withdrawing from others, but they are less likely to become aggressive. Both males and females typically rate their *quality of life* as lower than that of their peers (Pope & Snyder, 2004; Slifer et al., 2004). Psychosocial functioning of individuals with clefts often improves after further surgery, but the positive outlook may be short-lived due to unrealistic expectations of the surgery (Topolski, Edwards, & Patrick, 2005). Not all adolescents with clefts have significant psychosocial problems; still, it is important for parents to be aware of psychosocial challenges their adolescents may face and to know where to turn if problems arise (Persson, Aniansson, Becker, & Svensson, 2002).

Adults

Among adults, an indication of self-satisfaction and feelings of success in social interactions is their dating and marrying patterns. Several studies have reported that adults with repaired clefts marry later and less often than other adults. There also are more childless couples and fewer children per marriage (Yttri, Christensen, Knudsen, Bille, 2011). Individuals with repaired clefts tend to rely on extended family for support and social activities, often having just a few close friends. They tend to have a high rate of persistent dissatisfaction with their appearance, teeth, hearing, speech, and social life (Havstam, Laakso, Lohmander, & Ringsberg, 2011; Marcusson, 2002; Marcusson, Akerlind, & Paulin, 2001). However, Clifford (1987) and Hunt, Burden, Hepper, and Johnston (2005) reviewed the psychosocial literature on this area and concluded that individuals with repaired clefts generally assume a reasonable position in society and typically fall within the norms in their educational levels, employment, psychosocial adjustment, and social integration.

Although adults with repaired clefts generally are in the norms and mainstreams of society, there is strong agreement among cleft palate and craniofacial team members that the parents of children born with clefts would benefit from access to a psychologist and that children and adolescents, every 2 to 3 years, should receive a psychological consultation, particularly before and after each major surgery (Krueckeberg, Kapp-Simon, & Ribordy, 1993; Pope & Ward, 1997; Strauss, 1991).

> **Application Question**
>
> Had you been born with a cleft or other physical anomaly that you knew you could pass on to your children, would it influence your decision about marrying? About having a child? About having more than one child?

CHAPTER SUMMARY

There are a variety of clefts that can occur, with some affecting just the lip, others affecting the hard palate, and still others affecting just the soft palate. The severest kind of cleft occurs when all three structures are involved. A submucous cleft occurs when there is a defect in the hard palate in the absence of an actual opening into the nasal cavity. Velopharyngeal incompetence is the inability to achieve adequate separation of the nasal cavity from the oral cavity by velar and pharyngeal action, resulting in hypernasal resonance.

Many infants have difficulty feeding and children have middle ear infections and dental anomalies. Resonance disorders caused by velopharyngeal incompetence are the hallmark of a cleft palate. Speech and language problems are common for children with clefts.

Management of children with cleft lip and palate requires an interdisciplinary team approach. The goal of surgical closure of the palate is to establish an intact division between the oral and the nasal cavities, including a fully functional velopharyngeal system. Most children with cleft palates need therapy to improve their articulation or phonological development, as well as general expressive language abilities. During the first year, the primary speech pathology concerns are feeding and the development of the prerequisites for verbal communication. For the next couple of years, language development is the primary focus. The preschool and school-age years usually require the SLP to focus on articulation and phonological development and expressive language development.

A baby born with a serious facial disfigurement sets in motion an array of emotions in everyone related to or involved with the newborn. Elementary school children have significantly greater dissatisfaction with their appearance, less success in school, and greater general unhappiness and anxiety than other children. Adolescent males and females with repaired clefts typically rate their quality of life as lower than that of their peers. Adults with repaired clefts tend to have a high rate of persistent dissatisfaction with their appearance, teeth, hearing, speech, and social life. However, individuals with repaired clefts generally assume a reasonable position in society and typically fall within the norms in their educational levels, employment, psychosocial adjustment, and social integration.

STUDY QUESTIONS

Knowledge and Comprehension

1. What is velopharyngeal incompetence (VPI)?
2. What is hypernasality?
3. Define *interdisciplinary team* and list the essential (core) members of a cleft palate team.
4. What are the primary concerns of the speech-language pathologist during the child's first year?
5. What are some of the parental reactions that may be expected when first seeing their baby's cleft?

Application

1. How can a cleft lip cause articulation problems?
2. Why is it important to evaluate the receptive and expressive language of a child who has a cleft lip, cleft palate, or both?
3. Explain three of the noninstrumental tests a speech pathologist might use during an evaluation of a child for velopharyngeal incompetence.
4. Why is a speech-language pathologist always in an evaluation process when working with individuals who have cleft palates?
5. As a clinician, how can being aware that parents may "externalize" their reactions to various professionals help you better work with their frustrations and anger?

Analysis/Synthesis

1. Explain the similarities and differences between hypernasality and nasal emission.
2. Discuss the similarities and differences between hypernasality and hyponasality.
3. Discuss the differences in emphasis of the speech-language pathologist's work during the first years and those of preschool through school age.

4. How does the focus of counseling change from the initial work with the parents to later work with the child and adolescent?

5. Explain why the cleft palate team members may need to continue their involvement into a person's adulthood.

REFERENCES

Al Jamal, G., Hazza, A., Rawashdeh, M. (2010). Prevalence of dental anomalies in a population of cleft lip and palate patients. *The Cleft Palate-Craniofacial Journal, 47*(4), 413–420.

American Cleft Palate–Craniofacial Association (1996). The cleft and craniofacial team. Available at http://www.acpa-cpf.org.

Antonelli, P., Jorge, J., & Feniman, M. (2011). Otologic and audiologic outcomes with the Furlow and von Langenbeck with intravelar veloplasty palatoplasties in unilateral cleft lip and palate. *The Cleft Palate-Craniofacial Journal, 48*(4), 412–418.

Asimov, L. (1982). *Asimov's biographical encyclopedia of science and technology* (2nd ed.). Garden City, NY: Doubleday.

Baylis, A. L., Munson, B., & Moller, K. (2011). Perceptions of audible nasal emission in speakers with cleft palate: A comparative study of listener judgement. *The Cleft Palate-Craniofacial Journal, 48*(4), 399–411.

Berger, Z. E., Hons, D., & Dalton, L. J. (2011). *Coping with a cleft: Factors associated with psychological adjustment of adolescents with a cleft lip and palate and their parents.* The Celft Palate-Craniofacial Journal, *48*(1), 82–90.

Blakely, R. W., & Brockman, J. H. (1995). Normal speech and hearing by age 5 as a goal for children with cleft palate: A demonstration project. *American Journal of Speech-Language Pathology, 4*, 25–32.

Bradbury, E., & Hewison, J. (1994). Early parental adjustment to visible congenital disfigurement. *Child Care Health and Development, 20*(4), 251–266.

Broder, H. L., Smith, F., & Strauss, R. (1994). Effects of visible and invisible orofacial defects on self-perception and adjustment across developmental eras and gender. *Cleft Palate–Craniofacial Journal, 31*, 429–436.

Broen, P., Devers, M., Doyle, S., Prouty, J. M., & Moller, K. (1998). Acquisition of linguistic and cognitive skills by children with cleft palate. *Journal of Speech, Language, and Hearing Research, 41*, 676–687.

Carlisle, D. (1998). Feeding babies with cleft lip and palate. *Nursing Times, 94*(4), 59–60.

Chapman, K. L. (2011). The relationship between early reading skills and speech and language performance in young children with cleft lip and palate. *The Cleft-Palate Craniofacial Journal, 48*(3), 301–311.

Chapman, K. L. (1993). Phonologic processes in children with cleft palate. *Cleft Palate–Craniofacial Journal, 30*, 64–71.

Chapman, K. L., & Hardin, M. A. (1992). Phonetic and phonological skills of two-year-olds with cleft palate. *Cleft Palate–Craniofacial Journal, 29*, 435–441.

Chapman, K. L., Hardin-Jones, M. A., & Halter, K. A. (2003). The relationship between early speech and later speech and language performance for children with cleft lip and palate. *Clinical Linguistics and Phonetics, 17*(3), 173–197.

Chung, C. S., & Kau, M. C. (1985). Racial differences in cephalometric measurements and incidence of cleft lip with or without cleft palate. *Journal of Craniofacial Genetics and Developmental Biology, 5*, 341–349.

Clifford, E. (1987). *The cleft palate experience: New perspectives on management.* Springfield, IL: Charles C Thomas.

Collett, B. R., & Speltz, M. L. (2006). Social–emotional development of infants and young children with orofacial clefts. *Infants and Young Children, 19*(4), 262–291.

Collier, P. F. (1910). *Oath and law of Hippocrates.* Available at http://www.medword.com/hippocrates.html.

Coy, K., Speltz, M. L., & Jones, K. (2002). Facial appearance and attachment in infants with orofacial clefts: A replication. *Cleft Palate–Craniofacial Journal, 39*, 66–72.

Depars, J., Peters, C., Borghini, A., Pierrehumbert, B., Habersaat, S., et al. (2011). Impact of a cleft lip and/or palate on maternal stress and attachment representations. *The Cleft Palate-Craniofacial Journal, 48*(4), 419–424.

Diehl, S. R., & Erickson, R. P. (1997). Genome scan for teratogen-induced clefting susceptibility in the mouse: Evidence of both allelic and locus heterogeneity distinguishing cleft lip and cleft palate. *Proceedings of the National Academy of Science, 94*, 5231–5236.

Dolger-Hafner, M., Bartsch, A., Trimbach, G., Zobel, I., & Witt, E. (1997). Parental reactions following the birth of a cleft child. *Journal of Orofacial Orthopedics, 58*(2), 124–133.

Doyle, W. J., Cantekin, E. I., & Bluestone, C. D. (1980). Eustachian tube function in cleft palate children. *Annals of Otology, Rhinology, and Laryngology Supplement, 89*(3, Pt. 2), 34–40.

Elder, R. A. (1995). Individual differences in young children's self-concepts: Implications for children with cleft lip and palate. In R. A. Elder (Ed.), *Developmental perspectives on craniofacial problems.* New York, NY: Springer-Verlag.

Endriga, M. C., Jordan, J., & Speltz, M. L. (2003). Emotion self-regulation in preschool children with and without orofacial clefts. *Journal of Developmental and Behavioral Pediatrics, 24*(5), 336–344.

Ericson, A., Kallen, B., & Westeholm, P. (1979). Cigarette smoking as an etiologic factor in cleft lip and palate. *American Journal of Obstetrics and Gynecology, 135*, 348–351.

Fallowfield, L., & Jenkins, V. (2004). Communicating sad, bad, and difficult news in medicine. *Lancet, 363*(9405), 312–319.

Farrall, M., & Holder, S. (1992). Familial recurrence pattern analysis of cleft lip with or without cleft palate. *American Journal of Human Genetics, 50,* 270–277.

Flasher, L. V., & Fogle, P. T. (2012). *Counseling skills for speech-language pathologists and audiologists* (2nd ed.). Clifton Park, NY: Delmar Cengage Learning.

Garrett, J. D., & Deal, R. E. (2002). Endoscopic and perceptual evaluation of velopharyngeal insufficiency and hypernasality. *Journal of Medical Speech-Language Pathology, 19,* 194–200.

Golding-Kushner, K. J. (2001). *Therapy techniques for cleft palate speech and related disorders.* Clifton Park, NY: Delmar Cengage Learning.

Ha, S., & Kuehn, D. P. (2011). Temporal characteristics of nasalization in speakers with and without cleft palate. *The Cleft Palate-Craniofacial Journal, 48*(2), 134–144.

Hardin-Jones, M., Chapman, K., & Scherer, N. J. (2006). Early intervention in children with cleft palate. *ASHA Leader, 11*(8), 8–9, 32.

Havstam, C., Laakso, K., Lohmander, A., & Ringsberg, K. C. (2011). *Taking charge of communication: Adults' descriptions of growing up with a cleft-related speech impairment.* The Cleft Palate-Craniofacial Journal, 48(6), 717–726.

Hodgkinson, P., Brown, S., Duncan, D., Grant, C., McNaughton, A., Thomas, P., & Mattick, C. (2005). Management of children with cleft lip and palate: A review describing the application of a multidisciplinary team working in this condition based upon the experiences of a regional cleft lip and palate centre in the United Kingdom. *Fetal and Maternal Medicine Review, 16,* 1–27.

Hunt, O., Burden, D., Hepper, P., & Johnston, C. (2005). The psychological effects of cleft lip and palate. *European Journal of Orthodontics, 27*(3), 274–285.

International Perinatal Database of Typical Oral Clefts Working Group (IPDTOC). (2011). Prevalence at birth of cleft lip with or without cleft palate: Data from the IPDTOC. *The Cleft Palate-Craniofacial Journal, 48*(1), 66–81.

Khoury, M., Gomez-Farias, J., & Mulinare, J. (1989). Does maternal cigarette smoking during pregnancy cause cleft lip and palate in offspring? *American Journal of Diseases in Children, 143,* 333–337.

Koepp-Baker, H., & Harkins, C. (1936). *The [cleft palate] child we have forgotten.* Philipsburg, PA: The Women's Club of Philipsburg.

Koren, G., Pastuszak, A., & Ito, S. (1998). Drugs in pregnancy. *New England Journal of Medicine, 338,* 1128–1137.

Krueckeberg, S., Kapp-Simon, K., & Ribordy, S. (1993). Social skills of preschool children with and without craniofacial anomalies. *Cleft Palate–Craniofacial Journal, 30,* 475–481.

Kuehn, D. P., & Henne, L. J. (2003). Speech evaluation and treatment for patients with cleft palate. *American Journal of Speech-Language Pathology, 12,* 103–109.

Kuehn, D. P., & Moller, K. T. (2000). Speech and language issues in the cleft palate population: The state of the art. *Cleft Palate–Craniofacial Journal, 37*, 348–383.

Kummer, A. W. (2008). Cleft palate and craniofacial anomalies: Effects on speech and resonance (2nd ed.). Clifton Park, NY: Delmar Cengage Learning.

Kwan, W. M., Abdullah, V. J., Liu, K., van Hasselt, C. A., & Tong, C. F. (2011). Otitis media with effusion and hearing loss in Chinese children with cleft lip and palate. *The Cleft Palate-Craniofacial Journal, 48*(6), 684–689.

Lazarus, D., Hudson, D., van Zyl, J., Fleming, A., & Fernandes, D. (1998). Repair of unilateral cleft lip: A comparison of five techniques. *Annals of Plastic Surgery, 41*(6), 587–594.

Liedman-Boshki, J., Lohmander, A., Persson, C., Lith, A., & Elander, A. (2005). Perceptual analysis of speech and the activity in the lateral pharyngeal walls before and after velopharyngeal flap surgery. *Scandinavian Journal of Plastic and Reconstructive Surgery and Hand Surgery, 39*, 22–32.

Marcusson, A. (2002). Facial appearance in adults who had cleft lip and palate treated in childhood. *Scandinavian Journal of Plastic and Reconstructive Surgery and Hand Surgery, 35*(1), 16–23.

Marcusson, A., Akerlind, I., & Paulin, G. (2001). Quality of life in adults with repaired complete cleft lip and palate. *Cleft Palate–Craniofacial Journal, 38*(4), 379–385.

Middleton, G., & Pannbacker, M. (1997). *Cleft palate and related disorders*. Bisbee, AZ: Imaginart International.

Millard, T., & Richman, L. C. (2001). Different cleft conditions, facial appearance, and speech: Relationship to psychological variables. *Cleft Palate–Craniofacial Journal, 38*, 68–75.

Mitchell, L. E., & Risch, H. (1992). Mode of inheritance of nonsyndromic cleft lip with or without cleft palate: A reanalysis. *American Journal of Human Genetics, 51*, 323–332.

Moller, K., & Glaze, L. (2009). Cleft lip and palate: interdisciplinary issues and treatment (2nd ed.). Austin, TX: Pro-Ed.

Murthy, J., Sendhilnathan, S., Hussain, A. (2010). *Speech outcomes following late primary palate repair*. The Cleft Palate-Craniofacial Journal, *47*(2), 156–161.

Pamplona, M., & Ysunza, A. (1999). Active participation of mothers during speech therapy: Improved language development of children with cleft palate. *Scandinavian Journal of Plastic and Reconstructive Surgery, 33*, 1–6.

Pamplona, M., Ysunza, A., & Uriostegui, C. (1996). Linguistic interaction: The role of parents in therapy for cleft palate patients. *International Journal of Pediatric Otorhinolaryngology, 37*, 17–27.

Pannbacker, M. (1975). Oral language skills of adult cleft palate speakers. *Cleft Palate Journal, 12*, 95–106.

Persson, M., Aniansson, G., Becker, M., & Svensson, H. (2002). Self-concept and introversion with cleft lip and palate. *Scandinavian Journal of Plastic and Reconstructive Surgery and Hand Surgery, 36*(1), 24–27.

Peterson-Falzone, S. J. (1989). Compensatory articulations in cleft palate speakers: Relative incidence by type. Proceedings of the International Congress on Cleft Palate and Related Craniofacial Anomalies, Jerusalem, Israel.

Peterson-Falzone, S. J., Hardin-Jones, A., & Karnell, M. P. (2010). *Cleft palate speech* (4th ed.). St. Louis, MO: Mosby.

Pillemer, F. G., & Cook, K. V. (1989). The psychosocial adjustment of pediatric craniofacial patients after surgery. *Cleft Palate Journal, 26*(3), 201–207.

Pope, A. W., & Snyder, H. T. (2004). Psychosocial adjustment in children and adolescents with a craniofacial anomaly: Age and sex patterns. *Cleft Palate-Craniofacial Journal, 42*, 4–12.

Pope, A. W., & Ward, J. (1997b). Self-perceived facial appearance and psychosocial adjustment in preadolescents with craniofacial anomalies. *Cleft Palate-Craniofacial Journal, 34*, 396–401.

Prokhorov, A. V., Perry, C., Kelder, S., & Klepp, K. (1993). Lifestyle values of adolescents: Results from the Minnesota Heart Health Youth Program. *Adolescence, 28*, 119–127.

Rahimov, F., Jugessur, A., & Murray, J. C. (2012). Genetics of nonsyndromic orofacial clefts. *The Cleft Palate-Craniofacial Journal, 49*(1), 73–91.

Ramstad, T., Ottem, E., & Shaw, W. (1995). Psychosocial adjustment in Norwegian adults who had undergone standardized treatment of complete cleft lip and palate. *Scandinavian Journal of Plastic and Reconstructive Surgery, 29*, 251–257.

Redford-Badwal, D. A., Mabry, K., & Frassinelli, J. D. (2003). Impact of cleft lip and/or palate on nutritional health and oral-motor development. *Dental Clinics of North America, 47*(2), 305–317.

Richman, L. C., & Millard, T. (1997). Cleft lip and palate: Longitudinal behavior and relationships of cleft conditions to behavior and achievement. *Journal of Pediatric Psychology, 22*, 487–494.

Rosenblatt, C. B. (1995). Effects of folate deficiency on embryonic development. *Braillieres Clinical Hematology, 8*(3), 617–637.

Salas-Provance, M. (2012). Counseling in a multicultural society. In L. V. Flasher & P. T. Fogle, *Counseling skills for speech-language pathologists and audiologists* (2nd ed.). Clifton Park, NY: Delmar Cengage Learning.

Salas-Provance, M. B., Kuehn, D., & Marsh, J. (2003). Phonetic repertoire and syllables characteristics of 15-month-old babies with cleft palate. *Journal of Phonetics, 31*, 23–38.

Sampson, P. D. (2000). On categorization in analyses of alcohol teratogenesis. *Environmental Health Perspectives, 108*, 421–428.

Sanders, C. (1998). Gender difference in bereavement expression across the life span. In K. Doka & J. Davidson (Eds.), *Living with grief: Who we are, how we grieve.* Washington, DC: Hospice Foundations of America.

Scherer, N. J., & D'Antonio, L. L. (1997). Language and play development in toddlers with cleft lip and/or palate. *American Journal of Speech-Language Pathology, 6*(4), 48–54.

Sekhon, P., Ethunandan, M., Mrkus, A., Krishnan, G., & Rao, C. (2011). Congenital anomalies associated with cleft lip and palate: An analysis of 1623 consecutive patients. *The Cleft Palate-Craniofacial Journal, 48*(4), 371–378.

Slade, P., Emerson, D. J., & Freedlander, E. (1999). A longitudinal comparison of the psychological impact on mothers or neonatal and 3-month repair of cleft lip. *British Journal of Plastic Surgery, 52*, 1–5.

Slifer, K., Amari, B., Diver, T., Hilley, L., Beck, M., Kane, A., & McDonnel, S. (2004). Social interaction patterns of children and adolescents with and without oral clefts during a videotaped analogue encounter. *Cleft Palate-Craniofacial Journal, 41*, 175–184.

Slifer, K., Pulbrook, M., Amari, B., Vona-Messersmith, M., Cohen, J., Ambadar, Z., Beck, M., & Piszczor, R. (2006). Social acceptance and facial behavior in children with oral clefts. *Cleft Palate–Craniofacial Journal, 43*(2), 226–236.

Snyder, H. T., Bilboul, M. J., & Pope, A. W. (2005). Psychosocial adjustment in adolescents with craniofacial anomalies: A comparison of parent and self-reports. *Cleft Palate–Craniofacial Journal, 42*, 5–16.

Strauss, R. P. (1985). Culture, rehabilitation, and facial birth defects: International case studies. *Cleft Palate Journal, 22*(1), 56–62.

Strauss, R. P. (1991). Culture, health care, and birth defects in the United States: An introduction. *Cleft Palate Journal, 27*(3), 275–278.

Strauss, R. P., Sharp, M., Lorch, S., & Kachalia, B. (1995). Physicians' communication of "bad news"—Parent experiences of being informed of their child's cleft lip/palate. *Pediatrics, 96*(1), 82–89.

Sulprizio, S. L. (2010). *The source for cleft palate and craniofacial speech disorders*. East Moline, IL: LinguiSystems.

Taub, P. J., & Lampert, J. A. (2011). Pediatric craniofacial surgery: A review for the multidisciplinay team. *The Cleft Palate-Craniofacial Journal, 48*(6), 670–683.

Topolski, T. D., Edwards, T. C., & Patrick, D. L. (2005). Quality of life: How do adolescents with facial differences compare with other adolescents? *Cleft Palate–Craniofacial Journal, 42*, 1, 19–24.

Turner, S. R., Rumsey, N., & Sandy, J. R. (1998). Psychological aspects of cleft lip and palate. *European Journal of Orthodontics, 20*(4), 407–415.

Vanderas, A. P. (1987). Incidence of cleft lip, cleft palate, and cleft lip and palate among the races: A review. *Cleft Palate Journal, 24*(21), 216–225.

Van Staden, F., & Gerhardt, C. (1995). Mothers of children with facial cleft deformities: Reactions and effects. *South American Journal of Psychology, 25*(1), 39–46.

Warschausky, S., Kay, J., Buchman, S., Halberg, A., & Berger, M. (2002). Health-related quality of life in children with craniofacial anomalies. *Plastic and Reconstructive Surgery, 110*(2), 409–41.

Yttri, J. E., Christensen, K., Knudsen, L. B., & Bille, C. (2011). Reproductive patterns among Danish women with oral clefts. *The Cleft Palate-Craniofacial Journal, 48*(5), 601–607.

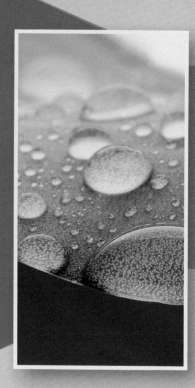

CHAPTER 11
Neurological Disorders in Adults

LEARNING OBJECTIVES

After studying this chapter, you will:

- Know the etiologies of neurogenic communication disorders and the various types of strokes.
- Be able to discuss the common characteristics of the aphasias.
- Be familiar with cognitive disorders caused by closed and open head injuries.
- Know the common characteristics of right-hemisphere syndrome.
- Understand basic information about dementia and Alzheimer's disease.
- Be familiar with principles of assessment of aphasia and cognitive disorders.
- Be able to discuss general principles of therapy for aphasia and cognitive disorders.
- Be familiar with the emotional and social effects of neurological disorders on patients and their families.

KEY TERMS

activities of daily living (ADLs)
agrammatic (agrammatism)
agraphia
alexia (acquired dyslexia)
Alzheimer's disease (AD)
aneurysm
anomia
anomic aphasia
anosognosia
aphasia (dysphasia)
arteriosclerosis

atherosclerosis
attention impairments
autopsy (postmortem)
board and care home
Broca's aphasia
cerebral embolism (embolus)
cerebral hemorrhage (hemorrhagic stroke)
cerebral thrombosis (thrombus)
chronic traumatic encephalopathy (CTE)

circumlocution
closed head injury (CHI) (nonpenetrating brain injury)
cognitive disorder
coma
computerized tomography (CT) scan
concussion
contrecoup injury
cortical atrophy
custodial care
degenerative disease

KEY TERMS continued

dementia
edema
expressive aphasia
family therapy
fluent aphasia
functional outcomes
global aphasia
high blood pressure
(hypertension)
incontinence
infarction (necrosis)
integrate (integration)
jargon aphasia
literal or phonemic
paraphasia
loss of consciousness
(LOC)
magnetic resonance
imaging (MRI)
mental status
examination
metastasis
neologism

neuritic (senile) plaques
neurofibrillary tangles
neuropsychologist
nonfluent aphasia
occlusive (ischemic)
stroke
open head injury (OHI)
perseverate/
perseveration
persistent vegetative
state (PVS)
positive emission
tomography (PET)
postconcussion
syndrome (PCS)
post-traumatic stress
disorder (PTSD)
premorbid
prognosis
prosody (prosodic)/
melody (melodic)
prosopagnosia
quality of life

receptive aphasia
residential care facility
right-hemisphere
syndrome
senility
spontaneous recovery
stroke (cerebrovascular
accident, CVA)
toxin
transient ischemic attack
(TIA)
traumatic brain injury
(TBI) (head trauma,
acquired brain injury
[ABI])
tumor (neoplasm)
vegetative state
verbal or semantic
paraphasia
visual–spatial
impairments
Wernicke's aphasia
working memory

CHAPTER OUTLINE

Introduction
Etiologies of Neurogenic Speech, Language, Cognitive,
and Swallowing Disorders
Strokes (Cerebrovascular Accidents)
Traumas
Tumors
Toxins
Degenerative Diseases and Disorders
The Aphasias
Classifications and Terminology Associated with the
Aphasias
Fluent and Nonfluent Aphasia Classification System
Major Types of Aphasia
Principles of Assessment of Aphasia
Multicultural Considerations
General Principles of Therapy
Cognitive Disorders
Traumatic Brain Injury
Right-Hemisphere Syndrome
Dementia
Emotional and Social Effects of Neurological Disorders
Chapter Summary
Study Questions
References

INTRODUCTION

Neurological disorders may occur at any age, but most commonly occur in people over 65 years of age. With improved medical care and the increasing "graying of America," there is an increase in individuals with neurological disorders. Speech-language pathologists work with individuals who have neurological impairments in settings such as hospitals (acute care, subacute care, and convalescent [sometimes called a *nursing home, skilled nursing facility—SNF,* or *long-term care facility—LTC*]), inpatient and outpatient clinics, rehabilitation centers, home health care, private practices, and university clinics.

ETIOLOGIES OF NEUROGENIC SPEECH, LANGUAGE, COGNITIVE, AND SWALLOWING DISORDERS

Neurogenic communication and swallowing problems have many possible etiologies. The causes vary somewhat by age group; for example, young adults are more likely to have traumatic brain injuries from motor vehicle accidents (MVAs) or altercations, and older individuals are more likely to have strokes, brain tumors, or degenerative disorders. Understanding the causes of patients' speech, language, cognitive, and swallowing problems can be helpful in both assessment and treatment. However, we base therapy not on just the neurological cause of the communication or swallowing impairments but on the signs and symptoms we see during our assessment and ongoing work with patients. In some cases our assessment and therapy may be initiated before we are able to obtain a clear medical or radiological cause of a patient's disorders. Also, our prognosis for an individual patient's rehabilitation and recovery is based more on what we see during our assessment and treatment than what may be predicted based on a neurologist's or radiologist's findings (Cherney, 2004; Davis, 2007; Huckabee & Pelletier, 2003; LaPointe, 2005; Murray & Clark, 2006; Papathanasiou, Coppens, & Potagas, 2012). Many patients make progress far beyond what might be predicted based on the cause and extent of neurological damage, and some make less progress.

Strokes (Cerebrovascular Accidents)

Strokes or **cerebrovascular accidents (CVAs)** are the third-leading cause of death in the United States and the world for people over 45 years of age, with the first- and second-leading causes of death being heart attacks and cancer. The average age to have a first stroke is approximately

stroke (cerebrovascular accident, CVA)

A disruption of blood supply to the brain caused by an occluded (blocked) artery or an artery that has.

67 years. Men have a higher risk for stroke, with an incidence of 1.25 times higher than that of women; however, women are more likely to die from stroke (of every five deaths caused by stroke, two are men and three are women) (American Heart Association, 2012 [Note: the American Stroke Association is a division of the American Heart Association].

Nearly 150,000 people in the United States die from strokes each year, with about 600,000 survivors experiencing various forms and degrees of speech, language, cognitive, swallowing, and physical impairments affecting all parts of their bodies (strokes are the leading cause of disability in the United States). Approximately 85% of stroke survivors are able to return to their prestroke living environment with various levels of permanent impairments, and about 15% of survivors must be admitted to long-term care facilities (Goldstein, 2009; American Heart Association 2012).

The number of strokes in the United States has been increasing from approximately 550,000 per year in the 1970s to about 730,000 per year in the 1990s. The reasons for this increase are uncertain, although they may be related to dietary and stress factors (American Heart Association, 2012). A physiological manifestation of stress is **high blood pressure (hypertension)**, which causes increased susceptibility to strokes.

Strokes result in brain damage because of the disruption of blood flow that prevents oxygenated blood and nutrients from reaching areas of the brain. This can result in a range of problems, from *localized lesions* (relatively small damaged areas) to widespread, diffuse damage. Strokes can occur in any area of the central nervous system: the brain, cerebellum, brainstem, and even spinal cord. The *site* (location) and size of the lesion are what generally determine the characteristics and extent of neurological damage. Beyond the stroke itself, edema of brain tissue can develop that increases pressure inside the brain, causing further damage.

Since the 1990s, the National Stroke Association and the American Heart Association have attempted to increase public awareness about the eminent dangers of strokes by calling them *"brain attacks."* This term was adopted because of the public's awareness of the need for immediate medical attention for heart attacks. People who have heart attacks are susceptible to strokes because the same vascular problems that occur in heart attacks can cause brain attacks.

Numerous risk factors predispose a person for a stroke; for example, being male, smoking, being overweight, a fatty diet, lack of exercise, heavy alcohol consumption, diabetes mellitus, high blood pressure, getting older, family history of stroke or heart attack, and lack of regular health checkups. Risk factors for strokes are also risk factors for heart attacks (American Heart Association, 2012) (see Figure 11–1).

Occlusive (Ischemic) Strokes

An **occlusive (ischemic) stroke** means that an area of the brain is deprived of blood because of a blocked (*occluded*) artery. Occlusive strokes make up about 80% of the strokes in people. If the occlusion

high blood pressure (hypertension)

A common disorder in middle age and later (although now often being seen in obese children and young adults) in which blood pressure is chronically above 140 over 90 mm Hg (120/80 is considered normal).

occlusive (ischemic) stroke

A partial or complete blockage (occlusion) of a cerebral artery, causing decreased blood supply to brain tissue.

Application Question

Considering your age and gender, what risk factors might you have for a stroke or heart attack? What do you do regularly to decrease your risk factors?

It is important for everyone to know warning signs of stroke. If you become aware of any of the following symptoms in yourself or another person, emergency medical care is essential:

 Sudden numbness or weakness of the face, arm, or leg, especially on one side of the body

 Sudden confusion or difficulty speaking or understanding

 Sudden difficulty seeing in one or both eyes

 Sudden difficulty walking, dizziness, and loss of balance or coordination

 Sudden, severe headache with no known cause

A quick test to recognize if a person is having a stroke uses the acronym **F.A.S.T.:**

 Face: Ask the person to smile. A stroke can cause one side of the face to droop. Abrupt dimming of vision and a sudden, severe headache with no known cause are also warning signs.

 Arms: Ask the person to raise both arms. If one arm drifts downward or it cannot be raised, a stroke may be causing weakness, numbness, or paralysis. Individuals may also have a loss of balance or a sudden fall.

 Speech: Ask the person to repeat a simple sentence. Listen for slurred words and trouble speaking or understanding speech.

 Time: If the person has any symptoms, call 911 immediately. Time is of the essence!

Figure 11–1

General warning signs of stroke and F.A.S.T.

Adapted from the American Stroke Association, 2012; and Kothari, Pancioli, Liu, Brott, & Broderick, 1999.

---

infarction (necrosis)

A localized area of necrotic (dead) tissue resulting from lack of blood supply and oxygen to the tissue.

transient ischemic attack (TIA)

An episode of cerebral vascular insufficiency with partial occlusion of a cerebral artery by atherosclerotic plaque or an embolus; disturbances of vision in one or both eyes, dizziness, weakness, numbness, dysphasia, or unconsciousness may occur; TIA (sometimes called "ministroke") usually lasts a few minutes, and in rare cases symptoms may continue for several hours.

lasts for more than 3 minutes, death (**infarction, necrosis**) of brain tissue is likely. In addition, swelling (edema) of brain tissue develops around the area damaged from the stroke, compressing and causing temporary or permanent damage to more brain tissue. **Transient ischemic attacks (TIAs)** (sometimes called "*ministrokes*") are episodes of cerebral vascular insufficiency with partial occlusion of a cerebral artery by atherosclerotic plaque or an embolus. The symptoms vary with the site and degree of occlusion (Mosby, 2009).

Even the Strong Have Strokes

On February 6, 2005, Tedy Bruschi led the New England Patriots to a 24–21 victory in Super Bowl XXXIX, with six solo tackles and a timely fourth-quarter interception against the Philadelphia Eagles. But 10 days later, at 4 a.m. on February 16, Bruschi awoke with a severe headache, his left arm and leg numb, and loss of vision in his left visual field. After an emergency trip to Massachusetts General Hospital, a CT scan revealed that Bruschi had sustained a stroke caused by a blood clot. However, on October 30, 2005, following months of rehabilitation, Bruschi was back on the football field as a Patriot. That day he made 10 tackles in a win over Buffalo and was named the National Football League's Comeback Player of the Year for the 2005 season.

Cerebral Thrombosis (Thrombus)

A **cerebral thrombosis (thrombus)** occurs when an artery in the brain gradually becomes blocked by debris in the blood. Fatty substances accumulate over decades on the lining of arterial walls. This causes a buildup of atherosclerotic plaque, which may lead to **atherosclerosis**, a type of **arteriosclerosis** (hardening of the arteries). Eventually, 50%–100% of an artery may be blocked. With increased blockage, blood flow decreases to the areas of the brain the artery supplies (see Figure 11–2). The person's functioning may slowly deteriorate over many years, but the person may not have any acute symptoms that alert the need for medical attention until there is a complete blockage. By that time, the person has a dramatic change in functioning and there may be considerable deterioration of tissue in some areas of the brain.

Cerebral Embolism (Embolus)

A **cerebral embolism (embolus)** occurs when a fragment of material travels through the circulatory system and reaches a small artery in the brain, where it occludes a blood vessel. At the location of the occlusion, the embolus begins to function as a thrombus. A variety of material may form as an embolus from most locations in the body (e.g., fragment of atherosclerotic plaque, piece of a blood clot, or tumor material). Many cerebral emboli are associated with coronary artery disease (Mosby, 2009).

Cerebral Hemorrhage

Cerebral hemorrhages (hemorrhagic strokes) account for approximately 20% of strokes. Hemorrhages are the result of a rupture of a blood vessel. People with chronic high blood pressure are most susceptible to hemorrhagic strokes (see Figure 11–3). During a cerebral hemorrhage, blood is forced into the brain tissue and destroys it (blood is toxic to brain tissue). Besides the death of neurons, the blood forms a

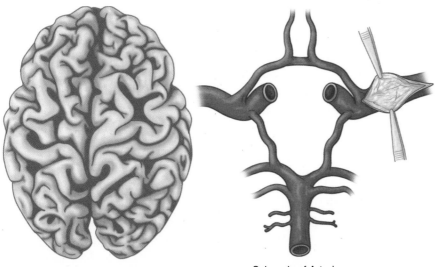

Atrophy of the Brain in Arteriosclerosis

Sclerosis of Arteries
in the Base of the Brain

cerebral thrombosis (thrombus)

An abnormal condition in which a clot (thrombus) develops within a blood vessel.

atherosclerosis

A common disorder characterized by yellowish plaques of cholesterol and other lipids (fats) in the inner layers of the walls of arteries; often associated with tobacco use, obesity, hypertension, diabetes mellitus, and aging.

arteriosclerosis

A common disorder characterized by thickening, hardening, and loss of elasticity of arterial walls as a result of build-up of atherosclerotic plaque, leading to decreased blood supply.

cerebral embolism (embolus)

An abnormal condition in which a blood clot, piece of tumor, or other material (embolus) circulates in the bloodstream until it becomes lodged in a cerebral blood vessel, causing an occlusion; at the location of the occlusion, the embolus begins to function as a thrombus.

cerebral hemorrhage (hemorrhagic stroke)

The result of a blood vessel under pressure rupturing and sending blood into the brain tissue; hemorrhages may be arterial, venous, or capillary.

Figure 11–2

Atherosclerotic plaque and arteriosclerosis.

© Cengage Learning 2013.

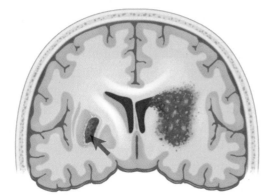

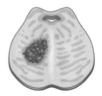

(b)   Cerebellar Hemorrhage

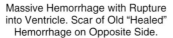

Figure 11–3

Cerebral hemorrhages may occur in different locations in the (a) brain, (b) cerebellum, or (c) brainstem.

© Cengage Learning 2013.

(a)   Massive Hemorrhage with Rupture into Ventricle. Scar of Old "Healed" Hemorrhage on Opposite Side.

(c)   Pontine Hemorrhage

mass (like a clot) that can create pressure on surrounding brain tissue, causing further neurological symptoms that are remote from the area of the hemorrhage. Cerebral hemorrhages are a medical emergency of the highest degree (Broderick, Adams, & Barsan, 1999).

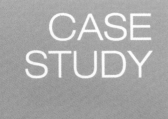

CASE STUDY

Kirk Douglas's Stroke of Luck

A stroke can occur in anyone, regardless of who we are or what we do. In 1994, Kirk Douglas, the famous actor (whose son is another famous actor, Michael Douglas), sustained an occlusive stroke in his left hemisphere. After discharge from the hospital, he received rehabilitation treatment, including speech therapy in his home. Before Douglas's stroke, the Academy of Motion Picture Arts and Sciences had voted to award him an Oscar for Lifetime Achievement. He worked with his speech-language pathologist to be ready to appear on stage in front of 2,000 of his peers and millions of television viewers.

On Oscar night, Douglas was introduced by director Steven Spielberg. Douglas later wrote:

I thought of my speech therapist: "Pause . . . breathe . . . swallow . . . articulate." I started slowly: "I see my four sons. They're proud of the old man." The audience laughed. They understood me! I spotted my wife sobbing. I held up the Oscar. "Anne, this belongs to you. I love you." I paused, took a deep breath and swallowed. "Thank you for 50 wonderful years in the wonderful world of moviemaking." I bowed, thunderous applause engulfing me. I couldn't believe it. They really understood me! ■

Adapted from Douglas, 2002.

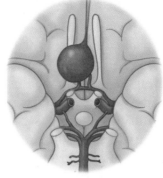

(b) Aneurysm of Anterior Cerebral Artery

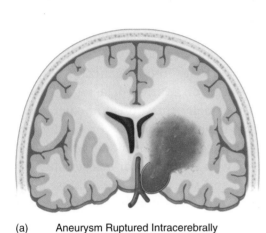

(a) Aneurysm Ruptured Intracerebrally

Figure 11–4

A cerebral aneurysm: (a) aneurysm ruptured intracerebrally and (b) aneurysm in anterior cerebral artery.

© Cengage Learning 2013.

An **aneurysm** is a bulging of an artery at its weakest point (much like a chain is only as strong as its weakest link; an artery is only as strong as its weakest point). The walls of the aneurysm are stretched and thinned, increasing the likelihood of hemorrhaging when a person's blood pressure is unusually high (see Figure 11–4).

Multicultural Considerations

Ethnicity and culture appear to have roles in the prevalence of strokes and aphasia. Behind these two factors may lay differences in socioeconomic status and health. However, data on ethnicity and cultural differences for health problems of all kinds, including strokes, are both limited and inconsistent.

Some data are seen as generally reliable. For example, African Americans have a higher incidence of high blood pressure than other populations in the United States and are, therefore, more susceptible to strokes (Singh, Cohen, & Krupp, 1996). In fact, African American men and women are nearly twice as likely to have strokes as the Caucasian population. Mexican Americans have a higher incidence of strokes compared to the non-Hispanic white population. African Americans and Hispanic Americans tend to have strokes younger than the Caucasian population. African American males have the highest death rates from strokes, and Hispanics and American Indians and Alaskan Natives have the lowest. The risk factors for strokes are generally the same for all ethnic and cultural populations—that is, high blood pressure, smoking, high cholesterol, obesity, poor diet, high-sodium diet, lack of exercise, alcohol consumption, and diabetes (American Heart Association, 2012).

aneurysm

A localized dilation of a blood vessel wall, resulting in the thinning of the wall at that site (much like a balloon being blown up) and increasing the likelihood of hemorrhaging, especially with high blood pressure.

Recovery from Strokes

Most people make their greatest gains in **spontaneous recovery** (physiological healing of the brain) during the first few weeks or months after a stroke. The majority of speech and language recovery occurs during the first six months post onset; however, additional but slower recovery may continue for years after (Code, 2001).

Each patient has a limited capacity for reorganizing the brain circuitry, and the limitations are based on a variety of factors; for example, a patient's chronological age (usually, the younger the person, the better the **prognosis**); physical health (a person who is physically healthy without serious organ damage from an accident or illness has a better prognosis than a person who is not well or has serious organ damage); and the site (location) and size of the lesion. Most people who have had strokes have some residual problems with their speech, language, cognitive functioning, or a combination of these. Many individuals have difficulty returning to their previous employment, others become somewhat housebound, and some must be admitted to long-term care facilities.

Traumas

Traumatic brain injury (TBI) (also called *acquired brain injury* or ABI) has its highest incidence in the 15- to 24-year-old age group. It is the leading cause of death of people under 35 years of age and the leading cause of neurological disability of people under the age of 50. About one in three people are left with permanent disabilities; consequently, many individuals who sustain a TBI must cope with communicative and cognitive difficulties for the greater part of their adult lives (Guerrero, Thurman, & Sniezek, 2000).

Approximately one-half to two-thirds of all head traumas are caused by motor vehicle accidents, and many of these are alcohol related, particularly with younger drivers. Assaults that are often related to alcohol or drugs (particularly in the young male adult population) and falls (in the older population) account for most other TBIs. The frontal lobes are the most commonly damaged area of the brain in TBIs (see Figure 11–5). Males are nearly twice as likely to receive TBIs as females (Guerrero, Thurman, & Sniezek, 2000; Tate, McDonald, & Lulham, 1998).

Closed Head Injury (CHI) (Nonpenetrating Brain Injury)

Closed head injuries (nonpenetrating brain injuries) are the most common type of head injury in the civilian population. In CHIs, the skull receives a severe impact and may be fractured, but it is not penetrated. The most common causes of CHIs in adults are motor vehicle accidents and assaults. In CHIs, damage is usually caused either by a blunt object (e.g., the head hitting the windshield of a vehicle) or by a sudden stopping of the head's movement in a particular direction (e.g., the head

---

spontaneous recovery

The physiological healing of the brain's damaged tissue, including reduction of cerebral edema, development of collateral blood vessels, and rerouting of neural pathways.

prognosis

A prediction of the probable course, duration, recovery, or termination of a disease or disorder; a prediction of the outcome of a proposed course of treatment, its effectiveness and duration, and the individual's progress.

traumatic brain injury (TBI) (head trauma, acquired brain injury [ABI])

An acquired injury to the brain caused by an external force and resulting in partial or total functional disability, including psychosocial impairment; applies to both closed and open head injuries, affecting speech, language, cognition, psychosocial behavior, and physical functioning.

closed head injury (CHI) (nonpenetrating brain injury)

Severe impact to the skull, often with a blunt object such as the windshield of a vehicle or a bat, or the head striking the ground after a fall; the skull may be fractured but is not penetrated (e.g., by a bullet).

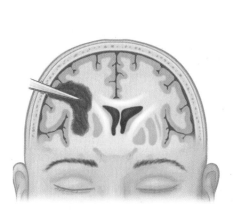

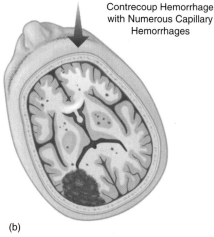

Impact

Contrecoup Hemorrhage with Numerous Capillary Hemorrhages

(a)   Direct Trauma (Stab Wound)   (b)

Figure 11-5

Traumatic brain injuries can occur in countless ways, including (a) direct trauma such as a stab wound causing an open head injury or (b) closed head injury from a motor vehicle accident that may result in contrecoup hemorrhage.
© Cengage Learning 2013.

hitting the ground during a fall). The sudden stopping of the head's momentum sets off a cascade of physiological events. Closed head injuries sometimes result in **contrecoup damage** (pronounced "contra-coo") in which there is damage to the brain at both the site of impact and the opposite side because the brain "flows" and causes intense compression (see Figure 11-5). After a CHI, the brain tissue swells, causing sustained compression of the neurons and damaging them further. The edema may not subside for several days to weeks, during which time the person will present as more severely impaired than after the edema has diminished (Kochanek, Clark, & Jenkins, 2007; Tate, McDonald, & Lulham, 1998).

In motor vehicle accidents, *whiplash injury* often occurs at the same instant as the brain damage because of the rapid forward and backward or rotational movement of the head. Whiplash injuries damage the cervical vertebrae or their supporting ligaments and muscles. Whiplash injuries also can damage the brainstem, resulting in weakness or paralysis of the muscles of the speech systems causing in dysarthria and/or dysphagia (see Chapter 12), as well as bodily impairments.

Mild Traumatic Brain Injury (mTBI)

More than two-thirds of all head injuries are classified as mild, where there is **concussion** but no **loss of consciousness (LOC)** (lack of awareness and wakefulness), or no more than 30 minutes of LOC (other medical criteria are used as well). There is an increased awareness of concussions that occur in sports, causing **chronic traumatic encephalopathy (CTE)**. At the high school level, 15% of injuries among athletes are concussions, with some athletes sustaining more than one concussion in the same year. High school football is the most likely sport for males to receive concussions, followed by soccer and ice hockey. For females, high school soccer and lacrosse are the most likely sports to receive concussions (Meechan, d'Hemecourt, Collins, & Comstock, 2011).

contrecoup injury

In closed head injuries damage to the brain occurring on the opposite side of the trauma site; for example, when an impact to the right frontal side of the skull results in brain damage on the left posterior side.

concussion

Mild traumatic brain injury caused by a violent jarring or shaking that often occurs during a closed head injury and results in at least a brief loss of consciousness.

loss of consciousness (LOC)

Impaired responsiveness, usually caused by diffuse brain dysfunction or damage to the brainstem and the reticular activating system; duration is often used as a measure of traumatic brain injury severity.

chronic traumatic encephalopathy (CTE)

A degenerative brain disease caused by repeated brain traumas (particularly concussions) that results in behaviors similar to Alzheimer's disease.

CASE STUDY

**computerized
tomography (CT) scan**

A radiographic technique to
visualize body tissue not able to be
seen on standard X-ray images;
formerly called computerized axial
tomography (CAT) scan.

**magnetic resonance
imaging (MRI)**

An imaging study that does not
expose the patient to radiation
and often provides images with
sharper detail than those from
computerized tomography (CT)
scans; medical imaging based on
the resonance of atomic nuclei in
a strong magnetic field.

Haitham

Haitham was a 26-year-old man referred by a physician to a speech-language pathologist in private practice. He was a civil engineer who had been born and raised in Amman, Jordan, and his first language was Arabic. Haitham sustained a TBI when he was 23 years old during a motor vehicle accident. **Computerized tomography (CT) scan** and **magnetic resonance imaging (MRI)** of his head revealed multiple brain traumas with diffuse axonal damage and cerebral edema. Haitham was in a coma for 8 months and after recovering consciousness was transferred to a rehabilitation center in Amman where he received physical, occupational, and speech therapy. Eighteen months after the motor vehicle accident he was flown to London, England, where he was seen at a neurological rehabilitation center as an outpatient. A **mental status examination** by a **neuropsychologist** revealed that Haitham remained at considerable risk for emotional difficulties, particularly when the somewhat unrealistic goals he had set for himself could not be realized (i.e., returning to his work as a civil engineer).

Haitham eventually came to California with his mother to live with a relative and to continue receiving speech, language, and cognitive therapy. Evaluation of Haitham by the speech-language pathologist revealed severe dysarthria, mild-to-moderate receptive and expressive aphasia, and severe cognitive impairments that interfered with independent functioning in a consistently safe manner in the home and community. He worked with the therapist twice weekly for several months, making significant gains in most areas, and then returned to his home in Amman, Jordan. Haitham remained unrealistic about his potential to return to his previous work as a civil engineer. ■

**mental status
examination**

A structured interview and
observations conducted by a
psychologist or neuropsychologist
of a patient's orientation,
attention, concentration, memory,
language comprehension and
expression, visual–spatial skills,
abstraction abilities, general
cognitive functioning, and
insight into problems to provide
direction for cognitive-linguistic
rehabilitation that is typically
provided by a speech-language
pathologist.

Because most concussions do not result in loss of consciousness, they are typically more difficult to detect and can be under-diagnosed in athletes (Moser, Iverson, Echemendia, et al., 2007).

Postconcussion syndrome (PCS) is a constellation of symptoms seen in some patients with mild traumatic brain injury, including headache, poor concentration, short-term memory deficits, and affective disturbances (e.g., anxiety, depression, and irritability). However, when loss of consciousness occurs and is prolonged (hours to years) the person is comatose and the length and depth of the **coma** has some prognostic implications for long-term recovery. Patients who have longer and deeper comas generally have a poorer recovery than patients who have shorter and lighter comas (Guthrie, Mast, McQuaid, & Pavlakis, 1999; Johnson & Jacobson, 2007). The term **vegetative state** differs from coma; whereas there is neither awareness nor wakefulness in coma, in a vegetative state a patient may have some minimal level of wakefulness but has not regained awareness (i.e., there is no observable cognitive function).

Persistent vegetative state (PVS) is applied to individuals who survive extensive and irrevocable brain damage but are highly unlikely ever to achieve higher functioning above a vegetative state (Giacino & Whyte, 2005; Hirsch, 2005; Golper, 2010).

Even when head injuries are mild, there are often long-lasting subtle impairments, including difficulty concentrating under distracting conditions (e.g., reading with a television on) or multitasking (trying to do more than one task at a time, such as preparing a meal while talking with someone, or driving—the ultimate challenge in multitasking). Individuals who have had mild traumatic brain injuries often have ongoing difficulty with attention, memory, and higher-level cognitive functioning, particularly when there is frontal lobe damage. Motivation is frequently impaired, and these individuals often have increased anxiety, depression, and irritability (Iverson, Lange, Gatz, & Zasler, 2007; McDonald, 2007; Ponsford, 2004; Sohlberg & Mateer, 2001).

People with mild TBIs are usually discharged from the acute-care hospital after only a short stay, and they may receive some outpatient rehabilitation. However, their real impairments often do not become apparent until they try to return to work and find that they cannot easily perform at the same level as they did before their TBI. Problems also start developing at home. Because people with brain injuries cannot perform at their **premorbid** level on the job, they may be demoted or lose their jobs, causing financial strain on the family. Marital relationships often deteriorate. The individuals may feel guilty that they cannot be the same husband or wife or father or mother they were before the accident. If they are able to maintain a job, they come home exhausted with little or no reserve energy for family life. Resentment may build up within the family because injured people prefer to rest rather than do family activities on weekends. Old friends may begin to stay away because injured people often lose interest or are unable to continue activities they had enjoyed all of their lives. As rehabilitation specialists, we need to always keep in mind that the effects of neurological damage on individuals affect everyone with whom they are associated (Flasher & Fogle, 2012; McDonald, 2007; Tanner, 2007).

Open Head Injury (OHI)

Open head injuries (OHI) are the result of the skull and brain being penetrated either by severe impact or by projectiles (e.g., bullets, fragments of glass, or shrapnel from explosions). In many cases, there is a single trajectory (path) of the projectile (e.g., bullet), and it is mainly the tissue damaged along the path that causes the *cognitive-linguistic impairments* we see. Patients with OHIs often continue to have significant impairments the rest of their lives. In civilian life, OHIs occur less often than CHIs.

War Wounds

Traumatic brain injuries may cause CHIs or OHIs, and the injuries are often different from typical TBIs in civilian life (Lew, Poole, Alvarez, &

---

neuropsychologist

A Ph.D. psychologist specialized in the area of practice in clinical psychology and neurogenic disorders who assesses cognitive functioning, discriminates between psychiatric and neurological conditions, distinguishes among different neurological conditions, and predicts the course of a patient's recovery; however, most of the cognitive-linguistic therapy is provided by SLPs.

postconcussion syndrome (PCS)

A constellation of symptoms seen in some patients with mild traumatic brain injury, including headache, poor concentration, short-term memory deficits, and affective disturbances (e.g., anxiety, depression, and irritability).

coma

A prolonged period of unconsciousness in which a patient has minimal, if any, purposeful responses to stimuli.

vegetative state

A condition in which a person may have some minimal level of wakefulness but has not regained awareness (i.e., they lack observable cognitive function).

persistent vegetative state (PVS)

A medical diagnosis made only after numerous neurological and other tests that, due to extensive and irrevocable brain damage, a patient is highly unlikely ever to achieve higher functioning above a vegetative state.

premorbid

In medicine, the wellness or functioning of a patient before a significant illness or injury.

Personal Story — Vietnam

As a combat medic in Vietnam in 1969, I knew how uncomfortable and heavy steel helmets were after wearing them for many hours every day and night. I encouraged men to wear their helmets at all times while on the lines or on patrols, but some men chose not to. I saw many men receive head wounds from rifle fire and shrapnel from mortars and rockets that could have been prevented or at least lessened if they had been wearing their helmets. Fortunately, in later wars (e.g., Iraq and Afghanistan) the new helmet material is lighter yet stronger and helmets are worn more consistently because of comfort—and because the soldiers are following strict orders to wear them. This information is particularly important for clinicians who will work in VA hospitals and will see many men and women with war wounds. ■

Application Question

Do you know anyone who had a mild traumatic brain injury or concussion? Were there any differences in how they were as people before and after the head injury?

open head injury (OHI)

Head injury in which the skull and brain are penetrated by a severe impact or by a projectile (bullet, fragment of glass, or shrapnel from an explosion).

post-traumatic stress disorder (PTSD)

A set of symptoms after exposure to a psychologically extreme traumatic stressor that involves intense fear, horror, or helplessness; symptoms include persistent reexperiencing of the traumatic event or events, avoidance of stimuli associated with the trauma, and symptoms of increased arousal (*hypervigilance*).

Moore, 2005). In war wounds, the open head injuries are usually more extensive (partly because the high-velocity bullets from military weapons result in powerful shock waves in the brain, causing more diffuse damage) and the individuals often have multiple severe injuries throughout their bodies, including their face and neck. In civilian life, war wounds are seen in explosions, including terrorist attacks. In all cases, the medical goal is to keep the person alive. Once the person is *stabilized* (physiological and metabolic processes of equilibrium in the body), rehabilitation can begin. Some SLPs and Auds work in Veterans Administration (VA) hospitals where they see terrible wounds in men and women. In some cases, soldiers may be discharged from a VA hospital and moved to a community hospital closer to the soldier's home where rehabilitation can continue. Clinicians need to be aware that these patients may be a "different" type of patient compared to those injured in civilian life (Flasher & Fogle, 2012).

Post-traumatic stress disorder (PTSD) is a problem that can affect combat veterans (whether or not they were physically wounded) in both subtle and obvious ways the rest of their lives. However, providing therapy for veterans is often a pleasure because they are disciplined and motivated, they have a joy of life (perhaps because they have seen so much loss of life), and they appreciate all that is done for them (Fogle, 2009b).

Tumors

Tumors (neoplasms) may grow in the brain and cause various communication, cognitive, and swallowing problems. The sites and sizes of tumors determine the impairments that develop in individuals. Tumors are abnormal masses of tissue that cause compression and displacement of

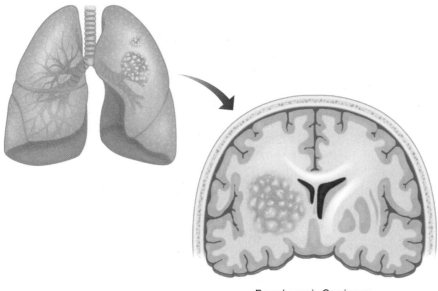

Bronchogenic Carcinoma
Metastasizing to Brain

Figure 11–6

Tumors may metastasize to the brain from other areas of the body.

© Cengage Learning 2013.

brain tissue unassociated with the specific site of the tumor. Tumors may be either *primary* (originating in the brain) or *secondary* (originating elsewhere in the body and then traveling to the brain). For example, a tumor may originate in the lungs (the primary tumor), and then cells from that tumor can **metastasize** (travel or spread) by way of the bloodstream to other areas of the body, such as the CNS (see Figure 11–6). Tumors may be either *benign* (not cancerous) or *malignant* (cancerous).

Toxins

SLPs sometimes work with patients who have neurological disorders caused by various toxins, some of which are preventable. **Toxins** are substances that poison or cause inflammation of the CNS. Probably the most commonly used toxic substance is alcohol. Years of excessive alcohol consumption can have severe effects on the CNS. Besides alcohol, many other toxins are self-administered as "recreational" drugs that can have lifelong effects on the nervous system and the person's quality of life. Many patients with neurological damage from various toxins have poor prognoses for significant improvement because much of their brain can be affected, leaving little "healthy" brain tissue available to be used for rehabilitation.

Degenerative Diseases and Disorders

Neurogenic communication disorders may be caused by **degenerative diseases** that affect structures and functions and cause progressive deterioration over time. Degenerative diseases can affect speech, language, cognition, swallowing, hearing, and balance. Examples of degenerative diseases that SLPs see clinically that result in cognitive-linguistic

tumor (neoplasm)

Any abnormal growth of new tissue, either benign or malignant, caused by aberrant increases in the rate of cell reproduction.

metastasis/metastasize

The process by which tumor cells travel or spread to distant parts of the body.

toxin

A substance that poisons or causes inflammation of tissue, including in the central nervous system.

degenerative disease

Any condition that causes gradual deterioration of normal body functions.

"I Wanted To See What Would Happen."

During a graduate internship at Rancho Los Amigos Hospital in Southern California, I was asked by my supervisor to accompany him to a local convalescent hospital to assess a 19-year-old man. The patient had taken an overdose of a drug and was left with severe neurological damage sufficient to cause him to remain hospitalized for the rest of his life. I asked him (probably inappropriately) why he did it, and he answered, "I wanted to see what would happen." As clinicians, we sometimes see individuals who, in a moment of reckless abandon, alter their lives forever. ■

impairments are the dementias (including Alzheimer's disease) (see Cognitive Disorders) and motor speech disorders such as amyotrophic lateral sclerosis (ALS, or Lou Gehrig's disease), Parkinson's disease, and myasthenia gravis (see Chapter 12).

THE APHASIAS

aphasia (dysphasia)

An acquired language impairment resulting from neurological damage in the absence of cognitive, motor, or sensory impairments.

cognitive disorder

Impaired ability to process and use incoming information for memory, organization of information, reasoning, judgment, and problem solving for adequate functioning in activities of daily living, including a person's work. A diagnostic term implies that a certain set of characteristics apply to a patient.

receptive aphasia

Difficulty comprehending verbal, written, and/or gestural language.

expressive aphasia

Difficulty formulating verbal, written, and/or gestural language.

Numerous definitions of **aphasia (dysphasia)** have been used by various authors. Brookshire, in his earlier writings (1992, p. 1), provided a relatively simple but useful definition by saying that "Aphasia is a deficit in language processing that may affect all input modalities (auditory, visual, and tactile) and all output modalities (speaking, writing, and gesturing)." Code (2012) defines aphasia as an acquired language impairment resulting from neurological damage in the absence of **cognitive disorders** or motor and sensory impairments. Most SLPs use the term *aphasia* even though patients typically have impaired or disordered language (*dysphasia*) rather than a complete loss of language.

Classifications and Terminology Associated with the Aphasias

Classifications and terminology influence the way speech-language pathologists communicate with other SLPs, PTs, OTs, physicians, nurses, third-party payers (e.g., Medicare and insurance companies), and with patients and their families (Threats & Worrall, 2004). Although each patient is different, there are sufficient similarities so that we can use classification systems and diagnostic terms that communicate to other professionals of the basic impairments of the person. A diagnostic term implies that a certain set of characteristics apply to a patient.

The two classifications used specifically for aphasia are: **receptive aphasia** and **expressive aphasia**. That is, a person's language impairments may be narrowed down to difficulty understanding what is being communicated (auditory, reading, or gestural comprehension), difficulty expressing what the person wants to communicate (verbal, written, or gestural expression), or both. The receptive and expressive aphasia classification is roughly equivalent to the *fluent* (receptive) and *nonfluent* (expressive) classification system.

Fluent and Nonfluent Aphasia Classification System

Speech fluency is an important concept for understanding aphasia syndromes; therefore, the **fluent** and **nonfluent aphasia** classification system was devised. The **prosodic** or **melodic** characteristics of speech are the primary distinguishing factors for fluent and nonfluent aphasia. Fluency, when referring to the aphasias, does not connote stuttering (disfluency), although the concept of speech that flows easily (fluent) versus speech that has hesitations and repetitions (nonfluent) is the origin of the concept as it relates to aphasia (LaPointe, 2005).

Fluent aphasias are often associated with lesions posterior to the fissure of Rolando (central sulcus), primarily in and around the language areas in the temporal lobe of the left hemisphere *(perisylvian region)*. Patients with fluent aphasia typically have **auditory comprehension** impairments, difficulty comprehending written information, omission of important nouns, verbs, and adjectives in sentences, and syntactic errors; however, their speaking rate is relatively normal (100–200 words per minute), with normal phrasing (5–8 words per phrase or sentence), and they have relatively normal articulation, inflections, and intonation. Nonfluent aphasias are associated with lesions anterior to the fissure of Rolando, primarily in or around Broca's area in the premotor strip of the left frontal lobe. Nonfluent aphasia is characterized by relatively good auditory and reading comprehension, but difficulty initiating speech and saying the first sound or syllable of a word, reduced rate of speech (less than 50 words per minute), unusual effort when speaking, and omission of *functor* words (e.g., *a, an, the*).

Fluent aphasias include *Wernicke's aphasia, anomic aphasia, conduction aphasia*, and *transcortical sensory aphasia*. Nonfluent aphasias include *Broca's aphasia, transcortical motor aphasia*, and *global aphasia*. The *Boston Classification System* (Goodglass, Kaplan, & Barresi, 2001) has been particularly influential in our understanding of the different types of aphasia and the likely areas of neurological damage (see Figure 11–7).

Major Types of Aphasia

Each type of aphasia has its own characteristics. However, depending on the site and size of the lesion, many patients have two or more types of aphasia, making a simple or clear diagnosis difficult.

fluent aphasia

Aphasia that results from damage to posterior regions of the cortex (i.e., temporal or temporal-parietal lesions) characterized by language with normal pauses and articulation but with frequent syntactic errors, paraphasias, and circumlocutions.

nonfluent aphasia

Aphasia that results from damage to anterior cortical regions (i.e., frontal lobe lesions) characterized by sparse, perseverative language with disturbed prosody, misarticulations, errors in syntax, and a reduction in phrase length.

prosody (prosodic)/ melody (melodic)

The qualities of stress and intonation in the voice that are influenced by the pitch, loudness, and duration of individual speech sounds.

auditory comprehension

The ability to understand spoken language at the single word, phrase, simple sentence, complex sentence, paragraph, and conversational speech levels.

Application Question

A single word can conjure up numerous memories (auditory, visual, tactile, and even taste and smell), associations, thoughts, and feelings. For just a moment, think about the word *mother*. What images, memories, experiences, associations, thoughts, and feelings start coming to mind? Which modalities and lobes of your brain are you using?

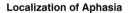

Localization of Aphasia

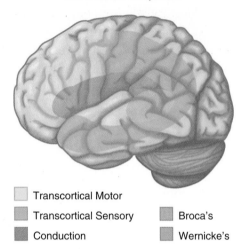

Transcortical Motor
Transcortical Sensory — Broca's
Conduction — Wernicke's

Figure 11-7

General areas of damage
for fluent and nonfluent
aphasia.
© Cengage Learning 2013.

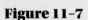

Wernicke's aphasia

A fluent aphasia characterized
by impaired comprehension,
integration of information, and
formulation of language caused
by damage to the perisylvian
regions in or around Wernicke's
area in the posterior superior
left temporal lobe (auditory
association cortex).

**alexia (acquired
dyslexia)**

Impaired ability to read as the
result of neurological damage.

Wernicke's Aphasia

A German neurologist, Karl Wernicke (1848–1905), in 1874 was the first to describe the location of damage and the symptoms of what was later to be called **Wernicke's aphasia** (Geshwind, 1965). Wernicke's aphasia is a fluent aphasia caused by damage to the perisylvian regions in or around Wernicke's area in the posterior superior left temporal lobe (i.e., the *auditory association cortex*). Wernicke's aphasia is characterized by impaired auditory comprehension, integration, and formulation of language (LaPointe, 2005).

Impaired Auditory Comprehension

Impaired auditory comprehension (minimal to profound) is a hallmark characteristic of Wernicke's aphasia (Caspari, 2005; LaPointe, 2005; Morris & Franklin, 2012). Patients often have significant difficulty understanding single words, following simple directions, and understanding conversation. They have increasing difficulty at all levels when there is background noise, conversation, or visual distractions. To comprehend information or a conversation, a variety of areas in the brain may be actively involved to understand individual words, unique combinations of words in a sentence to convey a message, tone of voice, facial expressions, and body language of the speaker. In essence, *integration* (cognition) is the core of both comprehension and formulation of language. A person's expressive language may be the result of a combination of impaired comprehension and integration of information.

Patients with aphasia often have comprehension problems in more than the auditory modality; typically, they have equal or more severe impairments with reading comprehension (**alexia** or **acquired dyslexia**) (Webb, 2005). Patients may have difficulty associating sounds with letters, recognizing and naming letters, and reading and comprehending individual words, sentences, and paragraph-length information. It is important for SLPs to diagnose and document reading problems of patients. In addition to reading, patients also may have difficulty comprehending other people's gestural and body language. Overall, for many patients there is no intact input modality.

Communication Techniques That May Help a Person Better Understand You

- Have the person watch your face as you speak.
- Speak clearly, but do not exaggerate your articulation or facial expressions—use a natural tone of voice and inflection as you would talk to any normal adult.
- Have short pauses between sentences to give the person a little more time to process the information.
- If the person asks you to repeat something or looks quizzically at you, repeat what you said verbatim and in the same tone of voice so that he does not have to try to compare and comprehend different words or different voice inflections.
- If the person still does not understand, change just a few words that may help him comprehend.
- Writing a word or sentence may help the person understand.
- Avoid becoming frustrated when a person does not understand—he is doing the best he can, and his lack of understanding is always harder on him than it is on anyone else.

Impaired Integration of Information

To **integrate** information (process it at various levels of depth and relate it to information stored in other modalities), numerous areas of the brain need to become actively involved (remember that all processing is occurring at the neuronal and synaptic levels of the brain). Other terms for *integration* are *cognitive processing, cognition,* or *thinking;* that is, the brain's manipulation of stimuli in various lobes and areas to use it. Comprehension and integration cannot be separated—they are occurring in the brain simultaneously and in multiple areas.

Impaired Formulation of Language

Patients with aphasia often have a variety of language-formulation problems, the most common of which is **anomia** (Martin, 2012; Raymer, 2005). Anomia goes by several terms that are more descriptive than the technical diagnostic term; for example, *naming impairments, word-finding problems, word-recall deficits,* and *word-retrieval difficulties* (note that *impairments, deficits, difficulties,* and *problems* are interchangeable). Anomia is often one of several expressive language impairments seen in patients who have aphasia.

Anomia can range from mild to profound, including difficulty remembering a person's own name. When patients cannot name an object, they may try to talk about it or describe it (**circumlocution**), perhaps hoping that listeners will name it for them. People with aphasia experience

integrate (integration)

The process of combining into a complete and functional whole; combining and processing information from the various input modalities to store, attach meaning, and respond.

anomia

Impaired ability to retrieve (remember) names of people, places, or things, as well as to retrieve other parts of speech (e.g., verbs and adjectives) while speaking.

circumlocution

Description or "talking around" something when the specific word cannot be recalled.

Personal Story   A Medical–Legal Case

Because of my work in *forensic* speech-language pathology (work with attorneys and courts on legal cases that involve speech, language, cognition, and swallowing) (Fogle, 2000; Fogle, 2003; Fogle, 2006), I receive requests from attorneys around the country to evaluate legal documents of individuals who have had speech-language and swallowing therapy to make various determinations about communicative, cognitive, and swallowing competence.

An attorney from another state contacted me asking if I would review all available medical and rehabilitation documentation on a 72-year-old man who had sustained a left-hemisphere CVA. The patient was diagnosed by an SLP as having receptive and expressive aphasia (including reading impairments), cognitive impairments, and dysphagia (swallowing problems). One hour before undergoing a modified barium swallow study (see Chapter 12, Swallowing Disorders/Dysphagia), the patient was asked by his adult son to sign a significant change in his will. A few days after the modified barium swallow study, the patient died and there was a legal dispute about the change in the will. The legal questions being asked were, "Was the patient able to read and comprehend the changes in his will?," and "Was he cognitively competent to make an informed decision?" After careful review of the patient's entire medical chart, reports, and documentation (including the SLP's reports and daily therapy notes), I determined that the patient was not able to read and comprehend such a complex legal document or cognitively competent to make an informed decision. I wrote an extensive report that supported my conclusions, which was used in the final determination of the case. The case was eventually settled out of court, and I was later contacted by the attorney who informed me about the legal decisions. The patient's wife won the case and the changed will was "thrown out," allowing her to remain the beneficiary of her husband's estate. ■

---

literal (phonemic paraphasia)

Sounds and syllables that are correctly articulated but may be extraneous, transposed, or substituted, usually with the preservation of the vowels and intended number of syllables in a word (e.g., tar for car); often occurring in both speech and writing.

difficulty remembering words whenever they try to communicate, and some people begin to avoid communicating because of embarrassment and frustration.

The language (both spoken and written) of patients with aphasia is often filled with various paraphasias. **Literal** or **phonemic paraphasias** are substitutions of unintended sounds for intended sounds in words; for example, *mat* for *cat* and *hairblane* for *airplane*. (LaPointe, 2005, provided the following literal paraphasia of a former mortician who had aphasia. The mortician attempted to explain a proverb by saying, "Don't put all your eggs in one *casket*.") **Verbal** or **semantic paraphasias** are word errors in which the erred word is often semantically related to the intended word; for example, *salt* for *pepper* and *mother* for *wife*. (LaPointe also provided the following verbal paraphasia of one of his patients who was trying to give his clinician a compliment, "You are very *begoing* today, Nancy.") **Neologisms** are another form of paraphasia in which a person combines consonants and vowels that sound like they could be words and even uses inflection to give them emotional meaning; for example, *bingtema* and *hitican*. A patient using neologisms or other paraphasias may be unaware of the errors and continue talking as though he is making complete sense, which is referred to as **jargon aphasia**. Patients with aphasia may use a variety of paraphasias and actual meaningful words in a sentence, along with appropriate prosody and inflection, so that listeners may get the gist of what is being communicated.

In addition to impaired verbal expression, most patients with aphasia have even more difficulty communicating in writing—**agraphia**. The combination of alexia and agraphia is common (McNeil & Tseng, 2005; Mortensen, 2004; Papathanasiou & Csefalvay, 2012). As with their speech, writing may be copious but meaningless. Such patients write using paraphasias (phonemic, semantic, neologistic, and jargon) and circumlocutions and have syntactic errors.

Anomic Aphasia

Some patients may have primarily a persistent and severe naming (word retrieval) problem when other areas of their language are relatively intact (e.g., auditory comprehension). These patients may be said to have **anomic aphasia**. Anomia is the most common residual symptom of people who have had any type of aphasia (Boyle, 2004; Martin, 2012). Individuals with anomic aphasia have frequent and often severe difficulty remembering most classes of words, not just nouns (names); for example, verbs and adjectives often elude them (Freed, Celery, & Marshal, 2004). Reading comprehension is usually fairly good, but they have significant difficulty describing what they read because of the word-finding impairment.

Broca's Aphasia

Broca's aphasia was first described in 1863 by Paul Broca (1824–1880), a French neurosurgeon (he called the impairment *aphemia*) after studying the impaired speech and language of several patients, followed by autopsies of their brains after death (one patient became known as "Tan" because that was the only word he could say) (Berker, Berker, & Smith, 1986). The site of lesion that impaired the speech and language of these patients was in the lower posterior region of the left frontal lobe in the premotor cortex (premotor strip), the area that later became known as *Broca's area*. However, since that time it has been discovered that damaged cortex around Broca's area also may cause signs and symptoms of Broca's aphasia (Kearns, 2005).

verbal (semantic paraphasia)

Unintended substitution of one word for another word that is often semantically related to the intended word (e.g., *sister* for *brother* and *horse* for *dog*); often occur in both speech and writing.

neologism

A form of paraphasia in which a person combines consonants and vowels that sound like they could be words and uses inflection to give them emotional meaning; for example, *bingtema* and *hitican*.

jargon aphasia

Continuous but unintelligible speech with various combinations of literal and verbal paraphasias and neologisms, with little or no conveying of information; often with the speaker having little awareness of the problem and occurring in both speech and writing.

agraphia

An acquired disorder of writing resulting in difficulty writing letters, words, and sentences.

anomic aphasia

A disorder whose primary feature is persistent and severe difficulty retrieving names of people, places, and objects, as well as all classes of words (e.g., verbs and adjectives).

Application Question

What strategies do you use when you cannot remember a word, for example, on an exam?

CASE STUDY

A Nurse's Aphasia

A male nurse in his early 40s had a CVA that resulted in receptive and expressive aphasia, cognitive impairments, and right-side hemiparesis (weakness on one side). He received physical therapy, occupational therapy, and speech therapy at the acute-care hospital and in the rehabilitation unit. After being discharged from rehabilitation, he learned that because of his impairments he had lost his job at the convalescent hospital where he had worked for several years. He was unmarried and had difficulty taking care of himself in his small apartment, but he was determined to be as independent as possible.

He began therapy at a university speech-language clinic and worked diligently and consistently for several semesters. His goal and motivation were always to return to nursing. He even brought in nursing textbooks to use as part of his therapy. The client made significant improvement during his semesters in the clinic, although he continued having difficulty with auditory comprehension, verbal expression, and cognition, as well as right-side hemiparesis and balance problems. He eventually became more realistic about returning to nursing work. He stopped attending therapy when he had accepted and adjusted to his communication problems and his new self. As SLPs, we need to keep in mind that clients and patients will sometimes remain in therapy only until they reach their personal goals or have accepted their limitations, even though they may have potential for further improvement. ■

Broca's aphasia

A nonfluent expressive aphasia characterized by agrammatic language with omissions of articles, conjunctions, prepositions, plurals, possessives, and verb morphemes and auxiliary verbs; speech is often limited to high-frequency content words, making it sound telegraphic; apraxia of speech, dysarthria, or both often coexist.

agrammatic (agrammatism)

Impairment of the ability to produce words in their correct sequence and with all necessary morphemes.

Patients with Broca's aphasia often have right-side weakness (*paresis, hemiplegia*) or complete loss of movement (*paralysis, hemiplegia*) of the face (including the articulators) because the damage around Broca's area also can affect the *precentral gyrus* (motor strip controlling the face and articulators). These patients also may have paresis or paralysis of the right arm and hand and of the leg and foot.

Many patients with Broca's aphasia have problems with auditory comprehension, although not as severe as that of patients with fluent aphasias. They have particular difficulty understanding syntactical morphemes and structures (e.g., *-ing, -ed, have been*) and relational words (e.g., *heavier–lighter*), much like their difficulty using grammatical structures.

Patients with Broca's aphasia often use **agrammatic** expressive language because they tend to omit the grammatical function (*functor*) words such as articles (*the, a, an*), conjunctions (e.g., *and, but*), prepositions (e.g., *in, out, on, off*), plurals and possessives (*-s, -'s*), verb morphemes (e.g., *-ing, -ed*), and auxiliary verbs (e.g., *have, has, is, are, was, were*). The expressive language of these patients often sounds *telegraphic* (i.e., language that is condensed so that only the most essential words and morphemes are used—much like the language used in a telegram) (Kearns, 2005; Marshall, 2012).

Patients who have Broca's aphasia without other complications tend to have a relatively good prognosis. However, Broca's aphasia often occurs with the motor speech disorders of apraxia of speech, dysarthria, or both. Patients with multiple diagnoses often have *"guarded" prognoses*, that is, there is considerable uncertainty in the potential for significant recovery.

The speech of patients with Broca's aphasia is often slow and effortful because of trial-and-error groping for the intended articulatory movements. Such patients frequently use substitutions, omissions, and repetitions of sounds with little consistency in their errors. Patients have increasing difficulty as the length of a word becomes longer (e.g., *live— lively—liveliest*).

Patients with Broca's aphasia commonly have difficulty with both reading and writing. Their oral reading is effortful and nonfluent. They may understand the content words (e.g., nouns, verbs, and adjectives) easier than the syntactical morphemes and structures (much like their auditory comprehension abilities). Their writing, like their speech, is slow, laborious, and halting. Their written language is similar to their spoken language—that is, agrammatic (Kearns, 2005).

Global Aphasia

Global aphasia is a combination of fluent and nonfluent aphasia and is generally considered the most severe form of aphasia. Global aphasia is usually caused by occlusion of the left middle cerebral artery, causing diffuse damage to the temporal, frontal, and parietal lobes. The occlusion can severely impair all language processing and speech production. Patients have severe impairments of comprehension, integration, and formulation of language in all modalities, as well as significant cognitive impairments. They may have apraxia of speech, resulting in severe difficulty with planning articulatory movements. They also may have severe weakness in the speech systems (respiratory, phonatory, resonatory, and articulatory), causing profound distortions of speech (dysarthria). The prognosis for these patients is often poor because of the extent of the neurological damage and the severity of the combination of disorders (Collins, 2005; Portagas, Kasselimis, & Evdokimidis, 2012).

Cognitive Impairments Associated with Aphasia

Patients with receptive, expressive, or both types of aphasia also may have cognitive impairments. People use more than just their left hemisphere when comprehending, integrating, and formulating language. People use language when consciously thinking (cognition); therefore, when individuals have aphasia, they will likely have some level of difficulty with the various components of cognition (Portagas, Kasselimis, & Evdokimidis, 2012).

global aphasia

A severe-to-profound aphasia resulting from a diffuse lesion involving portions of the left temporal, frontal, and parietal lobes that is characterized by severely impaired receptive and expressive language in all input and all output modalities, with motor speech disorders of apraxia of speech, dysarthria, or both.

Principles of Assessment of Aphasia

When working in hospitals or other medical settings, assessment of patients with neurological damage usually follows a general format. After the SLP receives the referral (*consult*) from the patient's physician, she reads the patient's medical chart that is usually located at the nurses' station. Reviewing all parts of the chart is essential to understand as much as possible about the patient.

After reviewing the medical chart, the clinician interviews the patient and obtains a case history. Speaking with family members can be helpful to add to or corroborate information the patient has provided. The interview is the initiation of the evaluation and the clinician should note the patient's hearing acuity (a formal hearing evaluation may be needed later), assess the speech systems (respiratory, phonatory, resonatory, articulatory), and evaluate receptive and expressive language abilities. In many cases, some cognitive assessment may be appropriate. The purpose of an assessment is always to identify and document general and specific strengths and impairments using relevant functional items so that a diagnosis can be made and a treatment program can be developed and implemented (Helm-Estabrooks & Albert, 2004; Larkins, Worrall, & Hickson, 2004; Murray & Clark, 2006). The following are the most commonly assessed areas of patients with neurological disorders (note that these areas apply to most individuals with communication impairments, regardless of etiology):

Receptive language abilities

- Hearing acuity (with and without hearing aid devices)
- Visual acuity (with and without glasses or contacts)
- Pointing to objects or pictures named by the clinician
- Answering simple to complex questions
- Following simple to complex spoken directions
- Answering questions about spoken discourse
- Following conversational speech

Expressive language abilities

- Evaluation of the speech systems (respiratory, phonatory, resonatory, articulatory)
- Naming common objects (*confrontation naming*)
- Providing the verb (action) associated with common objects
- Providing the word that commonly completes a phrase spoken by the clinician (*responsive naming*; e.g., salt and _____)
- Word fluency (e.g., naming all the animals the patient can think of in 1 minute)
- Repeating words, phrases, and sentences of different lengths spoken by the clinician
- Producing automatic speech (e.g., days of the week or months of the year)

- Producing a sentence using a word provided by the clinician
- Describing what is happening in a picture
- Engaging in conversation (*discourse*)

Ability to communicate nonverbally (through body language)

- Imitation of common facial expressions and gestures
- Following simple commands for facial expressions and gestures

Reading abilities

- Matching pictures, letters, and geometric forms
- Matching printed words to pictures
- Reading aloud printed numbers, letters, words, phrases, and sentences
- Verbally answering printed questions
- Silently reading a paragraph or story and verbally answering questions about it

Writing abilities

- Copying geometric forms, letters, and words
- Writing letters, words, and sentences spoken by the clinician
- Writing biographical information (e.g., name, age, phone number, address, and names of close relatives)
- Writing names of common objects and their functions
- Formulating and producing written narratives

Multicultural Considerations

Assessment and treatment of patients from diverse ethnic, cultural, and linguistic backgrounds present significant challenges for clinicians because most tests have not included a representative number of people from diverse backgrounds in their standardization (Edwards & Bastiannse, 2007; Penn, 2007). Moreover, standardized aphasia tests have not been systematically translated into other languages. Some SLPs are bilingual (usually English and Spanish); however, most clinicians struggle to assess patients in any language other than English (Tonkovich, 2002).

Interpreters and translators can help by removing many of the language barriers between clinicians and patients; however, something is often "lost" in the interpretation or translation from the clinician to the patient and from the patient back to the clinician (Kayser, 2006; Wallace 1997). Centeno (2005) and Hegde and Davis (2010) present several suggestions for clinicians working with individuals from varied ethnic, cultural, and linguistic backgrounds:

- If the use of a standardized instrument is necessary even though it may not be totally appropriate for a given patient, interpret the test results cautiously, considering the patient's ethnic, cultural, and linguistic background.

- While working with certain ethnocultural groups, beliefs about health, illness, disability, and disorders, as well as medical care and rehabilitation, may need to be explored because beliefs affect motivation to seek and continue services.
- If possible, consult with another SLP who belongs to the same or a similar ethnocultural background as the patient.
- Avoid multicultural stereotyping and consider whether your own ethnic, cultural, and linguistic background is influencing your interactions with and assessment of the patient.

General Principles of Therapy

Successful treatment of individuals with neurological disorders is based on numerous and complex interacting factors, including the following:

- *Age of the patient*—Usually the younger, the better.
- *Premorbid language and literacy skills*—The higher the level of premorbid language and literacy, the better.
- *Nature of neuropathology (size and site of lesion)*—The smaller the lesion in a less crucial area, the better.
- *Severity of the impairments*—The less severe, the better.
- *General physical health*—The healthier the patient, the better.
- *Timing of therapy*—The sooner therapy is initiated, the better.
- *Length of therapy*—Generally, the lengthier and more extensive the therapy, the better.
- *Intensity of therapy*—Within reasonable limits, the more intensive (the number of hours per week) of therapy, the better.
- *Appropriateness and effectiveness of therapy goals and procedures*—The more appropriate and effective, the better.
- *Family involvement*—The more supportive and willing to take direction from the clinician, the better.

Clinicians mainly use the *restorative* or the *compensatory* approach when treating individuals with neurological impairments (Ben-Yishay & Diller, 1993; Code, 1991). The restorative approach focuses on improving the underlying processes that are impaired. For example, when patients have word-finding problems, improving their word-finding abilities (e.g., teaching strategies to recall words, not just teaching single words) will likely help them develop functional communication more than trying to recall individual words. Clinicians can enlist conversational partners (e.g., family and friends) to help support patients' attempts to interact and communicate (Fogle, 2009a; Kagan, Black, Duchan, Simmons-Mackie, & Square, 2001). *Aphasia Couples Therapy* (ACT) (Boles, 2009) empowers spouses and other caregivers to become involved in a practical way in the care and therapy of their loved one in ADLs outside of the clinic.

A compensatory approach may be used to provide strategies for persistent language deficits. For example, patients with severe word-finding problems who have not benefited significantly from a restorative approach may need to be taught to use gestures or a communication board to communicate their basic wants, needs, thoughts, and feelings (see Chapter 13, Augmentative and Alternative Communication).

Therapy Goals and Rationales

Therapy goals are determined by the assessment results, the clinician's observations of the patient during the interview and evaluation, and the goals the patient identifies for herself. The bottom line is always to improve the person's **quality of life** (Fogle & Reece, 2006; Hilari & Byng, 2001; Murray & Clark, 2006). The clinician's goals for the person and the person's goals for himself need to be in agreement, and therapy should be designed to meet those goals. This encourages shared decision making with a client-focused treatment approach (Cruice, Worrall, & Hickson, 2000).

We need to have good rationales for our therapy goals, and it is essential to consider the **functional outcomes** that will most benefit the patient (Code & Muller, 1995; Fogle, 2009a; Helm-Estabrooks & Albert, 2004). The rationales for functional outcomes answer the question, What are we going to do in therapy that will have direct effects on the patient's ability to communicate? That is:

- In the hospital setting with medical and rehabilitation staff
- In the home, performing **activities of daily living (ADLs)**
- In the community
- On the job (if he returns to work)

Clinicians also need to ask, Will an insurance company or Medicare reviewer recognize that we are working on goals that will actually improve the person's daily functioning and quality of life and merit reimbursement?

COGNITIVE DISORDERS

Cognitive disorders are seen in many individuals with neurological disorders from various etiologies. Three of the most common etiologies are traumatic brain injuries (TBIs), right-hemisphere damage, and the dementias. Cognitive impairments create some interesting and challenging behaviors that need to be understood and managed by individuals who are working and living with these individuals.

Traumatic Brain Injury

The nature or type of head injury an individual has can significantly affect the symptoms seen during assessment and therapy. It is important to carefully read the hospital medical chart for information on the type of head injury the patient sustained and any bodily injuries he may have. Head injuries are divided into two main classifications: closed head injuries (CHIs) and open head injuries (OHIs).

quality of life

A global concept that is difficult to measure but often is considered to involve a person's standard of living, personal freedom, and the opportunity to pursue happiness; a measure of a person's ability to cope successfully with the full range of challenges encountered in daily living; the characterization of health concerns or disease effects on a person's lifestyle and daily functioning.

functional outcomes

The results of treatment intended to clearly show a person's improved ability to communicate in the hospital setting with medical and rehabilitation staff; at home, performing activities of daily living (ADLs); in the community; and on the job (if the person returns to work).

activities of daily living (ADLs)

The normal activities and tasks people perform in the course of a day, such as ablutions (washing, bathing, brushing the teeth, toileting), dressing, and eating.

Cognitive Impairments Resulting from Traumatic Brain Injury

Traumatic brain injuries can result in numerous cognitive impairments. As with CVAs, the site and size of the lesion determine the symptoms seen (Constantinidou & Kennedy, 2012; Eslinger, Zappala, Chakara, & Barrett, 2007). Many patients with severe TBIs are initially in a comatose state.

Coma

Coma (prolonged period of unconsciousness) may occur with severe brain damage. The patient has minimal, if any, purposeful responses to environmental stimuli. When a patient is in a deep coma, he has no observable response to touch, pain, sound, or movement. In lighter stages of coma, the patient may respond with generalized body movements to strong stimuli. The length and depth of a coma is a fairly reliable indicator of eventual recovery. Patients with longer and deeper comas generally have a poorer recovery than patients with shorter and lighter comas (Mysiw, Fugate, & Clinchot, 2007).

Be Careful of What You Say

Clinicians (really, all people) need to be careful of what they say around patients who are comatose or semicomatose because some patients, when able to eventually communicate, have described both appropriate and inappropriate comments they had heard, understood, and remembered while in their comatose states.

Attention

Patients with damage to various areas of the brain may have impaired *attention* as seen in decreased readiness to respond to stimuli and difficulty with *selective attention* (attending to specific stimuli and ignoring others); *alternating attention* (shifting focus of attention between tasks); *divided attention* (responding simultaneously to more than one task); and *sustained attention* to a task for a reasonable length of time.

Memory

Memory is a complex and controversial area. Many models of memory have been developed within different disciplines (e.g., cognitive psychologists, neuropsychologists, and speech-language pathologists), each with its own preferred terminology (Loring, 1999). In general, patients with neurological disorders have impairments in the acquisition and retention of information (Constantinidou & Kennedy, 2012; McDonald, 2007; Moran & Gillon, 2004; Turkstra, 2001).

Orientation

Orientation is typically divided into four areas: person, place, time, and purpose (i.e., *oriented* ×4). This sequence roughly represents increasingly complex cognitive processing. Patients with TBIs often are disoriented to person (who and what the person is and what the person is doing); place (where the person is and the surrounding environment, including the room, building, city, state, and country); time (month, season, and year, and approximate time, day, and date); and purpose (understanding and being able to reason why something has occurred or is occurring) (Johnson & Jacobson, 2007).

Reasoning and Problem Solving

In all aspects of daily living and working, *abstract reasoning* and *problem solving* are important. Reasoning and problem solving are considered high-level thought processes that rely on all previously discussed cognitive functions; that is, a person has to have functional attention, memory, and be oriented × 4.

Reasoning involves drawing conclusions based on general knowledge or principles or forming solutions from information that supports a conclusion. Problem solving involves (1) recognition of a problem, (2) the ability to select a strategy to solve the problem, (3) the use of the strategy to solve it, and (4) evaluation of the outcome. Patients with neurological disorders, particularly those with right-hemisphere damage and TBIs, often have impaired abstract reasoning and problem solving (Constantinidou & Kennedy, 2012; Fogle, Reece, & White, 2008; Sohlberg & Mateer, 2001).

Executive Functions

Executive functions are controlled by the executive system, a nonspecific region of the prefrontal cortex. This area is thought to coordinate input from all other regions of the brain and, therefore, is important for coordinating and *actualizing* (making things happen) activities involved in cognitive processes (Ponsford, 2004). Executive functions refer to abstract thinking and our ability to (1) anticipate needs, (2) set goals to meet those needs, (3) plan strategies to achieve those goals, (4) implement those strategies, and (5) use feedback to determine the success of the plan and strategies. Executive functions are important in regulating our behaviors (including abstract reasoning and problem solving) and emotions (Chapey, 2008; Sohlberg & Mateer, 2001).

Individuals with executive function impairments have difficulty with ADLs in the home and community, including maintaining personal safety (Fogle, Reece, & White, 2008). They have difficulty in the work environment because they cannot anticipate what needs to be done, figure out ways to do it, and clearly determine that they accomplished what they wanted. Many people are in work environments where safety risks are always a concern and good executive functioning is essential. Executive functions, more than any other cognitive dimension, determine the extent of social and vocational recovery and the ability to live independently (McDonald, 2007; Ponsford, 2004).

Speech and Language Disorders

Along with cognitive impairments, patients with both CHIs and OHIs can have localized lesions that affect speech and language. This combination of impairments may occur for a couple of reasons. In both CHI and OHI, the left hemisphere's Broca's area, precentral gyrus, and Wernicke's area may be damaged, resulting in apraxia of speech, dysarthria, or classic aphasia symptoms. Language impairments, however, may be confused with problems caused by impaired attention, memory, and other cognitive processes. For example, comprehension disorders may be the result of attention and memory problems. In addition, it is difficult to clearly separate language and cognition during comprehension, integration, and formulation of language because many areas of the brain may need to be involved at any instant during communication.

Auditory comprehension abilities, anomia, pragmatics, and reading and writing problems are the most common language impairments seen in individuals with TBIs (McDonald, 2007; Murdoch & Theodoros, 2001). SLPs do not typically administer aphasia tests to patients with TBIs but recognize the possibilities of receptive and expressive language impairments during the interview and through the responses of patients during assessment of cognition.

General Principles of Assessment of Traumatic Brain Injury

Initially, some patients may be comatose or semicomatose and unable to respond to verbal or visual stimuli. However, for most patients during our assessments we often see that they are inconsistent, disorganized, disoriented, confused, restless, and irritable. Both formal and informal assessments of a patient with a TBI are needed to evaluate his cognitive, linguistic, and speech abilities (Murdoch & Whelan, 2007).

General Principles of Therapy for Traumatic Brain Injury

Therapy for patients with TBIs requires maximum teamwork with other medical and rehabilitation specialists. Patients often have unique medical complications, including external and internal injuries, cognitive-linguistic impairments, and behavioral disorders because of disinhibition. SLPs typically use the following approaches with patients who have TBIs: *environmental control, behavioral management, orientation therapy, cognitive retraining,* and *compensatory training.* The cognitive-linguistic approaches used by clinicians are usually determined by the stage of recovery or cognitive level of functioning of the patient.

SLPs may combine two or more approaches in any one therapy session to maximize the benefits of the therapy (Chapey, 2008; Murdoch & Whelan, 2007; Togher, 2007).

Environmental Control

Patients who are confused and agitated after TBIs are not responsible for their own behaviors; therefore, the professionals involved with these patients must try to make their environments stable, secure, and predictable. This helps minimize confusion and agitation and allows patients to use their cognitive energy to better manage themselves. This can be accomplished, in part, by having a consistent, organized daily routine. For example, meals can be served in the same location daily, and rehabilitation appointments can be scheduled at the same time, in the same place, and with the same therapists each day.

Behavioral Management

Behavioral management is used with environmental controls. Therapists attempt to increase adaptive behaviors and decrease maladaptive behaviors. Controlling the environment and reinforcing appropriate behaviors allow patients to begin to function more appropriately in structured environments. *Tangible reinforcements* are needed for these patients, for example, allowing patients to briefly listen to some favorite music or providing food reinforcement, such as a small bowl of ice cream for accomplishing a specific task.

Orientation Therapy

Most patients with TBIs are at least moderately disoriented to person, place, time, and purpose. Therapy is devised to help patients increase their orientation $\times$ 4, which also helps them increase their ability to manage themselves. For example, much repetition is needed to help patients realize and remember that they have weakness on one side of their body or that they must lock the brakes on their wheelchair before attempting to stand up.

Cognitive Retraining

In a sense, all rehabilitation involves cognitive retraining. However, more specifically, therapy is directed at increasing each of the components of cognition. Attention is often the first cognitive function targeted in therapy because that is the foundation of the rest of therapy; if the patient is not attending, he cannot receive maximum benefit from any therapy task. Increasing memory is needed for the patient to recall specific tasks, sequences, and behaviors, as well as important biographical information. Therapy to help patients redevelop their ability to organize information prepares them for problem-solving tasks for ADLs and to act in a reasonable and safe manner in their homes and communities. A collaborative approach is essential to help patients return to some level of functioning in the home, school, and/or work environments. Collaboration with family and friends who can help the patient carry over the rehabilitation program into the home and community environments is important for the patient to maximize his independence (Fogle, 2009a).

Compensatory Training

Few patients with moderate-to-severe TBIs return to their previous levels of functioning in their home, community, and work environments; therefore, they need to learn compensatory strategies to manage tasks that they could have managed independently premorbidly. For example, patients may be taught to keep daily notebooks with them to remind them of appointments or find a quiet room to be alone for a while if they begin to feel agitated.

Right-Hemisphere Syndrome

Recall from the discussion in Chapter 3, Anatomy and Physiology of Speech and Language, that the right hemisphere is particularly important in attention, orientation (e.g., self-awareness, where the person is, time of day, etc.), emotions, and cognition. Approximately half of all strokes and other neurological damage occur in the right hemisphere of the brain. **Right-hemisphere syndrome** is the result of a person having damage to the right hemisphere with impairments of its normal functions.

Cognitive Impairments

Right-hemisphere damage typically results in a variety of characteristics that comprise right-hemisphere syndrome, including several cognitive impairments (Blake, 2005; Myers, 2008). Right-hemisphere impairments are often subtle but may have profound effects on a person's daily life. Patients may be unaware of or do not appreciate the severity of their disorders (**anosognosia**). When a patient does not appreciate the severity of the impairments, the person may not be sufficiently motivated to work hard in therapy to make significant gains.

Visual–Spatial Impairments

Patients with right-hemisphere damage often have **visual–spatial impairments** and become disoriented and easily confused or lost, particularly in unfamiliar places such as the maze of hospital corridors or in grocery stores or shopping centers. When these patients are discharged from the hospital and are eager to begin driving, their visual–spatial impairments could prove to be life-threatening (Mackenzie & Paton, 2003; Tanner, 2007). These patients also may have difficulty recognizing familiar faces (**prosopagnosia**), including those of family members, medical personnel, and rehabilitation staff (e.g., they may not recognize you and may say they have never seen you before even though you have worked with them many times), however, they may recognize your voice.

---

right-hemisphere syndrome

Damage to the right hemisphere of the brain that can result in impairments of attention, visual–spatial abilities, orientation to person, place, time, and purpose, emotions, cognition, subtle to overt communication problems, and left-side neglect.

anosognosia

Decreased awareness of deficits or disabilities often seen in right-hemisphere damage; impairment of an individual's ability to relate to parts of his body.

visual–spatial impairments

Difficulty associating seen objects with their spatial relationships, that is, what is around the objects and the environment; often results in disorientation.

prosopagnosia

Difficulty recognizing familiar faces (including those of family members) and famous people.

Attention Impairments

Attention impairments occur with both right-hemisphere and left-hemisphere damage, but they are particularly noticeable in patients with right-hemisphere damage. Patients with attention impairments have difficulty staying focused on tasks and difficulty appropriately shifting attention from one task to another. Patients also may **perseverate**, that is, continue a thought or behavior after it is no longer appropriate.

Left-Side Neglect (Visual Hemi-inattention)

Neglect (i.e., lack of awareness and attention) of the left side of the body or space around the body is common in individuals who have right-hemisphere damage, particularly with damage to the parietal-temporal region (Davis, 2007). Individuals with *left neglect* tend to bump into things on their left, not notice food on the left side of the plate or tray, apply make-up on only the right side of the face, and draw only the right side of an object. Individuals also may have reading difficulties related to not attending to the left side of words or the left side of a page (*neglect dyslexia*), and, likewise, may have writing problems (*neglect dysgraphia*) where they have large margins on the left side of a page and use a right upward slant when writing words and sentences (Murray & Clark, 2006).

Communication Impairments

Subtle and sometimes overt receptive and expressive communication impairments are commonly seen in patients with right-hemisphere damage (Myers, 2008; Sohlberg & Mateer, 2001). These patients tend to be literal in their interpretation of messages, without realizing subtleties of meaning conveyed by choice of words, voice inflection, facial expressions, and body language. Metaphors (e.g., "The stars look like little diamonds in the sky."), idioms (e.g., "He kicked the bucket."), and proverbs (e.g., "Every cloud has a silver lining.") are often taken literally. People with right-hemisphere damage frequently violate the social and interactional aspects of communication (pragmatics), such as *turn-taking* (rambling on without regard to the listener), *topic maintenance* (frequent changes in the direction of conversation without regard to the topic of conversation), and *social conventions* (interrupting another person who is talking, not showing interest and respect for another's point of view, etc.). Patients typically interject irrelevant, tangential, and inappropriate comments into conversations. Their communication also may be devoid of emotion, have decreased prosody, and have an overall flat affect (Myers, 2008; Sohlberg & Mateer, 2001).

Individuals with right-hemisphere damage may have naming problems. They may be able to name several objects in a category (e.g., car, truck, and motorcycle), but have difficulty naming the category itself (e.g., transportation). When describing pictures, they may be able describe what they see but have difficulty giving a holistic view of what is occurring in the scene.

attention impairments

Difficulty staying focused on a task, difficulty appropriately shifting attention from one task to another, and dividing attention between auditory and visual stimuli.

perseverate/ perseveration

An automatic and often involuntary continuation of a thought or behavior after it is no longer appropriate.

General Principles of Assessment and Therapy for Right-Hemisphere Syndrome

Assessment for patients with right-hemisphere damage is similar to that of aphasia and cognitive disorders; however, assessments for attention and visual-perceptual disturbances are frequently included. Both formal and informal assessment procedures may be used. In general, we can apply the principles of therapy for aphasia and cognitive disorder to patients with right-hemisphere damage, with additional focus on the characteristics of this syndrome. Also, just as with patients with aphasia and cognitive disorders, we need to consider the functional outcomes and benefits for each patient's ADLs.

Dementia

Dementia is a medical term for a syndrome caused by a progressive neurological disease that involves intellectual, cognitive, communicative, behavioral, and personality deterioration that is *more severe* than would occur through normal aging (Mahendra & Hopper, 2012). Dementia is perhaps the most devastating cognitive problem associated with aging. **Senility**, however, refers to *normal loss* of cognitive functioning with advanced age. It is dementia, not senility that we are concerned about (American Psychological Association, 2000; Bourgeois, 2005; Pachalska, 2007).

Dementia has numerous causes and types, with Alzheimer's type being the most common cause. Two other causes and types of dementia include *vascular dementias* (the second most common cause) in which atherosclerosis in the brain develops from deposits of fats and other debris that form on the inside of arteries and partially or completely block the flow of blood. Blockages cause multiple occlusive strokes (*multi-infarct dementia*) and interruptions of blood flow to the brain. Dementia also may be a late-onset symptom of Parkinson's disease, with memory, judgment, reasoning, and speech most affected.

Alzheimer's Disease

Alzheimer's disease (AD) (dementia of the Alzheimer type, or DAT) is the most common and probably the best-known progressive dementia. Approximately one-half of individuals with dementia have Alzheimer's disease. Alois Alzheimer (1864–1915), a German professor of neuropsychiatry, described the behaviors of a 55-year-old woman who had been institutionalized for several years in an asylum for the insane in Frankfurt, Germany. She was disoriented, confused, severely demented, and used "perplexing language." Alzheimer performed the autopsy of her brain and discovered that she had extensive cortical tissue loss (**cortical atrophy**), as well as other neuronal cell changes that have become the hallmarks of the disorder. Alzheimer published his findings in 1906 and described the cognitive and behavioral characteristics, as well as the neuroanatomical changes of the patient (the term *Alzheimer's disease* was

---

dementia

A medical term for a syndrome caused by a progressive neurological disease that involves intellectual, cognitive, communicative, behavioral, and personality deterioration that is more severe than what would occur through normal aging.

senility

A medical term that refers to the normal loss of cognitive functioning with advanced age.

Alzheimer's disease (AD)

A disease that causes progressive dementia that usually begins after age 65 and in many cases is related to genetic factors that cause neuronal degeneration, cerebral atrophy, neurofibrillary tangles, neuritic plaques, white matter changes, and diminished neurotransmitters; characterized by decline in memory, intellect, disorientation, delusions, personality changes, and communication impairments.

cortical atrophy

Shrinkage and wasting away of cortical (brain) tissue that is common in dementia.

first used by another German psychiatrist in 1910 in honor of Alzheimer). Ironically, Alzheimer died of Alzheimer's disease at the young age of 51.

Alzheimer's disease tends be seen in women more than men because of their greater longevity, which puts them in older age groups with greater risks. Alzheimer's disease causes degenerative dementia characterized by slow onset with a progressive and deteriorating course. It is characterized by a decline in intellect, memory, communication, and personality. The DSM-IV-TR (APA, 2000) says the cognitive and intellectual impairments should be severe enough to interfere with social or occupational functioning.

Cortical atrophy may be observed through MRIs in people with Alzheimer's disease, as well as other forms of dementia. **Autopsy (postmortem)** examination of brain tissue is needed to reveal **neurofibrillary tangles** and **neuritic (senile) plaques** for a clear diagnosis of Alzheimer's disease. Various medical diagnostic tests (e.g., blood and urine) and brain imaging techniques on patients cannot definitively determine the existence of Alzheimer's disease. However, there are currently attempts to develop diagnostic criteria for Alzheimer's disease in individuals who are living by investigating *biomarkers* (indicators of disease) using various brain scans (e.g., MRI, **positive emission tomography [PET]**), as well as spinal taps that may reveal signs of neurological changes (De Meyer, Shapiro, & Vanderstichele, 2010).

Stages of Alzheimer's Disease

Alzheimer's disease is usually categorized into three stages: mild, moderate, and severe (also called early, middle, and late stages). Each stage has general characteristics that may not apply to all individuals. The signs and symptoms may overlap from one stage to the next, and some signs and symptoms may never occur in some individuals (Bayles & Tomoeda, 2007; Pachalska, 2007; Toner & Shadden, 2011).

Stage I: Mild Alzheimer's, Early-Stage Alzheimer's, Forgetfulness Stage

During the early stage, the warning signs of Alzheimer's disease are often subtle, which makes it difficult for the individual and family members to recognize that something is wrong. Some of the earliest signs and symptoms include: impaired **working memory**; difficulty completing familiar tasks; difficulty remembering common names; misplacing items in inappropriate places (e.g., putting a wallet in the refrigerator); sudden changes in mood or behavior for no apparent reason; showing an indifference to personal appearance; disorientation to place, time, and purpose; and becoming lost while driving on familiar streets.

During the mild stage, people may try to maintain regular routines at work, at home, and in the community. Their difficulties may be thought of as stress related, and they may become frustrated and angry with the increasing difficulties. They may begin to take out their frustration and anger on family, friends, and coworkers.

autopsy (postmortem)

A medical examination performed to determine or confirm the cause of death.

neurofibrillary tangles

Neuronal abnormalities seen in Alzheimer's disease where there are filamentous bodies (fine, threadlike fibers) in nerve cells, axons, and dendrites.

neuritic (senile) plaques

Neuronal abnormalities and degeneration seen in cortical and subcortical brain regions of people with Alzheimer's disease.

positive emission tomography (PET)

A computerized radiographic scanning technique that examines metabolic activity, blood flow, and biochemical activity of the brain and other body parts.

working memory

Temporary information storage that is limited in capacity and requires rehearsal; often thought of as "what is on your mind" at any given moment.

Personal Story — "That's—That's My Wife!"

I had been working in a convalescent hospital during the summer. One of my residents was Mr. McAdams, an 84-year-old man with cognitive-linguistic impairments. I had worked with him for several sessions when I learned from another staff member that his wife was in the residential care facility across the parking lot from the convalescent hospital we were in. I also learned that Mr. McAdams had probably not seen his wife in at least 2 months because no staff member had taken the time or effort to bring her to the convalescent hospital.

After working through the normal nursing and administrative channels to no avail to try to arrange a visit of Mrs. McAdams to see her husband, I took it upon myself to make all of the arrangements. The following day at 2 p.m., I rolled Mr. McAdams in his wheelchair into the empty dining room that was light and cheery and had little vases of flowers on the tables. I placed Mr. McAdams beside a table with two glasses of water on it and turned his chair to face the open door. I told him I would be back in a few minutes. I walked across the parking lot and found Mrs. McAdams in her room, where she had put on her best dress and had her hair and make-up done. She was beaming as I rolled her across the parking lot to the convalescent hospital where she would see her husband for the first time in more than 2 months.

When we got to the door of the dining room, Mrs. McAdams sat up straight and had a big smile on her face. I wheeled her directly to her husband and she had tears in her eyes. When Mr. McAdams could clearly see her, he said, "That's—that's my wife!" I placed Mr. and Mrs. McAdams beside one another in their wheelchairs. They started to hug and cry. I left the room and closed the door.

After that day, I brought Mrs. McAdams over to see her husband twice a week, sometimes during craft time so that they could work on crafts together. When it was time for me to leave the hospital at the end of the summer to return to teaching, I wrote in the patient care plan in Mr. McAdams's medical chart that his wife was to be brought over twice a week for visits. By having this officially written in his medical chart, it was then nursing's professional obligation to carry out the visits, along with all that was written in the patient's Care Plan. As speech-language pathologists, we can sometimes "go beyond the call of duty" and help people by simply being extra caring. ■

Depression is common in the forgetfulness stage, although it is often under-diagnosed and undertreated (Reynolds, Alexopoulos, & Katz, 2002). Although individuals in stage I could benefit from therapy that targeted their deteriorating cognitive functioning, few people receive help.

Stage II: Moderate Alzheimer's, Middle-Stage Alzheimer's, Confusion Stage

The warning signs of Alzheimer's disease are more apparent at the middle stage. Beyond obvious memory loss, the person is not thinking clearly or using good judgment. This is when family members are likely to take the person to see the doctor and the diagnosis of Alzheimer's disease is made. Some signs and symptoms of the moderate stage include: increased loss of working memory; significantly diminished vocabulary; conversation is increasingly empty, meaningless; loss of reading and writing ability; difficulty with tasks that require skilled movements, such as tying shoelaces or using utensils (see Figure 11-8); aggressiveness, outbursts of anger, or withdrawal; inappropriate public behavior; and hallucination or delusions.

At this stage, the person is not responsible for his personal safety and others need to monitor and manage any safety concerns (Fogle, Reece, & White, 2008). For example, the person should no longer be allowed to drive or have access to vehicle keys. Any firearms that may have been available to the person should be removed or locked up. The person

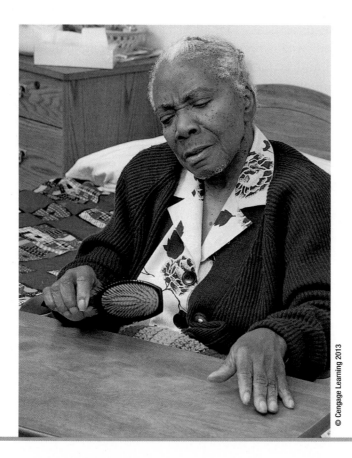

© Cengage Learning 2013

Figure 11-8

A patient with moderate Alzheimer's disease may forget how common objects are used and have problems with normal activities of daily living.

should be carefully watched when trying to cook or using any appliance that becomes hot, including irons and hairdryers. This is an emotionally trying time for the family, which needs to develop a new perspective of the relationship with the person with Alzheimer's disease. A "24-7" monitoring and caregiving approach needs to be established. An individual's independence is partly determined by the confidence caregivers have in the person's ability to act in a safe and reasonable manner. When the caregivers can no longer provide a safe environment and maintain a person's health and hygiene, placement in a convalescent or nursing home may need to be considered. Speech-language pathologists are often the professionals who educate and train family members and caregivers about strategies that are helpful for maximizing individuals' cognitive-linguistic abilities, as well as providing the safest environments for these individuals.

Stage III: Severe Alzheimer's, Late-Stage Alzheimer's, Terminal Stage

The progress of Alzheimer's disease to the severe stage may take a few years to many years. By this time, the person is no longer able to think and reason or consistently communicate wants and needs. The person likely needs maximum assistance for all ADLs, including dressing, eating, and toileting. Some signs and symptoms of the severe, late stage include: little or no memory; difficulty speaking and understanding simple sentences and individual words; expresses little or no emotion; minimal verbal discourse; difficulty recognizing others and sometimes himself in a mirror; needs assistance for all ADLs and personal care; and difficulty chewing and swallowing that results in loss of weight, dehydration, and risks for aspiration pneumonia (see Figure 11–9).

Individuals in stage III Alzheimer's disease are not candidates for speech and language therapy. Because of their frequent swallowing problems, many people with Alzheimer's disease develop aspiration pneumonia, which causes death more often than the Alzheimer's itself.

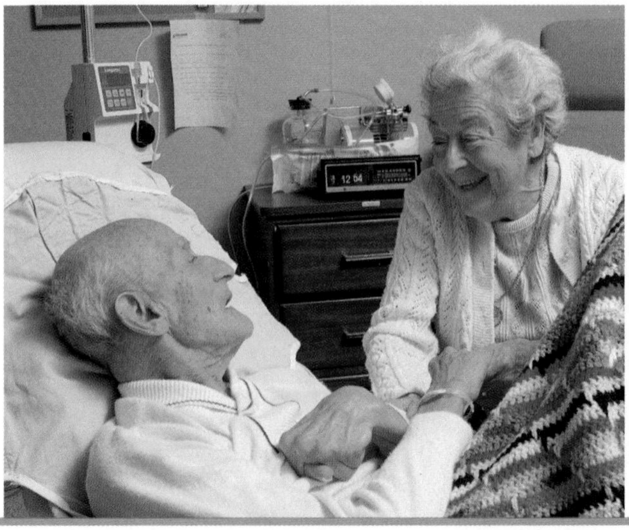

Figure 11–9

A convalescent hospital or nursing home may be the only option when the caregiver of an individual with dementia can no longer provide a safe environment or sufficient care.

© Cengage Learning 2013

Daisy

Some residents I work with in convalescent hospitals particularly touch my heart. Because few residents have anything to cuddle, hug, and "care for," many times I have given them little stuffed animals. Daisy was a resident I worked with who had both dementia and swallowing problems. She told me she liked little dogs. I found a cute little stuffed dog at a toy store, and just before I had to discharge Daisy from therapy I gave her the stuffed animal. She loved it. She began keeping it with her all of the time. Her dog "slept" with her at night and was on her lap or beside her when she was in her wheelchair. One day I had a nurse take a picture of us together, with her "pet" beside her (see Figure 11–10).

A couple of months after I returned to my fall teaching, I received a note from one of Daisy's daughters saying that Daisy had died. The family buried the little stuffed dog with her. Over the years, I occasionally thought about Daisy. Then in the fall of 2004, a new graduate student in my department (Vanessa) said that she recognized me as soon as she first saw me. Daisy was her great-grandmother and the student had seen the picture of Daisy and me together (it was also the last picture taken of Daisy alive). Vanessa told me about her visits with Daisy at the convalescent hospital when she was young and that "Daisy loved her speech therapist!" ▪

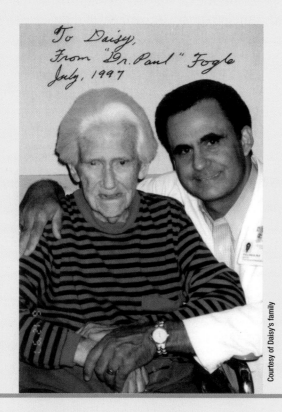

Courtesy of Daisy's family

Figure 11–10
The author with Daisy.

Death occurs, on average, about 8 to 10 years after the initial diagnosis of Alzheimer's disease by a physician.

General Principles of Assessment and Treatment of Cognitive-Linguistic Functioning of People with Dementia

The purpose of the speech-language pathologist's evaluation of individuals with dementia is not to diagnose dementia or Alzheimer's disease (although our evaluations may help confirm a diagnosis), but to assess their cognitive, linguistic, and swallowing abilities and from the assessment determine what, if any, therapy is appropriate. The actual diagnosis of dementia and Alzheimer's disease is made by physicians and psychologists.

People who are in the mild-to-moderate stages of Alzheimer's disease, and even some in the severe stage, may still be living at home, in a **board and care home**, or in a **residential care facility**. Family members and caregivers need to learn specific strategies for maximizing the abilities of individuals with dementia to communicate and function in their environments.

The speech-language pathology therapy goals for individuals with dementia (primarily those in stages I and II) are to help maximize their current cognitive-linguistic abilities and slow the inevitable deterioration of those abilities. Clinicians also need to help patients with awareness and problem solving for safety issues in the hospital and home environments (Fogle, Reece, & White, 2008). Much of what we do involves counseling and educating the caregivers (including family) on ways to manage and cope with the progressive cognitive and behavioral deterioration of the patient. The therapy goals, as with all individuals with neurological impairments, need to be functional—for both the patient and the caregivers. Ultimately we are trying to improve the quality of life of the patient and, by doing so, improve the quality of life of the people involved with the patient (Worrall & Hickson, 2003).

---

board and care home

A homelike environment where there may be a few to several elderly or physically impaired individuals residing and meals, laundry, and other services are provided.

residential care facility

Often a fairly large complex of small "apartments" where individuals or couples live; there is communal dining, and various services (e.g., security, trips to the mall, and outings) are provided to residents.

custodial care

Services and care of a nonmedical nature (e.g., bathing and feeding) provided long term, usually for convalescent and chronically ill patients.

incontinence

The inability to control or retain urination or defecation.

Alzheimer's Units

The question may be asked, What happens to people with advanced stage Alzheimer's disease or dementia? In the United States and most industrialized countries where health care is available from birth to end of life, these individuals may be placed in "Alzheimer's units" of specialized convalescent hospitals or care facilities. At this time in the progression of Alzheimer's disease or dementia, patients often need **custodial care** because of **incontinence** of bowel and bladder. They need protection from wandering away from the facility; therefore, the unit can only be entered or exited through a locked door. Psychosis also can occur as a secondary syndrome in Alzheimer's disease; therefore, patients often need protection from harming themselves and others (Palmer, Folsom, Bartels, & Jeste, 2002).

End-of-Life Care

End-of-life care is something many people think about as they get older: How do I want to be cared for in my final months, weeks, and days of life? Patients may choose either palliative care or hospice care. *Palliative care* is designed to relieve or reduce discomfort and pain, and patients may choose to pursue aggressive medical therapy aimed at curing a disease. Palliative care may continue for years to decades. *Hospice care* is normally intended for those who have a *life-limiting illness* (i.e., a *terminal condition*) where the prognosis is 6 months or less, should the disease follow a normal progression. Hospice care is family-focused care, and "family" is whomever the patient considers is family—not just blood relatives. Hospice care is interdisciplinary and may include physicians, nurses, social workers, chaplains, aides, and trained volunteers. Much of the care of the patient is pain management and attempts to maintain the patient's comfort and dignity (Jenko & Moffit, 2006; Roffi, 2007).

EMOTIONAL AND SOCIAL EFFECTS OF NEUROLOGICAL DISORDERS

Beyond the communication and cognitive impairments of individuals with neurological impairments, there are always emotional effects for both the patient and the family. As clinicians, we always need to keep in mind the entire person (and the family) with whom we are working, not just the disorder or disorders the person has. We need to place considerable importance on developing good, caring, working relationships with clients and families, without which our therapy could not be carried out optimally. The clinician's understanding of the emotional and social effects on the patient and family can help during the evaluation of the patient and the sensitive time of discussing the results of the evaluation. Understanding and appreciating the emotional and social effects can help clinicians maintain empathy during the process of treatment. It also helps patients and families feel that the clinician understands the realities of the challenges the patient and family face (Flasher & Fogle, 2012; Sander, 2007).

When an individual has a neurological injury, it often sets into motion a chain of events for the patient and family. Initially, after a neurological insult, a person may be comatose or semicomatose and, therefore, not aware of significant changes in his communication and cognitive functioning. However, when awareness emerges, the person begins to realize that he is not only having difficulty communicating, remembering, and recognizing other people but also may have obvious bandages and scars on his body, face, and head from a motor vehicle accident or neurosurgery after a stroke. His self-image (self-concept) takes a blow, and mental confusion may add to his lack of understanding of why he is in the hospital with tubes entering and exiting his body (e.g., a nasogastric tube for feeding and a catheter for urinary excretion).

The person with the neurological impairment has an immediate alteration of his self-image; the family does also. Family members likely will see themselves in a passive role during the medical treatment to keep their loved one alive and to minimize the brain damage. Like the impaired person, family members will feel fear and confusion. The experience is likely nothing they can relate to: a family member being rushed to the hospital; anxious time in an emergency room; admission to the hospital, possibly to a critical care unit; possible neurosurgery and wondering if it will be successful; weeks to months of rehabilitation; and having a loved one's levels of functioning altered forever.

Family systems theory and family-centered service delivery models are particularly applicable to individuals and families when a neurological disorder has occurred. When an individual in a family has a neurological impairment, the family system as a whole is affected. Elisabeth Kübler-Ross's five *stages of grief* (denial, anger, bargaining, depression, and acceptance) apply to their experiences. In addition to the emotional effects of the neurological impairment on the patient and family, social and financial effects add to the distress of each person (Flasher & Fogle, 2012; Roberts, 2011).

CHAPTER SUMMARY

This chapter on neurological (neurogenic) disorders in adults has covered an extensive amount of information on a challenging population of individuals that many speech-language pathologists work with full-time in acute-care hospitals, outpatient clinics, subacute hospitals, convalescent hospitals, rehabilitation centers, home health care, and private practices.

Strokes are the most common cause of neurological disorders in adults and they can occur at any age, not just in older adults. The two main types of strokes are occlusive and hemorrhagic. The site and size of the stroke usually determine the symptoms seen. Other common causes of neurogenic disorders are traumatic brain injuries, tumors, toxins, and degenerative diseases and disorders. Aphasia is a common disorder after a stroke in the left hemisphere's temporal lobe in or around the perisylvian area. Aphasia is a deficit in language processing that affects all input modalities (auditory, visual, and tactile) and all output modalities (speaking, writing, and gesturing). Aphasia is generally classified as receptive aphasia (difficulty with auditory comprehension) and expressive aphasia (difficulty formulating and verbally expressing language). Wernicke's aphasia is a fluent aphasia characterized by impaired comprehension, integration, and formulation of language; Broca's aphasia is a nonfluent aphasia with symptoms of impaired initiation of sound sequences, restricted grammar, and vocabulary that limits verbal expression to high-frequency content words (nouns, verbs, and adjectives). Patients with global aphasia have severely impaired receptive and expressive language in all input and output modalities. Assessment of aphasia involves evaluating a patient's auditory reception and verbal expression language abilities, as well as reading and writing abilities.

Therapy focuses on strengthening the impaired modalities with an emphasis on functional communication in activities of daily living.

Cognitive disorders are typically the result of traumatic brain injuries, right-hemisphere syndrome, and dementia. Patients with TBIs often have a variety of cognitive impairments affecting their attention, memory, orientation, reasoning, and problem-solving abilities. Patients with TBIs can be some of the most challenging people speech-language pathologists work with. Therapy often includes environmental control; behavioral management techniques; orientation to person, place, time, and purpose; cognitive retraining; and compensatory retraining.

Right-hemisphere syndrome is characterized by decreased awareness of deficits, visual–spatial impairments, attentional impairments, decreased awareness of emotions of other people, and cognitive impairments. Patients with right-hemisphere damage also may have communication impairments, including both receptive and expressive language disorders.

Dementia involves declining cognitive and social abilities that are more severe than what would occur through normal aging. Alzheimer's disease is the most common and best-known form of dementia. Alzheimer's disease has three commonly recognized stages, each with increasingly severe symptoms. The SLP's goals are to maximize the patient's current cognitive-linguistic abilities and slow the inevitable deterioration of those abilities, and help with their swallowing problems.

Regardless of the cause or severity of the neurological disorder, we are always working with a person and the person's family. Individual who have neurological injuries often awaken to discover that they are not the person they were a moment before the injury. They may not have the physical, communication, or cognitive abilities that they had relied on every minute of their lives. Both patients and their families typically go through the stages of grief—denial, anger, bargaining, depression, and, hopefully, acceptance of their new circumstances. Neurological damage takes a major toll on the person and all the people the individual associates with.

STUDY QUESTIONS

Knowledge and Comprehension

1. What are five warning signs of stroke?

2. Define receptive aphasia and expressive aphasia.

3. Discuss any three cognitive impairments that may be seen with a traumatic brain injury.

4. What are some of the interacting factors that may affect successful treatment of patients with neurological disorders?

5. What is the difference between dementia and senility?

Application

1. Why is it important to know the warning signs of stroke when working with patients of any age, but particularly those at risk for stroke?

2. What are the general areas that are normally evaluated when assessing a patient with a neurological impairment?

3. Why do important areas for therapy include a patient's awareness and problem-solving abilities for safety issues in the hospital and home?

4. What are any five general principles of therapy for aphasia?

5. Why is it important to understand the emotional and social effects of a neurological disorder on a patient and the family?

Analysis/Synthesis

1. Why is a speech-language pathologist's therapy based on her own evaluation more than on the neurological cause of the communication impairment?

2. In Wernicke's aphasia, how could impaired auditory comprehension contribute to problems with integration and formulation of language?

3. Discuss the similarities and differences between closed and open head injuries.

4. Discuss the stages of Alzheimer's disease that would most benefit from therapy.

5. Why is it important to always keep in mind functional outcomes when working with patients?

REFERENCES

American Heart Association. (2005). *Heart disease and stroke statistics: 2005 update.* Dallas, TX: American Heart Association. Available at http://www.strokeassociation.org.

American Psychological Association. (2000). *Diagnostic and statistical manual of mental disorders* (DSM-IV-TR) (4th ed., text rev. ed.). Washington, DC: APA.

Bayles, K. A., & Tomoeda, C. K. (2007). *Cognitive-communicative disorders of dementia: Definition, diagnosis, and treatment.* San Diego, CA: Plural Publishing.

Ben-Yishay, Y., & Diller, L. (1993). Cognitive remediation in traumatic brain injury: Update and issues. *Archives of Physical Medicine and Rehabilitation, 74,* 204–213.

Berker, E. A., Berker, A. H., & Smith, A. (1986). Translation of Broca's 1865 report: Localization of speech in the third frontal convolution. *Archives on Neurology (Chicago), 43,* 1065–1072.

Blake, M. L. (2005). Right hemisphere syndrome. In L. LaPointe (Ed.), *Aphasia and related neurogenic language disorders* (3rd ed.). New York, NY: Thieme.

Boles, L. (2009). *Aphasia couples therapy (ACT) workbook.* San Diego: Plural Publishing.

Bourgeois, M. S. (2005). Dementia. In L. LaPointe (Ed.), *Aphasia and related neurogenic language disorders* (3rd ed.). New York, NY: Thieme.

Boyle, M. (2004). Semantic feature analysis treatment for anomia in two fluent aphasia syndromes. *American Journal of Speech-Language Pathology, 13*(3), 236–249.

Broderick, J. P., Adams, H., & Barsan, W. (1999). Guidelines for the management of spontaneous intracerebral hemorrhage. *Stroke, 30,* 905–915.

Brookshire, R. (1992). *Introduction to neurogenic communication disorders* (4th ed.). Minneapolis, MN: Brookshire.

Caspari, I. (2005). Wernicke's aphasia. In L. LaPointe (Ed.), *Aphasia and related neurogenic language disorders* (3rd ed.). New York, NY: Thieme.

Centeno, J. (2005). Working with bilingual individuals with aphasia: The case of a Spanish–English bilingual client. *Perspectives on Communication Disorders and Sciences in Culturally and Linguistically Diverse Populations. ASHA, Division 14, 12*(1), 2–5.

Chapey, R. (Ed.). (2008). *Language intervention strategies in adult aphasia and related neurogenic disorders* (5th ed.). Baltimore, MD: Lippincott Williams & Wilkins.

Cherney, L. R. (Ed.). (2004). *Clinical management of dysphagia in adults and children.* Gaithersburg, MD: Aspen.

Code, C. (1991). *Aphasia therapy: Studies in disorders of communication.* Clifton Park, NY: Delmar Cengage Learning.

Code, C. (2001). Multifactorial processes in recovery from aphasia: Developing the foundations for a multilevel framework. *Brain and Language, 77,* 25–44.

Code, C. (2012). Significant landmarks in the history of aphasia and its therapy. In I. Papathanasiou, P. Coppens, & C. Potagas (Eds.). *Aphasia and related neurogenic communication disorders.* Burlington, MA: Jones & Bartlett Learning.

Code, C., & Muller, D. (Eds.). (1995). *The treatment of aphasia: From theory to practice.* Clifton Park, NY: Delmar Cengage Learning.

Collins, M. (2005). Global aphasia. In L. LaPointe (Ed.). *Aphasia and related neurogenic language disorders* (3rd ed.). New York, NY: Thieme.

Constantinidou, F., & Kennedy, M. (2012). Traumatic brain injury in adults. In I. Papathanasiou, P. Coppens, & C. Potagas (Eds.). *Aphasia and related neurogenic communication disorders*. Burlington, MA: Jones & Bartlett Learning.

Cruice, M., Worrall, L., & Hickson, L. (2000). Quality of life measurement in speech pathology and audiology. *Asia Pacific Journal of Speech, Language and Hearing, 5*, 1–20.

Davis, G. (2007). Aphasiology: *Disorders and clinical practice*. Boston, MA: Allyn and Bacon.

De Meyer, G., Shapiro, F., & Vanderstichele, H. (2010). Diagnosis-independent Alzheimer disease biomarker signature in cognitively normal elderly people. *Archives of Neurology, 67*, 949–956.

Douglas, K. (2002). *My stroke of luck*. New York, NY: William Morrow.

Edwards, S., & Bastiannse, R. (2007). Assessment of aphasia in a multicultural world. In M. Ball & J. S. Damico (Eds.). *Clinical aphasiology: Future directions: A festschrift for Chris Code*. London: Psychology Press, Taylor & Francis Group.

Eslinger, P., Zappala, G., Chakara, F., & Barrett, A. (2007). Cognitive impairments after TBI. In N. Zasler, D. Katz, & R. Zafonte (Eds.). *Brain injury medicine: Principles and practice*. New York, NY: Demos Medical Publishing.

Flasher, L. V., & Fogle, P. T. (2012). *Counseling skills for speech-language pathologists and audiologists* (2nd ed.). Clifton Park, NY: Delmar Cengage Learning.

Fogle, P. T. (2000, February). Forensic speech-language pathology: A practical guide for the expert witness. In *ADVANCE for speech-language pathologists and audiologists*. King of Prussia, PA: Merion Publications.

Fogle, P. (2003). A practical guide for the expert witness. *Vital Resources for Medical-Legal Solutions, 4*(6), 2.

Fogle, P. (2006). Forensic speech-language pathology: Court testifying as an expert witness. Paper presented at New Zealand Speech Therapy Association Convention, Canterbury, New Zealand.

Fogle, P. T. (2009a). Cognitive Rehabilitation: Collaborative Brain Injury Intervention. Paper presented at the Asia Pacific Society for the Study of Speech, Language, Hearing Conference, Honolulu, HI, July 2009.

Fogle, P. T. (2009b, March). Being a veteran and speech-language pathologist. *Advance for Speech-Language Pathologists and Audiologists*. King of Prussia, PA. Merion Publications.

Fogle, P. T., & Reece, L. (2006). *Classic aphasia therapy stimuli*. San Diego, CA: Plural Publishing.

Fogle, P. T., Reece, L., & White, J. (2008). *The source for safety: Cognitive retraining for independent living*. East Moline, IL: LinguiSystems.

Freed, D., Celery, K., & Marshall, R. C. (2004). Effectiveness of personalized and phonological cueing on long-term naming performance by aphasic subjects: A clinical investigation. *Aphasiology, 18*(8), 743–757.

Geshwind, N. (1965). Wernicke's contribution to the study of aphasia. *Cortex, 3,* 449–463.

Giacino, J., & Whyte, J. (2005). The vegetative and minimally conscious states: Current knowledge and remaining questions. *Journal of Head Trauma Rehabilitation, 20,* 30–50.

Goldstein, L. B. (Ed.). (2009). *A primer on stroke prevention and treatment: An overview based on the American Heart Association/ American Stroke Association Guidelines.* New York, NY: Wiley-Blackwell.

Golper, L. A. (2010). *Medical speech-language pathology: A desk reference* (3rd ed.). Clifton Park, NY: Delmar Cengage Learning.

Goodglass, H., Kaplan, E., & Barresi, B. (2001). *The Boston diagnostic aphasia examination* (3rd ed.). Philadelphia, PA: Lea & Febiger.

Guerrero, J., Thurman, D., & Sniezek, J. (2000). Emergency department visits associated with traumatic brain injury: United States, 1995–1996. *Brain Injury, 14,* 181–186.

Guthrie, E., Mast, J., McQuaid, M., & Pavlakis, S. (1999). Traumatic brain injury in children and adolescents. *Child and Adolescent Psychiatric Clinics of North America, 8,* 807–826.

Hegde, M. N., & Davis, D. (2010). *Clinical methods and practicum in speech-language pathology* (5th ed.). Clifton Park, NY: Delmar Cengage Learning.

Helm-Estabrooks, N., & Albert, M. L. (2004). *Manual of aphasia and aphasia therapy* (2nd ed.). Austin, TX: Pro-Ed.

Hilari, K., & Byng, S. (2001). Measuring quality of life in people with aphasia: The stroke specific quality of life scale. *International Journal of Language & Communication Disorders, 36,* 86–91.

Hirsch, J. (2005). Raising consciousness. *Journal of Clinical Investigation, 115*(5), 1102–1112.

Huckabee, M. L., & Pelletier, C. A. (2003). *Management of adult neurogenic dysphagia.* Clifton Park, NY: Delmar Cengage Learning.

Iverson, G., Lange, R., Gatz, M., & Zasler, N. (2007). Mild traumatic brain injury. In M. Zasler, O. Kats, & R. Zafonte (Eds.). *Brain injury medicine: Principles and practice.* New York, NY: Demos Medical Publishing.

Jenko, M., & Moffit, S. (2006). Transcultural nursing principles: An application to hospice care. *Journal of Hospice and Palliative Nursing, 8*(3), 172–180.

Johnson, A. F., & Jacobson, B. H. (2007). *Medical speech-language pathology: A practitioner's guide* (2nd ed.). New York, NY: Thieme.

Kagan, A., Black, S. E., Duchan, J. F., Simmons-Mackie, N., & Square, N. (2001). Training volunteers as conversation partners using "supportive conversation for adults with aphasia" (SCA): A controlled trial. *Journal of Speech, Language, and Hearing Research, 44,* 623–638.

Kayser, H. (2006). Service delivery issues for culturally and linguistically diverse populations. In R. Lubinski, L. E. Golper, & C. Frattali (Eds.), *Professional issues in speech-language pathology and audiology* (3rd ed.). Clifton Park, NY: Delmar Cengage Learning.

Kearns, K. P. (2005). Broca's aphasia. In L. LaPointe (Ed.), *Aphasia and related neurogenic language disorders* (3rd ed.). New York, NY: Thieme.

Kochanek, P., Clark, R., & Jenkins, L. (2007). Traumatic brain injury: Pathobiology. In M. Zasler, O. Kats, & R. Zafonte (Eds.). *Brain injury medicine: Principles and practice.* New York, NY: Demos Medical Publishing.

LaPointe, L. L. (2005). Mixed metaphors. *Journal of Medical Speech-Language Pathology, 13*(3), vii–viii.

Larkins, B., Worrall, L., & Hickson, L. (2004). Use of multiple methods to determine items relevant for a functional communication assessment. *New Zealand Journal of Speech-Language Therapy, 59,* 13–18.

Lew, H. L., Poole, J. H., Alvarez, S., & Moore, W. (2005). Soldiers with occult traumatic brain injury. *American Journal of Physical Medicine and Rehabilitation, 84*(6), 393–398.

Loring, D. (Ed.). (1999). *International neuropsychological society dictionary of neuropsychology.* Oxford: Oxford University Press.

Mackenzie, C., & Paton, G. (2003). Resumption of driving following stroke. *Aphasiology, 17*(2), 107–122.

Mahendra, N., & Hopper, T. (2012). Dementia and related cognitive disorders. In I. Papathanasiou, P. Coppens, & C. Potagas (Eds.). *Aphasia and related neurogenic communication disorders.* Burlington, MA: Jones & Bartlett Learning.

Marshall, J. (2012). Disorders of sentence processing in aphasia. In I. Papathanasiou, P. Coppens, & C. Potagas (Eds.). *Aphasia and related neurogenic communication disorders.* Burlington, MA: Jones & Bartlett Learning.

Martin, N. (2012). Disorders of word production. In I. Papathanasiou, P. Coppens, & C. Potagas (Eds.). *Aphasia and related neurogenic communication disorders.* Burlington, MA: Jones & Bartlett Learning.

McDonald, S. (2007). The social and neuropsychological underpinnings of communication disorders after severe traumatic brain injury. In M. Ball & J. S. Damico (Eds.). *Clinical aphasiology: Future directions: A festschrift for Chris Code.* London, England: Psychological Press, Taylor & Francis Group.

McNeil, M. R., & Tseng, C. H. (2005). Acquired neurogenic agraphias: Writing problems. In L. LaPointe (Ed.), *Aphasia and related neurogenic language disorders* (3rd ed.). New York, NY: Thieme.

Meechan, W. P., d'Hemecourt, P., Collins, C., & Comstock, R. (2011). Assessment and management of sport-related concussions in United States high schools. *American Journal of Medicine, 20*(10), 2311–2318.

Moran, C., & Gillon, G. (2004). Working memory influences on traumatic brain injury: A tutorial. *New Zealand Journal of Speech-Language Therapy, 59*, 4–12.

Morris, J., & Franklin, S. (2012). Disorders of auditory comprehension. In I. Papathanasiou, P. Coppens, & C. Potagas (Eds.). *Aphasia and related neurogenic communication disorders*. Burlington, MA: Jones & Bartlett Learning.

Mortensen, L. (2004). Perspectives on functional writing following acquired brain impairment. *Advances in Speech-Language Pathology, 6*(1), 15–22.

Mosby. (2009). *Mosby's dictionary of medicine, nursing, & health professions* (8th ed.). St. Louis, MO: Mosby Elsevier.

Moser, R., Iverson, G., Echemendia, R., Lovell, M., Schatz, P., et al. (2007). Neuropsychological evaluations in the diagnosis and management of sports-related concussions. *Archives of Clinical Neuropsychology, 22*, 909–916.

Murdoch, B. E., & Theodoros, D. G. (2001). *Traumatic brain injury: Associated speech, language and swallowing disorders*. Clifton Park, NY: Delmar Cengage Learning.

Murdoch, B. E., & Whelan, B. (2007). Assessment and treatment of speech and language disorders in TBI. In N. Zasler, D. Katz, & R. Zafontel (Eds.). *Brain injury medicine: Principles and Practice*. New York, NY: Demos Medical Publishing.

Murray, L. L., & Clark, H. M. (2006). *Neurogenic disorders of language: Theory driven clinical practice*. Clifton Park, NY: Delmar Cengage Learning.

Myers, P. S. (2008). Communication disorders associated with right hemisphere brain damage. In R. Chapey (Ed.). *Language intervention strategies in adult aphasia and related neurogenic disorders* (5th ed.). Baltimore, MD: Lippincott Williams & Wilkins.

Mysiw, W., Fugate, L., & Clinchot, D. (2007). Assessment, early rehabilitation intervention, and tertiary prevention. In N. Zasler, D. Katz, & R. Zafontel (Eds.). *Brain injury medicine: Principles and Practice*. New York, NY: Demos Medical Publishing.

Pachalska, M. (2007). Progressive language and speech disorders in dementia. In M. Ball & J. S. Damico (Eds.). *Clinical aphasiology: Future directions: A festschrift for Chris Code*. London, England: Psychology Press, Taylor & Francis Group.

Palmer, B., Folsom, D., Bartels, S., & Jeste, D. (2002). Psychotic disorders in late life: Implications for treatment and future directions for clinical services. *Generations: Journal of the American Society of Aging, 26*(1), 39–43.

Papathanasiou, I., Coppens, P. & Potagas, C. (Eds.). (2012). *Aphasia and related neurogenic communication disorders.* Burlington, MA: Jones & Bartlett Learning.

Papathanasiou, I., & Csefalvay, Z. (2012). Written language and its impairments. In I. Papathanasiou, P. Coppens, & C. Potagas (Eds.). *Aphasia and related neurogenic communication disorders.* Burlington, MA: Jones & Bartlett Learning.

Penn, C. (2007). Cultural dimensions of aphasia: Adding diversity and flexibility to the question. In M. Ball & J. S. Damico (Eds.). *Clinical aphasiology: Future directions: A festschrift for Chris Code.* London: Psychology Press, Taylor & Francis Group.

Ponsford, J. (2004). *Cognitive and behavioral rehabilitation: From neurobiology to clinical practice.* New York, NY: Guilford Press.

Portagas, C., Kasselimis, D. S., & Evdokimidis, I. (2012). Elements of neurology essential for understanding the aphasias. In I. Papathanasiou, P. Coppens, & C. Potagas (Eds.). *Aphasia and related neurogenic communication disorders.* Burlington, MA: Jones & Bartlett Learning.

Raymer, A. M. (2005). Naming and word-retrieval problems. In L. LaPointe (Ed.), *Aphasia and related neurogenic language disorders* (3rd ed.). New York, NY: Thieme.

Reynolds, C., Alexopoulos, G., & Katz, I. (2002). Geriatric depression: Diagnosis and treatment. *Generations, Journal of the American Society of Aging, 26*(1), 28–31.

Roberts, S. D. (2011). Patient- and family-centered care: Today's standard of care delivery. *CSHA Magazine, 41*(1), 6–7.

Roffi, B. (2007, February). End-of-life care. *Advance for Nurses.* King of Prussia, PA: Merion Publications.

Sander, A. (2007). A cognitive-behavioral intervention for family members of persons with TBI. In N. Zasler, D. Katz, & R. Zafonte (Eds.). *Brain injury medicine: Principles and practice.* New York, NY: Demos Medical Publishing.

Singh, R., Cohen, S. N., & Krupp, R. (1996). Racial differences in cerebrovascular disease. *Neurology, 46*(Supplement 21), A440–A441.

Sohlberg, M. M., & Mateer, C. A. (2001). *Introduction to cognitive rehabilitation theory and practice* (2nd ed.). New York, NY: Guilford Press.

Tanner, D. C. (2007). *Surviving traumatic brain injury and communication disorders: A professional and family guide.* San Diego, CA: Plural Publishing.

Tate, R. L., McDonald, S., & Lulham, J. L. (1998). Traumatic brain injury: Severity of injury and outcome in an Australian population. *Journal of Australia and New Zealand Public Health, 22*, 11–15.

Threats, T., & Worrall, L. (2004). Classifying communication disability using the ICF. *Advances in Speech-Language Pathology, 6*(1), 53–62.

Togher, L. (2007). Traumatic brain injury rehabilitation: Advanced communication perspectives. In M. Ball & J. S. Damico (Eds.). *Clinical aphasiology: Future directions: A festschrift for Chris Code.* London, England: Psychology Press, Taylor & Francis Group.

Toner, M. A., & Shadden, B. B. (2011). *Aging and communication: For clinicians by clinicians* (2nd ed.). Austin, TX: Pro-Ed.

Tonkovich, J. D. (2002). Multicultural issues in the management of neurogenic communication and swallowing disorders. In D. E. Battle (Ed.), *Communication disorders in multicultural populations* (3rd ed., pp. 233–265). Boston, MA: Butterworth-Heinemann.

Turkstra, L. S. (2001). Treating memory problems in adults with neurogenic communication disorders. *Seminars in Speech and Language, 22*(2), 147–155.

Wallace, G. L. (1997). Working with interpreters and translators. In G. L. Wallace (Ed.), *Multicultural neurogenics: A resource for speech-language pathologists providing services to neurologically impaired adults from culturally and linguistically diverse backgrounds.* San Antonio, TX: Communication Skill Builders.

Webb, W. G. (2005). Acquired dyslexia: Reading disorders associated with aphasia. In L. LaPointe (Ed.). *Aphasia and related neurogenic language disorders* (3rd ed.). New York, NY: Thieme.

Worrall, L. E., & Hickson, L. M. (2003). *Communication disability in aging: From prevention to intervention.* Clifton Park, NY: Delmar Cengage Learning.

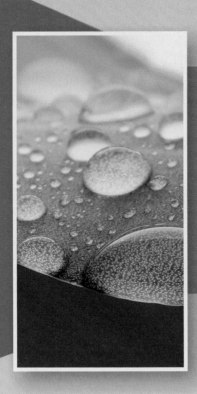

CHAPTER 12
Motor Speech Disorders and Dysphagia/ Swallowing Disorders

LEARNING OBJECTIVES

After studying this chapter, you will:

- Know the essentials of motor speech disorders—dysarthria and apraxia.
- Be familiar with principles of assessment of dysarthria and apraxia of speech.
- Be able to discuss general principles of therapy for dysarthria and apraxia of speech.
- Understand the essentials of dysphagia.
- Recognize the need for a team approach to dysphagia.
- Be able to explain each of the four phases of swallowing.
- Be able to discuss disordered swallowing in each of the four phases.
- Understand essential procedures for evaluating adults with swallowing disorders.
- Be able to describe treatment of adults with swallowing disorders.
- Be familiar with the emotional and social effects of motor speech disorders and swallowing disorders on patients and their families.

KEY TERMS

amyotrophic lateral sclerosis (ALS, Lou Gehrig's disease)
anarthria
apraxia of speech (speech apraxia, verbal apraxia, acquired apraxia)
aspiration
aspiration pneumonia

automatic speech
autonomy
bioethics
differential diagnosis
dysarthria
dysphagia (swallowing disorder)
enteral feeding

INTRODUCTION

Dysarthria, speech apraxia, and dysphagia are frequently seen as problems in the same patient (Duffy, 2005; Duffy, 2006; Logemann, 1998). Dysarthria is a neurological speech disorder that is a result of weakness, paralysis, or inability to coordinate the articulatory, resonatory, phonatory, and/or respiratory systems. All of these systems also are important in swallowing. Speech apraxia is the result of an impaired ability to plan, sequence, coordinate, and initiate motor movements of the articulators, which also can affect voluntary initiation of swallowing. The same neurological insults (e.g., CVAs, TBIs, degenerative diseases) that cause dysarthria and apraxia can cause dysphagia. This is not only true for adults, but also true for children (Morgan & Skeat, 2010; Morgan, Mageandran, & Mei, 2010).

MOTOR SPEECH DISORDERS

Disordered speech is sometimes the first sign of neurological disease. Because speech is normally such an automatic process, a sudden disturbance requires immediate attention. Darley, Aronson, and Brown (1975) estimated that for every second a person is talking, approximately 140,000 neuromuscular contractions and relaxations occur in the speech production muscles (i.e., muscles of the respiratory, phonatory, resonatory, and articulatory systems).

Motor speech disorders result from neurological impairments affecting the motor planning, programming, neuromuscular control, execution of speech, or a combination of these. They include the dysarthrias and apraxia of speech. Motor speech disorders have a sensory component and should be thought of as *sensorimotor*, not just motor, in character (Duffy, 2005; Weismer, 2006). Motor speech disorders often accompany aphasia, cognitive impairments, or both when the lesion is extensive; however, motor speech disorders can occur alone.

Dysarthria

Dysarthria is a general term for a collection of speech disorders characterized by weakness in the muscles that control respiration, phonation, resonation, and articulation (see Figure 12–1). The weakness may have a minimal-to-profound effect on all speech systems, depending on the site and size of the lesion or lesions. In general, the **range of motion (ROM)**, strength, coordination, and rate of muscle movement may be affected in each of the speech systems, which have an overall affect on the prosody of speech (Duffy, 2005; Weismer, 2006; Yorkston, Beukelman, Strand, & Hakel, 2010). Individuals with severe dysarthria may have no

motor speech disorders

Neurological impairments that affect the motor planning, programming, neuromuscular control, and/or execution of speech and include the dysarthrias and apraxia of speech; they typically have a sensory component and should be thought of as sensorimotor disorders.

dysarthria

A group of motor speech disorders caused by *paresis* (weakness), *paralysis* (complete loss of movement), or incoordination of speech muscles as a result of central and/or peripheral nervous system damage that may affect respiration, phonation, resonation, articulation, and prosody; dysarthric speech sounds "mushy" because of distorted consonants and vowels.

range of motion (ROM)

For speech, the limits the mandible can open and close, the lips can protrude and retract, and the tongue can protrude and retract, elevate and lower, and move side to side (*lateralize*).

- *Respiration*—Low intensity and speech that is limited to short phrases caused by decreased respiratory support
- *Phonation*—Breathy phonation caused by unilateral or bilateral vocal fold paresis or paralysis (weakness)
- *Resonation*—Hypernasality caused by weak movement of the soft palate leading to velopharyngeal incompetence
- *Articulation*—Distorted, imprecise consonants caused by weakness and incoordination of the mandible, lips, and tongue

Figure 12-1

Speech dimensions of dysarthria.

Adapted from Duffy, 2005.

functional intelligible speech, and many of these individuals would benefit from augmentative and alternative communication (AAC) systems.

Dysarthria may have the same etiologies as aphasia and cognitive disorders (e.g., CVAs, TBIs, tumors, toxins, degenerative diseases, and others). Sometimes, however, dysarthria has no clearly identifiable cause. Of the two motor speech disorders (apraxia and dysarthria), dysarthria is the more prevalent, primarily because a variety of areas in the CNS and PNS may be damaged and result in dysarthria (Duffy, 2005; Weismer, 2006).

Neuromuscular Disorders Commonly Associated with Dysarthria

Certain neuromuscular conditions or disorders are commonly associated with dysarthria. Some of these conditions may be seen in relatively young adults; however, in general, the older a person becomes, the more susceptible the person is to neurological diseases and disorders that may result in dysarthria (Golper, 2010).

Parkinson's Disease

Parkinson's disease (PD) is caused by a gradual deterioration of certain nerve centers in the brain that are important in the delicate balance of chemicals needed for transmission of nerve impulses for control of movement of the body, including the articulators. Arms and legs become stiff and do not swing or move in a smooth manner because opposing muscles (e.g., biceps and triceps in the arms) are contracting simultaneously. The face may become masklike with little expression, although the person has all of the same emotions as before the Parkinson's disease. A common symptom of Parkinson's disease is **tremors at rest**, for example tremors of the hands or head when the person does not consciously move them. Speech-language pathologists become involved with these individuals when their Parkinson's disease begins to affect their speech, swallowing, or both. Dysarthria is the speech disorder associated with the disease (McAuliffe, Ward, & Murdoch, 2007).

Application Question

Have you ever listened to a person who was drinking alcohol and becoming progressively drunk? The slurred speech of some people who have been drinking is similar to that of some individuals with dysarthria.

tremors at rest

Tremors that occur when the head, limbs, hands, or fingers are not intentionally being moved; when movement is initiated, the tremors subside until the body part is again no longer moving.

Michael J. Fox

The actor Michael J. Fox (recall the *Back to the Future* movies) has suffered from Parkinson's disease for many years, including when he was the star of the television series *Spin City*. He was able to hide his Parkinson's disease from the viewing audience by constantly being in motion, which he incorporated into the character he played. When his Parkinson's disease became so severe that he could not make his movements appear to be part of a normal functioning person, he made his problem known publicly. Since then, he has been an important advocate and spokesperson for research into Parkinson's disease. (Note: Mr. Fox has not yet developed any noticeable dysarthria.)

myasthenia gravis

A neuromuscular disorder more commonly seen in women than men; characterized by chronic fatigue and muscle weakness, especially in the facial and articulatory muscles, resulting in dysarthria.

amyotrophic lateral sclerosis (ALS, Lou Gehrig's disease)

A rare, rapidly progressive degenerative disease of motor neurons that control movement of all muscle systems, including the speech systems.

anarthria (anarthric)

The complete inability to articulate or speak that is usually caused by brain lesions or damage to peripheral nerves that innervate the articulatory muscles.

Myasthenia Gravis

Myasthenia gravis is a disease that affects women twice as often as it affects men, with an incidence of approximately 1 in 10,000. The disease often begins in women in their 30s, and in men the onset is usually in their 60s. Symptoms of myasthenia gravis appear first and most noticeably in the face. The eyelids begin to droop, double vision occurs, and weakness in the articulators causes slurred speech (dysarthria), dysphonia, and difficulty swallowing (Chang, Lee, & Kuo, 2004). The arms and legs may be affected, making it difficult to comb the hair or stand without being wobbly. A key diagnostic feature is decreasing muscle function with use and easy fatigability. With medication, some transmission of nerve impulses can be restored, but myasthenia gravis cannot be cured.

Amyotrophic Lateral Sclerosis

Amyotrophic lateral sclerosis (ALS) is commonly called *Lou Gehrig's disease* (named after the famous New York Yankee's baseball player who retired in 1939 because of ALS after playing 2,130 consecutive games). ALS is a rare, rapidly progressive degenerative disease of the motor neurons that control movement of all muscle systems, including the speech systems. ALS usually begins in middle age, with the age of initial symptoms occurring as early as the 40s and as late as the 70s. Males are affected more often than females. Death usually occurs within 5 years from wasting of the body, with pneumonia typically being the final illness. There is no known medical treatment.

Every physical function of the body can be affected, including breathing, swallowing, speaking, and walking (Hillel et al., 1989). Speech-language pathologists are likely to see patients with ALS for swallowing disorders, speech disorders, or both. As the disease progresses, the speaking rate of most patients diminishes. During the last years or months of life, they experience a severe communication disorder, with some individuals being **anarthric**.

TABLE 12-1 Characteristics of the Six Types of Dysarthrias

TYPE	DISEASE/DISORDER CHARACTERISTICS	SITE OF LESION	SPEECH CHARACTERISTICS
Spastic	Pseudobulbar palsy	Upper motor neuron	Imprecise articulation, slow rate, harsh voice quality
Ataxic	Cerebellar or Friedrich's ataxia	Cerebellum	Phoneme and syllable prolongation, slow rate, abnormal prosody
Flaccid	Bulbar palsy, myasthenia gravis	Lower motor neuron	Audible inspiration, hypernasality, nasal emission, breathiness
Hyperkinetic	Huntington's chorea, dystonia	Extrapyramidal system	Imprecise articulation, prolonged pauses, variable rate, impaired prosody
Hypokinetic	Parkinson's disease	Extrapyramidal system	Monoloudness, monopitch, reduced intensity, short rushes of speech
Mixed	Multiple sclerosis, amyotrophic lateral sclerosis	Multiple motor systems	Dependent on motor systems affected

Adapted from Gillam, Marquardt, & Martin, 2000.

Multiple Sclerosis (MS)

Multiple sclerosis (MS) is a debilitating disease in which the body's immune system slowly destroys the protective sheath (*myelin*) that covers the nerves. This interferes with the communication between the brain and the muscles and organs of the body. MS is most often seen in females between 20 and 40 years of age whose families originated in northern Europe, but it can occur at any age. Signs and symptoms of MS vary depending on the nerve fibers affected and may include numbness or weakness in one or more limbs, tingling or pain in parts of the body, tremors and lack of coordination or unsteady gait, fatigue, dizziness, and partial or complete loss of vision. Over time, speech, language, cognition, and swallowing may be affected. In the early stages of the disease individuals typically experience exasperation of symptoms that are followed by partial or complete remission. There is no known cure for MS, although medical management can modify the course of the disease and treat its symptoms.

Types of Dysarthrias

Six types of dysarthria have been described in the literature (Darley et al., 1975; Duffy, 2005; Weismer, 2006): spastic dysarthria, ataxic dysarthria, flaccid dysarthria, hyperkinetic dysarthria, hypokinetic dysarthria, and mixed dysarthria (see Table 12-1).

General Principles of Assessment of Dysarthria

A diagnosis of a motor speech disorder is made after a thorough evaluation of a patient's motor speech abilities. Sometimes evaluation results are unambiguous and a clear diagnosis can be made. More commonly, there are several possible interpretations and the clinician has to rank the possibilities. The process of narrowing possibilities and reaching conclusions about the nature of a deficit is known as **differential diagnosis**. A thorough evaluation of the speech systems (respiratory, phonatory, resonatory, and articulatory) is completed, with emphasis on the oral mechanism. Careful visual, auditory, and even tactile perceptual evaluations are essential, with emphasis on the auditory. Perceptual evaluations are the "gold standard" for clinical differential diagnosis, judgments of severity, many decisions about management, and assessment of functional change (Duffy, 2005; Weismer, 2006; Yorkston et al., 2010).

General Principles of Therapy for Dysarthria

The primary goal of speech therapy for dysarthria is to maximize the effectiveness, efficiency, and naturalness of communication (Swigert, 2010; Yorkston et al., 2010). Depending on the severity of the dysarthria, patients and clinicians together may choose different approaches. For example, patients with mild dysarthria may focus on efficient and natural-sounding speech; patients with moderate dysarthria may choose to work on speech intelligibility and efficiency (i.e., manageable physical effort); and for those with severe dysarthria, the emphasis may be on effective and efficient alternative means of communication (Duffy, 2005).

Speech pathologists treat dysarthria by using *behavioral management*, with its primary goal to maximize communication (McAuliffe, 2006; Weismer, 2006). When improving speech intelligibility is the focus of therapy, clinicians attempt to reduce the patient's impairments by increasing physiological support for speech; for example, modifying or improving posture and increasing range of motion, muscle tone, strength, and rate of movement. *Drill* (the systematic practice of specially selected and ordered exercises) is a foundation of therapy. Patients with motor speech disorders must speak to improve their speech. When speech muscles are not exercised sufficiently, muscle strength may further decline (this is similar to general body deconditioning when patients are confined to bed) (Covertino, Bloomfield, & Greenleaf, 1997). When speaking, patients need to make speech highly conscious so that their focus is on being heard and understood rather than on how quickly they can communicate their messages.

Apraxia of Speech

Apraxia of speech (speech apraxia, verbal apraxia, acquired apraxia) is caused by damage in the region of the posterior inferior left frontal lobe in or around Broca's area (Duffy, 2005; Yorkston et al., 2010).

---

differential diagnosis

The process of narrowing possibilities and reaching conclusions about the nature of a deficit.

apraxia of speech (speech apraxia, verbal apraxia, acquired apraxia)

A deficit in the neural motor planning and programming of the articulatory muscles for voluntary movements for speech in the absence of muscular weakness; primarily interferes with articulation and prosody.

The most common cause of apraxia of speech is stroke. The important motor functions of Broca's area are planning and programming for voluntary movements of the articulators. Speech apraxia is the result of an impaired ability to plan, sequence, coordinate, and initiate motor movements of the articulators. When only Broca's area is damaged, the speech errors are not the result of weakness; however, when the adjacent precentral gyrus or the pyramidal tract also is damaged, weakness can contribute to impaired speech intelligibility. A patient may have both speech apraxia and dysarthria (to be discussed in more detail later).

Characteristics of Apraxia of Speech

The characteristics of apraxia of speech were first described by Darley et al. (1975), and further described by Wertz, LaPointe, and Rosenbek (1991):

- Articulation errors are not the result of muscle weakness or paralysis.
- Articulation errors are highly variable.
- Sound errors are more often substitutions than distortions, omissions, or additions.
- Consonant errors are more common than vowel errors.
- Errors occur most often on the initial consonant of words.
- Consonant clusters (e.g., /bl, sp, st, tr/) are more likely to be in error than single consonants.
- Errors increase with increasing word length (i.e., number of sounds and syllables).
- There are trial-and-error "gropings" for the correct placement of the articulators to produce sounds, causing the person to look like he is working hard or struggling to talk.
- Front-of-the-mouth sounds (e.g., /b, d, z/) are more likely to be correct than back-of-the-mouth sounds (e.g., /k, g, ch, sh/).
- There are "islands" of fluent, error-free words, phrases, and sentences amid effortful, struggling speech.

Individuals with severe apraxia of speech may be able to say a few "stock" (*stereotypic*) phrases, such as "I'm fine. How are you?," or even "I know what I want to say, but I can't say it," or "I know I want to say 'I work in construction,' but I can't say it." In the last instance, the person actually says automatically and effortlessly the very word, phrase, or sentence that could not be said when intentionally trying to say it. Once the patient is able to volitionally say the word or phrase correctly, he usually thinks that he will be able to say it again without difficulty, but his next attempt may be as difficult and off target as his first attempt (Duffy, 2005; Weismer, 2006; Yorkston et al., 2010).

One of the hallmark characteristics of apraxia of speech is its inconsistency. Patients may be able to say complex, multisyllabic words and

Personal Story — Profanity

One of my patients at a university medical center was the wife of a professor. She always had been known by her family and friends as a rather demure and proper lady who never used profanity. However, after having a stroke and developing moderate-to-severe speech apraxia, many of her attempts to communicate were punctuated with a variety of scatological words and other profanities. Her family and friends were surprised and she was embarrassed, saying that she sounded like a "drunken sailor." Fortunately, as her speech apraxia diminished, so did her profanity. ■

automatic speech

Over-learned sequences of words that can be recited without much conscious thought, such as counting to 10; saying the days of the week, months of the year, and the alphabet; and singing some songs (e.g., the birthday song).

oral apraxia (nonverbal apraxia, facial apraxia, buccofacial apraxia)

Difficulty with volitional nonspeech movements of the articulators (e.g., puffing the cheeks, clicking the tongue, protruding the tongue, whistling, or smiling).

then may have difficulty with simple, single-syllable words. They often can say sequences of **automatic speech**, such as counting to 10 and saying the days of the week or the months of the year. However, when a patient is trying to say *Thursday,* for example, he may not be able to say it alone, so he gets a "running start" by starting with *Sunday* and when he reaches *Thursday* he stops and says, "That's it." Many people also can sing very familiar songs (e.g., the birthday song) even though they may have difficulty saying "happy birthday." Another fairly common characteristic of speech apraxia is the ability to fluently use profanity and strings of profane words (even individuals who claim to never use profanity may spontaneously and almost uncontrollably use profane words). This automatic and difficult-to-control behavior is embarrassing to some individuals.

Patients with a pure speech apraxia (i.e., no aphasia or cognitive disorders) typically recognize their errors and try to repair them, but to their chagrin the harder they try the more difficult it is for them to say their intended words. Patients often become frustrated and angry with themselves. Individuals with severe apraxia may begin to avoid talking and feel that the effort and embarrassment are not worth trying to communicate.

Patients with speech apraxia also may have **oral apraxia (nonverbal apraxia, facial apraxia, buccofacial apraxia)**. They have difficulty with nonspeech movements of their articulators; for example, intentionally blowing through the lips, clicking the tongue, protruding the tongue, whistling, and smiling. They have effortful groping of the articulators or inconsistent trial-and-error attempts. They usually are confused, frustrated, embarrassed, and sometimes even amused by their difficulty with seemingly easy tasks. However, these same individuals may automatically and spontaneously do any of these movements and be unaware they just performed them (Duffy, 2005; Yorkston et al., 2010).

Limb Apraxia

The articulators are not the only muscles in the body that may be apraxic. *Limb apraxia* (considered the result of damage to the posterior region of the frontal lobe, particularly the left frontal lobe near Broca's area) is seen when a patient cannot perform volitional movements of an arm, hand, or fingers. Limb apraxia is typically more severe with the hand and fingers than with the arm. For example, a patient is likely to have more difficulty showing you how to snap his fingers, flip a coin, or wind a watch than showing you how to salute or drink from a glass. This symptom is important to speech-language pathologists because when a patient has a moderate-to-severe speech apraxia, we cannot rely on the patient having sufficient control of finger movements to write what he cannot say. In addition to writing being nonfunctional, teaching a patient to use finger spelling or a complex sign system such as *American Sign Language* (ASL) may not be practical. However, a sign system such as *American Indian Hand Talk (Amerind)* (Skelly, 1979), which relies on somewhat universal "natural gestures" (e.g., raising the fingers to the mouth as if eating to represent *hunger, food,* or *eat*) may be functional for the person to learn for basic communication.

General Principles of Assessment of Apraxia of Speech

As with dysarthria, a thorough evaluation of the speech systems is completed. When an apraxia of speech is suspected, the patient's speech and oral mechanism are the target of the evaluation. The previously described signs and symptoms are noted and, when appropriate, a diagnosis of apraxia of speech is made. Many patients have combinations of other impairments, such as dysarthria, aphasia, cognitive disorders, and dysphagia.

General Principles of Therapy for Apraxia of Speech

The primary goal of therapy for apraxia of speech is to maximize the effectiveness, efficiency, and naturalness of communication. Therapy focuses on restoring or compensating for impaired functions, as well as helping the person emotionally adjust to the loss of abilities that cannot be restored. *Behavioral intervention* is at the heart of therapy for apraxia of speech (Duffy, 2005; Weismer, 2006; Yorkston et al., 2010).

Therapy for individuals with apraxia of speech should start as early as possible. The various approaches to therapy emphasize carefully selecting the stimuli (functional words) the clinician wants the patient to work on during any one session, an orderly progression of therapy tasks (generally from easiest to hardest), and the use of intensive and systematic drill (practicing repeatedly).

Many individuals with apraxia of speech benefit from watching their face and articulators in a mirror while they are talking. The visual feedback helps compensate for their lack of awareness of where their articulators are and where they want to move them. Apraxia therapy often uses a multimodality approach.

CASE STUDY

John: A Speech-Language Pathologist with Aphasia and Apraxia of Speech

John, a prominent retired speech-language pathologist, had surgery on his lower esophageal valve to help manage his severe gastric reflux. The surgery was successful; however, while in his hospital room resting, he had an occlusive stroke that resulted in severe receptive and expressive aphasia and speech apraxia (global aphasia). He received the amount of speech, physical, and occupational therapy his insurance authorized and was then discharged home. John's wife, Ginger, contacted a speech-language pathologist who taught the courses in neurological disorders in adults and motor speech disorders at a university about an hour away. Ginger wanted to discuss John's problems and try to "make sense" of them.

As a speech-language pathologist, John certainly knew what aphasia and apraxia were, but because of the severity of his aphasia, he could understand little of what was said to him and could communicate only minimally his wants, needs, thoughts, and feelings. The speech-language pathologist decided to show John and Ginger a professionally produced videotape that was made to help laypeople understand strokes, aphasia, and motor speech disorders. The video showed a variety of stroke survivors talking about their problems. While John and Ginger watched the video with the speech-language pathologist, one or the other would occasionally and excitedly point to the television and say, "That's it! That's it!" The video was able to help them see and understand from other survivors' perspectives the problems John was experiencing.

Because of the distance the couple lived from the university, the speech-language pathologist referred them to a university speech-language clinic that was closer to them and had a stroke support group that met weekly. John became a regular member of that group for several years and, although his recovery **plateaued** (still at a severe "global" level), he continued with the group because he enjoyed being around other people that he could relate to. ■

plateau

A patient's general leveling off of improvement in rehabilitation, after which gains are slower and less easily documented; often the reason for discharging from rehabilitation.

dysphagia (swallowing disorders)

Difficulty swallowing that occurs when impairments affect any of the four phases of swallowing (oral preparatory, oral, pharyngeal, or esophageal); puts a person at risk for aspiration of food and/or liquid and potential aspiration pneumonia.

DYSPHAGIA/SWALLOWING DISORDERS

Dysphagia refers to difficulty swallowing (*deglutition* [L. *deglutire,* to swallow]) that occurs when impairments affect any of the four phases of swallowing (oral preparatory, oral, pharyngeal, or esophageal) and put a person at risk for **aspiration**—food, liquid, or both entering the larynx, trachea, and lungs—and potential **aspiration pneumonia**. It is the area of rehabilitation that speech-language pathologists have most recently encompassed. Dysphagia is not part of communication, but it is intimately connected to the speech systems (respiratory, phonatory, resonatory, and articulatory) that serve verbal communication. Speech-language pathologists are recognized by the medical community as the professionals most knowledgeable and directly responsible for the evaluation and treatment of dysphagia (Corbin-Lewis, Liss, & Sciortino, 2005; Miller & Groher, 2005). Dysphagia assessment and treatment are within our scope of practice (see ASHA's "Scope of Practice for Speech-Language Pathologists" on their website, www.asha.org).

Dysphagia requires a team approach, with the speech-language pathologist typically the coordinator or head of the team (Davies, Taylor, MacDonald, & Barer, 2001; Homer, 2003; Leonard & Kendall, 2008; Swigert, 2007). Team members may include (in alphabetical order): a *dentist* for making dental appliances and dentures; a *dietician* or *nutritionist* who checks the patient's daily intake of liquids and food and tries to make the various food textures as palatable (edible) as possible and makes certain the patient is receiving adequate nutrition for maintaining and improving health; various *family* members who may be involved with feeding the patient and making decisions about the level of care a patient may be able to return to; a *gastroenterologist* for evaluating esophageal problems and inserting nasogastric and stomach feeding tubes; a *neurologist* for assessing and treating some aspects of the patient's neurological impairments; *nurses* who can manage the patient's day-to-day medical needs and inform the team members about a patient's medical changes; an *occupational therapist* for helping with positioning the patient for meals and assessing and managing the patient's ability to retrieve food from a plate and bring it to the mouth; an *otolaryngologist* to examine laryngeal function; a *pharmacist* for providing information about side effects of the patient's medications that may influence swallowing adversely; a *physical therapist* who assesses and manages postural problems and finds the best wheelchair for the patient; one or more *physicians* who are managing the patients medical problems; a *pulmonologist* who can assess respiratory functions and treat respiratory problems such as aspiration pneumonia; a *radiologist* for performing and helping read modified barium swallowing studies; a *respiratory therapist* who can carry out various respiratory treatments, sometimes several times a day; and a *social worker* who is involved in patient advocacy and works with insurance companies, Medicare, and other third-party payers (see Figure 12–2).

The work of SLPs with patients who have dysphagia is in some ways the most challenging and high-risk work we do because a patient's physical health (indeed, life) may be determined by our evaluation, correct diagnosis, and appropriate management of the swallowing disorder (Logemann, 1998; Murry & Carrau, 2006). Beyond basic academic course work on dysphagia during graduate training, there must be considerable hands-on training during hospital internships and additional training through professional workshops and seminars to become competent to work independently with patients who have swallowing disorders. It is essential that clinicians develop the skills outlined by ASHA (2000a; 2000b;

aspiration

A term in reference to material (food, liquid, saliva, etc.) penetrating the larynx and entering the airway below the true vocal folds; food or liquid entering the lungs rather than the stomach after the swallow.

aspiration pneumonia

An acute inflammation of the lungs caused by foreign material (e.g., food or liquid) entering the lung tissue and resulting in infection; alveolar and bronchiole congestion with substances discharged from the alveolar walls as a protection against foreign material.

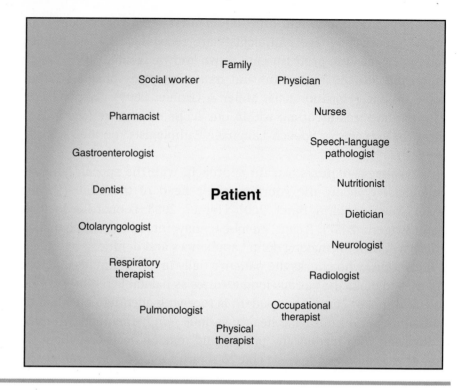

Figure 12-2

Potential members of a dysphagia team.

© Cengage Learning 2013.

2002; 2004a; 2004b) for providing services to patients and clients with dysphagia:

- Identify people at risk for dysphagia.
- Conduct and interpret clinical assessments of oral–pharyngeal and respiratory functions related to feeding.
- Conduct and interpret instrumental-based evaluations of swallowing.
- Develop intervention strategies (i.e., safe feeding recommendations, swallowing precautions, and therapeutic interventions).
- Document care and discharge planning.
- Provide education, counseling, and training to patients and all other relevant individuals (e.g., family and health professionals).

Causes of Dysphagia

Swallowing disorders may occur at any age—from newborns to the end of life. Essentially, the same neurological causes of motor speech disorders and cognitive disorders in children and adults may cause dysphagia. However, in addition to neurological etiologies, cancer (lingual, oral, pharyngeal, and laryngeal) may cause swallowing problems. The treatment of these cancers (surgical removal, radiation, chemotherapy) also may cause or contribute to swallowing impairments. Side effects of some medications may cause swallowing problems. Muscle relaxants may affect muscle tone of the swallowing muscles (Carl & Johnson, 2006). HIV and AIDS in children and adults are associated with dysphagia

(Crary & Groher, 2003; Finley, Clifton, Stewart, Graham, & Worsley, 2001; Huckabee & Pelletier, 2003).

Speech-language pathologists work with dysphagia in all clinical settings, plus home health care. In a U.S. study of acute care hospital patients, it was found that approximately one-third of patients with new strokes have dysphagia (Teasell, Foley, Fisher, & Finestone, 2002). Dysphagia has become the primary focus of the acute care hospital work for speech-language pathologists in Australia and England (Armstrong, 2003; Code & Heron, 2003). In some hospitals, speech-language pathologists become known as *swallowing therapists* more than speech pathologists. School-based SLPs are increasingly finding that their caseloads include children with medical complications and even swallowing problems, particularly those with orthopedic handicaps (e.g., cerebral palsy) (Ratner, 2006; Kurjan, 2000; Rempel & Moussavi, 2005).

THE NORMAL SWALLOW

To understand when a patient has a swallowing problem, we must first understand the anatomy and physiology of a normal swallow. What we take for granted every time we unconsciously swallow is the complex interaction of several muscle groups with split-second timing to allow us to effortlessly, automatically, and safely carry out one of the most mundane functions of our bodies. People generally swallow approximately 600 times a day (we even automatically swallow our saliva during sleep), which is almost 220,000 times a year. If we multiply that by, say, 50 years, it means that the average 50-year-old person has swallowed automatically and mostly unconsciously more than 10 million times. Each swallow has four phases (stages): (1) oral preparatory phase, (2) oral phase, (3) pharyngeal phase, and (4) esophageal phase. Patients may have difficulty with any or all of the phases and even specific problems within each portion of a phase (Corbin-Lewis et al., 2005; Kendall, 2008; Logemann, 1998).

Oral Preparatory Phase

All of our senses come into play during the oral preparatory phase—that is, vision, hearing (e.g., the sound of food cooking or popcorn popping), touch, smell, and taste (Fogle, 1998). The oral preparatory phase may be considered to begin with a person's cognitive level of awareness that food or drink is available to be consumed. The next cognitive process is to decide how to bring the food or liquid to the mouth. Once food enters the mouth, it must be chewed sufficiently to prepare it to be swallowed (it is referred to as a *bolus* [Gk. *bolos,* lump] when it is in the mouth). How we chew and how long we chew depends on the temperature of the food and the size, texture, and consistency of the bite. As we prepare the food inside our mouth, we tighten our cheeks slightly to prevent food

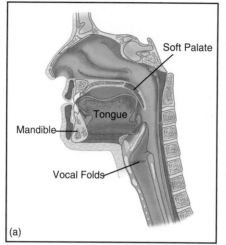

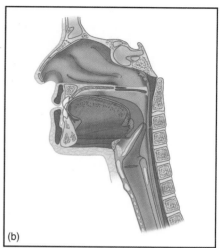

(a)

Soft Palate

Tongue

Mandible

Vocal Folds

(b)

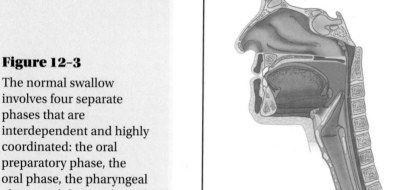

(c)

(d)

Figure 12-3

The normal swallow involves four separate phases that are interdependent and highly coordinated: the oral preparatory phase, the oral phase, the pharyngeal phase, and the esophageal phase. This series demonstrates a lateral view of bolus propulsion during the swallow: (a) The tongue begins the voluntary initiation of the swallow; (b) this triggers the pharyngeal swallow; (c) the bolus moves to the vallecula; (d) the tongue base then moves anteriorly and the pharyngeal walls begin peristalsis; and (e) the bolus moves to the cervical esophagus and the cricopharyngeal region.

© Cengage Learning 2013.

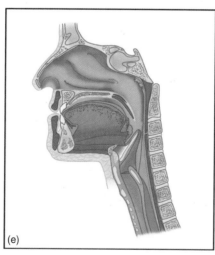

(e)

from lodging between our gums (*gingiva*) and our cheeks. We also pull the soft palate down firmly against the base of the tongue to prevent food from falling past the tongue into the open airway. We use our tongue to move the food around inside our mouth and between our teeth to chew the food (see Figure 12–3).

Oral Phase

The oral phase begins when we stop chewing and the tongue tip elevates to touch the alveolar ridge. The food is on top of the tongue and the tongue quickly sweeps back, pulling the food to the back of the mouth and toward the pharynx. The soft palate moves up to make contact with the posterior pharyngeal wall to prevent food from accidentally entering the nasal passage (*nasal regurgitation*). The oral phase normally takes 1 second.

Pharyngeal Phase

Passage of food through the pharynx and into the esophagus occurs during the pharyngeal phase of swallowing. Four physiological responses occur during the pharyngeal phase. First, as the bolus flows over the base of the tongue, there is a squeezing action (*peristalsis*) caused by contraction of the muscles in the pharynx that helps move the bolus downward. Second, the thyroid cartilage of the larynx rises, which causes the epiglottis to drop down over the opening into the larynx to shield it and prevent food or liquid falling into the open airway (*aspiration*), and initiates the opening of the *upper esophageal valve* (UEV) so the bolus can enter the esophagus. Third, the true and false vocal folds adduct tightly, which provides two more levels of protection (defense) from food or liquid entering the trachea. And fourth, the upper esophageal sphincter at the top of the esophagus relaxes and opens, allowing the bolus that has flowed around the epiglottis to enter into the esophagus. All of the pharyngeal phase normally takes 1 second.

Esophageal Phase

When the bolus passes the upper esophageal sphincter, the sphincter closes and the peristaltic squeezing action of the esophageal muscles carries the bolus to the *lower esophageal sphincter* at the bottom of the esophagus, which then briefly opens to allow the bolus to enter the stomach. When the bolus has passed, the sphincter again closes to prevent gastric contents from reentering the esophagus. The esophageal phase may take 8 to 20 seconds.

DYSPHAGIA—DISORDERED SWALLOWING

Individuals may have problems in any or all four of the phases of swallowing, and a problem at an earlier phase may cause a problem during a later phase (Corbin-Lewis et al., 2005; McCulloch & Jaffe, 2006). When thinking about swallowing disorders, it is helpful to organize your thinking by considering each phase in sequence.

Application Question

Try swallowing one or two sips of water. What do you notice? When you are going to eat some food, think about each of the four phases of swallowing. What do you notice?

Oral Preparatory Phase Problems

Many patients have decreased cognition because of neurological damage from a stroke or head trauma. Some patients have impaired awareness and do not realize that there is food in front of them or what to do with it if they are aware. Some patients, particularly those with TBIs, are impulsive and will take dangerously large bites of food and keep putting more spoonfuls into their mouths before adequately chewing (*masticating*) and swallowing the previous bites. Patients also may have weak mandible, lip, and tongue muscles that make it difficult to hold food in their mouths and to chew and control it adequately.

Oral Phase Problems

This phase involves the final movement of the bolus to the posterior oral cavity on its way to the pharynx. If the lips do not have a good seal, *anterior spillage* (drooling) may occur. When there is a poor posterior seal between the soft palate and the base of the tongue, food or liquid may spill over the base of the tongue before the swallow is initiated (*premature spillage*). A weak tongue, particularly the tip, will cause discoordinated and impaired posterior movement of the bolus to the back of the mouth. *Pocketed food* between the cheek and the gums (*sulcus*) may leave *residue* or *stasis* (food that is not cleared and swallowed). In some patients, the force used to propel the bolus is insufficient and the bolus will not move efficiently through to the next phase.

Pharyngeal Phase Problems

Numerous problems may occur in this phase. There may be a *delayed swallow response* from a few seconds to many seconds after the patient attempts to swallow. Timing and coordination of the oral–pharyngeal structures may be impaired. The soft palate may be too weak to close the velopharyngeal port to prevent material from entering the nasal passages. Muscles that raise the larynx may be weak causing the epiglottis not to drop down to cover the open airway, causing *penetration*, and the upper esophageal valve may not open, preventing food or liquid entering the esophagus. The true and false vocal folds may not have strong closure, allowing material that may enter the larynx to pass below the vocal folds (aspiration).

Patients with swallowing disorders may not have normal sensation in the laryngeal region, and material may penetrate the larynx without a protective cough or choking occurring, resulting in **silent aspiration**. That is, material enters the larynx, passes below the vocal folds, and moves down the trachea into the lungs without the patient having any sensation of something in the airway. Without sensation, there are no protective maneuvers such as coughing and choking (Ramsey, Smithard, & Kalra, 2003; Murry & Carrau, 2006). Other individuals may attempt to cough, but the cough is too weak to be protective and effective; therefore, the material is able to pass below the vocal folds into the trachea and down into the lungs.

silent aspiration

Penetration of food or liquid (including saliva) into the larynx and passing below the vocal folds without a protective cough or choking occurring.

Esophageal Phase Problems

Esophageal problems may be the result of the upper esophageal sphincter not opening at the precise time or not remaining open for the entire bolus to flow through. Slow or absent *esophageal peristalsis* may not carry the bolus through the esophagus in an efficient and complete manner, causing discomfort or pain in the chest and leaving residue on the esophageal walls that can cause infection. In some patients, the lower esophageal valve (LEV) does not sufficiently relax to allow the food in the esophagus to flow into the stomach causing *achalasia* (abnormal constriction of the lower portion of the esophagus). **Gastroenterologists** are the medical professionals who treat esophageal disorders.

gastroenterologist

A physician who specializes in diseases of the gastrointestinal tract.

DIAGNOSIS OF DYSPHAGIA

When an SLP begins her day at a hospital, she may be given a physician's order to "evaluate and treat" a particular new admission for swallowing problems. These medical orders should be taken care of as soon as possible because in some instances a patient's meals may be held up until the SLP can make a decision about swallowing safety. Also, legally the clinician has a certain window of time to complete an assessment and written report. The SLP is a hospital's main resource on swallowing function and disorders, and nurses and other medical staff members follow the SLP's recommendations. Referrals to a speech-language pathologist to evaluate a patient's swallowing typically are based on three general areas of concern:

- The patient appears to be at risk for aspirating food or liquid based on the medical diagnosis.
- Difficulties have been observed related to feeding and the intake of food or liquid.
- The patient appears not to be taking in adequate nourishment (Cherney, 2004; Logemann, 1998; Swigert, 2007).

Bedside (Clinical) Swallow Evaluation

The evaluation of a patient who may have dysphagia begins with a careful review of the patient's medical chart. The next step is screening the patient, which includes interviewing the patient to understand her perceptions of the problem and to determine whether the patient has a sufficiently strong protective cough to clear food or liquid from the airway. A multistep clinical or "bedside" evaluation is performed, including an oral-mechanism examination with careful observation of the anatomy and physiology of the articulatory structures, the *symmetry* of the structures (i.e., are both left and right sides equal in dimension and function), volitional movements, range of motion, strength, and coordination of each articulator. The clinician needs to observe the patient drinking different consistencies or thicknesses of liquids (i.e., *regular* [thin], *nectar, honey,* and *pudding*) and foods of different textures (i.e., *regular* [normal diet with all textures], *mechanical soft* [food easily chewed into a cohesive bolus], and *puree* [blended food or baby-food texture] (Rodriquez & Borelli, 2003). Some signs and symptoms that a patient is at risk for aspiration and needs an *instrumental evaluation* are: coughing or choking during the evaluation, difficulty managing oral secretions, multiple attempts to swallow a bolus of food, and others. When there is risk for aspiration an instrumental evaluation is needed to clarify the kind of swallowing disorder the patient has (e.g., oropharyngeal) and the underlying physiological deficits. It is essential to document in the patient's medical chart all assessment procedures and results (ASHA, 2005a; Swigert, 2007).

Modified Barium Swallow Study

The **modified barium swallow study** (MBS study or MBSS; also known as a *videofluoroscopy swallow study,* or VFSS) is considered the "gold standard" instrumental evaluation for viewing the physiology of the swallow and determining the presence or absence of aspiration (see Figure 12–4). It is a *dynamic* (moving) imaging *radiographic* (x-ray) procedure to examine the process of swallowing; that is, a video recording of real-time movement of the bolus from entering the mouth to entering the stomach. The MBSS provides the most thorough information on the physiology of the swallowing process (ASHA, 2004a; Becker, McLeroy, & Carpenter, 2005; DeMatteo, Matovich, & Hjartarson, 2005). It is performed in the radiology (x-ray) suite with the speech-language pathologist and radiologist working as a team. The clinician presents to the patient various liquid consistencies that have been mixed with *barium* (a *radiopaque* substance that stops the passage of x-rays and is used to outline the interior of hollow organs, e.g., the esophagus) and food textures that have been

modified barium swallow study (MBSS)

A dynamic (moving) imaging radiographic (x-ray) procedure focusing on the mouth, pharynx, larynx, and cervical esophagus used to examine the process of swallowing; a video recording of real-time movement of a bolus from entering the mouth to entering the stomach.

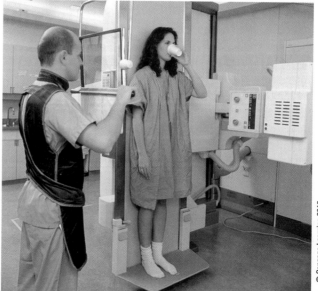

Figure 12–4

A radiologist conducting a modified barium swallow study with a patient.

© Cengage Learning 2013

coated with barium. The clinician carefully observes on the video screen the patient's oral preparatory, oral, pharyngeal, and esophageal phases of swallowing. Beyond diagnosing oropharyngeal dysphagia, the clinician also has the patient try various compensatory swallowing techniques to see which techniques allow for a safe and efficient swallow; for example, modified liquid consistencies and food textures, postural adjustments of the patient, and swallowing maneuvers. These techniques can later be trained during the dysphagia therapy (Swigert, 2007).

Fiberoptic Endoscopic Evaluation of Swallowing

Fiberoptic endoscopic evaluation of swallowing (FEES) is a procedure used to provide information about the pharyngeal phase of swallowing (ASHA, 2002a; Langmore, 2003). During the FEES procedure, the patient sits in a chair and a flexible endoscope with a light source (see Figures 9-10 and 9-11) is passed through the nasal passageway into the nasopharynx and down to just below the epiglottis. FEES studies are video-recorded for detailed analysis. A selected texture of food is dyed green (e.g., applesauce) to provide a clear color contrast from the laryngeal tissue and is given to the patient to chew and swallow. The laryngopharynx is viewed through the endoscope to determine whether food material remains in the pharynx, penetrates into the larynx, or is aspirated into the airway with or without attempts to clear the throat through coughing or choking (see Figure 12-5). The FEES procedure allows the clinician to view the movement of the vocal folds and the pharyngeal and laryngeal structures only before and after the swallow.

fiberoptic endoscopic evaluation of swallowing (FEES)

A procedure used to provide visual information about the pharyngeal phase of swallowing; a flexible endoscope is passed through the nasal passageway into the nasopharynx to view the laryngopharynx and the patient is asked to swallow food or liquid that has been dyed green for contrast.

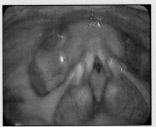

Courtesy of KayPENTAX

Figure 12-5

Fiberoptic Endoscopic Evaluation of Swallowing (FEES). Note the green colored applesauce on the right side of the larynx but not in the glottal region, i.e., there is no penetration into the airway.

TREATMENT OF DYSPHAGIA

A complete evaluation of dysphagia does not end at diagnosing a swallowing disorder in the oral or pharyngeal phases; in a sense, the clinician is reevaluating the patient during every therapy session. Treatment planning requires numerous careful decisions. The first decision is to choose a long-term functional goal based on the prognosis of the patient. *Long-term functional goal* refers to treatment results that improve a patient's swallowing ability in *natural environments* (home, community) or in a patient's future *lowest level of care* (e.g., skilled nursing facility). For most patients with dysphagia the long-term goals are "Patient will achieve safe and efficient swallowing to sustain adequate nutrition and hydration orally" or "Patient will be able to eat a regular diet safely" (Swigert, 2007). The emphasis in safety is important in many areas of our work with patients who have neurological disorders, but it is particularly important for patients who have swallowing problems (Fogle, Reece, & White, 2008).

As discussed previously, the SLP's decision to provide dysphagia therapy must be based on firm anatomical and physiological findings that indicate skilled intervention is necessary for a patient to eat safely and adequately to provide sufficient nutrition to maintain body weight.

Treating adults and children with dysphagia is interesting and challenging work. *Best practices* have been established and are continually refined for our treatment of dysphagia (ASHA, 2004b). In all therapy, clinicians need to consider **treatment efficacy**, which involves the extent to which an intervention can be shown to be beneficial under optimal (or ideal) conditions, and **treatment effectiveness**, which involves the extent to which services are shown to be beneficial under typical (or real-world) conditions (ASHA, 2004a, 2005; El Dib & Atallah, 2006; Frymark, Schooling, Mullen, et al., 2009; Logemann, 2004).

treatment efficacy

The extent to which an intervention can be shown to be beneficial under optimal (or ideal) conditions.

treatment effectiveness

The extent to which services are shown to be beneficial under typical (or real-world) conditions.

evidence-based practice

The quality of treatment that is measurable in terms of some form of functional outcomes and maintained in the face of cost-containment efforts.

Evidence-Based Practice

Evidence-based practice refers to quality of treatment that is measurable in terms of some form of functional outcomes and maintained in the face of cost-containment efforts. Evidence-based practice is an approach that deemphasizes both clinician intuition and unsystematic approaches to clinical care. It requires decisions to be made through a scientific process rooted in the examination of clinical research. Clinicians must be effective literature researchers and return to their academic roots. In this manner, clinical work may be supported with clinical evidence and literature (Lubinski, Golper, & Frattali, 2007).

Third-party payers (Medicare, health maintenance organizations [HMOs], etc.) do not want to know a test score; they want to know if a patient can be discharged, go home, recover, and return to work. Payers want those outcomes for the least amount of money and in the least amount of time. In other words, providers need to keep costs down, keep quality high, achieve maximum patient satisfaction, and be able to measure it and prove it. Health care delivery has become a process that balances costs and risks yet affords an acceptable outcome and level of quality (Lubinski, Golper, & Frattali, 2007).

For patients who have swallowing problems, therapy can include *compensatory treatment techniques, facilitation treatment techniques, compensatory and facilitation techniques, and diet modification techniques* (Swigert, 2007).

Compensatory Treatment Techniques

Compensatory treatment techniques help optimize a patient's ability to use his current swallowing abilities. The hospital staff and family may be taught to use these techniques when they are preparing or helping the patient to eat or drink.

Postural Techniques

Postural techniques are used to control the flow of the food or liquid bolus and reduce the risk of the patient's symptoms; for example, while attempting to swallow, tucking the chin downward or rotating the head to one side. Patients with communication and cognitive problems usually find postural techniques the easiest to learn (Leonard & Kendall, 2008; Murry & Carrau, 2006).

Food Placement

Food is normally placed in the midline of the tongue; however, some patients benefit from having food placed on the stronger side of the mouth, especially if it is food that needs to be chewed. Controlling bolus size is also important, usually limiting it to a small amount such as 5cc ($\approx$ 1 tsp.).

Facilitation Treatment Techniques

Facilitation treatment techniques are designed to improve the function of the swallowing mechanism and include techniques that help increase vocal fold adduction and teaching the patient to intentionally hold his breath just prior to and during the swallow, among other techniques. Oral-motor exercises for strengthening the muscles of the articulators have not been clearly effective for individuals with muscle weakness from dysarthria; however, there is indication they may be helpful for increasing muscle tone and strength to help improve swallowing (Clark, 2003; Hind, Nicosia, Roecker, Carnes, & Robbins, 2001; Murry & Carrau, 2006). Shaker (pronounced "shakeer") exercises help to increase laryngeal elevation and opening of the upper esophageal sphincter.

Compensatory and Facilitation Techniques

Compensatory and facilitation techniques are intended to help a patient's swallow become more functional. *Swallow maneuvers* try to bring aspects of the pharyngeal phase of the swallow into conscious awareness and voluntary control. A few swallowing maneuvers have been developed, a couple of which are the *supraglottic swallow* that is designed to close the airway at the level of the true vocal folds before and during the swallow, and the *effortful swallow* that is designed to increase posterior motion of the tongue base during the pharyngeal swallow phase (Cherney, 2004; Huckabee & Pelletier, 2003; Logemann, 1998). (Note: It is beyond the scope of this text to include descriptions of the various swallow maneuvers.)

Diet Modification Techniques

Diet modification techniques are often needed for patients with oral and/or pharyngeal phase swallowing problems (Logemann, 1998; Swigert, 2007). The National Dysphagia Diet Task Force (2002) standardized dietary modifications for patients based on a graded series of four levels of food textures and four levels of liquid consistencies (see Table 12-2). SLPs can choose which of the food textures and liquid consistencies they feel are best and safest for a particular patient who has dysphagia.

Although our treatment for dysphagia can be challenging, many patients benefit from the treatment and many can return to relatively

TABLE 12-2 Textures of Foods and Consistencies of Liquids

FOODS	LIQUIDS
Regular: No restrictions in foods but meats and some vegetables may be chopped; includes baked potatoes, rice, cooked or uncooked vegetables, fruits, fruit pies, cookies, cooked or dry cereals.	**Thin:** No restrictions.
Dysphagia advanced: Ground or chopped tender meat, potatoes (no skin), pasta, cooked vegetables, beans, canned fruits, apple slices (no peel), cookies, fruit pies, fried eggs, hot cereal.	**Nectar-like:** All liquids (including water) must be thickened to a nectar consistency; fruit nectars, V8 juice, eggnog.
Dysphagia mechanical soft: Ground or finely chopped tender meat with gravy, mashed potatoes with gravy, pasta, soft cooked vegetables, canned fruits, soft cookies, scrambled eggs, cooked cereals.	**Honey-like:** All liquids (including water) must be thickened to a honey consistency, usually with a commercial thickener.
Dysphagia pureed: Pureed meat, mashed potatoes with gravy, pureed vegetables, strained soups thickened to pudding consistency, pureed fruits, pudding, cooked cereals.	**Spoon-thick:** All liquids (including water) must be thickened to a pudding consistency, usually with a commercial thickener.

© Cengage Learning 2012.

normal eating and drinking. Early identification of and intervention for swallowing disorders reduce the risk of aspiration, shorten the hospitalization time, and improve quality of life. Overall, treatment for dysphagia has been reported to be cost effective compared to the cost of hospitalization and treatment of aspiration pneumonia (Evidence Reports/Technology Assessments, 1999; Johns Hopkins, 2000).

NPO (Nothing by Mouth)

Some patients have such severe swallowing disorders that they must be placed on **NPO (nothing by mouth)**, at least temporarily. NPO is a patient care instruction advising that the patient is prohibited from orally ingesting food, beverage, or medicine. Usually, after having swallowing therapy, patients are able to eat orally again. Patients who are on NPO may receive their nutrition through **enteral feeding**, which is the delivery of nutrition and hydration into the gastrointestinal (GI) tract by way of tube feedings through the nose (*nasogastric tube* [NG-tube]) or the stomach (*gastrostomytube* [G-tube]) (Johnson & Jacobson, 2007) (see Figure 12–6). Enteral feeding may be a temporary or permanent source of nutritional support. A common source of nutrition and hydration for patients on enteral feeding is the lactose-free nutrition supplement Ensure™ (Pediasure™ for children) that contains protein, carbohydrates, fat, vitamins, and minerals. Ensure™ and Pediasure™ can be purchased in local supermarkets and pharmacies.

NPO (nothing by mouth)

A patient care instruction advising that a patient is prohibited from orally ingesting food, beverage, or medicine; patients must receive nutrition through enteral feeding.

enteral feeding

The delivery of hydration and nutrition into the gastrointestinal (GI) tract by way of tube feedings through the nose or stomach.

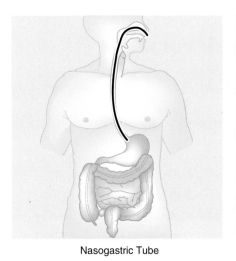

Nasogastric Tube

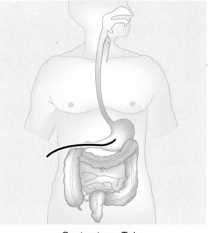

Gastrostomy Tube

Figure 12–6

Nasogastric tube (NG tube) and gastrostomy tube (G tube) feeding for patients who are NPO.

© Cengage Learning 2013.

CASE STUDY

Rachelle

Rachelle was a 29-year-old female and a single mother of three children. Rachelle had been in a motor vehicle accident while driving alone. She sustained a moderately severe head injury with contrecoup damage. The patient was impulsive, as well as confused and agitated. The speech-language pathologist's bedside evaluation revealed moderate receptive and expressive language impairments, severe cognitive impairments (which likely were contributing to her language problems), and significant impulsivity. She had bilateral weakness, worse on the left side of her body. There was moderate dysarthria affecting each of the speech systems. She had an adequate but not a strong protective cough. The bedside swallowing evaluation using a mechanical soft diet revealed an impaired oral preparatory phase as a result of impulsivity (trying to eat too fast) and discoordinated lingual movements with pocketing of food in the left lateral sulcus. She was not able to tolerate (manage) thin liquids but did well with nectar consistency. The oral phase was slow with poor posterior lingual movement. During the pharyngeal phase of swallowing, there was slow laryngeal elevation because of apparent weakened suprahyoid muscles. An MBSS confirmed the preceding findings and revealed residue on the left side pharyngeal wall likely caused by decreased pharyngeal peristalsis. She received a diagnosis of moderate oropharyngeal dysphagia and was considered a good candidate for swallowing therapy. With appropriate dysphagia and speech, language, and cognitive therapy, as well as physical and occupational therapy, Rachelle eventually was able to return home and to her job and support her family. ■

Personal Story

Multicultural Work Environments

In many of the hospitals where I have worked, numerous cultures were involved with the care of a single patient. In one hospital, an elderly female Vietnamese patient who had dysphagia did not understand or speak English. Her family routinely brought in food for her that was not appropriate for her dysphagia diet. Each person who tried to explain the potential risks to the patient and family spoke English with a different accent. The patient had a male Indian physician, several female and male Filipino nurses, female and male African American and Hispanic certified nursing assistants, and me, a Caucasian male speech-language pathologist from California. The patient and family may not have understood the message (i.e., no foods or liquids from home that are not of the right texture or consistency), or they made the choice to disregard the recommendations. As clinicians, we need to keep in mind that patients may receive medical care and treatment from a variety of cultures with different first languages, dialects, accents, and worldviews. Also, we need to remember that as speech-language pathologists we not only evaluate and treat patients from many cultures but work with professionals from many cultures. ■

Multicultural Considerations

All cultures have their own food preferences and unique ways of preparing foods. In addition, cultures have rituals around food and meals. There may be religious and dietary preference and taboos related to the use of special spices and food preparation practices, when and where meals are served, and even who is present during meals (some cultures have rigid rules as to whether both males and females can be present) (Shoemaker, 1997). Patients in hospitals are presented "institutional food" that the kitchen staff tries to make as nutritious and enjoyable as possible. However, many patients would agree that the food is often rather bland and not always appetizing or appealing.

For patients who are accustomed to "ethnic" foods because of their ethnic and cultural backgrounds, the hospital food presented may be totally foreign to them. A patient with dysphagia may be a visitor to this country or a long-time resident, but has not adopted the food choices and preparation methods of this country. The hospital kitchen staff cannot provide the desired ethnic foods for every person in the hospital who wants it; therefore, many patients are presented foods that are foreign and even distasteful to them.

Family members sometimes try to bring in food and drinks to a patient that they know their loved one will enjoy. This is a very caring and loving gesture; however, the food and drinks may be the wrong texture and consistency and cause the patient to cough, choke, or aspirate. Patients who have not eaten "real" food for a while may try to eat too fast and cause themselves swallowing problems. As clinicians, it is our job to educate both the patient and family about the hazards of feeding a patient foods and liquids that are unsafe (Provencio-Arambula, Provencio, & Hegde, 2006; Tonkovich, 2002).

EMOTIONAL AND SOCIAL EFFECTS OF MOTOR SPEECH DISORDERS AND DYSPHAGIA

Patients who have motor speech disorders are often very aware of the difficulty they have being understood and attempts to communicate can be fraught with frustration. Individuals may have only motor speech problems and little or no impairment of language or cognition. Some individuals, because of severe difficulty communicating verbally, will avoid verbal communication as much as possible—not wanting to place the burden of understanding on their listener and not wanting to embarrass themselves.

Adults who were very effective verbal communicators and may have even made their living based on their verbal skill, may find that without those skills they can no longer compete in the marketplace or enjoy socializing with colleagues, friends, and family. What they may have taken pride in for decades—their verbal skill—now eludes them and they feel isolated.

Food and eating have strong emotional significance for most people. Our thoughts about food and drink are typically based on acquiring and enjoying it, not on what damage it might do to our health (e.g., aspiration pneumonia or asphyxiation). Eating is a social function that people enjoy as a natural part of their lives. We "break bread together" as a way of establishing, building, and maintaining friendships and relationships. We raise a "toast" at weddings and other celebrations. We have our "comfort foods" and there is chocolate "to die for." People spend considerable time thinking about food: breakfast, midmorning snack, lunch, afternoon snack, dinner, evening snack, and maybe even a midnight snack. We have our favorite foods, meals, restaurants, coffee houses, bars, and pubs.

Eating alone or being fed by hospital staff takes away much of the enjoyment of eating, which can result in patients eating just enough to satisfy their hunger but not enough to get all of the nutrition and hydration they need (Fogle, 1998). What happens to people emotionally and socially when every bite of food and sip of liquid may bring on a "fit of coughing" or choking? How do they manage knowing that they may never again be able to swallow food without needing to consciously think about what they had spent their lives *not* thinking about? Does thinking about the mechanics of chewing and swallowing take away from the pure enjoyment of the taste and texture of food?

I have interviewed and discussed these concerns with numerous patients of mine in acute, subacute, and convalescent hospitals who had swallowing problems. Some of the following information is based on literature, and some of it comes from anecdotal reports from patients from their late teens into their 100s who have had dysphagia. So often when clinicians are working with patients with swallowing disorders, they focus on the anatomy and physiology of the swallowing problem and forget that there are genuine emotional and social concerns that may be helpful to discuss with their patients. The individuals we try to help are always *first* people and only *secondarily* patients or clients.

Quality of Life

A patient's quality of life is always the most important concern in patient care (Chen et al., 2001; Watt & Whyte, 2003). As clinicians and researchers, we are increasingly questioning what constitutes good quality of life from the patient's point of view. What we as professionals may think is good for patients may not be what they think is good for themselves, and ultimately they need to decide. We can inform, advise, and recommend, but they can demand. As clinicians we can provide information to patients about their swallowing problems and give our professional opinion about what we think is safest for their consumption of foods and liquids, but **bioethics** emphasizes that we must respect a patient's **autonomy** (Aiken, 2008; Beauchamp & Childress, 2008).

Food texture is important in the enjoyment of food. (Who would want pureed roast beef?) Decreasing the texture of food or increasing the *viscosity* (thickness) of liquids changes their flavor (Dahl, 2008; Matta, Chambers, Garcia, & McGowan-Helverson, 2006). Patients' complaints that foods do not taste the same when they are pureed are legitimate. Food has five inherent properties: appearance, aroma, flavor, texture, and nutrition. Only nutrition cannot be detected by the senses. It is the inherent qualities of food that we enjoy, and when these are lost (e.g., when finely chopped or pureed) many patients will decrease their consumption even though they understand the need for nutrition (Fogle, 1998).

Anxieties and Fears

Patients with dysphagia may experience anxieties and fears around eating. Examples include fear of: embarrassment in front of family and friends who visit during meal time; an acute or chronic illness (aspiration pneumonia), or even death because of aspiration; discomfort from suctioning of food or liquid out of the oral cavity, trachea, and lungs; never being able to eat their favorite foods (at least with a normal texture) and have normal thin liquids again (Ekberg et al., 2002; Flasher & Fogle, 2012).

Application Question

What are your comfort foods? How would you feel if the foods you need or crave for comfort were the very foods you could not have, particularly when you needed them most—when you are sick, anxious, or depressed?

bioethics

The attempt to understand and resolve ethical issues and problems in health care setting.

autonomy

Respect for the patient's right to determine his or her own choices in making health care decisions.

Mr. M and His Mittens

After beginning summer work in a skilled nursing facility, I was asked to evaluate an elderly gentleman for potential oral feeding. The patient had had a nasogastric tube (NG-tube) for several months and was wearing thick padded "mittens" on both hands as a restraint to prevent him from pulling out the NG-tube, which he had done many times before being required to wear the mittens. My evaluation revealed that he was not a safe oral feeder and that NPO was the safest method of feeding. He also had severe dysarthria and receptive and expressive aphasia. The patient's wife was present during my evaluation and shared her frustration and sadness about not being able to hold her husband's hand to comfort him because of the interference of the mittens. I suggested that a stomach feeding tube might be a consideration.

I wrote my evaluation results in the patient's medical chart with the recommendation to the physician for the placement of a gastric tube (G-tube). The physician denied my request, so I followed up and spoke with the physician. He told me that the patient was going to die soon and there was no need to change from an NG-tube to a G-tube. The patient's wife also spoke to the physician about wanting the change, but he would not be assuaged. As a speech-language pathologist, I was looking at the patient holistically rather than just physically. Had the patient received a G-tube months before, he could have had the comfort of his wife's hand on his, meeting both of their emotional needs. Sometimes we can only watch in sadness as medical decisions are made that we may feel do not take into consideration the patient as a whole person. ■

Stages of Grief

The stages of grief apply to dysphagia as well as other neurological disorders. Patients may begin with *denial* of their swallowing problem, possibly realizing that if they admit to it the SLP will take away their regular food and give them "baby food." When they realize they are having swallowing problems, they may become *angry* and displace the anger onto us and other people who are trying to help them. When their anger does not get them what they want (back on regular foods and liquids), they may try to *bargain* with the SLP, agreeing to do anything the clinician wants if she will just let them eat "real food" again. *Depression* may be partly the result of moving through the stages of grief, but it also may be compounded by the depression discussed previously. *Acceptance* is more a resignation of how things are and the realization that there are fewer episodes of coughing, choking, and pneumonia while on the new diet and when using the safe swallow techniques taught by the SLP.

When people lose lifelong natural abilities, they lose a sense of self. They have to readjust their self-images and self-concepts, and that takes time. Few patients receive counseling from any professional (including speech-language pathologists) about the emotional struggles they are dealing with around their swallowing problems (Ekberg et al., 2002). Most patients likely struggle in silence, complaining and grumbling sometimes but never "talking through" their sense of loss of who they were as a person.

CHAPTER SUMMARY

Motor speech disorders result from neurologic impairments affecting the motor planning, programming, neuromuscular control, execution of speech, or all of these. They include the dysarthrias and apraxia of speech. Motor speech disorders frequently accompany aphasia, cognitive impairments, and dysphagia; however, motor speech disorders can occur alone. *Dysarthria* is a general term for a collection of speech disorders characterized by weakness in the muscles that control respiration, phonation, resonation, and articulation. Apraxia of speech is the result of impaired ability to plan, sequence, coordinate, and initiate motor movements of the articulators in the absence of muscular weakness. Patients with speech apraxia also may have nonverbal oral apraxia.

Dysphagia refers to difficulty swallowing that occurs when impairments affect any of the four phases of swallowing (oral preparatory, oral, pharyngeal, or esophageal) that puts an individual at risk for aspiration of food and liquid and potential aspiration pneumonia. Dysphagia requires a team approach with numerous medical specialists; typically, the speech-language pathologist is the head of the team. Dysphagia is a major area of our work in hospitals, and children with swallowing disorders may be on the caseloads of school speech therapists. The same neurological causes of motor speech disorders and cognitive disorders can cause dysphagia, plus dysphagia may be caused by oral and laryngeal cancer.

Evaluation of patients with dysphagia includes a careful review of the medical chart, interview of the patient, a cursory assessment of the patient's speech, language, and cognitive functioning, an evaluation of the speech systems (respiratory, phonatory, resonatory, and articulatory), a bedside (clinical) evaluation of a patient's ability to tolerate various food textures and liquid consistencies, and possibly an instrumental evaluation such as modified barium swallow study (MBSS).

During treatment for dysphagia, the clinician works with the feeding environment, postural techniques, modifications of foods and liquids, oral motor exercises, and swallow maneuvers. Some patients are not able to tolerate any oral presentation of food and must be placed on NPO (nothing by mouth). These patients receive their nutrition and hydration through enteral (tube) feeding, either through the nose (nasogastric tube [NG-tube]) or through the stomach (gastric tube [G-tube]).

The quality of life of the patient is always the most important question in all aspects of patient care. Patients with swallowing problems have anxiety and fear about the possibility of choking or developing pneumonia. People with swallowing problems may become depressed, and they likely will go through the stages of grief.

STUDY QUESTIONS

Knowledge and Comprehension

1. Define dysarthria.
2. What are five characteristics of apraxia of speech?
3. Define dysphagia.
4. What is a modified barium swallow study (MBSS)?
5. Based on the National Dysphagia Diet, what are the four textures of food and four consistencies of liquids?

Application

1. Why is it important to evaluate each of the speech systems (respiratory, phonatory, resonatory, and articulatory) when differentially diagnosing dysarthria?
2. Why is it important to assess nonspeech movements of the articulators in patients who may have apraxia of speech?
3. Why would oral–pharyngeal (oropharyngeal) dysphagia be the most common diagnosis for a swallowing disorder?
4. Why is it essential to determine whether a patient has a protective cough during the evaluation?
5. Why is silent aspiration particularly dangerous for patients?

Analysis/Synthesis

1. Why might the severity of the dysarthria help determine the therapeutic approach?
2. Why is it important to consider the possibility of a limb apraxia in a patient who has apraxia of speech?
3. Why is it essential to have a thorough understanding of the process of normal swallowing in order to help patients with swallowing disorders?
4. What is evidence-based practice and why is it important to our profession?
5. What are the stages of grief and how do they relate to patients with dysphagia?

REFERENCES

Aiken, T. D. (2008). *Legal and ethical issues in health occupations* (2nd ed.). Philadelphia, PA: Saunders.

American Speech-Language-Hearing Association. (2000a). Clinical indicators for instrumental assessment of dysphagia. *ASHA Desk Reference, 3,* 225–233.

American Speech-Language-Hearing Association. (2000b). Skills needed by speech-language pathologists providing services to dysphagic patients/clients. *ASHA, 32*(Supplement 2), 7–12.

American Speech-Language-Hearing Association. (2002). Knowledge and skills for speech-language pathologists performing endoscopic assessment of swallowing functions. *ASHA* (Supplement 22), 107–112.

American Speech-Language-Hearing Association. (2004a). Preferred practice patterns for the profession of speech-language pathology. Available at ASHA website: preferred practice patterns for the profession of speech-language pathology.

American Speech-Language-Hearing Association. (2004b). Guidelines for speech-language pathologists performing videofluoroscopy swallowing studies. *ASHA* (Supplement 24), 77–92.

American Speech-Language-Hearing Association. (2005). Clinical guidelines for speech-language pathology services. *ASHA Leader,* May (6–7), 22–23.

Armstrong, E. (2003). Communication culture in acute speech pathology settings: Current issues. *Advances in Speech-Language Pathology, 5*(2), 137–143.

Beauchamp, T. L., & Childress, J. F. (2008). *Principles of bioethics* (6th ed.). Oxford, UK: Oxford University Press.

Becker, S., McLeroy, K., & Carpenter, M. A. (2005). Reliability of observations from modified barium swallow studies. *Journal of Medical Speech-Language Pathology,* June, 28–37.

Carl, L. L., & Johnson, P. R. (2006). *Drugs and dysphagia: How medications can affect eating and swallowing.* Austin, TX: Pro-Ed.

Chang, C., Lee, K., & Kuo, W. (2004). Dysphonia as the initial symptom of myasthenia gravis, *Journal of Otolaryngology, 33,* 57–59.

Chen, A., Frankowski, R., Bishop-Leone, J., Hebert, T., Leyk, S., Lewin, J., & Goepfert, H. (2001). The development and validation of a dysphagia-specific quality-of-life questionnaire for patients with head and neck cancer. *Archives of Otolaryngology Head and Neck Surgery, 127,* 870–876.

Cherney, L. R. (Ed.). (2004). *Clinical management of dysphagia in adults and children.* Gaithersburg, MD: Aspen.

Clark, H. M. (2003). Neuromuscular treatments for speech and swallowing. *American Journal of Speech-Language Pathology, 12,* 400–415.

Code, C., & Heron, C. (2003). Services for aphasia, other acquired adult neurogenic communication and swallowing disorders in the United Kingdom, 2000. *Disability and Rehabilitation, 25*(21), 1231–1237.

Corbin-Lewis, K. M., Liss, J. M., & Sciortino, K. L. (2005). *Clinical anatomy and physiology of the swallowing mechanism.* Clifton Park, NY: Delmar Cengage Learning.

Covertino, V., Bloomfield, S., & Greenleaf, J. (1997). An overview of the issues: Physiological effect of bed rest and restricted physical activity. *Medical Science and Sports Exercise, 29,* 187–194.

Crary, M. A., & Groher, M. E. (2003). *Introduction to adult swallowing disorders.* St. Louis, MO: Butterworth-Heinemann.

Dahl, W. J. (2008). *Modified texture food production: A manual for patient care facilities* (2nd ed.). Toronto, Ontario: Dietitians of Canada.

Darley, F. L., Aronson, A. E., & Brown, J. R. (1975). *Motor speech disorders.* Philadelphia, PA: W. B. Saunders.

Davies, S., Taylor, H., MacDonald, A., & Barer, D. (2001). An interdisciplinary approach to swallowing problems in acute stroke. *International Journal of Language & Communication Disorders, 36,* 357–368.

DeMatteo, C., Matovich, D., & Hjartarson, A. (2005). Comparison of clinical and videofluoroscopic evaluation of children with feeding and swallowing difficulties. *Developmental Medicine and Child Neurology, 47,* 149–157.

Duffy, J. R. (2005). *Motor speech disorders: Substrates, differential diagnosis, and management* (2nd ed.). St. Louis, MO: Elsevier Mosby.

Duffy, J. R. (2006). Apraxia of speech in degenerative neurological disease. *Aphasiology, 20*(6), 511–527.

Ekberg, O., Hamdy, S., Woisard, V., Wuttge-Hannig, A., & Ortega, P. (2002). Social and psychological burden of dysphagia: Its impact on diagnosis and treatment. *Dysphagia, 17*(2), 139–146.

El Dib, R. P., & Atallah, A. N. (2006). Evidence-based speech, language, and hearing therapy and the Cochrane Library's systematic reviews. *Sao Paulo [Brazil] Medical Journal, 124*(2), 51–54.

Evidence Reports/Technology Assessments. (1999). *Diagnosis and treatment of swallowing disorders (dysphagia) in acute-care stroke patients.* Rockville, MD: ECRI Health Technology Assessment Group.

Finley, R., Clifton, J., Stewart, K., Graham, A., & Worsley, D. (2001). Prediction of aspiration in patients with newly diagnosed untreated advanced head and neck cancer. *Archives of Otolaryngology Head and Neck Surgery, 127,* 975–979.

Flasher, L. V., & Fogle, P. T. (2012). *Counseling skills for speech-language pathologists and audiologists* (2nd ed.). Clifton Park, NY: Delmar Cengage Learning.

Fogle, P. T. (1998). Preparing a feast for the senses. *Advance for Speech-Language Pathologists and Audiologists, 8,* 14–16.

Fogle, P. T., Reece, L., & White, J. (2008). *The source for safety: Cognitive retraining for independent living*. East Moline, IL: LinguiSystems.

Frymark, T., Schooling, T., Mullen, R., Wheeler-Hegland, K., Ashford, J., McCabe, D., Musson, N., & Hammond, C. (2009). Evidence-based systematic review: Oropharyngeal dysphagia behavioral treatments: Part I – Background and methodology. *Journal of Rehabilitation Research & Development, 46*(2), 175–184.

Golper, L. A. (2010). *Medical speech-language pathology: A desk reference* (3rd ed.). Clifton Park, NY: Delmar Cengage Learning.

Hillel, A., Miller, R., Yorkston, K., McDonald, E., Norris, R., & Konikow, N. (1989). Amyotrophic lateral sclerosis severity scale. *Neuroepidemiology, 8,* 142–150.

Hind, J., Nicosia, M., Roecker, E., Carnes, M., & Robbins, J. (2001). Comparison of effortful and non-effortful swallows in healthy middle aged and older adults. *Archives of Physical Medicine and Rehabilitation, 82,* 1661–1665.

Homer, E. M. (2003). An interdisciplinary team approach to providing dysphagia treatment in the schools. *Seminars in Speech and Language, 24,* 215–234.

Huckabee, M. L., & Pelletier, C. A. (2003). *Management of adult neurogenic dysphagia*. Clifton Park, NY: Thomson Delmar Learning.

Johns Hopkins. (2000). Help when it's hard to swallow. *Johns Hopkins Medical Letter, Health After 50, 11*(12), 6–7.

Johnson, A. F., & Jacobson, B. H. (2007). *Medical speech-language pathology: A practitioner's guide* (2nd ed.). New York, NY: Thieme.

Kendall, K. (2008). Anatomy and physiology of deglutition. In R. Leonard & K. Kendall (Eds.). *Dysphagia assessment and treatment: A team approach*. San Diego, CA: Plural Publishing.

Kurjan, R. M. (2000). The role of the school-based speech-language pathologist serving preschool children with dysphagia. *Language, Speech, and Hearing Services in Schools, 31,* 42–49.

Langmore, S. E. (2003). Evaluation of oropharyngeal dysphagia: Which diagnostic tool is superior? *Current Opinions in Otolaryngology Head and Neck Surgery, 11,* 485–489.

Leonard, R., & Kendall, K. (2008). *Dysphagia assessment and treatment: A team approach*. San Diego, CA: Plural Publishing.

Logemann, J. A. (1998). *Evaluation and treatment of swallowing disorders* (2nd ed.). Austin, TX: Pro-Ed.

Logemann, J. A. (2004). Evidence-based practice. *Advances in Speech-Language Pathology, 6*(2), 134–135.

Lubinski, R., Golper, L. A., & Frattali, C. (2007). *Professional issues in speech-language pathology and audiology* (3rd ed.). Clifton Park, NY: Delmar Cengage Learning.

Matta, Z., Chambers, E., Garcia, J., & McGowan-Helverson, J. (2006). Sensory characteristics of beverages prepared with commercial thickeners used for dysphagia diets. *Journal of the American Dietetic Association, 106*(7), 1049–1054.

McAuliffe, M. J. (2006). Current approaches to the assessment and treatment of acquired dysarthria. New Zealand Speech-Language Therapists' Association Biennial Conference, Christchurch, New Zealand.

McAuliffe, M. J., Ward, E. C., & Murdoch, B. E. (2007). Intra-participant variability in Parkinson's disease: An electropalatographic examination of articulation. *Advances in Speech-Language Pathology, 9*(1), 13–19.

McCulloch, T. M., & Jaffe, D. (2006). Head and neck disorders affecting swallowing. *GI Motility*, May, 1–12.

Miller, R. M., & Groher, M. E. (2005). Speech-language pathology and dysphagia: A brief historical perspective. *Dysphagia, 8*(3), 180–184.

Morgan, A. T., Mageandran, S. D., & Mei, C. (2010). Incidence and clinical presentation of dysarthria and dysphagia in the acute setting following pediatric traumatic brain injury. *Child: Care, Health and Development (Special Edition on Traumatic Brain Injury), 36*(1), 44–53.

Morgan, A. T., & Skeat, J. (2010). Evaluating service delivery for speech and swallowing problems following pediatric brain injury: An international survey. *Journal of Evaluation in Clinical Practice, 17*(2), 275–281.

Murry, T., & Carrau, R. L. (2006). *Clinical management of swallowing disorders* (2nd ed.). San Diego, CA: Plural Publishing.

National Dysphagia Diet Task Force. (2002). *National dysphagia diet: Standardization for optimal care.* Washington, DC: American Dietetic Association.

Provencio-Arambula, M., Provencio, D., & Hegde, M. N. (2006). *Treatment of dysphagia in adults: Resources and protocols—a bilingual manual.* San Diego, CA: Plural Publishing.

Ramsey, D. J., Smithard, D. G., & Kalra, L. (2003). Early assessment of dysphagia and aspiration risk in acute stroke patients. *Stroke, 34,* 1252–1257.

Ratner, N. B. (2006). Evidence-based practice: An examination of its ramifications for the practice of speech-language pathology. *Language, Speech, and Hearing Services in Schools, 37,* 257–267.

Rempel, G., & Moussavi, Z. (2005). The effect of viscosity on the breath–swallow pattern of young children with cerebral palsy. *Dysphagia, 20*(2), 108–112.

Rodriquez, L., & Borelli, M. (2003). *Dysphagia screening: A training resource pack.* New York, NY: John Wiley & Sons.

Shoemaker, A. (1997). Religious and cultural issues in dysphagia treatment. *Advance for Speech-Language Pathologists & Audiologists, 10,* 19.

Skelly, M. (1979). *American gestural code based on universal American Indian hand talk.* New York, NY: Elsevier.

Swigert, N. B. (2007). *The source for dysphagia* (3rd ed.). East Moline, IL: LinguiSystems.

Swigert, N. B. (2010). *The source for dysarthria* (2nd ed.). East Moline, IL: LinguiSystems.

Teasell, R., Foley, N., Fisher, J., & Finestone, H. (2002). The incidence management and complications with medullary strokes to a rehabilitation unit. *Dysphagia, 17,* 115–120.

Tonkovich, J. D. (2002). Multicultural issues in the management of neurogenic communication and swallowing disorders. In D. E. Battle (Ed.). *Communication disorders in multicultural populations* (3rd ed.). Boston, MA: Butterworth-Heinemann.

Watt, F., & Whyte, M. N. (2003). The experience of dysphagia and its effect on the quality of life of patients with esophageal cancer. *European Journal of Cancer Care, 12*(2), 183–193.

Weismer, G. (2006). *Motor speech disorders.* San Diego: Plural Publishing.

Wertz, R. T., LaPointe, L. L., & Rosenbek, J. C. (1991). *Apraxia of speech in adults: The disorder and its management.* Clifton Park, NY: Delmar Cengage Learning.

Yorkston, K. M., Beukelman, D. R., Strand, E. A., & Hakel, M. (2010). *Management of motor speech disorders in children and adults* (3rd ed.). Austin, TX: Pro-Ed.

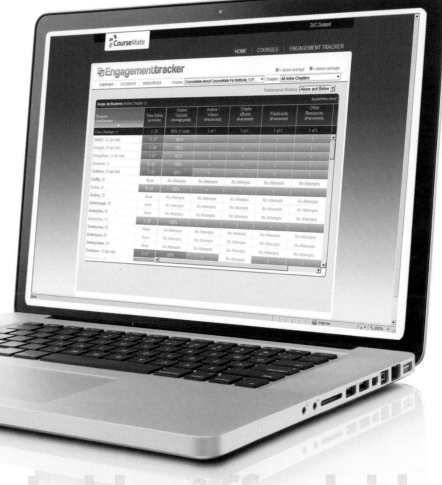
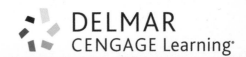

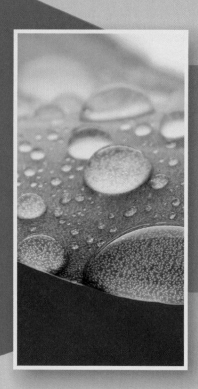

CHAPTER 13

Special Populations with Communication Disorders

LEARNING OBJECTIVES

After studying this chapter, you will:

- Understand the essentials of intellectual disabilities.

- Be familiar with Down syndrome.

- Know the common characteristics of autism and pervasive developmental disorders.

- Be able to discuss attention deficit/hyperactivity disorders (AD/HD, ADD).

- Be familiar with auditory processing disorders (APD).

- Understand the essential information about traumatic brain injury in children.

- Be able to discuss cerebral palsy and its various types.

- Be familiar with augmentative and alternative communication (AAC).

KEY TERMS

adaptive behavior

attention deficit/hyperactivity disorder (AD/HD, ADD)

auditory processing disorder (APD)/central auditory processing disorder (CAPD)

augmentative and alternative communication (AAC) or assistive technology (AT)

autism

autism spectrum disorder (ASD)

bruxing

cerebral palsy (CP)

communication (conversation) board

contracture

developmental disability (DD)

Down syndrome

echolalia

generalization

hypertonicity (hypertonic)

KEY TERMS continued

hypotonicity (hypotonic)

idiosyncratic language

infantile (primitive) reflex

intellectual disability (ID)

intelligence

intelligence quotient (IQ)

mutism

neural plasticity

occupational therapist (OT)

oral reflex

orthopedic

pervasive developmental
disorders (PDD)

physical therapist (PT)

psychophysiological
(psychosomatic) disorder

savant syndrome

seizure (epilepsy, convulsion)

sensory–motor (sensorimotor)
integration

stereotyped movements

CHAPTER OUTLINE

INTRODUCTION

Speech-language pathologists and audiologists may find certain clinical populations particularly interesting and challenging to work with and choose to specialize in assessment and treatment of these populations. To develop expertise in these areas, clinicians need considerable continuing education and training that is offered through ASHA, state, and other organizations. This education and training may include cross-training with other professionals, such as physical and occupational therapists.

Increasingly, SLPs and Auds are working with children who have complex medical problems (sometimes referred to as *medically fragile children*). Clinicians who work in public schools now need knowledge of numerous syndromes and other developmental and medical complications that can contribute to or cause a variety of communication disorders. This chapter provides essential information on special populations of children and adults who have communication and cognitive disorders associated with other disabilities. For some of these individuals, verbal communication is not realistic and augmentative and alternative communication methods are needed.

INTELLECTUAL DISABILITIES

An **intellectual disability (ID)** is a disability characterized by significant limitations in *intellectual functioning* (learning, reasoning, problem solving) and **adaptive behavior** that are apparent before the age of 18. An intellectual disability is under the umbrella term, **developmental disability (DD)** (American Association on Intellectual and Developmental Disabilities, 2010). The term "mental retardation" is generally avoided nowadays when referring to individuals with developmental or intellectual disabilities. For example, what was formerly titled the American Association on Mental Retardation (AAMR) is now the American Association on Intellectual and Developmental Disabilities (AAIDD).

An individual's intellectual functioning is measured by tests of **intelligence** to obtain an **intelligence quotient (IQ)**. Intellectual disability is diagnosed when IQs are below 70 (with 100 being considered the mathematical average). *Mild* intellectual disability is considered as 50 to 70 ($\approx$90% of DD); *moderate* disability falls in the range of 35 to 49 ($\approx$6% of DD); *severe* disability from 20 to 34 ($\approx$3% of DD); and *profound* disability below 20 ($\approx$1% of DD). Children with developmental disabilities are sometimes referred to as *special needs* or *exceptional* children

---

intellectual disability (ID)

A disability characterized by significant limitations in intellectual functioning (learning, reasoning, problem solving) and adaptive behavior that are apparent before the age of 18.

adaptive behavior

The ability to act as independently and responsibly as other people of the same age and cultural background in everyday social and practical skills; includes conceptual skills (e.g., language and money concepts), social skills (e.g., following rules and pragmatics), and practical skills (e.g., dressing appropriately and work skills).

developmental disability (DD)

An umbrella term that relates to some childhood disabilities and includes intellectual disability, physical disabilities (e.g., cerebral palsy or epilepsy), and disabilities that may be both intellectual and physical (e.g., Down syndrome).

(e.g., Special Olympics). According to the World Health Organization (2001), the prevalence of intellectual disability is believed to be between 1%–3% worldwide, with higher rates in developing countries because of the higher incidence of injuries and anoxia around birth and early childhood neurological damage, in part because of poor nutrition. Intellectual disabilities occur about twice as often in males than in females. Numerous syndromes have developmental disabilities as a prominent characteristic, including Down syndrome.

A syndrome is a complex of signs and symptoms resulting from a common etiology. A few examples of syndromes that may significantly affect communication and cognitive development include (1) *Down syndrome* (discussed later); (2) *fetal alcohol syndrome* (FAS) (characterized by prenatal and postnatal growth retardation, facial abnormalities, heart defects, joint and limb abnormalities, and intellectual impairment); and (3) *Asperger's syndrome* (a pervasive developmental disorder with similarities to autistic disorder, characterized by severe impairment of social interactions and by restricted interests and behaviors, although speech, language, and cognitive development may be near normal). Many syndromes, including those mentioned here, also include mild to severe speech, language, and cognitive delays or disorders.

American Association on Intellectual and Developmental Disabilities

The American Association on Intellectual and Developmental Disabilities (AAIDD (formerly known as the American Association on Mental Retardation [AAMR]), was founded in 1876 and is an international multidisciplinary association of professionals. Since 1921, the association has had the responsibility of defining intellectual disability and providing information and support to individuals with developmental disabilities and their families, as well as professionals.

Language Delays and Disorders

Children with intellectual disabilities typically have both receptive and expressive language delays and disorders. They generally understand single words better than sentences because the syntax may be confusing for them. They understand concrete information better than abstract information. They understand speech better when the rate is slightly slower than normal and pauses between sentences are slightly longer than normal. In general, the "rule of fives" is helpful when communicating in sentences with individuals with intellectual delays; that is, use five-letter words (i.e., one- or two-syllable words) in five-word sentences (i.e., simple declarative or interrogative sentences).

Expressive language is usually one of the most impaired areas for children with intellectual disabilities. Individuals with intellectual disabilities commonly have limited vocabularies and some difficulty

intelligence

A global construct involved in the collective capacity to act purposely, think rationally, and deal effectively with the environment.

intelligence quotient (IQ)

An estimate of intellectual status based on an index determined by dividing the *mental age* (MA) in months by the *chronological age* (CA) in months and reducing the result to a percentage; 100 is considered the mathematical average.

recalling words they have used frequently. Their vocabularies tend to be filled with concrete words (things they can see, hear, or touch) and basic verbs to describe the most common actions of nouns. They have limited synonyms for words and difficulty describing characteristics of objects (e.g., size, color, shape, texture, composition), so they tend to repeat a specific word (until they are emphatic) because they cannot provide another word with the same meaning or describe what they are talking about. Depending on their level of intellectual disability, they may communicate in single words, simple sentences, or even complex sentences.

Pragmatics for most individuals with intellectual disabilities are a problem. They often do not initiate conversation, so they have fewer peer interactions than would be normal. When they do initiate conversation, they tend to use *imperative sentences* (sentences that give demands or make requests). They often have difficulty appreciating a listener's "personal space" and may move an uncomfortable distance toward the listener (Adams, Lloyd, Aldred, & Baxendale, 2006; Farmer & Oliver, 2005).

These individuals (both children and adults) may be aware when listeners do not understand them and may attempt conversational repairs by repeating what they have said. However, because of their limited vocabulary, they seldom can go beyond repetition. **Generalization** of language skills taught in therapy is often limited. Children with intellectual disabilities may be able to demonstrate their improved use of language in the clinical setting but may not be able (perhaps not remember) to use these skills in other settings.

Speech

Speech intelligibility problems are common among children and adults with intellectual disabilities because of articulation and phonological disorders. There also may be a motor component such as apraxia or dysarthria. In general, the severity of speech intelligibility depends on the degree of intellectual disability; that is, the more severe the intellectual disability, the more severe the articulation problems. Many children with intellectual disabilities also have hearing losses, which contribute significantly to their speech impairments (Martin & Clark, 2009).

Down Syndrome

Down syndrome is the most common chromosomal cause of developmental (both intellectual and physical) disabilities, with an estimated 1 in every 800 to 1,000 infants born with this condition. A woman's chances of giving birth to a child with Down syndrome increases with age. For a woman 25 years old, the chance is 1 in 1,250; for a 35-year-old woman, it is 1 in 400; and for a 40-year-old woman, it is 1 in 100. Intellectual disability levels are typically in the mild to moderate range. Their speech and language delays may range from mild to severe, with many at the moderate level.

Application Question

If you have had interactions with individuals who have intellectual disabilities, what pragmatic problems have you noticed during the interactions?

generalization

The transfer of learning from one environment (e.g., therapy room or classroom) to a natural environment (e.g., home or community).

Down syndrome

A common chromosome disorder due to an extra chromosome number 21 (trisomy 21) that results in intellectual disability, small head, small ears, flat face with upward slant of the eyes, and abnormal physical development.

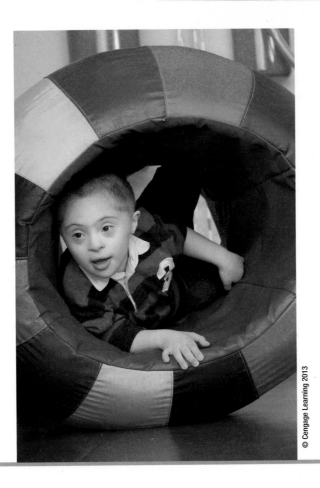

© Cengage Learning 2013

Figure 13-1

Facial features of someone with Down syndrome.

Hearing loss is common, both conductive and sensorineural. Down syndrome has distinctive physical characteristics, including a small head, small ears, flat face, and upward slanting eyes. Many children with Down syndrome are happy, affectionate, and easygoing (see Figure 13–1). Many go to school, learn to read and write, find jobs, and live relatively independent or semi-independent lives (Mayo Clinic, 2009).

Speech and Language

Children with Down syndrome have inconsistent and distorted speech that may be attributed to *hypotonicity* (weakness) and delayed motor development. They usually develop most sounds of other children but at a slower rate. Children with Down syndrome often have *macroglossia* (an abnormally large tongue) that can interfere with articulation because the tongue fills the oral cavity, not allowing normal range of movement and precise articulation points.

Children and adults with Down syndrome have language comprehension roughly equivalent to their mental age. Their vocabulary comprehension is usually better developed than their comprehension of syntax. In general, their comprehension abilities exceed their expressive language and speech abilities. These children often show relatively good language development during infancy and toddlerhood, particularly when involved in early-intervention programs. However, after this age,

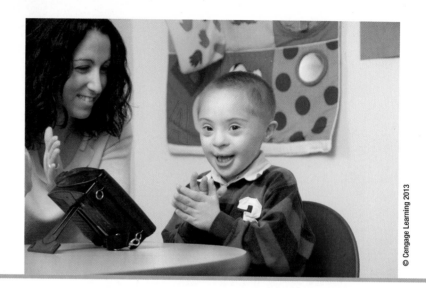

© Cengage Learning 2013

Figure 13-2

Children with Down syndrome are often a joy to work with.

autism (autistic disorder)

A highly variable neurodevelopmental disorder in the broad *autism spectrum disorders* (ASD), which is in the still broader group of *pervasive developmental disorders*. Autism is a lifelong complex behavioral syndrome that appears by 3 years of age, with children having a markedly absent interest in social interactions and relationships; severely impaired communication skills; and repetitive, stereotyped movements; and restricted interests that are often obsessive or fixated.

autism spectrum disorder (ASD)

A range of developmental disorders from mild to severe, with autism being the most severe form.

pervasive developmental disorder (PDD)

Serious multiple developmental impairments typically diagnosed in children before the age of 3 and occurs in males approximately four times as often as in females; autism spectrum disorders are the more severe extreme.

their rate of language learning continues at a slower pace into the early school years (see Figure 13-2). Many children appear to plateau in their language development around 8 years of age or as late as adolescence, with further development primarily in vocabulary.

AUTISM AND PERVASIVE DEVELOPMENTAL DISORDERS

Autism (autistic disorder) falls within the broader diagnostic category of **autism spectrum disorder (ASD)**, which in turn is within the still broader diagnostic category of **pervasive developmental disorder (PDD)** (see Figure 13-3). Autism was first described in the literature in 1943 (Kanner, 1943). Until the 1970s, Kanner and other mental health experts believed that autism was an emotional or psychiatric disorder generally attributed to environmental influences in the child's home, with the parents—unfairly—being held responsible for their child's disorder. Since the 1970s, autism has been viewed as a developmental disorder rather than an emotional disorder (American Psychiatric Association, 2000). It is now considered a developmental disability that has a genetic or unknown origin and is present from birth. The prevalence of autism is about 1–2 per 1,000 people worldwide; however, the Center for Disease Control and Prevention (CDC) reports approximately 9 per 1,000 children (≈1 in 110) in the United States are diagnosed within the autism spectrum disorder. The number of children diagnosed with autism has increased dramatically since the 1980s, partly due to changes in diagnostic practice; however, it is not certain whether the actual prevalence has significantly increased (Newschaffer, Croen, Daniels, et al., 2007; Tonge, 2002).

Autism is described as a complex behavioral syndrome that appears by 3 years of age with children having (1) a markedly absent interest in social interactions and relationships; (2) severely impaired communication skills; and (3) repetitive, **stereotyped movements**, combined with

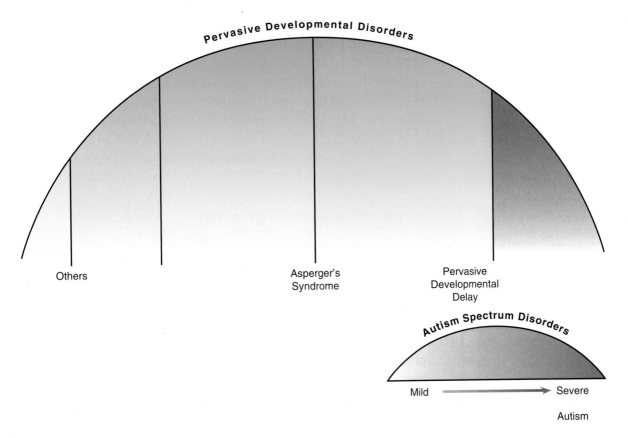

Figure 13-3

Pervasive developmental disorders.

© Cengage Learning 2013.

restricted interests that are often obsessive or fixated. Some individuals demonstrate extraordinary skills, such as memory for numbers or being able to mentally calculate dates (**savant syndrome**) (Heaton & Wallace, 2004). Early symptoms often appear by 18 months of age, such as lethargy, preferring solitude, or being highly irritable (Kupperman, 2006).

Numerous problems associated with autism have been reported, including intellectual deficiencies in approximately three-quarters of all children, with most cases at the moderate level (IQ 35–49). Most individuals have poor physical coordination and seizures occur in approximately one-third of individuals (seizures can deteriorate motor coordination). Individuals who are autistic often have *hyposensitivity* or *hypersensitivity* to certain stimuli; for example, they may be oblivious to heat, cold, or pain but show extreme distress when they are touched unexpectedly. Some show *hyperacusis* (abnormal intolerance for normal environmental sounds), for example, having a catastrophic reaction to a person's whispering but not reacting to very loud noises. They tend to prefer sounds they produce themselves, such as unusual vocalizations or teeth grinding (**bruxing**).

Many individuals have self-stimulating behaviors, for example twisting or twirling objects in front of their face (particularly shiny objects), spinning, rocking, hand flapping, toe walking, sniffing objects,

stereotyped movements

Persistent and inappropriate mechanical repetition of actions, body postures, or speech patterns, often seen in autism.

savant syndrome

The co-occurrence with autism of unexpected or unusual high-level skills with generally limited intelligence (e.g., mathematical calculations, days and dates in history or the future, or remarkable memory for unrelated information).

bruxing

A compulsive, unconscious clenching and grinding of the teeth, especially during sleep or as a mechanism for releasing tension during periods of extreme stress in waking hours.

repetitive feeling of the texture of materials, and attachment to and carrying around unusual objects. Some children have frequent self-injurious behaviors, such as self-biting, scratching, hitting, and head banging. However, of all the unusual and bizarre behaviors of children with autism, the two most common identifying behaviors are a marked lack of awareness of the existence of feelings of others and a persistent preoccupation with parts of objects (Dominick, Davis, Lainhart, Tager-Flushberg, & Folstein, 2007; Johnson & Myers, 2007; Reece & Challenner, 2006; Turner-Brown, Lam, Holtzclaw, Dichter, & Bodfish, 2011).

Speech and Language

The receptive language abilities of children within the ASD and PDD categories are generally similar to their mental age; for example, a 5-year-old child may have a mental age of 2 years. However, the comprehension abilities of any one child in the spectrum at any specific moment are particularly difficult to determine because of inconsistent or absent responses to both test and normal stimuli. That is, a child may understand what was said but not respond accurately or appropriately.

Approximately 50% of children with autism are considered nonverbal, with *selective* or *elective* **mutism** occurring in some cases; however, children who are nonverbal do not necessarily try to compensate with gestures or mime. Children with autism who are verbal are well known for their abnormal verbal behavior (Reed, 2010; Richard, 2008; Tager-Flusberg & Caronna, 2007). Children with PDDs tend to be more verbal than children within the autism spectrum, depending on their severity levels. One of the most striking verbal traits of children who are autistic is **echolalia**—the automatic repeating of words, phrases, or sentences said to them or to someone else. Although these children may repeat what is said, they often do it without normal accompanying facial expressions and gestures.

Although children with autism do not appear to have significant difficulty understanding pronouns, they have particular difficulty using pronouns correctly. They often make errors in gender (*he* for *she, him* for *her*) and singular and plural (*it* for *they* and *them*). They often use *you* to refer to themselves and *I* or *me* to refer to others.

The expressive language of some children with autism may be grammatically adequate but have unusual or bizarre semantics and pragmatics. They often use **idiosyncratic language**; that is, their choice of words and use of words in sentences have unique meanings, which may or may not be interpretable to a listener (e.g., "They're having a meal and then they're finishing and *siding the table*,"—interpreted as "clearing the table," and "He's seriously wounded like *cutes and bloosters*,"—interpreted as "cuts and bruises"). Sometimes they use *neologisms* (e.g., "She's *bawcet*,"—interpreted as "She's bossy") (Volden & Lord, 1991, p. 118).

Impaired pragmatics, social deficits, and inappropriate behaviors are hallmark characteristics of children with autism. The following behavioral characteristics are adapted from the American Psychiatric

mutism

The inability or unwillingness to speak; usually used in reference to voice disorders where an individual may use selective or elective mutism, that is, unconsciously or consciously not be able to use voice or speak.

echolalia

The automatic and involuntary repetition of another person's utterance that is normal for 18–24-month-old children, but which also can occur at later ages (including adulthood) in individuals who are autistic or have neurological damage.

idiosyncratic language

An individual's choice of words and use of words in sentences that have their own unique meaning, which may or may not be interpretable to a listener.

Association's *Diagnostic and Statistical Manual of Mental Disorders, 4th edition, Text Revision* (DSM-IV TR) (2000): nonverbal and verbal behaviors that include inadequate or inappropriate eye gaze, facial expressions, and general body language; general lack of initiating verbal interaction; frequent inappropriate whispering; unusual fluctuations of loudness; limited pitch range resulting in monotonous speech; excessive nasal resonance; voice inflections not in agreement with their meaning; repetition of television commercials verbatim; difficulty pointing to or showing objects to their parents; difficulty or inability to "read" the mood, needs, or intentions of others; and mechanical imitation of other people's actions or voices.

The speech of children in the autism spectrum or who have PDDs is generally intelligible but sounds much like the mental age of the child. There are frequent distortions of consonants in their speech throughout their lives. Overall, it is not their speech intelligibility that makes them difficult to understand but their idiosyncratic language and inappropriate speech inflections and pragmatics that leave listeners confused and bewildered.

ATTENTION DEFICIT DISORDERS

Attention deficit/hyperactivity disorder (AD/HD) was first described in 1845 by Heinrich Hoffman, a German physician who wrote texts in medicine and psychiatry. Hoffman also wrote children's books, with one titled *The Story of Fidgety Philip* that was translated into English and which accurately described a boy with characteristics of AD/HD. However, it was not until Sir George F. Still published a series of lectures that he presented to the Royal College of Physicians in England in 1902 that described a group of impulsive children with significant behavioral problems that AD/HD began to be accepted as a true disorder (Still, 1902). Attention deficit disorders are not new problems.

The DSM-IV TR (2000) is the standard and authoritative source for U.S. practitioners, researchers, and others in the field of mental disorders. The DSM-IV TR provides definitions, criteria, descriptions, and prevalence information for *attention deficit/hyperactivity disorder*. "ADD," as it is often written, is a broad syndrome relating to individuals who demonstrate three primary problems: inattention, impulsivity, and hyperactivity. *Inattention* refers to difficulty either in selecting what to attend to or in keeping attention focused as long as necessary to perform an age-appropriate task. *Impulsivity* means that the individual has difficulty properly controlling or regulating behavior. *Hyperactivity* relates to excesses in physical movement, especially excesses that have a purposeless, poorly directed, or driven quality. Approximately 3%–5% of school-age children in the United States have ADD, and boys are approximately four times more likely to have the problem than girls. Risk factors for ADD include being male, a possible hereditary component, and pregnancy and birth complications. ADD occurs in a heterogeneous population

attention deficit/ hyperactivity disorder (AD/HD, ADD)

A broad syndrome relating to children who demonstrate three primary problems: inattention, impulsivity, and hyperactivity.

of children and adults and from all family economic and educational backgrounds.

The DSM-IV TR states that the following four conditions must be met for a child to be diagnosed with attention deficit/hyperactivity disorder:

- Presence of a minimum number of symptoms (six or more) of inattention, hyperactivity–impulsivity, or both (see the complete symptom list in the DSM-IV TR, 2000)
- Presence of symptoms for 6 months or longer
- Presence of symptoms before 7 years of age
- Impaired functioning in two or more settings caused by ADD symptoms (usually home and school)

Barkley (2006), a professor of psychiatry and neurology, says attention is a global construct that is difficult to define; however, the construct includes:

- Arousal (becoming alert)
- Selective attention (choosing what to attend to)
- Sustained attention (staying focused)
- Short-term (working) memory (seconds to minutes)
- How much information can be attended to or processed at one time

Barkley says that children with ADD are distractible because they become bored with a task much sooner than normal children. Once they become bored, which may take only seconds, they shift their attention to something else.

Frequent Coexisting Disorders with Attention Deficit Disorders

Language disorders and ADD often coexist. The DSM-IV TR criteria for diagnosis of ADD include several behaviors that SLPs would assess as receptive language impairments and pragmatic problems. Children diagnosed by psychologists, psychiatrists, or pediatricians as having ADD would benefit from evaluations by SLPs to determine whether these children also have receptive and/or expressive language disorders and then to receive appropriate therapy (Schonwald & Lechner, 2006; Tetnowski, 2004).

ADD and **auditory processing disorders (APD)** coexist, making it difficult for these children when they are attending to clearly understand what is being said (Bellis, 2002, 2003; Stach, 2010). Learning disabilities also are a common problem for children with ADD and they are often referred to as "academic underachievers." ADD is estimated to co-occur in 20%–50% of children with learning disabilities, depending on how the disorders or disabilities are defined or assessed. Children's learning disabilities extend to reading and writing problems (Byrnes, 2008).

auditory processing disorder (APD)/central auditory processing disorder (CAPD)

A disorder in children and adults who have difficulty using auditory information to communicate and learn; may affect their abilities to listen, understand speech, develop language, and have academic success.

An ADD Support Group   *Personal Story*

My wife, a registered nurse (RN), and I ran a support group for three years for parents of children with ADD, APD, and learning disabilities. We met every other Wednesday evening in a high school classroom. (When I do seminars around the United States on ADD and APD, I tell the speech-language pathologists, audiologists, psychologists, teachers, and parents who attend that I speak from three perspectives: an academic who studies the problems, a therapist who works with children who have these problems, and a parent with a child [now adult] with these problems.) We had many parents who came to the support group almost in panic, saying, "My child was just diagnosed with ADD! What is ADD?" Other parents who had known about their children's problems for years would share (sometimes commiserate) stories about the trials of family life with a child (or two) who has ADD, APD, a learning disability, or a combination of these. We talked about strategies to help our children and ways for parents to cope with the sometimes unusual challenges they present. With enough of the right kinds of support (family, educational, psychological, and if needed, pharmacological), many of these children become productive and often unusually creative adults. ■

Some children with ADD have co-existing anxiety, depression, or both. If the anxiety and depression are treated, the child will be better able to manage the daily challenges that accompany ADD. Additionally, effective treatment of ADD can have a positive effect on anxiety and depression because these children are better able to succeed academically and in their family and social lives (Wilens, Biederman, & Spencer, 2002). Effective treatment often includes a multimodality approach: (1) behavioral intervention, (2) educational intervention, (3) psychological (counseling) intervention, and (4) medical (pharmacological) intervention. Children who have ADD grow up to be adults who have ADD, and the effects on their personal and occupational or professional lives can be incalculable (Wender, 2000).

AUDITORY PROCESSING DISORDERS

The term *auditory processing disorder (APD)* refers to children and adults who have difficulty using auditory information to communicate and learn (Jerger & Musiek, 2000). The auditory processing problems occur during different listening tasks and are made worse in noisy environments. APDs are associated with difficulty listening, understanding speech, developing language, and learning. APDs have been recognized by audiologists and speech-language pathologists for more than 50 years; however, it has only been since the 1990s that APDs have taken a prominent role in the work of many speech-language pathologists (ASHA, 1995; Bellis, 2003; Musiek & Chermak, 2007; Richard, 2004).

Factors Commonly Associated with Auditory Processing Disorders

Several factors are commonly associated with people who are diagnosed with an auditory processing disorder (Bellis, 2003; Geffner & Ross-Swain, 2007; Kelly, 2001; Musiek & Chermak, 2007; Richard, 2001):

- APD occurs in a heterogeneous population of children and adults and from all family economic and educational backgrounds.
- There is a complex of symptoms with no two children having precisely the same problems to the same degree.
- Most children have normal hearing, but there is typically a history of middle ear infections and *upper respiratory infections* (colds, flu, and sinus allergies).
- Children and adults with APD typically have difficulty understanding what is being said when there is background noise, for example, in noisy classrooms and work environments.
- They have difficulty following multipart directions.
- Children are often considered underachievers by teachers and parents.

A history of middle ear infections is the problem most consistently associated with APDs in children (middle ear infections will be discussed in some detail in Chapter 14, Hearing Disorders in Children and Adults). Middle ear infections also are associated with phonological disorders, language disorders, learning disabilities, and reading problems. These problems often require the services of speech-language pathologists and audiologists (Geffner & Ross-Swain, 2007; Hay & Flynn, 2004; Musiek & Chermak, 2007; Richard, 2001).

As mentioned previously, to complicate matters APD and ADD can coexist (Bellis, 2002, 2003; Stach, 2010). Determining which is the primary problem and which is the secondary problem is not easy. Ideally, when a child has problems with auditory processing and attention, both problems are diagnosed and treated. However, because it is often difficult to obtain a clear diagnosis of either APD or ADD, children who have both of these problems are fortunate if they receive a diagnosis of one or the other disorder and get appropriate follow-up treatment (Geffner & Ross-Swain, 2007). Stach (2010) states that it is necessary to have the combined efforts of an audiologist and speech-language pathologist during the diagnosis and treatment of APD.

Auditory Processing and Attention Deficit Disorders Beyond the United States

In 2004, I was invited by two separate organizations to Singapore to speak about auditory processing disorders and attention deficit disorders. The May conference was organized for parents of children who had been diagnosed with either APD or ADD (about 90% of the population in Singapore is Asian, but almost 100% of the people speak English as well as their primary language—Chinese, Malaysian, and others). I was surprised to be speaking to more than 200 Asian parents about problems that I had thought were primarily American.

In August, I returned to present an all-day seminar to the Speech-Language-Hearing Association of Singapore, titled "Evaluation and Treatment of APD/ADD/ADHD: A Cognitive-Linguistic Approach." I learned from the speech-language pathologists and audiologists present that they had received their professional training in various countries, including Australia, England, India, New Zealand, and Poland. The audiologist from India said that she had an entire academic course on auditory processing disorders and that APD is a recognized disorder in that country. The SLPs all stated that in whatever country they were from or wherever they received their training, ADD/ADHD and APD were increasingly being recognized, diagnosed, and treated. ■

Children with APD, ADD, or both may have cascading problems that result in various other difficulties. Either APD or ADD may contribute to language disorders and learning disabilities. Some children with learning disabilities develop emotional reactions, such as anxiety, depression, or both, as a result of their difficulties in school. Some children also may develop **psychophysiological (psychosomatic) disorders**, such as headaches, gastrointestinal problems, or both (Egger, Costello, Erkanli, & Angold, 1999; Santalahti, Aromaa, Sourander, Helenius, & Piha, 2005). As speech-language pathologists and audiologists, we must recognize the often pervasive effects of APD and ADD on the lives of children and their families. When we are helping children increase their auditory processing and attentional abilities, we may also be helping with other areas of their lives. Figure 13–4 is a model of how APD, ADD/ADHD, language disorders, learning disabilities, some psychological disorders, and some psychophysiological disorders may interact.

psychophysiological (psychosomatic) disorder

A disorder with physical signs and symptoms that have a psychological origin, often with common ailments such as tension headaches, gastrointestinal disorders, or both that are attributed to psychological stress.

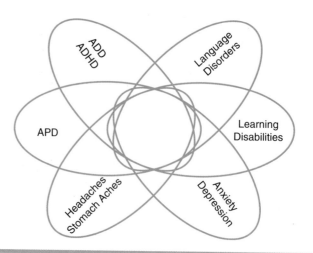

Figure 13-4

APD, ADD/ADHD, language disorders, learning disabilities, psychological disorders, and psychophysiological disorders may interact.

© Cengage Learning 2013.

TRAUMATIC BRAIN INJURY IN CHILDREN

Pediatric traumatic brain injury (TBI) (head trauma) can occur at any age, from newborns through adolescents. Infants may be dropped, may fall, or be abused; children have bicycle accidents, sports injuries, and unbelievable other ways of being injured; adolescents get into altercations and are beaten or shot; and any age may be in motor vehicle accidents (MVAs) (most TBIs in all ages are from MVAs) (Krause, 1995).

Shaken Baby Syndrome

One of the most tragic causes of pediatric TBI is shaken baby syndrome. Shaken baby syndrome is a condition of whiplash-type injury (which often damages the brainstem) caused by violent shaking. Damage ranges from bruises on the arms and trunk where the infant was firmly grasped to retinal hemorrhages in the eyes, seizures, intracranial bleeding from tearing of cerebral blood vessels, coma, and death (Mosby, 2009).

TBIs are particularly tragic because children may be normal one instant and the next instant severely impaired in all ways for the rest of their lives. Children and adolescents are especially susceptible to TBIs because of normal childhood impulsiveness and lack of awareness or concern about *cause and effect* (i.e., "If I do this, this is what could happen").

Speech, Language, Cognitive, and Swallowing Disorders

Depending on the location and severity of brain damage, a variety of speech, language, cognitive, and swallowing problems may be present (Blosser & DePompei, 2003; Lebby & Asbell, 2007; Savage & Callahan, 2003; Ylvisaker, 1998). A child may have apraxia, dysarthria, or both affecting speech intelligibility (see Chapter 5, Articulation and Phonological Disorders in Children). Receptive and expressive language problems

Being an Emergency Medical Technician in Ambulances

During my years of work as an emergency medical technician (EMT) in ambulances in Southern California, I saw countless infants, children, and adolescents who were injured in sometimes unbelievable ways. Many had multiple injuries to their bodies, in addition to their heads (especially in MVAs). In emergency work the goals are to keep the person alive by maintaining an open airway, stop profuse bleeding, splint broken bones, and prevent further injury during transportation to a hospital emergency room. That is not always easy with injured children who are crying and hysterical.

Because of remarkable advances in emergency care, more children are surviving serious traumas, which also means that the work of the rehabilitation team is that much more complex and challenging. The rehab team sees the children who have survived and been "cleaned up." We need to appreciate, however, that somebody had to extricate the children out of crushed automobiles, stop the bleeding, bandage the injuries, splint the broken bones, and transport the children to the next level of care. ■

(see Chapter 6, Language Disorders in Children) are commonly seen in children with traumatic brain damage. Both language and cognitive disorders that result from TBI can result in learning problems and behavioral problems (see Chapter 11, Neurological Disorders in Adults). Dysphagia may be present that causes a child to have difficulty swallowing foods and liquids and may require a feeding tube (see Chapter 12, Motor Speech Disorders and Dysphagia/Swallowing Disorders).

Generally, children with mild TBIs have good recovery, with the brain's **neural plasticity** likely being a significant factor. However, children with moderate to severe brain damage tend to experience long-term speech and language deficits, particularly in word-finding abilities. Children with moderate to severe brain injuries have more diffuse neuronal and axonal damage, which may affect the amount of neural plasticity potential (Chapman, Gamino, Cook, et al., 2009; DePompei, 2010).

The most devastating problems, however, are the cognitive impairments, including attention, memory (immediate or working memory, recent memory, and long-term memory), orientation (to person, place, time, and purpose), reasoning, judgment, and problem solving. The cognitive impairments affect intellectual abilities and academic performance. Children with such impairments are often placed in special education classes or one grade lower than before the head injury (Babikian & Asarnow, 2009; Chapman, 2006; Gamino & Chapman, 2009).

neural plasticity

The brain's ability to reorganize itself throughout life by forming new neural connections. Neural plasticity allows neurons to compensate for injury and disease and to adjust their activities in response to new situations or to changes in their environment.

Behavioral Effects of Traumatic Brain Injury

Beyond the speech, language, and cognitive impairments seen in children with TBIs, various behavioral effects can interfere with rehabilitation, resocialization, and success upon reentry into school. Clinicians need to be aware that there is a natural progression of behavioral changes throughout the recovery period, which may take months to years (Feeney & Ylvisaker, 2008; Lebby & Asbell, 2005; Turkstra, Williams, Tonks, & Frampton, 2008; Yeates & Taylor, 2006; Yen & Wong, 2007).

Children with TBIs often are not aware of the seriousness of their impairments and may try to do things they are not physically or cognitively capable of, which puts them at risk for additional injuries (e.g., riding a bicycle or driving a vehicle). They are often more impulsive and lack awareness of cause and effect than they were before the trauma, again putting themselves at risk for more injuries. (The person most likely to have a head injury is the person who already has had a head injury.) Their pragmatic skills are frequently severely impaired, and they may become verbally abusive to their family, caregivers, and rehabilitation staff. They often have difficulty getting along with even their best friends, which can cause the end of friendships. They eventually may feel isolated and despondent. However, over time, many of the more normal behaviors of these children begin to reemerge. They typically have to develop new friendships, often with children one or two years younger than themselves because they now relate better to those ages (Hawley, Ward, Magnay, & Mychalkwiw, 2004; Turkstra, et al., 2008).

CEREBRAL PALSY

cerebral palsy (CP)

A developmental neuromotor disorder that can occur prenatally, natally, or perinatally and result in a *nonprogressive* (does not worsen over time), permanent motor function disorder; dysarthria affecting all speech systems is the most common speech problems.

Cerebral palsy (CP) is the neuromotor impairment that is the most frequent cause of dysarthria in children. Cerebral palsy is one of the more common disorders caused by central nervous system damage in newborns, with an incidence of about 1 in 500 children in developed (industrialized) countries. However, because of increased survival rates of low-birth-weight infants, there has been an increase in the prevalence of cerebral palsy in these countries since the mid-1970s (Pharoah, Platt, & Cooke, 1996). The incidence of cerebral palsy may be even higher in developing countries than in developed countries because of poor prenatal care and inadequate medical care following cerebral infection (e.g., meningitis) and *febrile convulsions* often caused by malaria in infants, and TBIs in children of all ages (Stanley, Blair, & Alberman, 2000; Winter, Autry, Boyle, & Yeargin-Allsopp, 2002).

Causes of Cerebral Palsy

Cerebral palsy may be caused by damage to the central nervous system at different times in the *prenatal* (before birth), *natal/perinatal* (during birth), or *postnatal* (during childhood) history of the child. Some children

"Something Changed"

Personal Story

A local physician called me to ask if I would work with his 2-year-old son who recently had been diagnosed with severe spastic quadriplegic cerebral palsy. During my first meeting with the mother and father in their home, I interviewed them and asked questions about Samuel's (Sammy's) prenatal, natal, and postnatal history. The mother told me that the pregnancy was going well with no complications and then at 6 months she felt "something changed." She did not know what had changed, and her obstetrician could not detect anything that had gone wrong, but still the mother felt there was something "different" about the baby.

The labor and delivery were normal, and the newborn's birth weight was within normal limits, but his muscle tone was somewhat below normal. He had an Apgar score of 6 (moderate distress) at 1 minute and a score of 7 (borderline distress) at 5 minutes. Sammy's initial growth was normal, but muscle tone was abnormal. Sammy was not officially diagnosed with cerebral palsy until he was almost 2 years old (pediatricians and pediatric neurologists are often "conservative" when making a diagnosis of cerebral palsy). I worked with Sammy for almost 3 years twice a week in his home, typically on the living room floor or with him on his *incline board*, in his *corner chair*, or in his special wheelchair. A team approach was used and I consulted and interacted regularly with both a physical therapist and an occupational therapist. Sammy eventually entered a school for children with **orthopedic** disabilities, where he could receive further physical, occupational, and speech therapy. ■

orthopedic

A branch of health care concerned with the prevention and correction of disorders of the musculoskeletal systems of the body; an *orthopedist* is a physician who specializes in orthopedics.

may have damage that occurs at more than one time in their developmental history. Individuals who sustain damage to the brain (e.g., TBI) in later childhood, before anatomical and physiological maturation of the brain is complete, can have *acquired cerebral palsy*.

Some of the prenatal causes of cerebral palsy include mothers who take illegal drugs before pregnancy, during pregnancy, or both. *Fetal intracranial hemorrhages* (rupture of a blood vessel in the brain, cerebellum, or brainstem during gestation) are fairly common in preterm infants weighing less than 1,500 grams (≈3½ pounds). Infants born with various respiratory problems are also more likely to have intracranial hemorrhages (Wood, Marlow, Costeloe, et al., 2001).

A natal/perinatal cause of cerebral palsy is *fetal distress* (i.e., a compromised condition of the fetus during labor). When the heart is not beating normally, insufficient blood and oxygen reach the brain. Fetal distress may occur during a *breach delivery* (buttocks first) or *precipitous* (very rapid) *delivery*. *Traumatic forceps deliveries* are now rare because *cesarean sections* are performed more often to prevent the need for forceps (Mosby, 2009).

Traumatic brain injuries (falls, MVAs, assaults [e.g., shaken baby syndrome]) are the most common postnatal causes of cerebral palsy. Hypoxic and anoxic conditions such as *near drowning* are also common causes. Another postnatal cause is neurological diseases such as *encephalitis,* which is an inflammatory condition of the brain that can be caused by *lead poisoning* (most often caused by eating flakes of lead paint, as occurs in some children who live in dwellings painted with lead-based paints).

Classifications (Types) of Cerebral Palsy

Cerebral palsy may be classified by the muscle tone of the limbs. Some children with cerebral palsy have too much muscle tone (**hypertonicity**), making voluntary movements difficult, whereas other children have too little muscle tone (**hypotonicity**), making it difficult to maintain posture, balance, and grasp. Children may have a combination of hypertonicity in their limbs and hypotonicity in their trunks, with weak back, chest, and abdominal muscles (weak trunk muscles are associated with impaired respiratory support).

Another classification method relates to the limbs *involved* (affected or impaired). When one side of the body is affected, it is referred to as *hemiplegia;* when only the legs are involved, it is called *paraplegia;* when only one limb is involved, it is *monoplegia* (rare); when three limbs are involved, it is *triplegia* (rare); and when all four limbs are involved, it is *quadriplegia.* The most common classification system includes spastic type, athetoid type, ataxic type, and mixed type.

Spastic Type

Spastic (Gk. *spastikos,* drawing in) *cerebral palsy* (*spasticity*) is the most common form of the disorder (60%–70% of the cerebral palsy population). The most common symptom is increased muscle tone (hypertonicity) of flexor muscles (e.g., biceps), resulting in stiff, inflexible muscles and joints. Individuals have jerky, abrupt, rigid, and slow, labored movements. **Infantile (primitive) reflexes** (brainstem and midbrain level reflexes) are often present long after they should have been "overridden" by higher cortical areas of the brain. Some individuals develop **contractures** as a result of an *agonist* muscle (e.g., bicep of the arm) being in a constant, strong state of contraction that stretches and weakens an *antagonist* muscle (e.g., tricep of the arm).

Usually both sides of the body are involved, but often one side is more involved than the other. The person's arms, legs, and feet are rotated inward. The heels of the feet are pulled up, causing the person to be a "toe walker." One or both arms are raised with the wrists flexed (pulled down). The head may be drawn back and rotated to one side with the neck and back arched posteriorly (*extensor thrust pattern*). The mouth

hypertonicity/hypertonic

Excessive tone or tension in a muscle or muscle group (e.g., bicep or back muscles).

hypotonicity/hypotonic

Weak or absent tone or tension in a muscle or muscle group (e.g., tricep or abdominal and chest muscles).

infantile (primitive) reflex

Inborn behavioral patterns that develop during intrauterine life, are present at birth and are automatic, uncontrolled movements that normally disappear (become "integrated"—inhibited by higher centers in the brain) by about 6 months of age.

contracture

An abnormal, usually permanent condition of a muscle group (e.g., bicep and muscles of the forearm) characterized by flexion and fixation of the limb that may be caused by shortening of muscle fibers; in severe cases, the bone (e.g., humerus [upper arm]) may develop an abnormal curvature.

is usually open because the head is pulled back and the mandibular muscles are weak, resulting in *anterior spillage* of saliva (drooling). The facial muscles look tense and strained.

Athetoid Type

Athetoid (Gk. *athetos,* not fixed) *cerebral palsy* (*athetosis*) occurs in 20%–30% of the cerebral palsy population. It is a neuromuscular condition characterized by slow, writhing, "wormlike," continuous, and involuntary movements of the extremities. The feet and knees are often rotated inward, causing the person to walk on the outer edges of the feet and making balance difficult. The arms are flexed and the fingers are extended back at an awkward angle. The head is drawn back and rotated to one side. The person has to look down and to one side to see forward. An open mouth with drooling and the tongue protruding are common. Athetoid movements are often exaggerated when the person is excited or emotionally upset.

Ataxic Type

Ataxic (Gk. *ataxia,* without order) *cerebral palsy* (*ataxia*) occurs in 5%–10% of the cerebral palsy population. Ataxia is seen as an impaired ability to coordinate movements and maintain balance. The person keeps his legs spread wide in an attempt to maintain balance, resulting in an awkward, abnormal gait. He may push his head forward while his arms are drawn backward in a further effort to maintain balance. His arm and hand movements are clumsy, awkward, and uncoordinated. He often moves his arms and hands in the wrong direction and is continually correcting or overcorrecting his movements. His muscles are generally hypotonic and weak.

Mixed Type

Some children have symptoms of more than one of the common types of cerebral palsy, particularly if there is extensive neurological damage. The most common combination is spasticity and athetosis, with varying degrees of each type. Other combinations are also possible.

Speech, Language, Cognitive and Swallowing Problems

Most children and adults with cerebral palsy have speech impairments, primarily dysarthria. Because all speech systems may be involved simultaneously, the speech of many of these individuals is moderately to severely unintelligible. Sounds that require tongue-tip movements are usually most affected because of the rapid and fine coordinated movements required for speech. In addition, many children with cerebral palsy also have swallowing difficulties because of the weak and poorly coordinated swallowing mechanism.

Personal Story   The Tokyo Taxi

In 1969 I had a military leave to Tokyo, Japan. Among my memories is an incident that occurred on a rainy spring day on a busy city street. I happened to watch a man who had obvious cerebral palsy and was drenched from the rain (he could not hold an umbrella over his head) try to get a taxi. A taxi eventually pulled up to let him in, but when the taxi driver saw the man's abnormal, and to him perhaps bizarre movements, he harshly closed the door on the man and sped away, leaving him standing in the rain experiencing one more indignity and rejection that was probably a part of his daily life. ∎

Children with cerebral palsy typically have receptive and expressive language delays or disorders, or both. Cognitive impairments are also common and they affect all areas of children's lives, including their ability to learn. Parents of children who have cerebral palsy commonly have difficulty getting them dressed and ready to take on outings, which means the children have fewer life experiences to learn language and develop cognition (Pennington & McConachie, 2001). In addition, children and adults may not interact and play normally with children who have cerebral palsy, causing countless missed normal language and social interactions, not just during childhood but throughout life. Most people in communities have had little experience with adults who have cerebral palsy. When people encounter an individual who has awkward or strange movements of the body, unusual facial contortions when trying to talk, and speech that is difficult to understand, a common reaction is confusion and sometimes even fear. The individual with moderate to severe cerebral palsy does not lead a normal life, or at least a life that most other people would want to lead.

Associated Problems

Most children and adults with cerebral palsy have various other problems or impairments, including intellectual disabilities, hearing impairments, visual impairments, and seizure disorders (Reed, 2010; Workinger, 2005). Children with cerebral palsy, therefore, require management of a variety of problems beyond speech. A team approach with a number of different professionals is essential in helping these children maximize their potential. (Historically, children and adults with cerebral palsy often were treated cruelly and even horrendously, being imprisoned and chained because it was felt that their abnormal movements and speech indicated they were possessed by demons.)

Intellectual Disabilities

Intellectual disabilities occur in approximately 75% of individuals with cerebral palsy. However, about 25% of individuals with cerebral palsy have normal or even superior intellectual abilities (Surveillance of Cerebral Palsy in Europe, 2002). It is difficult to measure the intellectual functioning of most children with cerebral palsy because their impaired speech intelligibility interferes with examiners' (usually psychologists) accurate understanding of responses. Likewise, their arm and hand co-ordination impairments affect their ability to demonstrate intellectual capacities on the performance portions of IQ tests.

Seizure Disorders

Seizure (epilepsy, convulsion) disorders occur in almost 45% of individuals with cerebral palsy (Workinger, 2005). A seizure may be *tonic* (a temporary state of constant involuntary muscle contraction) or *clonic* (rapid, alternating involuntary contraction and relaxation of muscles); *unilateral* (one side) or *bilateral* (both sides); and *focal* (localized or limited to one area or region of the body), or *generalized* (all or most of the body involved). Antiseizure medications are used to prevent seizures. It is important for clinicians to be aware of a client's history of seizures because a seizure may occur during an evaluation or therapy. Clinicians need to learn (usually in a first aid course) how to recognize and assist an individual having a seizure.

Evaluation and Treatment of Cerebral Palsy

Cerebral palsy is a complex neuromuscular disorder that requires a team of professionals specialized in the evaluation and treatment. Evaluations by **physical therapists (PTs), occupational therapists (OTs)**, and speech-language pathologists are extensive and ongoing. Evaluations by PTs and OTs include the central nervous system's primitive reflexes that are normal in infants up to approximately six months of age, and beyond that are considered abnormal. SLPs assess the **oral reflexes** such as the *rooting reflex* (triggered when an infant's cheek is touched or stroked, causing the infant to turn his head and open his mouth for nursing) and *sucking* and *swallowing reflexes*. Because abnormal primitive reflexes throughout the body may affect speech development, the information gained by the physical and occupational therapists' evaluations is crucial to the SLP; likewise, the SLP's information is important to the physical and occupational therapists.

The physical therapist is usually the lead member of the treatment team. The PT can provide important information about the best postures and positions for the child to be in during various therapy tasks. *Neurodevelopmental therapy* (NDT) is a commonly used approach for treatment of cerebral palsy (originally known as the Bobath method, named after Karl and Berta Bobath, a physician and a physical therapist in England who pioneered the method [Bobath & Bobath, 1952, 1967]). Neurodevelopmental therapy emphasizes the inhibition or integration of primitive postural patterns and promotes the development of normal

seizure (epilepsy, convulsion)

A hyperexcitation of neurons in the brain that causes a sudden, sometimes violent, involuntary series of contractions of groups of muscles.

physical therapist (PT)

A rehabilitation specialist who is licensed to evaluate and treat developmental and physical impairments through the use of special exercises or other modalities to assist individuals to maximize independence and mobility, self-care, and functional skills necessary for daily living.

occupational therapist (OT)

A rehabilitation specialist who is licensed to evaluate and treat developmental, physical, and cognitive impairments that interfere with functional independence for daily living and work skills by facilitating the development of **sensory–motor (sensorimotor) integration**, perceptual functioning, and neuromuscular functioning.

oral reflex

Infantile primitive reflexes that are present at birth or soon after that are specifically designed to assist the infant in finding and obtaining oral nutrition; for example, the *rooting reflex*, *sucking reflex*, and *swallowing reflex*.

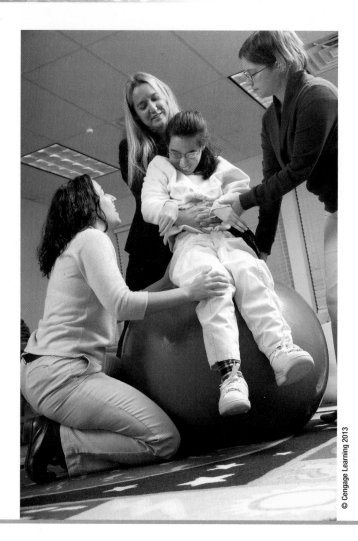

© Cengage Learning 2013

Figure 13-5

Children with cerebral palsy need to be correctly positioned during therapy.

sensory–motor (sensorimotor) integration

The ability to take information (*stimuli*) in through the senses of vision, hearing, touch, taste, and smell, and to combine the information with previously stored memories to develop a coherent concept or appropriate motor response.

postural reactions and achievement of normal muscle tone. Speech therapy initially focuses on *prespeech* abilities—that is, helping the child develop the ability to control and "override" primitive oral reflexes that are interfering with functional articulator movements for speech development (see Figure 13-5).

Many children and adults who cannot develop functional oral communication are able to use various augmentative and assistive devices to communicate. Despite their sometimes severe difficulty with communication and their substantial movement disorders, most children and adults with cerebral palsy appear to be generally happy individuals who are perhaps surprisingly accepting of their physical limitations (although, no doubt, they have many times of frustration and aggravation). My experience with every child and adult with cerebral palsy whom I have worked with clinically or gotten to know personally has consistently shown me that people with even severe challenging physical and communication handicaps can have joyful personalities and be magnanimous in the face of adversity. They are an inspiration to those of us who sometimes complain about the challenges in our own lives.

AUGMENTATIVE AND ALTERNATIVE COMMUNICATION (AAC)

Augmentative and alternative communication (AAC), also known as **assistive technology (AT)**, is any approach designed to support, enhance, or supplement the communication of individuals who are not independent verbal communicators in all situations. AAC is described in a document produced by the Augmentative and Alternative Communication (AAC) Special Interest Division 12 of ASHA (2005, p. 1) as follows:

> AAC refers to an area of research, clinical, and educational practice. AAC involves attempts to study and when necessary compensate for temporary or permanent impairments, activity limitations, and participation restrictions of persons with severe disorders of speech-language production and/or comprehension, including spoken and written modes of communication.

AAC is a multidisciplinary field in which individuals who use devices and their families, along with computer programmers, educators, engineers, linguists, occupational therapists, physical therapists, speech-language pathologists, and many other professionals, contribute to the knowledge and practice base (Beukelman & Mirenda, 2005; Schlosser, Wendt, Angermeier, & Shetty, 2005). AAC technology is developed and used internationally and there are members of the International Society for Augmentative and Alternative Communication (ISAAC) from more than 50 countries (Forbat, 2003).

AAC systems involve nonelectronic and electronic systems, and there are many advances in technology and new products every year. Children and adults who use AAC systems are sometimes referred to as individuals with *complex communication needs*. The AAC website hosted and updated regularly by the Barkley AAC Center at the University of Nebraska-Lincoln (http://aac.unl.edu) provides links to the websites of manufacturers and publishers in the AAC field.

The field of AAC incorporates three general areas of information: (1) *people* with disabilities who may benefit from AAC; (2) *processes,* such as messages, symbols, alternative access, assessment, and intervention; and (3) *procedures* developed to serve individuals with developmental disabilities who require AAC systems (Beukelman & Mirenda, 2005; Cook, 2011). We begin our discussion of the people, both young and old, who may use and benefit from augmentative and alternative communication.

augmentative and alternative communication (AAC) or assistive technology (AT)

Any approach designed to support, enhance, or supplement the communication of individuals who are not independent verbal communicators in all situations.

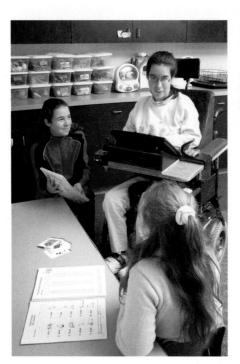
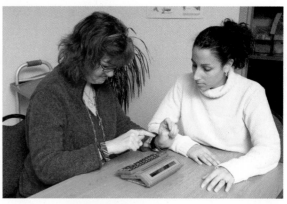
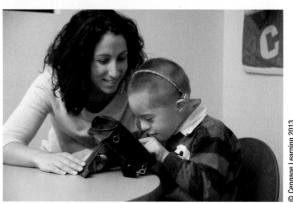

© Cengage Learning 2013

Figure 13–6

Individuals with a variety of developmental disabilities may benefit from AAC.

Children and Adults with Developmental and Motor Disabilities

Children and adults with a variety of severe physical and communication impairments may benefit from AAC, and some begin using assistive devices fairly early in life (see Figure 13–6). Children and adults with cerebral palsy are often the people who come to mind when thinking about who might benefit from AAC; however, individuals with severe apraxia of speech, intellectual disabilities, autism, and pervasive developmental disorders also may benefit (Harris, 2004; Johnston, Reichle, & Evans, 2004; Light & Drager, 2007; Sadao & Robinson, 2010; Wishart, 2010).

For children and adults to receive maximum benefits from sophisticated AAC systems, some level of literacy is essential. At a communication level, literacy skills improve the ability to participate in face-to-face interactions and allow individuals a means of self-expression and a way to develop personal independence. In addition, literacy skills provide access to educational and vocational opportunities, which can be limited due to the physical and communication impairments of these children and adults (Kent-Walsh & Rosa-Lugo, 2006; Sturm & Clendon, 2004). AAC can be mutually beneficial and mutually supportive for both communication and literacy development. That is, when individuals are able to use AAC to communicate, it can facilitate interactions with

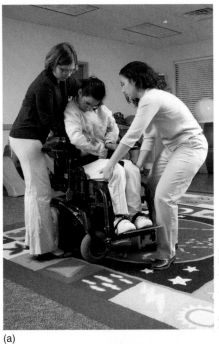

(a)

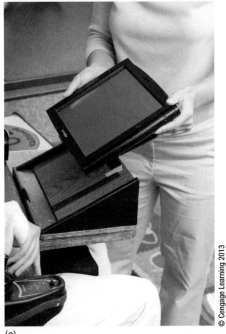

(c)

© Cengage Learning 2013

© Cengage Learning 2013

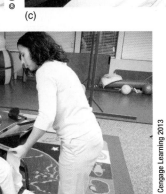

(b)

© Cengage Learning 2013

Figure 13-7

A team approach is necessary when fitting individuals with cerebral palsy with an AAC device: (a) A physical therapist and speech-language pathologist may work together to position a client in her wheelchair; (b) the speech-language pathologist places the tray that holds an AAC device; and (c) the speech-language pathologist then places the AAC device for the client to use.

parents and other caregivers, teachers, and others who are trying to help develop literacy skills. Likewise, developing literacy skills may allow children and adults to use more sophisticated AAC systems for better communication and may open the world of the Internet to them for educational growth, interpersonal communication, and entertainment (Poulson & Nicolle, 2004).

Children and adults with cerebral palsy have difficulty exploring the world on their own because of their motor dysfunctions. Because of their limited physical independence and speech impairments, they often are isolated from social environments. To become competent communicators, individuals with severe cerebral palsy need to acquire expressive symbolic and linguistic skills in communication modes within their own physical and cognitive limitations (Millar, Light, & Schlosser, 2006; Sutherland, Gillon, & Yoder, 2005) (see Figure 13–7).

Beukelman and Mirenda (2005) emphasize the need for a "balanced approach" to communication programs for people with severe expressive communication disorders. This means that emphasis on AAC

CASE STUDY

James

Samuel was a 37-year-old man who was living alone in the family home after his mother had died. An SLP in private practice was called by his aunt to help him obtain an assistive device. Samuel had already been assessed by a specialist in AAC, so the device had already been chosen for him; however, the specialist lived some distance from Samuel and could not continue working with him. Samuel had completed high school and had some community college education (cognitive functioning was not a problem). His communication impairment was severe dysarthria, plus he had ambulatory and moderate-to-severe general motor incoordination. He had an expensive powered wheelchair that he used when he left his home and went into the community.

The major challenge to acquiring the appropriate assistive communication device was the expense and the approval through various agencies for the payment of the device. It took months of reports, paperwork, and red tape to obtain the assistive device and the apparatus that allowed a connection to the client's wheelchair so that he could communicate with people when he was out in the community. Samuel was genuinely excited when the device and wheelchair attachments were all in place and working, and he was in his wheelchair ready to make his first excursion into the community on his own. It was a proud day, indeed. (Although the SLP had spent many hours involved with this client, he felt that it was appropriate to do the work pro bono [time and expertise donated]). ∎

needs should be balanced with motor development training, speech therapy, and academic instruction to maximize each person's overall potential. AAC systems may provide individuals an immediate ability to communicate their basic wants, needs, thoughts, and feelings; however, a systematic speech therapy program to train more complex skills may lay a firm foundation for developing more complex and balanced communication (Reichert Hoge & Newsome, 2002; Millar et al., 2006; Sadao & Robinson, 2010; Treviranus & Roberts, 2003).

Adults with Acquired Communication Disorders

Adults with acquired communication impairments (e.g., severe aphasia, apraxia, or dysarthria) from CVAs, TBIs, and other neurological disorders who are not able to develop functional speech and language can benefit from AAC. Other adults can benefit who have progressively deteriorating central and peripheral nervous system diseases, such as Parkinson's disease, amyotrophic lateral sclerosis (ALS),

Application Question

Have you ever tried to communicate with an adult who could not understand or speak effectively and did not have an AAC device? What did you do to try to make the person's communication easier?

Dorothy

Dorothy was a woman in her late 60s who had developed Parkinson's disease and had increasingly severe dysarthria. I was called by a daughter-in-law, Sharon, and asked to be her speech-language pathologist. I saw Dorothy twice a week in her home for many months. Initially, her speech was moderately dysarthric and I was able to help her maximize her intelligibility. However, the Parkinson's disease was stronger than her determination and therapy combined, and she began to deteriorate further. Emphasis in speech intelligibility changed from short phrases to two words and finally to single-word intelligible speech. Before she could no longer utter single words intelligibly, I helped her acquire an assistive device that allowed her to type, albeit slowly, messages that others could read; synthesized speech could also be heard. Eventually there was nothing more that I could do for Dorothy and I had to end therapy with her.

I did not hear from the daughter-in-law for several months. Then one day I received a telephone call from Sharon, letting me know that Dorothy had died. Sharon then asked if I would do the eulogy at Dorothy's funeral. I was humbled and honored to be asked to perform this important task at the funeral of such a prominent woman in the community. I agreed, and a few days later I was doing the eulogy at a funeral home chapel filled to standing room only, with people outside seated and listening to the service through a loudspeaker. However, not only was I to do the eulogy, I was told just before the service began that I would be "officiating" the service (i.e., introducing the singers and speakers, and leading all parts of the service). After the service was finished and all had gone well, I thought my job was over. Then the funeral home director told me that I would be conducting the graveside service as well—and that is what I did. Although I could have refused all that was asked of me, I felt it was important to accept the unusual requests and to step out of the role of a speech-language pathologist and into the role of a friend who the family felt they could rely on to perform a difficult task with dignity and equanimity. Sometimes a client comes back into our lives in unexpected ways and we have the choice to be of additional service. ■

multiple sclerosis, Guillain-Barré syndrome, or dementia (Armstrong, Jans, & MacDonald, 2000; Ball, 2003; Ho, Weiss, Garrett, & Lloyd, 2005; Purdy & Dietz, 2010). The AAC systems can be designed to accommodate each person's physical limitations. For these individuals, AAC can help them participate more fully in important life activities.

AAC SYSTEMS

Numerous areas need to be considered in an AAC assessment, including the person's positioning and seating, neuromotor impairments, motor capabilities, sensory and perceptual abilities (vision and hearing), communication abilities, cognitive abilities, functional symbols that can be used, and literacy skills. From the evaluation and understanding of the person—and some trial-and-error—the best AAC system can be developed (Reichert Hoge & Newsome, 2002).

Communication Boards

Communication (conversation) boards are the most widely used type of AAC system that are functional for many users in a variety of settings. They may be an apparatus, electronic device, or simple board upon which common communication symbols and messages are represented. They may be no-tech, low-tech, or sophisticated (and expensive) high-tech electronic devices. Basic communication boards typically have the alphabet, numbers 1–10, and a few key words and phrases a person can point to in order to communicate basic messages (see Figure 13–8). Some individuals use communication boards to "supplement" their speech. When a listener has not understood a verbal message, the individual can point to letters, numbers, words, or phrases to help the listener.

Because all communication involves symbols (spoken words are just arbitrary symbols [sounds] that represent whatever we say they represent), individuals employing AAC simply use a system of symbols different from that used by other people to communicate their messages. Representational symbols are some of the most common forms of communication used with AAC.

Photographs and Simple Illustrations

Simple black and white or color photographs or illustrations are excellent for representations of people, objects, and actions. Photographs for

communication (conversation) board

An apparatus or simple board upon which common communication symbols and messages (e.g., alphabet, numbers, pictures, symbols, and common words and expressions) are represented, allowing expressive communication by pointing or gazing; communication boards may be no-tech, low-tech, or sophisticated high-tech electronic devices.

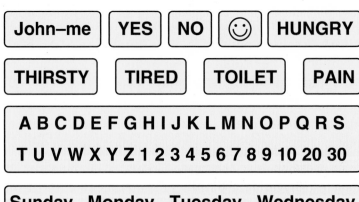

Figure 13–8

A simple, "no-tech" communication board.

© Cengage Learning 2013.

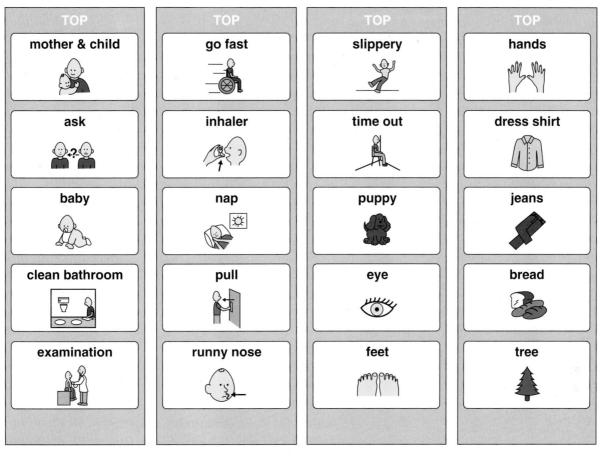

Figure 13-9

Examples of Picture Communication Symbols © (PCS) using Boardmaker™ software.

Source: The Picture Communication Symbols © 1981–2006 by Mayer-Johnson LLC. All rights reserved worldwide. Used with permission.

communication boards may be taken of people, objects, or locations in the client's environment or cut out of magazines, catalogs, advertisements, and so on. Users of AAC need to have sufficient visual acuity and visual perceptual abilities to recognize who or what is being shown in the photographs. No-tech communication boards can easily be made by clinicians by simply cutting out pictures, pasting or taping them to a piece of heavy stock paper or cardboard, and covering the board with a plastic protector.

Application Question

If you needed to use a simple communication board for a while, what would you like included on it?

Picture Communication Symbols

The Picture Communication Symbols© (PCS) developed by Johnson (1994) has more than 7,000 clear, simple black-and-white or color line drawings (including more than 500 verbs) that are available as Boardmaker™ software through Mayer-Johnson for both Windows and Macintosh (see Figure 13-9). The words displayed above the drawings are available in 24 languages and several that use non-Roman alphabets (e.g., Hebrew, Japanese, and Hmong).

Rebus Symbols

Rebus symbols are simple line drawings similar to the PCS. Rebus symbols were originally designed by Woodcock, Clark, and Davies (1968) to help nonhandicapped children read, but they were later developed in England for individuals with communication impairments (Van Oosterum & Devereux, 1985).

Applications for Smartphones and Pads

As smartphones and tablet computers (pads) become more common in the wireless market, so do applications for individuals with AAC needs (e.g., *Communicating Basic Needs App* for the iPod Touch, iPhone, and iPad). The proliferation of downloadable applications for smartphones has created opportunities for people with physical and cognitive limitations, including enhanced accessibility of mobile devices and expanded ability to engage in daily activities through the use of smartphones (Hallett, 2011; Steele & Woronoff, 2011). There is strong appeal for such applications because they would be relatively inexpensive downloadable "apps" when compared to dedicated AAC devices on the market.

Selection Techniques

The term *selection techniques* refers to the way a person who uses an AAC system selects or identifies items from the pictures, symbols, and words on a communication board. There are two basic selection methods, direct and scanning. Depending on the physical abilities of an individual, one or both methods may be used. For example, Figure 13–10 shows the Talara-32 system that is manufactured by Zygo Industries. This digital recording AAC device is designed for easy use and can be customized for both children and adults with wide ranging abilities and needs. The user can scan the numerous figures in the various overlays using the scanning mode that is best suited to the individual.

Most people using AAC systems use finger pointing or touch to indicate messages. More sophisticated and somewhat more challenging methods are headsticks and light pointers, including safe laser head pointers. Some people who do not have the motor control to point to

Figure 13-10

The Talara-32 AAC device.

Source: Courtesy of ZYGO-USA.

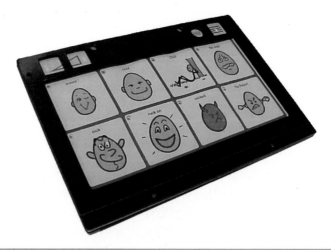

Steven

Steven is a typical 16-year-old adolescent who likes football, watching television, and talking to girls. He attends regular high school in Houston, Texas. Other than having severe spastic quadriplegic cerebral palsy, being in a powered wheelchair, and using an AAC device to communicate, Steven is normal. The AAC device doubles as his mode of vocal and written communication and a computer on which he can do his homework. He powers both the device and the head pointer system from his wheelchair battery. Steven makes maximum use of his AAC device and powered wheelchair to enjoy school and numerous activities. He socializes and feels most students in his school are his friends. He is planning to attend college and earn a degree in computer programming, hoping to help develop even more sophisticated AAC devices for other people. ■

individual symbols may use scanning devices. With a scanner, the person activates the electronic board and then when the desired symbol is highlighted indicates in some way that the symbol has been selected. This can be a slow, laborious process but still the most efficient method of communicating for some people (Bedrosian, Hoag, & McCoy, 2003).

CHAPTER SUMMARY

A intellectual disability is a disability that originates before 18 years of age and is characterized by significant limitations in intellectual functioning and adaptive behavior, and is under the umbrella term of developmental disability. Most children with intellectual disabilities have significant problems with speech and language, and essentially all have impairments of cognition. Down syndrome and autism are two of the best-known developmental disabilities. ADD/ADHD is a broad syndrome relating to children who demonstrate three primary problems: inattention, impulsivity, and hyperactivity. APD is a disorder in some children and adults who have difficulty using auditory information to communicate and learn that affects their abilities to listen, understand speech, develop language, and have academic success. Pediatric TBI can occur at any age, from newborns through adolescents. Depending on the location and severity of brain damage, a variety of speech, language, and cognitive problems may be present. Cerebral palsy is a developmental neuromotor disorder that can occur prenatally, natally, or perinatally and results in a nonprogressive, permanent motor function disorder. Cerebral palsy is the neuromotor impairment that is the most common cause of dysarthria in children.

Augmentative and alternative communication (AAC) systems involve nonelectronic and electronic systems that may be no-tech, low-tech, or high-tech devices. The field of AAC incorporates three general areas of information: (1) people, (2) processes, and (3) procedures. Children with a variety of severe physical and communication impairments may benefit from AAC, and some children begin using assistive devices fairly early in life. Adults who have congenital or acquired communication disabilities also benefit from AAC.

STUDY QUESTIONS

Knowledge and Comprehension

1. Define autism.

2. Describe the three primary problems that children with ADD demonstrate?

3. What are four factors that are often associated with auditory processing disorders?

4. Describe the behavioral effects of traumatic brain injury in children.

5. Discuss two problems that are associated with cerebral palsy.

Application

1. Why might it be valuable for speech-language pathologists working in various settings (e.g., schools, clinics, hospitals) to have a copy of the American Psychiatric Association's *Diagnostic and Statistical Manual of Mental Disorders, 4th edition, Text Revision* (DSM-IV TR)?

2. What are some of the behaviors you would look for that could indicate a child might be in the autism spectrum?

3. Discuss three examples of syndromes that may significantly affect communication and cognitive development.

4. How could speech, language, and/or cognitive problems caused by a TBI affect a child's learning?

5. Discuss the concept that people who use augmentative and alternative communication (AAC) systems need a "balanced approach" to communication.

Analysis/Synthesis

1. How can you apply information from the chapter on Language Disorders in Children to children with Down syndrome?

2. What could be the effects of an auditory processing disorder and an attention deficit disorder occurring in the same child?

3. How could you apply your knowledge about neurological disorders in adults (aphasia, traumatic brain injury, and cognitive disorders) to help you diagnose and treat children with traumatic brain injuries?

4. How can you apply information from the chapter on Motor Speech Disorders and Dysphagia/Swallowing Disorders to children who have cerebral palsy?

5. Why is some level of literacy essential for children to receive maximum benefits from sophisticated augmentative or alternative communication (AAC) systems?

REFERENCES

Adams, C., Lloyd, J., Aldred, C., & Baxendale, J. (2006). Exploring the effects of communication intervention for developmental pragmatic language impairments: A signal-generation study. *International Journal of Language and Communication Disorders, 41*(1), 41–65.

American Association on Intellectual and Developmental Disabilities. (2010). *Intellectual disability: Definition, classification, and systems of support* (11th ed.) Washington, DC: AAIDD.

American Psychiatric Association. (2000). *Diagnostic and statistical manual of mental disorders* (DSM-IV-TR) (4th ed., text rev. ed.). Washington, DC: APA.

American Speech-Language-Hearing Association. (1995). *Central auditory processing: Current status of research and implications for clinical practice. A report from the ASHA task force on central auditory processing.* Rockville, MD: ASHA.

American Speech-Language-Hearing Association. (2005). Roles and responsibilities of speech-language pathologists with respect to augmentative and alternative communication: Position statement. *ASHA* (Supplement 25).

Armstrong, L., Jans, D., & MacDonald, A. (2000). Parkinson's disease and aided AAC: Some evidence from practice. *International Journal of Language and Communication Disorders, 35*(3), 377–389.

Babikian, T., & Asarnow, R. (2009). Neurocogitive outcomes and recovery after pediatric TBI: Meta analysis of the literature. *Neuropsychology, 23*(3), 283–296.

Ball, H. (2003). AAC transitions for persons with ALS: A "classic" example. *ASHA Leader, 13,* 207.

Barkley, R. A. (2006). *ADHD: What do we know?* New York, NY: SR Publications.

Bellis, T. J. (2002). *When the brain can't hear: Unraveling the mystery of auditory processing disorder.* New York, NY: Atrira Books.

Bellis, T. J. (2003). *Assessment and management of central auditory processing disorders in the educational setting: From science to practice* (2nd ed.). Clifton Park, NY: Delmar Cengage Learning.

Beukelman, D. R., & Mirenda, P. (2005). *Augmentative and alternative communication: Supporting children and adults with complex communication needs* (3rd ed.). London, England: Paul H. Brookes.

Blosser, J. L., & DePompei, R. (2003). *Pediatric traumatic brain injury* (2nd ed.). Clifton Park, NY: Delmar Cengage Learning.

Bobath, K., & Bobath, B. (1952). The neuro-developmental treatment of spastic children. *British Journal of Physical Medicine, 5,* 87–94.

Bobath, K., & Bobath, B. (1967). The neuro-developmental treatment of cerebral palsy. *Journal of the American Physical Therapy Association, 47,* 1039–1041.

Byrnes, J. P. (2008). *Cognitive development and learning in instructional contexts* (3rd ed.). Boston, MA: Allyn and Bacon.

Chapman, S. B. (2006). Neurocognitive stall: A paradox in long term recovery from pediatric brain injury. *Brain Injury Professional, 3*(4), 10–13.

Chapman, S. B., Gamino, J. F., Cook, L. G., Hanten, G., Li, X., & Levin, H. S. (2009). Impaired discourse gist and working memory in children after brain injury. *Brain and Language, 97*, 178–188.

Cook, A. M. (2011). It's not about the technology, or is it? Realizing AAC through hard and soft technologies. *Perspectives on Augmentative and Alternative* Communication, *20*(2), 64–68.

DePompei, R. (2010, November). Pediatric traumatic brain injury: Where do we go from here? *The ASHA Leader.*

Dominick, K. C., Davis, N., Lainhart, J., Tager-Flushberg, H., & Folstein, S. (2007). Atypical behaviors in children with autism and children with a history of language impairment. *Journal of Developmental Disabilities, 28*(2), 145–162.

Egger, H., Costello, E., Erkanli, A., & Angold, A. (1999). Somatic complaints and psychopathology in children and adolescents: Stomach aches, musculoskeletal pains, and headaches. *Journal of the Academy of Child and Adolescent Psychiatry, 38*(7), 852–860.

Farmer, M., & Oliver, A. (2005). Assessment of pragmatic difficulties and socioemotional adjustment in practice. *International Journal of Language and Communication Disorders, 40*(4), 403–429.

Feeney, T. J., & Ylvisaker, M. (2008). Context sensitive cognitive-behavioral supports for young children with TBI: A second replication study. *Journal of Positive Behavioral Interventions, 10*(2), 115–128.

Forbat, L. (2003). Communicating without speech: Practical augmentative and alternative communication. *British Journal of Learning Disabilities, 31*(3), 140–144.

Gamino, J. F., & Chapman, S. B. (2009). Strategic learning in youth with traumatic brain injuy: Evidence for stall in higher-order cognition. *Topics in Language Disorders, 24*(3), 1–12.

Geffner, D., & Ross-Swain, D. (2007). *Auditory processing disorders: Assessment, management and treatment.* San Diego, CA: Plural Publishing.

Hallett, T. (2011, November). *IPods, IPads, & IPhones: Applications for teachers, supervisors, & researchers.* Paper presented at the American Speech-Language-Hearing Association convention, San Diego, CA.

Harris, M. D. (2004). Impact of aided language stimulation of symbol comprehension and production in children with cognitive disabilities. *American Journal of Speech-Language Pathology, 13*, 155–167.

Hawley, C., Ward, A. B., Magnay, A., & Mychalkwiw, W. (2004). Return to school after brain injury. *Archives of Disease in Childhood, 89*, 136–142.

Hay, E., & Flynn, M. (2004). Pediatric auditory processing disorder and its implications for speech-language therapists. *New Zealand Journal of Speech-Language Therapy, 59*, 35–39.

Heaton, P., & Wallace, G. L. (2004). The savant syndrome. *The Journal of Child Psychology and Psychiatry, 45*, 899–911.

Ho, K., Weiss, S., Garrett, K., & Lloyd, L. (2005). Effect of remnant and pictographic books on the communicative interaction of individuals with global aphasia. *Augmentative and Alternative Communication, 21*(3), 218–232.

Jerger, S., & Musiek, F. (2000). Report on the consensus conference on the diagnosis of auditory processing disorders in school-aged children. *Journal of the Academy of Audiology, 11*(9), 467–474.

Johnson, C. P., & Myers, S. M. (2007). Identification and evaluation of children with autism spectrum disorders. *Pediatrics, 12*0(5), 1183–1215.

Johnson, R. (1994). *The Picture Communication Symbols combination book.* Solana Beach, CA: Mayer-Johnson.

Johnston, S. S., Reichle, J., & Evans, J. (2004). Supporting augmentative and alternative communication use by beginning communicators with severe disabilities. *American Journal of Speech-Language Pathology, 13*(20), 1044–1058.

Kanner, L. (1943). Autistic disturbances of affective contact. *Nervous Child, 2*, 217–250.

Kelly, D. (2001). *Central auditory processing disorders: Identification and intervention.* Gaylord, MI: Northern Speech Services/National Rehabilitation Services.

Kent-Walsh, J., & Rosa-Lugo, L. (2006). Communication partner interventions for children who use AAC: Storybook reading across culture and language. *ASHA Leader, 11*(3), 6–7, 28–29.

Krause, J. F. (1995). Epidemiological features of brain injury in children: Occurrence, children at risk, causes and manner of injury, severity and outcomes. In S. Broman & M. Michel (Eds.), *Traumatic head injury in children.* New York, NY: Oxford University Press.

Kupperman, P. (2008). *The source for intervention in autism spectrum disorders.* East Moline, IL: LinguiSystems.

Lebby, P. C., & Asbell, S. J. (2005). *The source for traumatic brain injury: Children and adolescents.* East Moline, IL: LinguiSystems.

Light, J., & Drager, K. (2007). AAC technologies for young children with complex communication needs: State of the science and future research directions. *Augmentative and Alternative Communication, 23*(3), 204–216.

Martin, F. N., & Clark, J. G. (2009). *Introduction to audiology* (10th ed.). Boston, MA: Pearson.

Mayo Clinic. (2009). *Mayo Clinic family health book.* Rochester, MN: Mayo Clinic.

Millar, D., Light, J., & Schlosser, R. (2006). The impact of augmentative and alternative communication intervention on the speech production of individuals with developmental disabilities: A research review. *Journal of Speech-Language-Hearing Research, 49*, 248–264.

Mosby. (2009). *Mosby's medical, nursing, and allied health dictionary* (8th ed.). St. Louis, MO: Mosby.

Musiek, F. E., & Chermak, G. D. (2007). *Handbook of (central) auditory processing disorder: Vol 1. Auditory neuroscience and diagnosis.* San Diego, CA: Plural Publishing.

Newschaffer, C., Croen, L., Daniels, J., Giarelli, E., Grether, J., et al. (2007). The epidemiology of autism spectrum disorders. *Annual Review of Public Health, 28,* 235–258.

Pennington, L., & McConachie, H. (2001). Interaction between children with cerebral palsy and their mothers: The effects of speech intelligibility. *International Journal of Language and Communication Disorders, 36*(3), 371–393.

Pharoah, P., Platt, M., & Cooke, T. (1996). The changing epidemiology of cerebral palsy. *Archives of Disease in Childhood (fetal and neonatal ed.), 75,* 169–173.

Poulson, D., & Nicolle, C. (2004). Making the Internet accessible for people with cognitive and communication impairments. *Universal Access in the Information Society, 3*(1), 48–56.

Purdy, M., & Dietz, A. (2010). Factors influencing AAC usage by individuals with aphasia. *Perspectives on Augmentative and Alternative Communication, 19*(3), 70–78.

Reece, P. B., & Challenner, N. C. (2006). *The source for behavior management in autism.* East Moline, IL: LinguiSystems.

Reed, V. A. (2010). *An introduction to children with language disorders* (4th ed.) Boston, MA: Pearson Allyn and Bacon.

Reichert Hoge, D., & Newsome, C. A. (2002). *The source for augmentative alternative communication.* East Moline, IL: LinguiSystems.

Richard, G. J. (2001). *The source for processing disorders.* East Moline, IL: LinguiSystems.

Richard, G. J. (2004). Redefining auditory processing disorder: A speech-language pathologist's perspective. *ASHA Leader, 7*(March), 21.

Richard, G. (2008). Autism spectrum disorders in the schools. *The ASHA Leader, 13*(13), 26–28.

Sadao, K. C., & Robinson, N. B. (2010). *Assistive technology for young children: Creating inclusive learning environments.* Baltimore, MD: Brookes Publishing.

Santalahti, P., Aromaa, M., Sourander, A., Helenius, H., & Piha, J. (2005). Have there been changes in children's psychosomatic symptoms? A 10-year comparison from Finland. *Pediatrics, 115*(4), 434–442.

Savage, R. C., & Callahan, C. D. (2003). Review: Pediatric traumatic brain injury proactive intervention. *Journal of Head Trauma Rehabilitation, 18*(3), 303–304.

Schlosser, R. W., Wendt, O., Angermeier, K. L., & Shetty, M. (2005). Searching for evidence in augmentative and alternative communication: Navigating a scattered literature. *Augmentative and Alternative Communication, 21*(4), 233–255.

Schonwald, A., & Lechner, E. (2006). Attention deficit/hyperactivity disorder: Complexities and controversies. *Current Opinions in Pediatrics, 18*(2), 189–195.

Stach, B. A. (2010). *Clinical audiology: An introduction* (2nd ed.). Clifton Park, NY: Delmar Cengage Learning.

Stanley, F., Blair, E. & Alberman, E. (2000). *Cerebral palsies: Epidemiology and causal pathways.* London, England: Mac Keith Press.

Steele, R., & Woronoff, P. (2011). Design challenges of AAC apps on wireless portable devices for person's with aphasia. *Perspectives on Augmentative and Alternative Communication, 20*(2), 41–51.

Still, G. F. (1902). Some abnormal physical conditions in children: The Goulstonian lectures. *Lancet, 1,* 1008–1012.

Sturm, J., & Clendon, S. A. (2004). Augmentative and alternative communication, language, and literacy: Fostering the relationship. *Topics in Language Disorders, 24*(1), 76–91.

Surveillance of Cerebral Palsy in Europe. (2002). Prevalence and characteristics of children with cerebral palsy in Europe. *Developmental Medicine and Child Neurology, 44,* 633–640.

Sutherland, D., Gillon, G., & Yoder, D. (2005). AAC use and service provision: A survey of New Zealand speech language therapists. *Augmentative and Alternative Communication, 21*(4), 295–307.

Tager-Flusberg, H., & Caronna, E. (2007). Language disorders: Autism and other pervasive developmental disorders. *Pediatric Clinics of North America, 54*(3), 469–481.

Tetnowski, J. A. (2004). Attention deficit hyperactivity disorder and concomitant communicative disorders. *Seminars in Speech and Language, 25*(3), 215–223.

Tonge, B. J. (2002). Autism, autism spectrum and the need for better definition. *Medical Journal of Australia, 176*(9), 412–413.

Treviranus, J., & Roberts, V. (2003). Supporting competent motor control of AAC systems. In J. Light & D. Beukelman, *Communication competence for individuals who use AAC.* Baltimore, MD: Brookes.

Turkstra, L. S., Williams, W. H., Tonks, J., & Frampton, I. (2008). Measuring social cognition in adolescents: Implications for students with TBI returning to school. *NeuroRehabilitation, 23*(6), 501–509.

Turner-Brown, L. M., Lam, K., Holtzclaw, T. N., Dichter, G. S., & Bodfish, J. W. (2011). Phenomenology and measurement of circumscribed interests in autism spectrum disorders. *Autism, 15,* 437–456.

Van Oosterum, J., & Devereux, K. (1985). *Learning with Rebuses.* Black Hill, Ely, Cambridgeshire, England: WAEO, The Resource Centre.

Volden, J., & Lord, C. (1991). Neologisms and idiosyncratic language in autistic speakers. *Journal of Autism and Developmental Disorders, 21,* 109–130.

Wender, P. H. (2000). ADHD: *Attention-deficit hyperactive disorder in children, adolescents, and adults.* Oxford: Oxford University Press.

Wilens, T. E., Biederman, J., & Spencer, T. J. (2002). Attention deficit/hyperactivity disorder across the lifespan. *Annual Review of Medicine, 52,* 113–131.

Winter, S., Autry, A., Boyle, C., & Yeargin-Allsopp, M. (2002). Trends in the prevalence of cerebral palsy in a population-based study. *Pediatrics, 110,* 1220–1225.

Wishart, K. (2010). Clinical impressions of how young children use AAC at home and in child care settings: A Canadian perspective. *Perspectives on Augmentative and Alternative Communication, 19*(1), 21–28.

Wood, N. S., Marlow, N., Costeloe, K., Gibson, A., & Wilkinson, A. (2001). Neurologic and developmental disability after extremely preterm birth. *Obstetrics & Gynecology, 56*(1), 13–15.

Woodcock, R., Clark, C., & Davies, C. (1968). *Peabody Rebus reading program.* Circle Pines, MN: AGS Publishing.

Workinger, M. S. (2005). *Cerebral palsy resource guide for speech-language pathologists.* Clifton Park, NY: Delmar Cengage Learning.

World Health Organization. (2001). *International classification of functioning, disability, and health.* Geneva, Switzerland: WHO.

Yeates, K. O., & Taylor, G. H. (2006). Behavior problems in school and their educational correlates among children with traumatic brain injury. *Exceptionality, 14*(3), 141–154.

Yen, H. L., & Wong, J. T. (2007). Rehabilitation for traumatic brain injury in children and adolescents. *Annals, Academy of Medicine, Singapore, 36,* 62–6.

Ylvisaker, M. (1998). *Traumatic brain injury rehabilitation: Children and adolescents* (2nd ed.). Boston, MA: Butterworth-Heinemann.

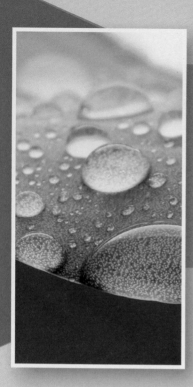

CHAPTER 14
Hearing Disorders in Children and Adults

LEARNING OBJECTIVES

After studying this chapter, you will:

- Be able to discuss the anatomy and physiology of the hearing mechanism.

- Understand hearing sensitivity and auditory nervous system impairments.

- Be familiar with newborn hearing screening.

- Understand the essentials of pure-tone and speech audiometry.

- Be able to discuss the essentials of amplification and assistive devices for individuals who are hearing impaired.

- Be familiar with aural rehabilitation.

- Appreciate that the Deaf culture has long been established in countries around the world.

- Understand the essentials of the emotional and social effects of hearing loss in children, adults, and their families.

KEY TERMS

acoustic trauma
(noise-induced
hearing loss)
adenoids (pharyngeal
tonsils)
admittance
air conduction
American Sign Language
(ASL)
assistive listening device
audiogram
audiometer
auditory brainstem
response (ABR)
auditory nervous system
impairment

auditory training
aural habilitation
aural rehabilitation
bone conduction
cerumen
cochlea
cochlear implant
compliance
conductive hearing loss
Deaf community
Deaf culture
differential threshold
Eustachian (auditory)
tubes
finger spelling

hearing aid
hearing sensitivity
impairment
hearing threshold
immittance audiometry
impedance
lipreading
manualism
manually coded English
masking
mastoiditis
Meniere's disease
middle ear
mixed hearing loss
oralism

KEY TERMS continued

CHAPTER OUTLINE

INTRODUCTION

The hearing mechanism is a system that takes physical energy and transforms it into chemical and electrical activity for us to hear the sounds in our environment. The auditory system includes the outer, middle, and inner ear structures and the auditory nervous system. Hearing loss is the most common of all physical impairments. The two major types of hearing impairments in children and adults are hearing sensitivity impairments and auditory nervous system impairments. Hearing screening of newborn infants is increasingly being performed in many hospitals. Hearing evaluations of children and adults attempt to determine the nature and extent of hearing loss. The evaluation information can provide important direction for rehabilitation. The goal of hearing rehabilitation is to limit the extent of any communication disorder that results from a hearing loss. Hearing aids and now cochlear implants may be used by individuals of most any age. Sign language (*manualism*) is a natural form of communication for many deaf children and adults when communicating among themselves. There are always emotional and social effects on children and adults who have a hearing loss.

ANATOMY AND PHYSIOLOGY OF THE HEARING MECHANISM

The hearing mechanism and auditory (L. *auditorius*, hearing) system are remarkable in both their simplicity and complexity. They take physical energy (i.e., acoustic air pressure waves) and transform it into chemical and electrical activity to allow us to hear the world around us. They continually monitor the environment for potential danger (e.g., the sound of footsteps behind you) while processing acoustic signals as complex as speech or music. (Note: Although the hearing mechanism is bilateral, descriptions usually refer to the singular, with most illustrations and models being of the right ear.)

Hearing is a distance sense unaffected by many barriers that interfere with sight, touch, smell, and taste. Sound can bend around corners with little distortion, and in many conditions it is possible to tell the direction of the source of the sound (*localization*). It is the millisecond difference between when a sound coming from the side reaches one ear and when it reaches the other ear that allows us to know from which direction it is coming. However, when a sound *reverberates* (reflects off of other surfaces), it is more difficult to distinguish the location of the source.

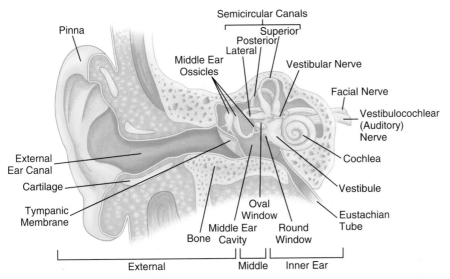

Figure 14-1

The human peripheral auditory system has three divisions: external, middle, and inner ear. The external ear consists of the pinna (auricle) and the external ear canal (external auditory meatus). The tympanic membrane (eardrum) closes off the medial end of the external ear canal. The middle ear is an air-filled cavity that contains the three middle ear ossicles. The middle ear cavity is connected to the nasopharynx by the **Eustachian tube**. The inner ear includes the cochlea, vestibule, and three semicircular canals. The cochlea contains the end organ for hearing. The vestibule and three semicircular canals contain the end organs for balance and motion detection.

© Cengage Learning 2013.

Eustachian (auditory) tube

A tube lined with mucous membrane that joins the nasopharynx and the middle ear cavity that is normally closed but opens during yawning, chewing, and swallowing to allow equalization of air pressure in the middle ear with atmospheric pressure.

The physical processing of acoustic (Gk. *akoustikos,* hearing) information occurs in three groups of structures, commonly known as the outer, middle, and inner ear (see Figure 14–1). Physiological processing begins in the inner ear and continues along the *auditory nerve* (VIII cranial nerve) to the central auditory nervous system.

Outer Ear

The **outer (external) ear** collects and resonates sound, assists in localizing the direction from which sound is coming, and helps protect the middle ear. The three main parts of the outer ear are the *auricle* (L. *auricula,* little ear) or pinna (L. *pinna,* feather; the cartilaginous portion you see), the *ear canal (external auditory canal),* and the outer surface of the **tympanic membrane (eardrum)**. The upper rim of the ear is the *helix* (Gk. coil), and the lower flabby portion is the *lobule* (Gk. *lobos,* lobe).

The external ear canal is a narrow channel or tube with a slight upward angle. It leads from an opening in the side of the temporal bone in the skull to the tympanic membrane, a distance of approximately 1 inch (2.5 cm) in adults. Rather than round, the canal is oval, with its height greater than its width. The canal contains sebaceous glands that secrete

outer (external) ear

The concave, somewhat funnel-like structure that collects, resonates, and directs sound waves to the tympanic membrane, assists in localizing the direction from which sound is coming, and helps protect the middle ear; composed of the auricle (pinna), ear canal, and outer layer of the tympanic membrane.

tympanic membrane (eardrum)

A thin, semitransparent membrane that separates the ear canal from the middle ear and transmits sound vibrations into the middle ear.

cerumen

A yellowish or brownish waxy secretion produced by ceruminous glands in the ear canal that protects the ear canal from intrusion by insects.

hearing threshold

In audiometry, the level at which a stimulus sound, such as a pure tone, is barely perceptible; usual clinical criteria demand that the level be just high enough for the subject to be aware of the sound at least 50% of the time it is presented.

middle ear

An air-filled chamber located within the temporal bone of the skull; beginning at the inner side of the tympanic membrane and attaching the ossicular chain to the oval window of the cochlea.

ossicular chain

The three small bones (ossicles) of the middle ear named after their basic shapes: *malleus*, for the mallet or hammer; *incus*, for the anvil; and *stapes*, for the stirrup.

cerumen (*sebum* or *earwax*), which helps discourage insects from entering the canal. Men tend to have hair near the opening of the canal, which also helps keep insects out. The length of the canal helps protect the tympanic membrane from trauma and keep it at a constant temperature and humidity. The ear canal directs sound to the tympanic membrane.

The tympanic membrane is a thin, nearly oval, semitransparent membrane with a vertical diameter of about 10 mm (a little less than 1/2 inch) that separates the ear canal from the middle ear and transmits sound waves (vibrations) into the middle ear. The tympanic membrane is fairly taut, like a drum, and it vibrates at the same rate (*frequency*) and magnitude (*intensity*) as the sound waves that reach it. It is an extremely efficient vibrating surface. Movement of one-billionth of a centimeter is sufficient to produce a **hearing threshold** response in normal-hearing individuals in the 800- to 6000-Hz range (i.e., the level at which a sound is just sufficient to produce a sensation—the person can barely detect the sound) (Harris, 1986).

Middle Ear

The **middle ear** is an air-filled chamber located within the temporal bone of the skull for protection (see Figure 14–2). It begins at the inner surface of the tympanic membrane and extends to the *oval window*. The entire middle ear, including the tympanic membrane, is lined with mucous membrane.

The middle ear contains the **ossicular chain**, which consists of three joined bones named after their basic shapes: the *malleus,* for the mallet or hammer; the *incus,* for the anvil; and the *stapes,* for the stirrup. The ossicles are suspended in the middle ear cavity and connect the tympanic membrane to the oval window of the *cochlea.* The ossicles provide a bridge between the tympanic membrane and the cochlea,

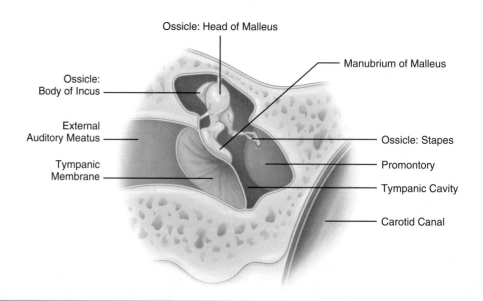

Figure 14–2

Tympanic membrane, middle ear, and ossicles.

© Cengage Learning 2013.

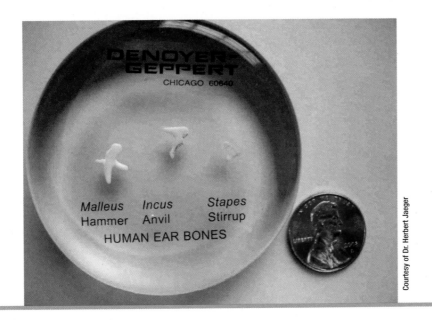

Courtesy of Dr. Herbert Jaeger

Figure 14–3

The size of the ossicles in relation to a penny (a penny is 20 mm [≈¾ inch] in diameter).

and they are set into vibration by the eardrum. Each of the ossicles is so delicately poised by its ligament connections within the middle ear that their collective function is unaltered by gravity when the head changes in position (Martin & Clark, 2012). The photograph in Figure 14–3 illustrates the size of the ossicles in relation to a penny. Vibrations of the tympanic membrane are conducted along the ossicular chain to the oval window of the cochlea. It is the action of the ossicles that provides the energy transformation for which the middle ear is designed.

The Eustachian Tubes

Air in the left and right middle ear cavities is kept at atmospheric air pressure by way of the Eustachian tubes. The Eustachian tubes lead from the middle ear to the nasopharynx at a downward angle of approximately 30 degrees in adults for a distance of about 35 mm (≈1¼ inches) (see Figure 14–1). In infants, the Eustachian tubes are shorter and in a more horizontal plane than they are in adults. The tubes are bone in the superior one-third and cartilage in the inferior two-thirds. The *orifices* (openings) of the Eustachian tubes are normally closed at the nasopharyngeal ends; however, they tend to remain open in infants until the age of about 6 months. They normally open with the oral and pharyngeal movements used during chewing, swallowing, yawning, and sneezing to allow air to enter the tubes and flow into the middle ear cavities, equalizing the atmospheric and middle ear pressure (*pressure equalization*) to maximize mobility of the tympanic membrane (recall from Chapter 12, Motor Speech Disorders and Dysphagia/Swallowing Disorders, that we swallow approximately 600 times a day, giving many opportunities for equalization of middle ear pressure, plus all of those provided by chewing). However, when atmospheric air pressure changes suddenly (e.g., going up or down in an elevator or ascending or descending in an airplane), the middle ear cavities will have relatively more or less pressure and

Valsalva maneuver

The procedure of closing the mouth and pinching the nostrils closed with the fingers and forcefully exhaling air, usually causing the Eustachian tubes to open and air to flow into the middle ear to equalize middle ear cavity air pressure with atmospheric air pressure, for example, when going up or down in an elevator or ascending or descending in an airplane, causing the ears to "pop"; any exhaling of air against tightly closed vocal folds, as when lifting heavy objects.

cochlea

The part of the inner ear containing the sensory mechanism of hearing; a spiral tunnel with 2¾ turns about 30 mm (about 1¼ inches) long, resembling a tiny snail shell.

vestibular system

The inner ear structures associated with balance and position sense, including the vestibule and semicircular canals of the vestibular mechanism, with interactions of the visual and **proprioceptive** systems and connection to the cerebellum.

proprioception/ proprioceptive

The sensation of body position and movement using sensory signals from muscles, joints, and skin.

a feeling of "fullness" in the middle ear can occur. The tympanic membrane is pressed outward as atmospheric air pressure decreases (ascending altitude) and pressed inward as atmospheric air pressure increases (descending altitude). A method of intentionally opening the Eustachian tubes is the **Valsalva maneuver**, where the mouth and nose are held closed while forcing air into the Eustachian tubes, causing the ears to "pop."

Flying and the Eustachian Tubes

Some people have had their eardrums rupture on airplane flights when their Eustachian tubes were not functioning normally because they were ill with an *upper respiratory infection* (URI) (common cold). They may have attempted to use the Valsalva maneuver to equalize the changing air pressure when they were ascending or descending, although without success, resulting in one or both tympanic membranes rupturing. Although this is relatively rare, anyone with an upper respiratory infection should give flying a second thought when their ears are "plugged up."

Babies unintentionally use the Valsalva maneuver when they start to cry when in an airplane that is ascending or descending. The loud crying causes the Eustachian tubes to open and equalize the middle ear cavity pressure with the changing air pressure inside the cabin of the plane. Once the plane has leveled out, the air pressure is stabilized and the baby is comfortable again.

Inner Ear

The inner ear consists of two important structures; the **cochlea** and the **vestibular system** (see Figure 14-4). The delicate cochlea is protected by being housed inside the temporal bone of the skull. The cochlea is the

Figure 14-4

The cochlea and semicircular canals are surrounded by the temporal bone for protection (view is looking from above down onto the cochlea and semicircular canals).

© Cengage Learning 2013.

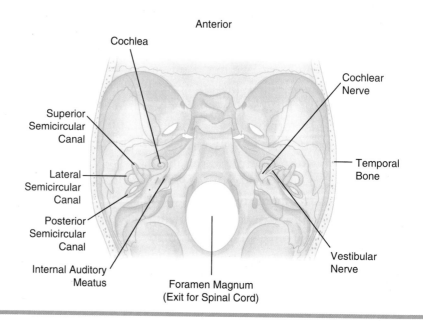

part of the inner ear that contains the sensory mechanism of hearing. It resembles a tiny snail shell with its 2¾-turn spiral tunnel and, uncoiled, is about 30 mm (about 1¼ inches) long. The cochlea is actually full size at the time of birth, which is important for the anatomical feasibility of **cochlear implants** in infants and young children. The cochlea has two fluid-filled tubes that are separated by the *basilar membrane*. The cochlea has over 15,000 tiny hair cells that are stimulated by movement of the cochlear fluid in response to sound.

The vibration of the stapes in the middle ear against the oval window of the cochlea creates motion of the fluid in the cochlea, resulting in stimulation of the hair cells that send neural impulses to the *auditory nerve* (*VIII cranial nerve*). Hair cells in different portions of the cochlea are stimulated by different frequencies of sound (higher frequencies are nearer the oval window and lower frequencies are farther from the oval window).

The Vestibular Mechanism

The vestibular mechanism of the inner ear acts as a motion detector and is affected by forces of gravity and inertia. The immediate entryway into the inner ear is the vestibule, which is filled with fluid. It is within the vestibular portion of the inner ear that the organs of equilibrium are housed. The vestibular system maintains a person's balance and interacts with the visual and proprioceptive systems that send their inputs to the cerebellum.

The vestibular mechanism's three *semicircular canals* contain fluid. Each semicircular canal lies at a different angle (plane), and as a person moves the head or body the fluid stimulates different portions of the semicircular canals, sending the sensation to the vestibulocochlear nerve (see Figure 14–5). When a person is tumbled around (e.g., in the ocean by heavy waves), the vestibular system becomes "confused" and

cochlear implant

A device that enables individuals with profound hearing loss to perceive sound through an array of electrodes that are surgically implanted in the cochlea and deliver electrical signals to the vestibularcochlear (VIII cranial) nerve, and an external amplifier that activates the electrode array.

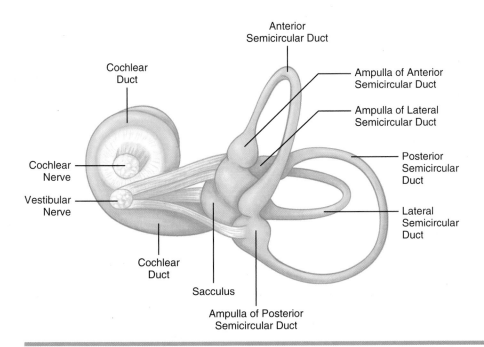

Figure 14–5

The semicircular canals of the vestibular mechanism.

© Cengage Learning 2013.

does not know which way is up (people have drowned because of that). Motion sickness (*kinesia*) is caused by erratic or rhythmic motions (such as in a boat or car) that stimulate the semicircular canals and can result in nausea, headache, and *vertigo* (a sensation of instability, loss of equilibrium, or spinning). Note: Some audiologists include in their practices *vestibular (balance) disorders*, although these disorders are beyond the scope of this text.

AUDITORY NERVOUS SYSTEM

The auditory nervous system is primarily an afferent system that sends neural (electrical) impulses from the cochlea to the auditory cortex in the temporal lobes of the brain. The hair cells have axons that leave the cochlea and form the cochlear branch of the vestibulocochlear nerve and synapse in the medulla of the brainstem. Approximately 75% of the impulses from the right ear are transmitted to the left hemisphere, and 75% of the impulses from the left ear are transmitted to the right hemisphere. The other 25% of impulses from each ear ascend to the *ipsilateral* (same side) hemisphere of the brain, allowing for *redundant pathways* (i.e., most information is sent to one hemisphere of the brain but some information also is sent to the other hemisphere). However, what is received in the right hemisphere must be sent by way of the corpus callosum to the temporal lobe in the left hemisphere for further auditory processing because in most people the left hemisphere is dominant for processing speech and language (Hixon, Weismer, & Holt, 2008; Seikel, King, & Drumright, 2010).

Central Auditory Nervous System

The central auditory nervous system has several synaptic junctions before reaching the primary auditory cortex (*Heschl's gyrus*) (see Figure 14-6)

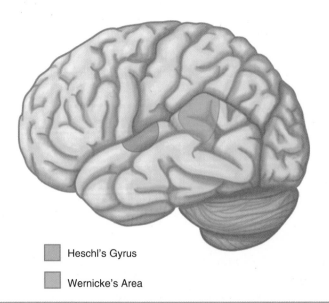

Figure 14-6

The primary auditory cortex (Heschl's gyrus) and Wernicke's area.

© Cengage Learning 2013.

Heschl's Gyrus

Wernicke's Area

in the temporal lobe of each hemisphere (Katz, Medwetsky, Burkard, & Hood, 2009). What begins as a pressure wave striking the tympanic membrane sets into motion a complex series of neural responses that spread throughout the auditory system. Processing of speech information occurs throughout the central auditory system, although its primary language processing occurs in the left temporal lobe. Recall from the section on language processing in Chapter 3, Anatomy and Physiology of Speech and Language, that auditory processing, auditory comprehension, and language processing involve numerous levels of skills that overlap and are essentially inseparable (Bellis, 2003; Geffner & Ross-Swain, 2007). Briefly, these skills include sensation, auditory attention, auditory discrimination, auditory association, auditory memory, and auditory cohesion.

HOW WE HEAR

The auditory system is able to both detect the smallest of pressure waves causing the faintest of sounds (*hearing sensitivity*) and discriminate minute changes in the nature of sound, such as pitch and intensity (*hearing acuity*). Hearing sensitivity involves hearing threshold and **differential threshold** (the smallest difference that can be detected between two auditory signals).

Stach (2010, p. 75) describes hearing in the following way:

differential threshold

The smallest difference that can be detected between two auditory signals.

> Our ability to hear relies on this very sophisticated series of structures that process sound. The pressure waves of sound are collected by the pinna and funneled to the tympanic membrane by the external auditory canal. The tympanic membrane vibrates in response to the sound, which sets the ossicular chain into motion. The mechanical movement of the ossicular chain then sets the fluids of the cochlea in motion, causing the hair cells on the basilar membrane to be stimulated. These hair cells send neural impulses from the VIII cranial nerve to the auditory brainstem. From the brainstem, networks of neurons act on the neuronal stimulation, sending the signals to the auditory cortex.

TYPES AND CAUSES OF HEARING IMPAIRMENTS

Hearing loss often has been called an "invisible condition" or "invisible handicap," yet its effect may be anything but invisible. The consequences of hearing loss may be seen in almost all aspects of a person's life.

Normal, everyday communication may be difficult or impossible as a consequence of hearing loss. A *communication handicap* involves the psychosocial disadvantages that result from hearing loss (Tye-Murray, 2009). The age of onset, type, and severity of the hearing impairment are the first considerations when working with an individual with a hearing loss. Because of hearing loss, a young child may have delays in development of speech, language, social skills, and educational achievement.

The term *impairment* is used to describe an abnormality in the structure or function of the ear. There are two primary types of hearing impairments in children and adults: hearing sensitivity impairments and auditory nervous system impairments. **Hearing sensitivity impairments** and *peripheral hearing loss* are the most common type of hearing loss (Bess & Humes, 2008; Martin & Clark, 2012). They are a reduction in the sensitivity of the auditory mechanism that results in sounds needing to be a higher intensity than normal before they can be heard by the listener. Auditory nervous system impairments are the result of reduced ability to hear sounds above the *hearing threshold* (the level at which a sound is barely detectable). **Auditory nervous system impairments** or *(central) auditory processing disorders* occur less often and individuals with them may have hearing sensitivity impairments concurrently, causing a dual auditory problem.

Incidence

Hearing loss is the most common of all physical impairments. Among infants and children, approximately 1 in every 22 newborns in the United States has some kind of hearing problem, and 1 in every 1,000 infants has a severe to profound hearing loss (ASHA, 2008a). Of school-age children, 83 out of 1,000 have an "educationally significant hearing loss" (National Information Center for Children and Youth with Disabilities, 2004). In a 2003–2004 study of 5,742 Americans ages 20 to 69 years, 16% (29 million) had hearing loss in one ear (9%) or both ears (7%). Men were 5.5 times more likely than women to have a hearing loss. Hearing loss prevalence occurred earlier among research participants who smoked, had noise exposure, or cardiovascular disease (Agrawal, Platz, & Niparko, 2008). The National Institute of Deafness and Communication Disorders (2002) reported that 54% of individuals over 65 years of age have some degree of hearing loss. In the Scandinavian countries of Denmark, Finland, Norway, and Sweden and in the United Kingdom, hearing loss also has a high incidence, with 20% in the general population having some degree of loss (Barton et al., 2001).

Hearing Sensitivity Impairments

When sound is not conducted normally through the outer ear, middle ear, or both, the result is a **conductive hearing loss**. When the sensory

---

hearing sensitivity impairment

The most common type of hearing loss; a reduction in the sensitivity of the auditory mechanism that results in sounds needing to be a higher intensity than normal before they can be heard by the listener.

auditory nervous system impairment

The result of reduced ability to clearly hear sounds above the hearing threshold; occurs less often than hearing sensitivity impairments, which may occur concurrently, causing a dual hearing problem.

conductive hearing loss

A reduction in hearing sensitivity because of a disorder of the outer or middle ear.

or neural cells or their connections within the cochlea are absent or are not functioning normally, a **sensorineural hearing loss** occurs. When both the conductive mechanism (outer ear, middle ear, or both) and the cochlea are not functioning normally, there is a **mixed hearing loss**. **Retrocochlear hearing loss** is a hearing disorder resulting from a *neoplasm* (tumor) or other lesion located on cranial nerve VIII or beyond in the auditory brainstem or cortex.

Conductive Hearing Loss

A decrease in the strength of a sound is referred to as *attenuation*. When a soft sound is attenuated because of poor conduction through the outer or middle ear, it may not have sufficient magnitude to reach the cochlea. A conductive hearing loss is easily experienced when you cover your ears tightly with your hands and try to listen to a conversation. Some words you hear clearly because they are spoken louder or there is more acoustic energy in the sounds of the words, other words may be misunderstood, and still other words are not heard at all.

Hearing Loss and the Outer Ear and the External Auditory Canal

Some disorders or malformations of the outer ear may occur that result in hearing loss, for example malformations of the *auricle (pinna)*. *Otic atresia* (Gk. *ous*, ear, *a-*, without, + *tresis*, opening) of the external auditory canal may occur where some or all of the canal is congenitally malformed or absent. Some otic atresias may occur because of traumas or severe burns. Otic atresia, unless surgically repaired, causes conductive hearing loss. Surgical procedures for correction of otic atresia are often successful, particularly when the cartilaginous portion of the canal and the tympanic membrane are normal.

　　External otitis (L. *externus*, outward, Gk. *ous*, ear, + *itis*, inflammation) is an infection that occurs in the skin of the external auditory canal. The condition is often seen in people who have had water trapped in their ear canals and is referred to as *swimmer's ear*. External otitis is usually caused by bacterial infection, but it can be caused by fungus (*otomycosis*). Itching is a common complaint with mild infections, and extreme pain often accompanies advanced infections. Edema of the ear canal may be present, but the canal usually is not completely occluded. There typically is not a noticeable loss of hearing during the infection. Medical treatment includes irrigating the ear canal with warm salt water, drying it carefully, and applying a topical antibiotic (Mosby, 2009).

　　Some people have copious amounts of cerumen that occludes the ear canal, creating a conductive hearing loss. However, when people try to remove the earwax themselves, they may end up pushing it further into the ear canal (*impacted cerumen*), even against the tympanic membrane. The cerumen needs to be properly removed. It is now within the

sensorineural hearing loss

A reduction in hearing sensitivity because of a disorder of the cochlea.

mixed hearing loss

A reduction in hearing because of a combination of a disordered outer or middle ear and inner ear.

retrocochlear hearing loss

A hearing disorder resulting from a *neoplasm* (tumor) or other lesion located on cranial nerve VIII or beyond in the auditory brainstem or cortex.

Application Question

Have you ever experienced a temporary conductive hearing loss? What was it like? What were some of your thoughts and feelings about it that you can recall?

scope of practice of audiologists who are specifically trained to perform this procedure (Wilson & Roeser, 1997).

Foreign bodies in the external ear canal are common, particularly in children. If something can fit into the ear canal, some child has probably gotten it stuck in there. In some cases, when an object has been in the canal for too long, swelling and infection may occur. Surgical removal of the foreign object under a microscope is sometimes required. When the external ear canal is occluded by a foreign object, there is a conductive hearing loss on that side.

Perforation (rupture) of the tympanic membrane can occur in many ways. Direct trauma from pointed objects such as hairpins during attempts to remove earwax has occurred. The tympanic membrane may be perforated by concussion from explosions or a hand clapped hard over the ear. The tympanic membrane also may be perforated when there is excessive buildup of fluid in the middle ear during a middle ear infection. Conductive hearing loss occurs with perforation of the tympanic membrane.

Hearing Loss and the Middle Ear

Several causes of middle ear problems result in hearing loss. The age of the person tends to determine the likely causes, with young children commonly having *otitis media* and *otosclerosis* being an adult problem. We discuss only the most common problems of the various ages.

Otitis Media (Middle Ear Infection) **Otitis media with effusion** (middle ear infection) is one of the most common disorders of the middle ear. Otitis media is any inflammation, infection, or both of the mucous membrane lining the interior of the middle ear, commonly with *purulent* (pus-producing) organisms resulting in *effusion* (fluid in the middle ear) (see Figure 14–7). Middle ear infections occur in almost 70% of children born in the United States before they are two years old, with many of these children experiencing more than one episode (Siegel & Bien, 2004). In a Chinese study of more than 3,000 children 3 to 6 years old, otitis media was present in almost 10% of the children (Chen, Lin, Hwang, & Ku, 2003).

Children who are exposed to tobacco smoke are more likely to have middle ear infections than other children (Kraemer et al., 1983). *Upper respiratory infections* (common colds), allergies, sinus infections (*sinusitis*), and sore throats caused by infections are also common contributors to otitis media. Often the infection is literally blown through the orifice of the Eustachian tube and into the middle ear by a stifled sneeze or by blowing the nose too hard (keeping the mouth open during sneezing and blowing the nose with just moderate force can help prevent forcing bacterial or viral infections into the Eustachian tube and middle ear).

Although otitis media is primarily a disease of childhood, it can occur at any age. When a Eustachian tube is infected, it becomes swollen, interfering with its middle ear pressure-equalization function. With a swollen Eustachian tube, the air inside the middle ear is trapped

otitis media with effusion

Any inflammation or infection of the middle ear; particularly common in childhood and often associated with a common cold, allergies, sinus infections, and sore throats; Eustachian tube malfunction typically is the physiological cause; effusion—the escape of fluid from tissue as a result of seepage.

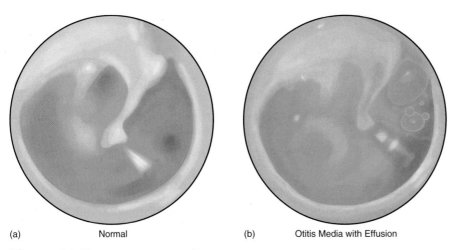

(a)   Normal   (b)   Otitis Media with Effusion

Figure 14–7

Illustrations of a normal tympanic membrane (a), and during an episode of otitis media with effusion (b). The normal membrane is sufficiently translucent that some underlying structures can be seen. The ear with otitis may show considerable redness, distention of the membrane, and the presence of fluid, ranging from clear to amber. Underlying structures are not typically visible as they are in the normal state.

© Cengage Learning 2013.

and begins to be absorbed by the mucosa (walls) of the middle ear cavity. This creates a slight vacuum effect (negative pressure) in the middle ear. The lining of the middle ear then becomes inflamed. If allowed to persist, fluid from the inflamed tissue begins to seep through the mucosal walls into the middle ear cavity (effusion). A conductive hearing loss results once this fluid is sufficient to impede normal movement of the tympanic membrane and ossicles. Harmful bacteria in the fluid can cause a middle ear infection.

Some behaviors of children with middle ear infections include irritability, difficulty hearing normal conversational levels, and turning up the television volume. As the infection worsens, children usually have elevated temperatures and are visibly ill. It is important for parents to take their child to a physician *as soon as possible* because by the time symptoms are apparent the infection may already have been present for a few days and a course of antibiotics may take a week to 10 days to be completed (recall from the discussion on "Auditory Processing Disorders" in Chapter 13 that middle ear infections are often associated with auditory processing disorders).

Medical treatment of otitis media is imperative, and without it there can be permanent damage to the middle ear structures. If the condition continues even further, the tympanic membrane may rupture (Klein, 2000). Pus that cannot find its way out of the middle ear may invade the *mastoid bone* (a protrusion of the temporal bone behind the outer ear), causing **mastoiditis**. Untreated mastoiditis can result in *meningitis* and sometimes death (Bess & Humes, 2008; Martin & Clark, 2012).

mastoiditis

An infection of one of the mastoid bones (just behind the ear) that is usually an extension of a middle ear infection, characterized by earache, fever, headache, and malaise; medical treatment may require intravenous antibiotics for several days, and residual hearing loss may follow the infection.

CASE STUDY

Jennifer

Jennifer was a 4-year-old girl when she experienced her first middle ear infection. She also suffered from allergies and began having occasional sinus infections, which may have contributed to the middle ear infections. The child's pediatrician treated her several bouts of otitis media with effusion with antibiotics and decongestants—common medical treatments. However, on one occasion the child had a severe reaction to the antibiotic, a derivative of penicillin, and had to be hospitalized for a few days. From that point, she could no longer have penicillin-derivative antibiotics because of a future life-threatening allergic reaction to them. The parents, both professionals in the medical field, took Jennifer to a local *otologist* (a physician who specializes in ear diseases and disorders) for placement of PE tubes. Over the next few years, Jennifer had six sets of PE tubes but continued to have allergies, sinus infections, and middle ear infections.

The parents began to feel that the adenoids might be the "culprits" in contributing to the middle ear infections, and they took Jennifer (now age 7) to an otolaryngologist who took x-rays of the nasopharyngeal region to determine the size of the adenoids. They were significantly enlarged and were occluding the opening of the Eustachian tubes and preventing normal aeration of the middle ear. The enlarged adenoids also prevented the child from being a normal nasal breather, forcing her to breathe through her mouth (an indication of enlarged adenoids is if a child cannot chew food with the mouth closed, even with repeated encouragement). The child was scheduled for an adenoidectomy and tonsillectomy in outpatient, short-stay surgery at a local hospital. The otolaryngologist did a postoperative visit with the parents and told them that Jennifer's adenoids were "the size of oysters." The removal of the adenoids took care of most of the middle ear infections, although the child later needed sinus surgery for more complete removal of sinus drainage to help end the sinus infections. A 3-year course of allergy shots helped take care of the chronic allergy problems that contributed to her sinus infections. As many parents learn, much of the ongoing expense of raising children is centered on the eyes (glasses and contacts), ears (middle ear infections), nose (allergies and sinus infection), and mouth (dental care and orthodontia). ■

Surgical Management for Otitis Media　When a child has had *recurrent otitis media* (usually a series of three to five middle ear infections in a 1-year period), many otolaryngologists or *otologists* (physicians who specialize in diseases and disorders of the ear) will consider surgical management. The primary purpose of surgery for patients with middle ear infections is to eliminate disease, and in some cases reconstruction of a damaged hearing mechanism is needed. The procedures are typically performed in an outpatient surgical setting and the patient is allowed to go home that same day.

Dormant Otitis Media

When the proper type and sufficient dosage of antibiotics are not used, the infection may move into a dormant state rather than being eliminated (*resolved*). Because the overt symptoms may disappear, the patient and family may assume that the otitis media has been cured. However, a few to several weeks later the patient may experience what seems like a new bout of otitis media, which is in reality an exacerbation of the same condition experienced earlier but allowed to lie dormant. Many patients discontinue their own antibiotic treatment when their symptoms abate, leaving some of the hardier bacteria alive. Then, when the condition flares up again, it is the result of a stronger strain, one less susceptible to medication (Martin & Clark, 2012). There is increasing concern among physicians and medical scientists about both children and adults having decreased benefits from antibiotics because of improper use of them and overreliance on them for a variety of illnesses, allowing some forms of bacteria to develop immunity to antibiotics (Lutter, Currie, Mitz, & Greenbaum, 2005; Samore et al., 2001).

A *myringotomy* (L. *myringa,* eardrum, + Gk. *temnein,* to cut) is performed in which a small surgical incision is made into the tympanic membrane to relieve pressure and release fluid or pus from the middle ear (see Figure 14–8a). A small suction device may be inserted through the incision to delicately suction out the fluid and pus. Antibiotics are given before and continued afterward to manage the infection (Mosby, 2009).

Following the myringotomy and cleaning of the middle ear, the otolaryngologist may insert a **pressure-equalizing (PE) tube** through the incision in the tympanic membrane (see Figure 14–8b and Figure 14–9). The tube is plastic, tiny, and hollow with a flange on each

pressure-equalizing (PE) tube

A small silicone tube inserted into the tympanic membrane following a myringotomy to equalize air pressure between the middle ear cavity and the atmosphere as a substitute for a nonfunctional Eustachian tube.

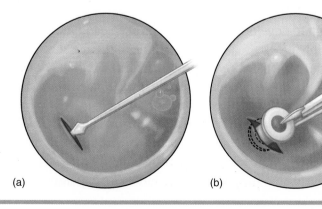

(a)   (b)

Figure 14–8

(a) A myringotomy incision. (b) A pressure-equalizing tube positioned through the tympanic membrane to allow middle ear ventilation.

© Cengage Learning 2013.

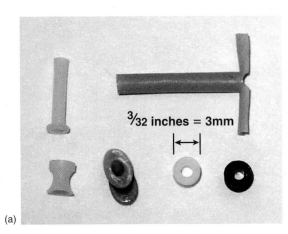

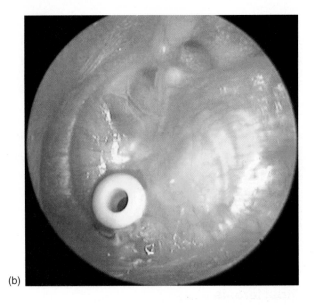

(a)

(b)

Figure 14–9

(a) Types of pressure-equalizing tubes. (b) Photo of a pressure-equalizing tube inserted in the tympanic membrane.

end that prevents the tube from falling into the middle ear or falling out of the tympanic membrane prematurely. The tube allows direct ventilation of the middle ear and functions as an artificial Eustachian tube to maintain normal middle ear air pressure. The tube may remain in place from several weeks to several months, after which time it *extrudes* (pushes out) naturally into the external auditory canal, usually without the child noticing. Newer-designed tubes may remain in place indefinitely.

Some children with middle ear infections have enlarged **adenoids (pharyngeal tonsils)** that may be occluding the openings to the Eustachian tubes and preventing aeration of the middle ear, leading to middle ear infections. Adenoids are made of *lymphoid tissue* (tissue that produces lymphocytes that are helpful in fighting infection) and are found in the *nasal–pharyngeal region* (on the pharyngeal wall above the soft palate, which does not allow them to be seen during an oral examination). They begin to develop about 6 months of age and may continue to grow and possibly block the passage of air from the nasal cavity into the pharynx, preventing nasal breathing and requiring mouth breathing (during an oral examination, clinicians should always determine whether a child is a nasal or mouth breather). Mouth breathing is a good indicator of enlarged adenoids. Another indicator of a child having enlarged adenoids is whether he has enlarged **palatine tonsils** (see Figure 3–10 for normal tonsils). Both the adenoids and the palatine tonsils normally have *atrophied* (decreased in size) and essentially disappeared by early adolescence.

Adenoidectomy and Tonsillectomy

Adenoidectomy and *tonsillectomy* are surgical procedures that may be performed because the adenoid tissue, tonsillar tissue, or both are enlarged, chronically infected, or causing obstruction. Normal adenoids may be *excised* (cut out) as a *prophylactic* (preventive) measure during a tonsillectomy. The surgery is performed under general anesthesia in children, but a local anesthesia may be used with adults. When the patient has recovered from the anesthesia, ice chips or clear liquids without a drinking straw may be offered (Mosby, 2009). Most of these procedures are now done in the outpatient surgical setting.

Otosclerosis

Otosclerosis is a common problem in adults and is typically hereditary (Chen et al., 2002). Otosclerosis occurs when there is growth of bony tissue around the footplate of the stapes that presses against the oval window, resulting in a conductive hearing loss. The otosclerosis prevents normal vibration and causes attenuation in the cochlea. Otosclerosis usually occurs bilaterally, although the two ears may not begin to be affected at the same time. It is a progressive disorder with onset ranging from mid-childhood to late–middle adulthood. Some individuals in early adolescence begin to notice some hearing loss. Women are more likely to be diagnosed with otosclerosis than men, and its onset is often related to pregnancy (Martin & Clark, 2012).

Auditory Nervous System Impairments

Auditory nervous system impairments may occur in the cochlea, auditory nerve and various synaptic junctions (*retrocochlear*), as well as in the primary auditory cortex (*Heschl's gyrus*) in the temporal lobe of each hemisphere. A problem at a lower level (e.g., cochlea) will send the distorted or errored neural impulses through the rest of the auditory system. Sensorineural hearing loss from cochlear disorders may arise from many causes. Newborns may have inherited disorders that affect the nervous system, as well as congenital malformations of the cochlea. Many disorders may occur at any age, such as infections, acoustic trauma, and *ototoxicity* (harmful effects of certain substances on the VIII cranial nerve or the organs of hearing and balance). *Presbycusis* is a common problem with aging.

Hearing Loss and Disorders of the Inner Ear

Abnormalities and diseases of the cochlea are probably the largest cause of sensorineural hearing impairments, with the delicate hair cells usually being involved. Although the hair cells are damaged, the auditory nerve

adenoids (pharyngeal tonsils)

Lymphoid tissue (tissue that produces lymphocytes, which are helpful in fighting infection) found on the pharyngeal wall in the nasal–pharyngeal region; begin to develop about 6 months of age and may continue to grow and possibly interfere with or occlude the openings of the Eustachian tubes; when enlarged, they may block the passage of air from the nasal cavity into the pharynx, preventing normal nasal breathing and requiring mouth breathing; sometimes removed to allow nasal breathing and help prevent middle ear infections.

palatine tonsils

Two almond-shaped masses of lymphoid tissue between the anterior and the posterior faucial pillars.

otosclerosis

Typically a hereditary condition that occurs when there is growth of bony tissue around the footplate of the stapes that presses against the oval window, resulting in a conductive hearing loss, and causing attenuation in the cochlea.

fibers connected to the hair cells often remain intact (this is an important fact with cochlear implants). When there is damage or abnormality in the cochlea, decreased hearing sensitivity is not the only symptom. Individuals often complain of difficulty understanding speech—more specifically, auditory discrimination problems. Drawing primarily from Martin and Clark (2012), and Stach (2010), the following discussions are based on ages of onset.

Prenatal Causes

Prenatal causes refer to adverse effects on the cochlea during embryological and fetal development, resulting in congenital hearing loss. Development of the external, middle, and inner ear takes place between the 4th and 8th weeks of gestation. Some infants have hereditary factors that predispose them to hearing loss. In some cases, there are associated genetic abnormalities that accompany the hearing loss, including skull, facial, and external ear deformities; cleft palate; visual disorders; abnormal skin pigmentation; thyroid disorders; disorders of the heart; musculoskeletal anomalies; cognitive disabilities; difficulty with balance and coordination; and a variety of sensorimotor impairments. In many cases, there may be a combination of genetic and in-utero environmental factors that come into play—that is, *multifactorial genetic considerations.*

Teratogens   As discussed in Chapter 10, Cleft Lip and Palate, teratogens are environmental substances or agents that result in malformations and anomalies of specific organs and systems that are undergoing rapid development in the embryo or fetus. Exposure to teratogens during these periods may result in major congenital anomalies. For example, exposure to teratogens between 21 and 27 days gestation is associated with anomalies of the external ear (Hayes & Northern, 1997). Exposure before the 3rd week of gestation may result in death and spontaneous abortion. There are numerous teratogens, such as drugs and alcohol, congenital HIV and AIDS, *rubella, cytomegalovirus* (CMV), *herpes simplex-type virus, toxoplasmosis,* and *congenital syphilis.*

Perinatal Causes

Perinatal causes of hearing loss are those that occur during the process of birth. Handicapping sensorineural hearing loss occurs in 2% to 4% of neonatal intensive care units (NICU) survivors (Amatuzzi, Northrop, Bento, & Eavey, 2005). Hearing loss in infants who were in NICUs is often associated with the identifiable disorders that caused the need for the NICU or treatment for the disorders, such as low birth weight and hypoxia. *Respiratory distress syndrome* (RDS; also called *hyaline membrane disease*) is the most common respiratory disease in premature infants. Infants who have RDS and become *septic* (generalized infection) are typically treated with antibiotics with potential **ototoxic** properties that place them at risk for hearing loss. *Congenital heart disease* (CHD) is among the most common birth defects; infants with congestive heart

ototoxic

Drugs that have harmful effects on the central auditory nervous system, including aspirin, aminoglycoside antibiotics, furosemide, and quinine.

disease often experience failure-to-thrive and feeding problems. Although CHD in newborns does not cause hearing problems, infants with CHD often have syndromes associated with hearing loss. Numerous central nervous system disorders may have hearing loss as one component of the disorder, including cerebral hemorrhage, hydrocephalus, and *neonatal seizures.* Any disorder that results in hypoxia may affect an infant's neurological status and hearing. Neurological dysfunction by itself does not affect hearing, but it can cause significant auditory processing, speech, and language development problems (Stach, 2010; Tye-Murray, 2009).

Postnatal and Childhood Causes

Postnatal causes of cochlear hearing loss are any factors occurring after birth. *Bacterial meningitis* may cause total deafness. Numerous childhood infections may affect hearing, such as *measles, mumps, chicken pox, influenza,* and *viral pneumonia.* Most virus-producing hearing losses are bilateral, except mumps. The body's natural reaction to infection is elevation of temperature; however, when fever becomes excessive, cellular damage can occur, including cells of the cochlea. Treatment of bacterial infections may necessitate use of ototoxic antibiotics. *Diabetes mellitus* and *kidney disease* have been implicated in sensorineural hearing loss. *Head traumas* may occur at any age and may result in both neurological disorders and hearing loss.

Older Children and Adults

Hearing loss in older children and adults has numerous causes, one of which is mostly preventable (i.e., noise-induced hearing loss). Most people are likely to have reduced hearing as they grow older (particularly after age 60); however, people can do many things to try to preserve their hearing. Hearing is usually one of the things in our lives that we do not think much about until we lose it.

Noise-Induced Hearing Loss and Acoustic Trauma

Noise-induced hearing loss and **acoustic trauma** dates back hundreds (thousands) of years. When World War II soldiers returned from battlefields with hearing impairments, this type of noise-induced hearing loss began attracting attention. Airports to construction sites, street repairs to lawn mowers, and even some large restaurants where you have to talk over the noise, create sustained loud noise, particularly for the workers (see Table 14–1). Noise-induced hearing loss can be temporary or permanent. Exposure to excessive sound results in a change in the threshold of hearing sensitivity. However, the length of time of exposure is also important; the longer the exposure level, the greater the possibility of damage to the hearing mechanism.

Acoustic trauma from a single exposure may cause permanent hearing loss. Gradual hearing loss from repeated exposure to excessive

noise-induced hearing loss

A permanent sensorineural hearing loss caused by exposure to excessive loud noise, often over long periods of time.

acoustic trauma

Damage to hearing from a transient, high-intensity sound.

TABLE 14-1   Decibel Levels of Common Sounds

DECIBELS	SOUND
130+	Jet takeoff, gunfire (pain threshold)
120+	Rock concert speaker sound, sandblasting, thunderclap, fireworks, pneumatic drill
110+	Dance club, snowmobile, powerboats, hammering metal
100+	Chain saw, bulldozer
90+	Subway trains, motorcycle, workshop tools (e.g., belt sander), lawn mower
80+	Heavy city traffic, factory noise, vacuum cleaner, garbage disposal, Niagara Falls
70+	Dog barking, noisy restaurant, busy traffic
60+	Ringing telephone, baby crying, alarm clock 2 feet away
50+	Quiet automobile 10 feet away
40+	Everyday conversation
30+	Quiet street at night with no traffic
20+	Whispered conversation
10+	Soft rustle of leaves, birds singing, dripping water faucet
0	Just audible sound

Based on data from: Northern & Downs, 2012; Van Bereijk, Pierce, & David, 1960; and the American Industrial Hygiene Association, 2007.

sound can damage or destroy the delicate hair cells in the cochlea. There is evidence that children and adolescents are suffering increased amounts of hearing loss from toys, phones, stereo systems, musical instruments, and a variety of other noise makers, some of which produce sound up to 155 dB, resulting in self-induced hearing loss (Nadler, 1997). Shargorodsky, Curhan, Curhan, and Eavy (2010) in an article on "Change in Prevalence of Hearing Loss in U.S Adolescents" in the *Journal of the American Medical Association* reported that 12- to 19-year-old U.S. adolescents had a 31% increase in hearing loss from 1988–1994 to 2005–2006, and that one in five adolescents had a hearing loss (6.5 million teens). The most likely cause of such an alarming increase in hearing loss among teens, as well as college students, is the use of MP3 players and earbuds that can present loud music to the ears without disturbing other people around the users (Hoover & Krishnamurti, 2010; Moore, 2010; Shafer, 2006).

The Author's Experience

Personal Story

During my military service in the U.S. Army, the many hours of training on the firing range with a variety of weapons (M16 rifles, 45-caliber pistols, M60 machine guns, M70 grenade launchers, and hand grenades) exposed me to countless sharp, very loud noises and explosions. Further training as a tank driver, with a 90-mm cannon firing directly over my head, exposed me to more painfully loud noise. During my time of service as a combat medic in Vietnam in 1969, not only did I need to fire many rounds with my M16 and an M60, but there were countless mortars and rockets that came in on us—sometimes like rain—with explosions all around. Our personnel would return fire with their "quad-4s" (four 50-caliber machine guns mounted on a turret) and various artillery (it is hard to describe the deafening sounds). Flying in noisy medevac (medical evacuation) helicopters (HU1s ["Hueys"]) with the side door off and insufficient ear protection added to the noise exposure. Realistically, protecting our hearing is not an important concern in combat—survival and doing our "job" are important. I now have some trouble hearing in my right ear—the side only inches from my weapons. I am a normal war veteran. Men and women who survive combat in all wars (currently and in the future) will likely suffer from some hearing loss. ■

What You Can Do to Protect Your Hearing

1. *Know which noises can cause damage.* Noises above 85 dB are most damaging. Whenever possible, avoid loud noises.

2. *Turn down the volume.* Today, many people play their TV sets, home and car stereos, and MP3 players unnecessarily loud (high school and college age are particularly inclined). Consider lowering the volume. When purchasing headphones, look for sets with volume limiters that keep the sound at safe levels. This is especially important when buying them for children and teenagers.

3. *Protect yourself.* Earplugs are inexpensive and come in a variety of types, sizes, and colors.

4. *Reduce your exposure.* Some situations are inherently noisy, but you can decrease the risk of noise-induced hearing loss by avoiding or limiting your time in loud restaurants and clubs. When riding motorcycles, personal watercraft, or other loud vehicles, limit the time you spend on them and wear ear protection.

5. *Remember your neighbors.* Noise from your personal recreation affects not only you but also everyone around you.

Based on information from the American Industrial Hygiene Association, 2007.

Hearing conservation programs can help protect workers from ongoing loud noises. The first line of defense against occupational noise is to diminish loud sounds at the source. Blocking noise with hearing protection devices such as earplugs or earmuffs can help the wearer—but only if they are worn correctly and when necessary. Noise-induced hearing loss is generally painless, progressive, permanent—and preventable. As speech-language pathologists and audiologists, part of our "mission" as professionals is to protect our hearing and to encourage others to protect theirs. Most people are going to lose some of their hearing sooner or later; there is no need for them to lose it sooner than they have to.

Tinnitus

Tinnitus is a subjective noise sensation that is often described as a ringing, roaring, or swishing in the ear that may be heard in one or both ears. Although tinnitus is more commonly associated with cochlear diseases, it can occur with some middle ear problems, including otosclerosis. The actual source of tinnitus within the auditory system is uncertain; it can likely rise from various sites, from the external ear to the auditory cortex (Sandlin & Olsson, 2000). It may be a sign of otosclerosis, acoustic trauma, Meniere's disease, presbycusis, or an accumulation of cerumen impinging on the eardrum or occluding the external auditory canal. It sometimes occurs for no reason. Many children with hearing loss requiring amplification experience some tinnitus (Gold, 2003). Tinnitus is common enough that tinnitus support groups have been formed in countries around the world (e.g., American Tinnitus Association, Australian Tinnitus Association, British Tinnitus Association, and Tinnitus Association of Canada—see the list of websites provided at the end of this chapter). Although tinnitus may not have a significant deleterious effect on hearing, it can affect concentration, sleep, education, employment, personal relationships, and social functioning. For some people, it may be socially debilitating (Davis & Refaie, 2000). Many treatments have been developed, but all have varying success.

Meniere's Disease

Meniere's disease is a common disorder with an unknown etiology that may involve both the cochlea and the vestibular system. Meniere's disease has a constellation of symptoms, including episodic *vertigo* (sensation of instability or rotation caused by disturbance in the semicircular canals of the inner ear), vomiting, tinnitus, pressure in the involved ear with a feeling of "fullness," and progressive, fluctuating, sensorineural hearing loss that is normally unilateral. The initial recommended medical treatment may be a change in diet, adherence to a low-sodium diet, diuretics, steroids, and/or other medications (Campbell, 2007).

Presbycusis

Presbycusis (also spelled *presbyacusis*) is a progressive hearing loss as a result of the aging process. Age takes its toll on the entire auditory system (actually, all bodily systems), including the tympanic membrane,

---

tinnitus

A subjective noise sensation, often described as a ringing, roaring, or swishing in the ear that may be heard in one or both ears; associated with a variety of hearing disorders in both adults and children; can affect concentration, sleep, education, employment, personal relationships, and social functioning, and sometimes is debilitating; treatment success varies.

Meniere's disease

A chronic disease of the inner ear characterized by recurrent episodes of vertigo, tinnitus, and sensorineural hearing loss may that be bilateral.

presbycusis

Hearing loss associated with old age, usually involving both a loss of hearing sensitivity and a reduction in clarity of speech.

ossicular chain, cochlea, and central auditory nervous system. Symptoms of presbycusis are usually seen by age 60. A common characteristic of presbycusis is difficulty understanding speech, although speech is usually more easily understood when it is slower rather than louder. Speech is also more difficult to understand when there is background noise. Some comments made by people with presbycusis (Pichora-Fuller, 1997) are:

- "I hear but I have trouble understanding."
- "I understand when it's quiet but have trouble in a group."
- "People seem to talk too fast; I need more time to make sense of what they're saying."
- "I don't know for sure when I hear correctly and when I don't."

Neural Disorders

Neural disorders can affect the auditory system. *Neuritis,* or inflammation of the auditory nerve, can cause temporary or permanent hearing loss. Multiple sclerosis and brainstem tumors can affect hearing function. *Neoplastic* growths, including carcinoma and various other types of tumors can affect the auditory system.

COMMUNICATIVE DISORDERS OF INDIVIDUALS WITH HEARING IMPAIRMENTS

Several variables affect the type and degree of communication disorders seen in hearing impaired individuals (Hull, 2009; Lee, 2012; Stach, 2010; Tye-Murray, 2009):

1. *Age*—Infants born with hearing impairments (congenital impairments) have more problems with communication than children who have already acquired speech and language.

2. *Severity*—Individuals of any age have more communication problems when the hearing loss is severe rather than mild.

3. *Configuration of the hearing loss*—*Low frequency* hearing loss will affect hearing some consonants and vowels (e.g., /z, v, b, d, m, n, l, i, u, e, o, ɔ/), *middle frequency hearing loss* will affect hearing other sounds (e.g., /a, æ, ʃ, tʃ, p, g, k/), and *high frequency loss* will affect still others (e.g., /f, θ, ð, s/) (see Figure 14–10).

4. *Type of hearing loss*—Individuals with conductive hearing losses may benefit from hearing aids in ways that individuals with sensorineural hearing losses may not.

5. *Beginning of professional care*—When a newborn is identified as having a hearing loss and professional care is initiated, the infant has a better opportunity for speech and language development than an infant who is not identified until 1 year of age or older. The younger and sooner children are identified and begin to receive

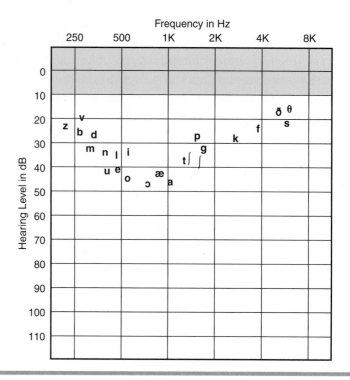

Figure 14-10

Generalized phonetic representations of speech sounds occurring at normal conversational levels plotted on an audiogram.

© Cengage Learning 2013.

comprehensive services, the better their opportunities to develop speech and language. Also, the more involved the parents are with their child's habilitation, the better the child's communication development will likely be.

6. *Presence of other handicaps*—Some children with hearing impairments also have other handicapping conditions, such as developmental delays and auditory processing disorders that compound the difficulty developing speech, language, and cognitive skills.

Speech

The sounds that cannot be heard well are the sounds most difficult to develop. Normal-hearing and normal-speaking individuals sometimes speak with a low intensity, making hearing conversation that much more difficult for individuals with hearing impairments. Final consonants are often spoken with such low intensity that there is barely a "hint" of the sound (e.g., the word *sound* may be spoken by many people so that it is heard more like *soun*). The person with a hearing impairment is unlikely to hear final consonants when there is little stress placed on them and, therefore, to produce them in conversation. Other sounds the person with a hearing impairment does not hear easily are also likely to be omitted, particularly unstressed sounds in blends; for example, *stream* may be heard as *stea*.

Individuals with severe hearing impairments often are confused about voiced and voiceless sounds (*cognates*) and substitute one for the other. For example, /p/ and /b/ may be inconsistently substituted for one another (e.g., *pat* becomes *bat* and *bat* becomes *pat*), as well as

/d/ and /t/ (e.g., *time* becomes *dime* and *dime* becomes *time*). Oral and nasal cognates are sometimes substituted, such as /m/ and /b/ (e.g., *meat* becomes *beat* and *beat* becomes *meat*). Children who develop some lipreading skills tend to recognize "visible" sounds more easily than "invisible" sounds (e.g., /p/ is easier to recognize than /k/).

Stress, speaking rate, breath control, pitch, and intensity (*suprasegmentals*) are common problems for children with significant hearing losses. They tend to have a distinct speech quality. Their speech often sounds breathy, labored, staccato, and arrhythmic. They may place equal stress on all syllables or stress syllables inappropriately (e.g., *baby* may have the stress on the second syllable, sounding like "bah-BEE") (Tye-Murray & Folkins, 1990). Children with severe-to-profound hearing losses typically speak slowly (approximately half the rate of normal-hearing children) and pause often, both within words and between words. Most children who are hard-of-hearing or deaf produce relatively few syllables per breath and use their breath inefficiently. They often let out more breath during connected speech than do children with normal hearing (Forner & Hixon, 1977). The voice quality of severely hearing impaired individuals is often unpleasant. Their pitch may sound excessively high or variable, or they may use a monotone. They often have pitch breaks, with the pitch abruptly changing from high to low. They often speak too softly or too loudly for the situation or environment, and their intensity may fluctuate inappropriately (Tye-Murray, 2009). (See Table 14–2 for more on hearing impairment levels.)

TABLE 14-2	Degree of Hearing Loss and Its Effects on Communication as Indicated by Pure-Tone Audiograms
HEARING LEVEL	**HEARING ABILITY**
Normal (-10 to 10 dB)	Can hear speech normally
Minimal (10 to 25 dB)	Has difficulty hearing faint speech in a noisy place
Mild (25 to 40 dB)	Has difficulty hearing faint or distance speech, even in a quiet environment
Moderate (40 to 55 dB)	Hears conversational speech only at a close distance
Moderately severe (55 to 70 dB)	Hears loud conversational speech
Severe (70 to 90 dB)	Cannot hear conversational speech
Profound (>90 dB)	May hear loud sounds; hearing is not the primary communication channel

Adapted from Stach, 2010.

Language

Regardless of which communication mode children with severe hearing impairments use (aural and oral or signing), most children who are profoundly deaf and who use hearing aids do not learn their native language well (Mahshie, Moseley, Scott, & Lee, 2006; Stiles, McGregor, & Butler, 2012; Vinson, 2011). Ninety percent of children with significant hearing loss are born to parents who have normal hearing. As a result, many children are not exposed to language early because they do not have access to the auditory signal and their parents have not learned sign language to communicate with these children (Tye-Murray, 2009). The grammar of adults with significant hearing loss is usually about the level of 8-year-old normal-hearing children, and their vocabulary development is normally at the fourth-grade level (Bamford & Saunders, 1985). We briefly look at form (syntax and morphology), content (semantics and vocabulary), and pragmatics (use).

Form

Children with hearing impairments tend to use primarily content words (nouns and verbs) and rarely use adverbs, prepositions, or pronouns. They often omit function words (*a, an, the,* etc.). They usually use short subject–verb–object sentences and rarely use compound or complex sentences. Their sentences often sound "telegraphic." Likewise, children with hearing impairments have difficulty understanding the compound and complex sentences used by normal-hearing people (Lee, 2012; Tye-Murray, 2009).

Content

Children with significant hearing losses consistently have weak vocabularies. Weak vocabularies typically mean poor understanding of basic concepts. They may, for example, understand and be able to use a word as a verb (e.g., *stand,* as in *stand up*) but not be able to use the same word as a noun (e.g., *stand,* as in *music stand* or *band stand*). They typically know and use few synonyms and antonyms. Understanding common idioms is a major problem for the hearing impaired. They understand and use concrete words more easily than abstract words (Lee, 2012; Tye-Murray, 2009).

Pragmatics

Children with hearing impairments often do not know how to initiate or maintain a conversation or how to repair breakdowns in communication. They have difficulty with turn-taking and changing topics. They often try to pretend that they are understanding when they are not and, therefore, have inappropriate responses (Tye-Murray, 2009).

Literacy

Children with significant hearing impairments have difficulty not only understanding and using oral language but also reading and writing.

This contributes significantly to their communication problems because they do not have a modality that they can use to clearly understand or communicate their wants, needs, thoughts, and feelings. As discussed in Chapter 7, Literacy Disorders in Children, learning to read and write is more challenging for children than learning to understand and use oral language. This is particularly true for children with hearing impairments.

Reading

Children who are hard of hearing or deaf and use hearing aids often have delays or differences with reading. The average reading and writing skills of high school students who are deaf are at a third- or fourth-grade level, which is barely adequate for reading a newspaper (Allen, 1986). Several interacting factors likely cause reading problems for children who are hearing impaired:

1. They have inadequate aural–oral language systems with deficits in vocabulary and compound and complex sentence structures that interfere with their ability to understand printed text.

2. Children with significant hearing losses do not develop an auditory basis for mapping sound to print (Golding-Meadow & Mayberry, 2001). When hearing impaired children do not have a normal phonological code, they have difficulty "sounding out words" in print that they are unfamiliar with.

3. Many children with hearing impairments do not have normal experiences with world knowledge (e.g., hearing and seeing TV news reports) with which to relate printed stories (e.g., newspaper articles). Many other factors, no doubt, are involved that affect children with hearing impairments abilities to read (Tye-Murray, 2009).

Writing

In general, poor syntax, vocabulary, and word spelling reflect the expressive language abilities of children and adults with hearing impairments. Their writing samples often contain syntactic errors such as omission of articles, inappropriate use of pronouns, and omission of bound morphemes (e.g., -'s and -ed). Most written sentences are simple subject–verb–object forms; rarely are there compound and complex syntactic structures. Synonyms, antonyms, and metaphors are seldom used. Topics are often introduced but not developed or elaborated. Writing narratives where there is a clear beginning, middle, and end to the story are difficult for children with hearing impairments. They are better at writing some factual details about a topic than explaining the theme or the main points of a topic (Shirin & Reed, 2005; Tye-Murray, 2009). Adults with hearing impairments commonly do not feel confident to write sentences to communicate with people who have normal hearing and literacy skills.

AUDITORY PROCESSING DISORDERS

Auditory processing disorders (APD) are mentioned briefly here because they are rather controversial among some audiologists, as they are among some speech-language pathologists; that is, not all of these professionals believe these disorders exist. The term *central auditory processing disorders* (CAPD) has been replaced by *auditory processing disorders* by most speech-language pathologists to emphasize the interactions of disorders at both the peripheral and the central sites without necessarily attributing difficulties to a single anatomical location (Bellis, 2003; Geffner & Ross-Swain, 2007; Jerger, & Musiek, 2000, Musiek & Chermak, 2007). Accurate diagnosis of auditory processing disorders requires a team approach and should include an audiologist, speech-language pathologist, psychologist, and educators. Auditory processing disorders were discussed in some detail in Chapter 13, Special Populations with Communication Disorders.

HEARING ASSESSMENT

The main purpose of a hearing evaluation is to define the nature and extent of the hearing impairment. From this information, decisions can be made about appropriate steps in the rehabilitation of the hearing disorder and handicaps that may result from the impairment. Several questions that need to be answered as part of a hearing evaluation include (Stach, 2010):

- Why is the person being evaluated?
- Should the person be referred for medical consultation?
- What is the person's hearing sensitivity?
- How well does the person understand speech?
- How well does the person process auditory information?
- Does the hearing impairment cause a hearing handicap?

People seek hearing evaluations by audiologists for various reasons. Parents want to find out if their child has a hearing problem. Older people seek evaluations to confirm their suspicion that they have developed a hearing problem. Adults may be referred to audiologists because of long-term noise exposure in the workplace or an accident with a view toward compensation for any hearing loss. Patients may be referred for audiological evaluations by otolaryngologists to determine the nature and extent of hearing impairments that result from active disease processes. Otolaryngologists will likely want audiological evaluations both before and after treating the disease process with drugs or surgery.

The fundamental purpose of an audiological evaluation is similar for most children and adults, although the specific focus of the evaluation can vary considerably depending on the nature of the individual and problem. We begin our discussion of hearing assessment at the beginning—with newborns.

Newborn Hearing Screening

Each year there are approximately 4 million babies born in the United States and an unknown number born around the world. Many children are born with significant hearing impairments but are not identified and provided with appropriate intervention. These children lose their ability to acquire fundamental speech, language, cognitive, and social skills required for later schooling and success in society. Early intervention for youngsters with hearing impairments is needed for them to develop communication skills on par with their normal-hearing peers (Vaughn, 2005; Yoshinaga-Itano & Gravel, 2001). Mohr, Feldman, Dunbar, et al. (2000), estimated that lifetime costs to society for individuals with prelingual (before speech development) onset of hearing loss exceeds $1 million, including costs of educational resources, reduced work productivity and earning capacity, social services (e.g., unemployment compensation), and other expenses and loss of income generating potential. The high cost associated with prelingual onset of severe to profound hearing impairment shows that interventions aimed at infants and children, such as early identification and aggressive medical and audiological intervention, can have a substantial payback.

Hearing screening is likely a low priority in many countries where the very survival of infants is the primary concern. Hearing screening may be a luxury in many nations, but it is becoming increasingly important in nations with the resources to provide the procedures. The challenge for the United States and many other countries is having qualified personnel who can perform the screening procedures accurately and reliably. Increasingly, hospitals are relying on supportive technicians and volunteers to carry out this important task. The use of supportive personnel for newborn screenings frees valuable time for audiologists whose efforts may be more meaningfully used for provision of follow-up, diagnostic, and intervention services (Katz, Medwetsky, Burkard, & Hood, 2009; Mahshie, Moseley, Scott, & Lee, 2006; Martin & Clark, 2009).

Newborn hearing screening did not become fairly common until the 1970s and 1980s for infants who were determined to be at risk for potential hearing impairment. Screening the hearing of newborn infants is now a routine procedure and compulsory in most states, and is both beneficial and justifiable. Hayes and Northern (1997) stated that the prevalence of significant hearing disorders in newborns may be as high as 6 in every 1,000 live births. Infants with low Apgar scores are considered at risk for hearing impairments. Some newborns may pass a hearing screening and still be at high risk for hearing loss; therefore, based on hereditary history, it is important to perform regular follow-up hearing screenings for at least several months (Mann, Cuttler, & Campbell, 2001). Detection of hearing loss in newborns may help alert medical professionals to the possibility of other complications. There appears to be a biological relationship between newborn hearing loss and other conditions, including *sudden infant death syndrome* (SIDS). Both may be caused by congenital deficiencies of certain important enzymes,

Application Question

If you are a parent, did your baby have a hearing screening before going home? If you are a possible future parent, would you request that your newborn have a hearing screening?

which can lead to a variety of disorders of other systems, such as vision, cardiopulmonary, and musculoskeletal, and a predisposition to infection (Walker, 2003).

Sudden Infant Death Syndrome (SIDS)

Sudden infant death syndrome (SIDS, formerly called *crib death*) is the unexpected and sudden death of an apparently normal and healthy infant that occurs during sleep and with no physical evidence of disease. It is the most common cause of death in children between 2 weeks and 1 year of age, with an incidence rate of 1 in every 300 to 350 live births in the U.S. The origin of SIDS is unknown, but multiple causes have been proposed. SIDS occurs most often in infants 2 to 4 months old, and in 95% of cases it occurs before 6 months of age. It is more common in infants born prematurely and most often occurs in the fall and winter months. SIDS is more prevalent in boys than girls and tends to occur more often among infants who have recently had a minor illness such as an upper respiratory infection. SIDS occurs more often among babies born to women who are in lower socioeconomic status groups, who are less than 20 years of age, who have at least one previous child, who begin prenatal care in the 3rd trimester, and/or who smoke, use drugs, or are anemic. SIDS is more common in infants who sleep in the prone (face down) or side-lying position; who have soft bedding, loose articles, or both in the sleeping environment; who are overheated (thermal stress); and who sleep with adults, especially on a sofa. There is a lower incidence of SIDS among breast-fed babies (Mosby, 2009).

> **Application Question**
>
> If you had an infant, what are some things you could do that could help prevent SIDS?

Newborn hearing screening requires the use of techniques that can be performed without active participation of the patient. One procedure that is frequently used is **auditory brainstem response (ABR)**, which is an electrophysiologic technique that involves attaching electrodes to an infant's scalp and recording electrical responses of the brain to sound. For screening purposes, the technique is often automated to limit testing interpretation errors (Stach, 2010).

auditory brainstem response (ABR)

An *electrophysiological response* (the relationship between electrical activity and biologic function, in this case, brain activity) to sound that consists of five to seven identifiable peaks that represent neural function of auditory pathways.

Pediatricians and Family Medicine (Practice) Physicians

Pediatricians and family medicine physicians are usually the first professionals to see a child with ear or hearing problems (Isaacson & Vora, 2003). The physician will take a thorough history and conduct a careful physical examination to diagnose and treat ear problems. The physical examination begins with visualization and palpation of the auricle and *periauricular* (around the auricle) tissue. A handheld *otoscope* (a device with a light source that permits visualization of the ear canal and eardrum) is used to examine the external auditory canal for *cerumen* (earwax), foreign bodies, and abnormalities of the canal skin (see Figure 14–11). The mobility, color, and surface anatomy of the tympanic

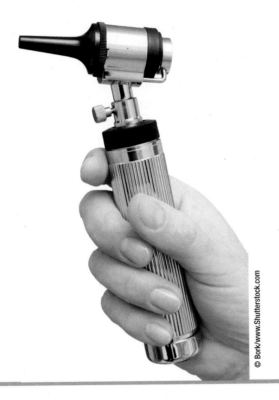

© Bork/www.Shutterstock.com

Figure 14-11

A handheld otoscope.

membrane are examined. A pneumatic bulb is used to test the movement of the tympanic membrane.

If the pediatrician or family medicine physician cannot treat or chooses not to treat the ear problem, she will likely refer the patient to an otolaryngologist for further evaluation and treatment. The otolaryngologist will likely perform many of the same examination techniques as the referring physician, plus others that he is more specialized in administering. Otolaryngologists often make referrals to audiologists for hearing evaluations.

Audiologists' Case History and Interview

Before evaluating pediatric or adult clients, audiologists typically gather a complete case history. A good case history guides an audiologist in several ways. It provides important information about the following:

- The patient's complaints about her hearing
- The family's complaints about the patient's hearing
- Whether the hearing problem is unilateral or bilateral
- Whether the problem is acute or chronic
- The duration of the problem
- What may be contributing to the hearing problem

Many audiologists use case history and questionnaire forms that can be completed by the patient or parents of a patient. Audiologists are sometimes the entry point into the health care system for individuals and it is important that they be knowledgeable about warning signs that indicate the need for a medical referral. For example, a patient's responses to questions about dizziness, numbness, weakness, tinnitus, and other signs indicate potential otological, neurological, or other medical problems. Experienced audiologists take advantage of the interview not only to obtain information from the client or patient but also to make important observations. For example, does the person have articulation or language problems, and is the person relying on lipreading to understand the audiologist? Getting a sense about how the person feels about a possible hearing loss helps the audiologist direct his counseling efforts (Mahshie et al., 2006).

Evaluating the Structures of the Outer and Middle Ear

Structural changes in the outer and middle ear can cause functional changes that result in hearing impairments. The auricle is inspected for shape, size, location on the head, and any visible abnormalities that may indicate possible syndrome involvement. Careful visual inspection of the external auditory canal can be done with an otoscope. The external ear canal is inspected for any obvious inflammation, obstruction from foreign objects, and excessive cerumen. The tympanic membrane is inspected for inflammation, perforation, or any other obvious structural abnormalities in structure. If disease processes are suspected, the patient should be referred for a medical assessment following the audiological evaluation.

Pure-Tone Audiometry

pure-tone audiometry

Audiometry using tones of various frequencies and intensities as auditory stimuli to measure hearing using both air conduction and bone conduction.

Pure-tone audiometry is built on the concept of tuning forks. Tuning forks are made of metal and are sometimes used by singers to match certain pitches or musicians to tune musical instruments (see Figure 14–12). A tuning fork produces a precise pitch and has a clear musical quality,

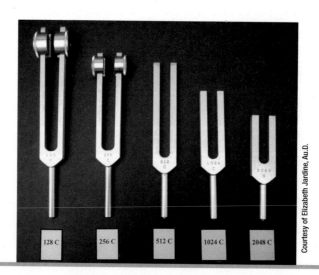

Figure 14–12

Tuning forks. The larger the tuning fork, the lower the frequency produced.

Courtesy of Elizabeth Jardine, Au.D.

usually corresponding to the musical scale of C. The tuning fork was used to test hearing more than a century ago, long before the development of audiometers.

Pure-tone audiometry uses tones of various frequencies and intensities as auditory stimuli to measure hearing and is performed with an **audiometer**, ideally in a sound-proof audiology booth (see Figure 14–13 and Figure 14–14). The purposes of pure-tone audiometry are to establish

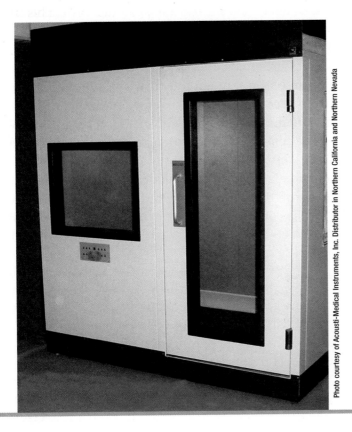

Photo courtesy of Acousti-Medical Instruments, Inc. Distributor in Northern California and Northern Nevada

audiometer

An electronic device designed to measure the sensitivity of hearing of pure-tone frequencies (*hertz*) and *intensities* (decibels); sounds are delivered to the ears either through earphones or *free field* (i.e., through loudspeakers in a testing environment with no reverberating surfaces) in an audiometry booth.

Figure 14–13

A commercial, double-room, sound-treated audiometric test booth.

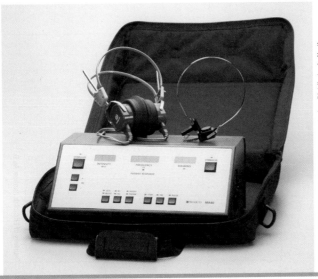

Photo courtesy of Acousti-Medical Instruments, Inc. Distributor in Northern California and Northern Nevada

Figure 14–14

Portable audiometers allow children and adults to be screened or tested away from sound-treated audiometric test booths.

hearing threshold sensitivity across the range of audible frequencies important for human communication, and to determine the lowest intensity that a person can "just barely hear"; that is, the *hearing threshold*. All newer audiometers are computerized with sophisticated microprocessors. To be accurate and reliable, audiometers need to be calibrated regularly by the manufacturer. Assessment reliability is based on the interrelationships among calibration of the equipment, test environment, patient performance, and experience of the examiner.

All audiometers can measure air conduction and bone conduction. **Air conduction** is the transmission of sound to the inner ear through the external auditory canal and the structures of the middle ear. Air-conduction thresholds are tested by transmission of sounds using earphones or free field through the outer and middle ear to determine auditory acuity (see Figure 14–14). **Bone conduction** is the transmission of sound to the inner ear through vibration applied to the bones of the skull. Bone conduction allows determination of the cochlea's hearing sensitivity while bypassing any outer or middle ear abnormalities. Bone conduction is tested by stimulation of the inner ear by placing a bone oscillator on the mastoid bone or forehead to determine whether a hearing loss is conductive, sensorineural, or mixed (i.e., both types) (see Figure 14–14).

Audiograms

Audiograms are graphs with a frequency-versus-intensity plot to show threshold sensitivity changes across the frequency range. *Audiometric frequencies* for conventional pure-tone audiometry are usually 250, 500, 1000, 2000, 4000, and 8000 Hz (see Figure 14–15).

air conduction

The transmission of sound to the inner ear through the external auditory canal and the structures of the middle ear.

bone conduction

Transmission of sound to the inner ear through vibration applied to the bones of the skull; allows determination of the cochlea's hearing sensitivity while bypassing any outer or middle ear abnormalities.

audiogram

A standard graph used to record pure-tone hearing thresholds with air- and bone-conduction thresholds graphed by frequency in hertz (Hz) and hearing level (HL) in decibels (dB).

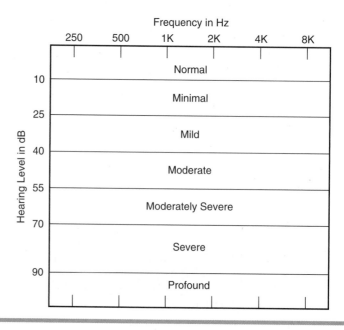

Figure 14–15

Degrees of hearing loss plotted on an audiogram.

© Cengage Learning 2013.

In clinical audiometry, intensity is expressed on a decibel scale relative to *average normal hearing*. The zero line running horizontally across the top of an audiogram is the sound intensity corresponding to average normal hearing at each of the test frequencies. Some people hear better than normal; therefore, –10 represents hearing at frequencies that a normal-hearing individual may not be able to hear. Pure-tone audiograms provide important information in several ways:

1. Audiograms indicate the degree of loss and its effects on communication. The effects on communication of a hearing loss may be considered the *functional results of the hearing loss;* that is, how the loss may affect a person's daily interactions with other people and the environment.

2. There are three basic shapes of loss on audiometric configurations. For example, a hearing loss may be the same at all frequencies and have a *flat configuration;* the degree of loss may decrease as the curve moves from the low-frequency region to the high-frequency region and have a *rising configuration;* or the loss may increase as the curve moves from the low-frequency region to the high-frequency region and have a *downward sloping configuration* (see Figure 14–16).

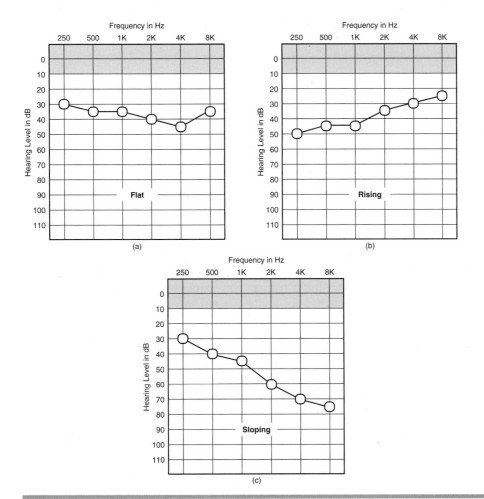

Figure 14–16

Three audiometric configurations: (a) flat, (b) rising, and (c) sloping.

© Cengage Learning 2013.

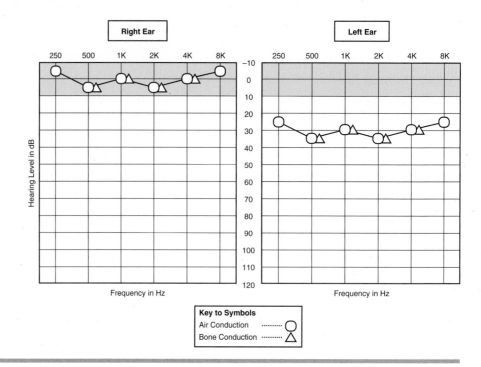

Figure 14–17

An audiogram representing asymmetrical hearing loss.

© Cengage Learning 2013.

3. The audiogram provides a measure of *interaural symmetry,* or the extent to which hearing sensitivity is the same in both ears or better in one than the other (see Figure 14–17).

4. The combination of air- and bone-conduction audiometry allows the differentiation of peripheral hearing loss into one of three types: conductive, sensorineural, or mixed (see Figure 14–18).

Masking

When two sounds are heard simultaneously, the intensity of one sound may be sufficient to cause the other to be inaudible. This change in the threshold of a sound caused by a second sound with which it occurs simultaneously is called **masking**. We all know what it is like not to hear someone speaking (or at least not clearly) because of background (*ambient*) noise. At such times, the background noise is *masking* (drowning out) the other person's speech. Light that has equal energy at all frequencies in the light spectrum is referred to as *white light.* This concept has been adapted to sound; that is, sound that has equal energy at all frequencies in the audible spectrum is referred to as *white noise.* Audiologists have various ways of using white noise as masking noise while performing pure-tone audiometry.

When an audiometric tone is presented to the test ear through an earphone at an intensity level that may cause the sound to "cross over" to the nontest ear, the nontest ear may allow the person to hear the sound. Whenever cross-hearing is suspected, it is necessary to remove the nontest ear from the test procedure to determine whether the original

masking

In audiology, the process that occurs when two sounds occur simultaneously and one sound is sufficiently loud to cause the other to be inaudible.

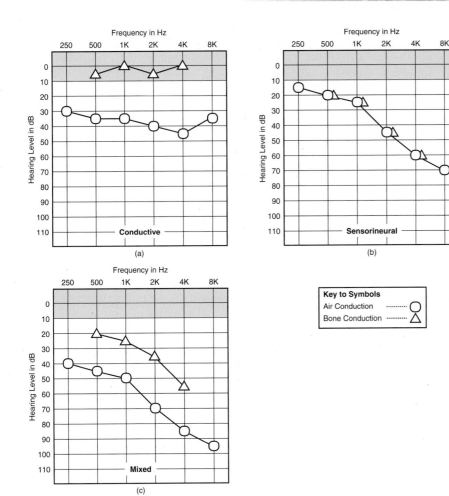

Figure 14-18

Audiograms representing three types of hearing loss: (a) conductive, (b) sensorineural, and (c) mixed.

© Cengage Learning 2013.

responses were obtained through the nontest ear and, if they were, what the true threshold of the test ear really is. This is accomplished by masking (Bess & Humes, 2008; Stach, 2010).

Speech Audiometry

Pure-tone audiometry provides valuable information about an individual's hearing; however, it does not yield clear insights into the degree of disability the individual has understanding speech. **Speech audiometry** uses the kinds of auditory signals present in everyday communication and, therefore, provides a more realistic assessment of how a hearing disorder might affect normal communication. Speech-language pathologists find that information obtained from speech audiometry is particularly helpful in planning therapy and client and family counseling (Bess & Humes, 2008; Mahshie et al., 2006; Martin & Clark, 2012). The influence of speech processing can be detected at all levels of the auditory system: middle ear, cochlea, auditory nerve, brainstem pathways, and auditory centers in the cortex. Speech audiometry is used to:

- Measure thresholds for speech
- Cross-check pure-tone sensitivity

speech audiometry

A key component of audiological assessment that uses auditory signals present in everyday communication; assessment involves, in part, the presentation of single-syllable words at a fixed intensity level above the threshold with the client aurally discriminating the sounds in the words to correctly say words aloud for the examiner to score.

tympanometry

A measurement of middle ear pressure that is determined by the mobility of the tympanic membrane as a function of various amounts of positive and negative air pressure in the external ear canal (the more positive or negative the air pressure in the external ear canal, the more the normal middle ear system becomes immobilized).

compliance

The ease with which the tympanic membrane and middle ear mechanism function.

impedance

The opposition of sound-wave transmission, which includes frictional resistance, mass, and stiffness, and is influenced by frequency.

immittance audiometry

A routinely used objective assessment of the functioning of the middle ear; a general term to describe measurements made of tympanic membrane impedance, compliance, or **admittance**.

admittance

The ease and flow of energy transmission through a system; the reciprocal of impedance.

- Quantify *suprathreshold* (above threshold) speech recognition
- Determine the range from most comfortable to uncomfortable loudness levels for an individual
- Determine the ability to recognize and discriminate speech sounds
- Assist in differential diagnosis
- Assess central auditory processing ability
- Estimate communicative function

A *speech threshold* is the lowest level at which speech can be detected or recognized; that is, the *speech awareness threshold* (SAT). A basic form of speech recognition testing involves the presentation of single-syllable words at a fixed intensity level above the threshold. The client has to hear and aurally discriminate the sounds in the words to correctly say the words aloud for the examiner to score. Differential diagnosis as to the location or locations in the auditory system in which the impairment is occurring can be determined from speech audiometry.

Tympanometry

Tympanometry is a measurement of middle ear **compliance** and **impedance** that is determined by the mobility of the tympanic membrane as a function of various amounts of positive and negative air pressure in the external ear canal. The tympanic membrane vibrates most efficiently when the pressure on both sides is equal (i.e., atmospheric air pressure). Tympanometry is performed using a *tympanometer,* which generally is part of **immittance audiometry** that performs immittance assessments (see Figure 14–19).

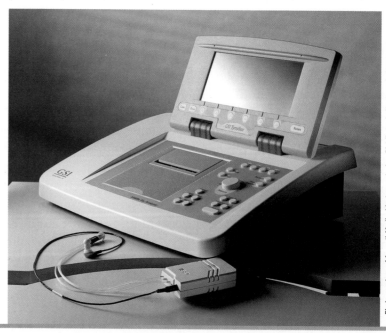

Figure 14–19

An immittance meter with insert earplugs (tips) for tympanometry.

During tympanometry assessment, an insert earplug is placed in one ear with a good seal obtained to prevent leakage of air pressure, creating a "closed system" with the earplug on one end of the canal and the tympanic membrane on the other. The tympanometer pumps air into the external ear canal to a particular level, creating a positive pressure against the tympanic membrane while measurements are taken by the tympanometer that reflect the compliance of the tympanic membrane (i.e., the ease of movement of the tympanic membrane under pressure). After the peak pressure and movement of the tympanic membrane are reached, the air pressure is decreased by the tympanometer and successive measurements are again taken. After the pressure in the external ear canal is again at atmospheric air pressure, the tympanometer creates negative pressure and additional compliance measurements are made. The purpose of tympanometry is to determine the point and magnitude of the greatest compliance of the tympanic membrane. These measurements are valuable in understanding the condition of the tympanic membrane and middle ear structures.

Evaluating the Functioning of the Cochlea and Auditory Nervous System

From the time acoustic stimuli reach the inner ear, what is transmitted to the brain is not "sound" but rather a series of *neuroelectrical* impulses. Measurement of the electrical responses generated within the cochlea establishes an objective measure of hearing sensitivity. *Electrocochleography* (ECoG) was developed to measure the electrical responses generated within the cochlea. In addition, whenever a sound is heard (perceived) by a person, there is some change in the ongoing electrical activity of the brain. Because electrical signals are transmitted extremely rapidly, they are measured in terms of milliseconds (one-thousandth of a second). *Auditory evoked potential audiometry* has been developed to extract the tiny voltages (*electrical potentials*) produced in the brain by acoustic stimulation. Discussion of electrocochleography or auditory evoked potential and electrophysiological testing methods is beyond the scope of this text. Refer to Bess and Humes (2008), Martin and Clark (2012), Stach (2010), or any other audiology introductory text for a discussion of these assessment procedures.

AMPLIFICATION FOR INDIVIDUALS WITH HEARING IMPAIRMENTS

Audiological habilitation (for children who did not have hearing prelinguistically) or *rehabilitation* (for children and adults who developed speech and language before losing their hearing) usually encompasses the diagnosis of hearing loss and the provision of listening devices, often with the emphasis on follow-up of **hearing aids** and less on communication strategies and speech perception training (Tye-Murray, 2009).

hearing aid

Any electronic device (usually battery operated) designed to amplify and deliver sound to the ear and consists of a microphone, amplifier, and receiver.

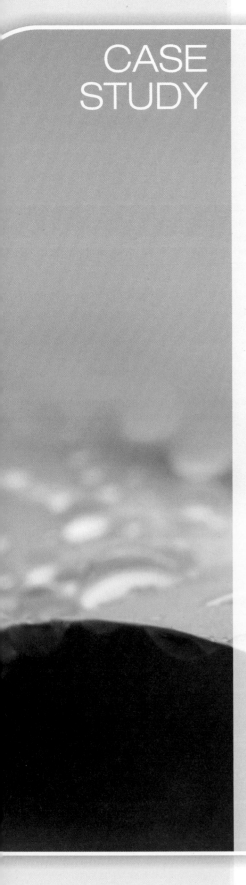

A Stroke and a Hearing Loss

A 23-year-old man sustained two hemorrhagic cerebrovascular accidents (CVAs) in an 18-month period. His first stroke involved the right temporal and parietal lobes and resulted in left arm and leg paresis. During his second stroke, he became confused and disoriented and began having seizures. His speech, language, and cognition were impaired, and for several days the patient had no hearing in either ear. During the 2nd week after the CVA, he began to hear loud sounds. Although he began to regain his hearing sensitivity, he could not understand conversational speech. About 6 months after the CVA, he could discern some speech in everyday situations, partly because of developing speechreading skills. Background noises were disturbing to him.

Computerized tomography (CT) scans and magnetic resonance imaging (MRI) revealed that both the right and the left hemispheres' Heschl's gyri and the temporal lobes were severely damaged by the two strokes. Audiological testing revealed profound central nervous system hearing losses bilaterally, likely caused by the severely damaged right and left Heschl's gyri. However, later pure-tone testing revealed fluctuating hearing losses bilaterally, and speech detection thresholds began to approach normal after several months. The patient did not begin to consistently understand single words until 14 months after the CVAs.

Long-term follow-up (over an 8-year period) indicated that this was a case of complete central deafness in that, initially, the patient could not perceive any environmental or speech sounds and had no response to standard pure-tone audiometric testing at the maximum output of the audiometer. The patient was young (23 years), which allowed him to benefit from plasticity of his brain for some recovery of auditory functions. Recovery of perception of environmental sounds (e.g., music) significantly preceded his ability to perceive speech sounds. The speech of familiar voices of people was more easily recognized than speech of unfamiliar speakers. As with many people who have impaired central auditory nervous systems, background noise, competing speech, and generally poor acoustics had a significant effect on his comprehension abilities. The partial recovery of this patient's central auditory nervous system was significantly enhanced by working with a speech-language pathologist on auditory identification and discrimination of speech sounds and adjusting the environment to decrease distracting background noises. Because of the long-term auditory rehabilitation, the efforts put forth by the patient, the speech-language pathologist, and the benefit of his young age and plasticity of his brain, the patient made significant progress in his communication abilities. (Adapted from Musiek, Baran, & Pinheiro, 1994.) ■

The fundamental goal of hearing rehabilitation is to limit the extent of any communication disorder that results from a hearing loss. The first step in reaching that goal is to maximize the use of *residual hearing.* That is, every effort is made to put the remaining hearing that a person has to its most effective use. Once this has been accomplished, treatment often proceeds with some form of aural rehabilitation (Mahshie, Moseley, Scott, & Lee, 2006; Stach, 2010; Tye-Murray, 2009). We begin our discussion where we began hearing assessment—with newborns.

Amplification for Infants

When an infant with a hearing impairment is identified before 3 months of age, the intervention process should begin before 6 months of age (Diefendorf, 2005; Yoshinaga-Itano & Gravel, 2001; Yoshinaga-Itano, Sedey, Coulter, & Mehl, 1998). This requires a comprehensive hearing evaluation as well as a team of professionals working closely with both the infant and the family (Munos, Nelson, Goldgewicht, & Odell, 2011). Over the course of a child's development, the professional team will likely include various pediatricians, otolaryngologists, audiologists, speech-language pathologists, early childhood specialists, social workers, counselors, educational psychologists, and special and regular educators. The head of the team is always the parents or primary caregivers— they are the ultimate determiners of what will or will not be done.

Federal law requires that when hearing loss is suspected in a newborn or young child, evaluation and early intervention services must be provided in accordance with the *Individuals with Disabilities Education Act (IDEA),* Part H (birth to 3 years of age) of Public Law 102-1119. The law provides for statewide, comprehensive, coordinated multidisciplinary, interagency programs of early intervention services for all children with disabilities and their families. In many cases, the professionals involved with the infant who has a hearing problem are more in tune to the reality of the problem than the parents.

The Role of the Parents and Family

Parent and family involvement with a newborn with a hearing impairment is crucial. The basic components related to early intervention include (1) counseling to support the parents' adaptation to the diagnosis and provide a forum in which they can express and work through their feelings; (2) fitting hearing aids to supplement the infant's impaired auditory reception; and (3) giving encouragement to early development of a rich symbolic communication system between the infant and the family (ASHA, 2008b; Bess & Humes, 2008; Tye-Murray, 2009).

Parental feelings must be considered and worked with before there can be successful intervention of the infant. Parents may not readily accept the diagnosis of a hearing loss or deafness of their baby. There may be few real signs of a hearing impairment and the parents must rely on the results of the audiologist's evaluation of the infant over several sessions. Most people have had no association with an audiologist and may not even know what an audiologist does. The parents now are expected to accept the diagnosis and take the recommendations from an unknown professional (and an unknown profession) that have turned their world upside down.

A family-centered treatment philosophy assumes that social support affects family functioning; the child's needs are best met by meeting the family's needs; and families have the right to retain as much control as they desire over the intervention process (Clark & English, 2004; Tye-Murray, 2009). We are, as always, working with the entire family constellation, and the person with the hearing loss is the center of the constellation.

Hearing Aids and Cochlear Implants for Infants and Young Children

Hearing aids or a cochlear implant should be considered and possibly provided as soon as the audiologist is firmly convinced that a hearing loss is present (Hayes & Northern, 1997; Katz, 2001; Mahshie et al., 2006). The evaluation and fitting of hearing aids is an ongoing process, and several changes may need to be made before the "final" fitting. In addition, if the infant or child has a progressive sensorineural loss, periodic monitoring and adjustments in aids will likely be required.

Binaural ear-level hearing aids are available in small sizes to fit behind the ears. The older, bulky body-type hearing aids with cord and external receiver are now seldom used. The newer aids are custom fitted and electronically tuned for the specific pattern of hearing loss identified for each ear. The audiologist may need to adjust the limit of the *gain* (the difference between the input signal and the output signal) of the hearing aids because aids that provide too much intensity (sound pressure level) may potentially cause further hearing loss. *Ear molds* can be made for an infant, but because of growth of the infant they need to be remade every few months.

Although it is the infant or young child who wears the hearing aids, it is the parents who are responsible for their care and daily use. The parents need to be willing and able to take on this critical responsibility (regretfully, not all parents are). Hearing aids and the batteries that power them are serious potential swallow hazards and careful monitoring of the infant and child is needed to be certain they are not ingested. In addition, parents or other caregivers need to be certain that the hearing aids are positioned correctly in the child's ear or ears, kept clean and dry, are in good working order, and have good batteries.

In addition to hearing aids, cochlear implants are the latest technology that has been developed to help young children with profound bilateral sensorineural hearing loss. Cochlear implants have been successfully used with children as young as 10 months of age (Hayes & Northern, 1997; Tomblin, Barker, Spencer, Zhang, & Gantz, 2005). For young children to be candidates for cochlear implants, they need to have normal intelligence, not have other handicaps that would contraindicate their use, and have dedicated family support (Cohen & Waltzman, 1996).

Application Question

What might be your reaction and feelings if you were a new parent and your infant was diagnosed as deaf or hard of hearing?

Application Question

If your infant or young child had to wear hearing aids, how might you prevent the child from accidentally swallowing an aid or battery?

Hearing Aids for Children and Adults

Attempts to amplify sound have existed as long as people have cupped their hands behind their ears to momentarily improve their hearing. What we consider primitive attempts at mechanical devices to improve hearing were "high tech" in their early days of development. Likewise, what we consider state-of-the-art now will someday be considered crude attempts at sophisticated technology. The advent of miniature batteries allowed behind-the-ear hearing aids and in-the-temple eyeglass hearing aids. The development of microbatteries and microprocessors allows in-the-ear aids and now aids completely in the ear canal. The following provides a basic understanding of hearing aids.

Components of Hearing Aids

A hearing aid is a miniature electronic amplifier that has three main components: a microphone, an amplifier, and a speaker (receiver). A battery is the power source and a volume adjuster (*gain control* or *attenuator*) allows the wearer to increase or decrease the hearing aid gain. The microphone is a vibrator that moves in response to the pressure waves of sounds in the environment (much like a person's tympanic membrane). The electrical signal is boosted by the amplifier and then delivered to the speaker. The speaker then converts the electrical signal back into an acoustic signal to be delivered to the person's eardrum.

Conventional Hearing Aids

Figure 14–20 shows the four most common styles of hearing aids used today:

- Behind the ear (BTE)
- In the ear (ITE)
- In the canal (ITC)
- Completely in the canal (CIC)

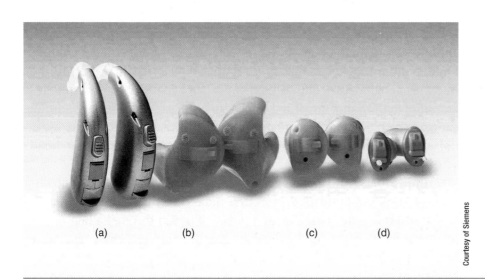

(a) (b) (c) (d)

Courtesy of Siemens

Figure 14–20

Four common types of hearing aids: (a) behind the ear (BTE), (b) in the ear (ITE), (c) in the canal (ITC), and (d) completely in the canal (CIC).

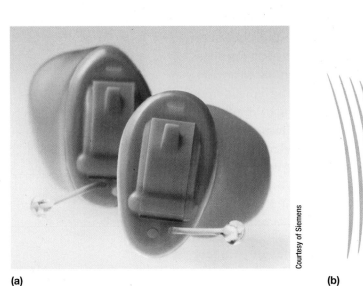

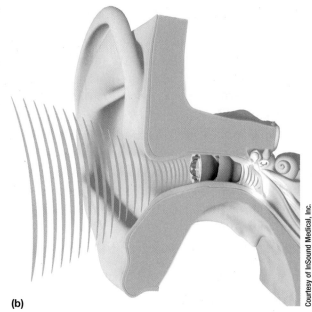

(a)   (b)

Figure 14-21

(a) A completely-in-the-canal (CIC) hearing aid. (b) The Lyric is the first hearing aid designed to fit deep in the ear canal and be invisible from the outside. It can be worn for up to three months without removal or replacement.

Application Question

If you had to wear a hearing aid, which type do you think you might prefer? Why?

A BTE hearing aid is worn over the ear and is held in place by a plastic "hook" that fits over the top of the ear. The amplified sound is delivered to the ear canal through a tube that leads to a custom-fitted ear mold. An ITE hearing aid is in a custom-fitted case that fits into the outer ear. An ITC hearing aid is a smaller version of an ITE, which fits mostly into the ear canal. A CIC hearing aid is an even smaller version of an ITE and is custom-fitted to sit 1 to 2 mm (approximately ¼ inch) inside the opening of the ear canal so that it is almost invisible.

The CIC type is the smallest and most inconspicuous hearing aid available at this time (see Figure 14-21). It is designed for mild-to-moderate hearing losses. The CIC aids have some advantages over larger aids. Because they sit completely in the ear canal, they receive the natural benefit of the auricle's collection and resonance properties that enhance sound in the higher frequencies, which is particularly helpful in understanding speech in background noise. Because CIC aids sit further into the ear canal, they allow better sound localization. They require less amplifier gain than a larger aid to produce the same amount of amplification, which also permits increased battery life. CIC aids reduce wind noise, improve ease of telephone use, and enhance listening with headsets (Martin & Clark, 2012; Strom, 2004).

Individuals who have incurred a sudden hearing loss following trauma or use of ototoxic drugs often benefit from auditory training to adjust to a radically altered listening state. Speech through a hearing aid may sound different from how they remember it, and they must learn to interpret what they hear. After successful fitting of a hearing aid, individuals benefit from support and training to maximize the benefits of the aid.

Assistive Listening Devices

Amplification systems other than conventional hearing aids have been designed for more specific listening situations. These devices are known as **assistive listening devices** (ALDs). Among the devices considered ALDs are personal amplifiers, telephone listeners, and frequency modulation (FM) systems. All of these systems are designed to enhance speech signals over background noise by use of a remote microphone. That is, rather than the microphone being built into the same case as the amplifier and receivers as it is in hearing aids, it is separated in some way to close the physical distance between the speaker and the listener.

Some individuals choose ALDs to supplement their hearing aids in certain situations, for example, in the workplace. Some people need ALDs just when talking on the telephone, watching television, or attending church. Others may benefit from these devices because of auditory processing disorders when they have difficulty understanding speech in background noise, for example, in a classroom.

A *personal amplifier (pocket talker)* consists of a microphone connected by a cord to a case about the size of a deck of cards that houses the battery, amplifier electronics, and volume control. The microphone is held by the person who is talking. Typically a set of lightweight headphones or earbud transducers are worn by the listener (see Figure 14–22). By separating the microphone from the amplifier, it can be moved close to the speaker's mouth, which enhances the signal-to-noise ratio (i.e., there is more speech signal and less background noise). Many speech-language pathologists working in hospital settings carry their own personal amplifiers when going to see a patient with a known hearing loss. Many patients with hearing losses do not have their hearing aids with them, or their hearing aids have been lost.

Telephone amplifiers are popular ALDs and are available in several forms (see Figure 14–23). Some telephone handsets have built-in amplifiers with a volume control. Many portable telephone amplifiers can be attached to any phone. Telephone receivers also can be adapted

assistive listening device

Amplification systems, other than conventional hearing aids, that are designed for specific listening situations (e.g., personal amplifiers, telephone amplifiers, personal text telephones, and personal FM systems).

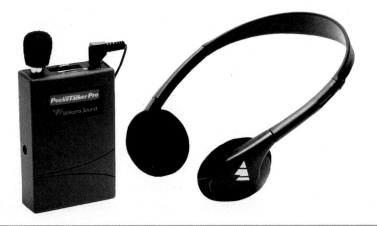

Courtesy of Williams Sound Corp.

Figure 14–22

A personal amplifier (pocket talker).

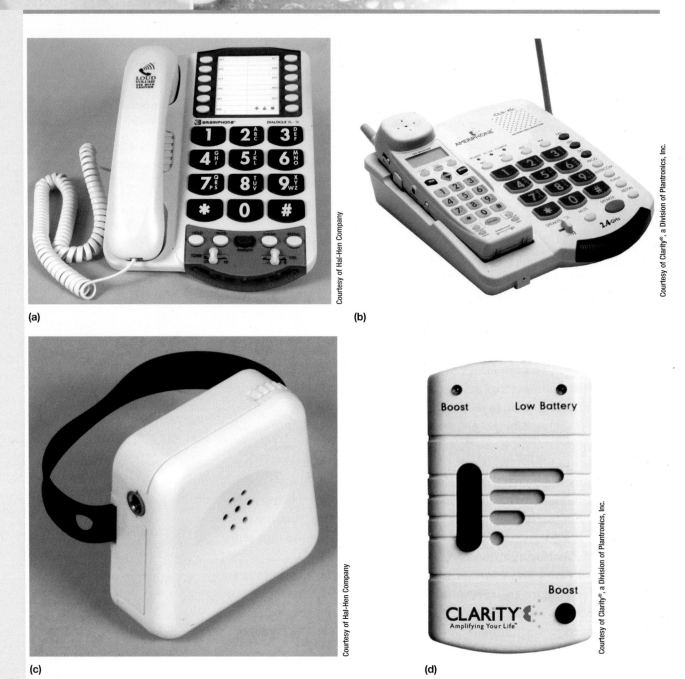

(a)
Courtesy of Hal-Hen Company

(b)
Courtesy of Clarity®, a Division of Plantronics, Inc.

(c)
Courtesy of Hal-Hen Company

(d)
Courtesy of Clarity®, a Division of Plantronics, Inc.

Figure 14-23

Examples of telephone amplifiers: (a) amplified telephone model XL-30, (b) built-in amplified telephone from Clarity®, (c) mini portable telephone amplifier, and (d) portable high-frequency amplifier.

to transmit over FM waves to a personal FM system. Telephones lines may be used to transmit text messages through a *personal text telephone* (TT) or *telecommunication device for the deaf* (TDD, also abbreviated TTY for teletypewriter) for a visual display of typed messages over the telephone, which are also available with printers (see Figure 14–24). *Text messaging* through cellular telephones is particularly easy and convenient for many hearing impaired individuals.

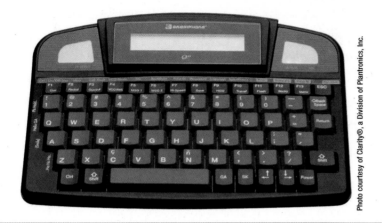

Photo courtesy of Clarity®, a Division of Plantronics, Inc.

Figure 14–24

The Ameriphone TTD is an example of a text telephone.

Personal FM systems consist of two parts, a microphone-transmitter and amplifier-receiver. The microphone is connected to, or is a part of, the case that contains the FM transmitter. The person who is talking (e.g., a teacher) wears the microphone and transmitter. Signals from the transmitter are sent to a receiver using FM radio waves. The listener wears the amplifier receiver, which acts like an FM radio and "picks up" the transmitted signal. The receiver is usually attached to the listener's ear by means of earphones or to hearing aid transmitter coils by means of a neck loop that transmits the signal. FM systems are particularly helpful for children with auditory processing disorders who find that normal classroom noises are distracting to them (Chermak & Musiek, 2007; Geffner & Ross-Swain, 2007; Tye-Murray, 2009). With the teacher wearing the microphone, the teacher's voice is no further away than her mouth from the child's ears. For individuals who also have hearing acuity problems, entire FM receiver systems can be integrated into conventional BTE or ITE hearing aids.

Other Assistive Devices for Hearing Impaired Individuals

Other assistive devices are available for hearing impaired people that do not amplify sound but add another modality to the stimulus; these include the following:

- *Closed captioning* provides written text to match the spoken words on a TV program.
- *Vibratory pagers* vibrate against the user to alert the person to an incoming telephone call that can be read as a text message.
- *Vibrating alarm clocks* have a vibrator that can be placed under the user's pillow.
- *Flashing alarm clocks* use a flashing lamp or strobe light to signal the alarm.
- A *doorbell signal* can be coupled to a lamp that flashes when the doorbell is rung.

Application Question

Have you ever spoken on the telephone with a person who is hard of hearing? What do you recall of the experience?

- A *smoke detector* can have a light that flashes a signal to alert for the presence of smoke.
- A *baby cry alert system* can have a flashing light with which a parent can be signaled if a baby begins to cry in another room.

These devices provide personal convenience for the hearing impaired, as well as some safety features for alerting of possible danger.

Cochlear Implants

Cochlear implants are the latest and most sophisticated devices to help children and adults with severe or profound bilateral hearing losses. Some individuals, however, benefit from having a cochlear implant in one ear while using a hearing aid in the other. Severe-to-profound deafness results from a loss of hair cell functioning in the cochlea. As a result, neural impulses are not generated and electrical activity in the auditory nerve is not initiated. Cochlear implants are designed to stimulate the auditory nerve directly.

The internal components of cochlear implants are the receiver and the electrode array. The surgery to insert a unilateral cochlear implant usually requires 2 to 3 hours and an overnight stay in the hospital. Under general anesthesia, a skin flap behind the auricle is elevated and a *partial mastoidectomy* performed (removing part of the mastoid bone directly behind the ear). The bone tissue removed makes room for the receiver component of the implant. The middle ear is entered, and the cochlea is opened. A tiny, flexible tube with an electrode array (up to 40 electrodes) is surgically implanted 22 to 24 mm (almost 1 inch) into the spiral tunnel of the cochlea (see Figure 14–25).

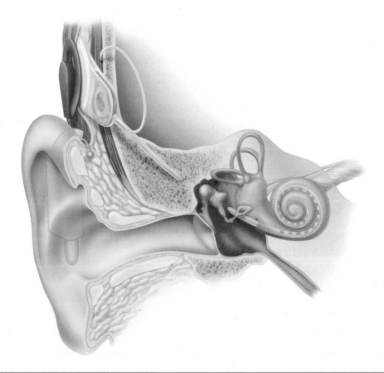

Figure 14-25

A view of the outer, middle, and inner ear, with an internal receiver and stimulator (electrode array) coiled in the cochlea.

Image courtesy of Cochlear Limited.

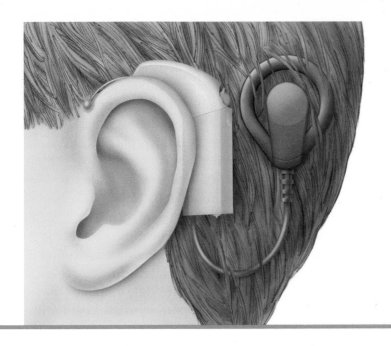

Figure 14-26

The external components with an ear-level speech processor and the transmitter, which is held in place by a magnet against the internal receiver. The transmitter is about the size of a nickel (20mm).

Image courtesy of Cochlear Limited.

The external components of a cochlear implant are similar to those of a conventional hearing aid (see Figure 14–26). The microphone is located in an ear-level device. Output from the microphone is routed to an amplifier that uses digital signal processing. The amplified signal is delivered to a receiver that sends signals to a transmitter coil. The transmitter coil has a magnet that holds it against the skin opposite the internal receiver. The signal is then transmitted electromagnetically across the skin. The receiver then transmits these signals to the proper electrodes in the array, where they can stimulate the intact auditory nerve fibers.

In sensorineural hearing impairments, although the hair cells are damaged, the auditory nerve fibers connected to the hair cells often remain intact. It is because of the intact auditory nerve fibers that cochlear implants can be successful. The nerve fibers can be stimulated to fire by applying the appropriate electrical currents using the cochlear implant. The actively propagated nerve impulses are sent through the auditory nerve and auditory pathway to the auditory cortex in the temporal lobe of the brain, where the impulses are interpreted as sound. Hearing success for the person improves with time and experience using a cochlear implant (Ertmer, 2005; Nicholas & Greers, 2003; Stach, 2010; Tye-Murray, 2009).

AURAL REHABILITATION

Aural rehabilitation is a broad term that involves intervention aimed at minimizing and alleviating the communication difficulties associated with hearing loss. It may include identification and diagnosis of hearing loss and communication handicaps, patient and family counseling and education, selecting and fitting amplification devices, communication

Application Question

If you were considering a cochlear implant for a hearing impairment, what questions might you ask the audiologist and the physician?

aural rehabilitation

A broad term that involves intervention aimed at minimizing and alleviating the communication difficulties associated with hearing loss; includes identification and diagnosis, patient and family counseling and education, selection and fitting amplification devices, communication training strategies, speech perception training, speech-language therapy, promotion of literacy, and educational management.

training strategies, speech perception training, speech-language therapy, promotion of literacy, and educational management (ASHA, 2008b). Aural rehabilitation not only includes assistance to improve or manage hearing loss but also includes emotional and social support for individuals with hearing loss and their families. For some people, a minor hearing loss can have significant, if not devastating, emotional and social effects on their lives, particularly if there is a rapid onset of loss with little time to adjust to it. For most older people, hearing loss is gradual and they make subtle adjustments to their losses until they or their family can no longer overlook or work around it (O'Neil, 2007).

Aural rehabilitation emphasizes three main areas: (1) understanding the individuals served by speech and hearing specialists; (2) providing them with appropriate professional support and counseling; and (3) maximizing their communication success in their everyday environments once they have received appropriate amplification (Mahshie et al., 2006; Tye-Murray, 2009). This portion of the chapter focuses on the third area.

Auditory Training

aural habilitation

Sometimes used synonymously with *aural rehabilitation*; intervention for people who have not developed listening, speech, and language skills; may include diagnosis of communication and hearing-related difficulties, speech perception training, speech and language therapy, manual communication, and educational management.

auditory training

Aural rehabilitation methods designed to optimize use of residual hearing by structured practice in listening, altering the environment, and use of hearing aids to increase sound awareness, sound discrimination, identification of words, and comprehension of spoken messages.

The goal of **aural habilitation** and **auditory training** for children with hearing loss is to develop their ability to recognize speech using auditory signals and to interpret auditory information (Tye-Murray, 2009). Auditory training helps children use their residual hearing to their maximum capability. Children should be fitted with appropriate amplification before starting an auditory training program. Hearing aids can enhance hearing, but the act of listening is a behavior that must be learned. In addition, auditory training will not change hearing sensitivity but will enhance a child's ability to use whatever sound is available. Children who are deaf since birth (*prelingual*) have no memory or concept of sound, but young children who acquire a hearing loss after developing some speech and language often have the concept and memory of sound, as well as some speech and language. The key elements to auditory training include detection, discrimination, identification, and comprehension (Hull, 2009).

Detection or Awareness of Sounds

Detection involves children becoming aware of sound and learning to attend to sounds. At the detection level, the child simply responds to the presence or absence of sound. For most hearing impaired children, this only occurs when there is adequate amplification. In addition, the parents play a crucial role in helping draw their child's attention to the linguistic and nonlinguistic sounds in the environment—for example, the mother pointing out to the child that he is hearing (as well as seeing) his daddy laugh or that the child is hearing the noisy blue jay bird in the backyard.

Discrimination of Sounds

Discrimination develops as children learn to perceive the differences in sounds. Suprasegmental discrimination of intensity, duration, pitch, and timing appear first. Discrimination allows children to tell whether auditory patterns are the same or different from others. How sounds differ and what sounds mean comes later in the child's development.

Identification of Sounds

Identification is the stage at which children can repeat or point to what sounds and words represent. Identification requires memory but not necessarily understanding of the sounds. It is when understanding accompanies memory that comprehension begins to develop.

Comprehension

Comprehension of speech and language is the most complicated stage of auditory development. Comprehension is a higher auditory skill level in which the child understands the meaning of spoken messages. Comprehension requires various areas of the brain to integrate the individual words in a message that express concepts that may require auditory, visual, tactile, smell, or taste sensory systems. For example, the word *popcorn* can conjure auditory sensations of the popping sounds; the visual sensations of the kernels before and after they pop; the olfactory sensation of freshly popped corn; the tactile sensations of warm popcorn in the hand and the feeling of crunching it between the teeth; and the taste sensations of delicious salted or buttered popcorn in the mouth.

Lipreading and Speechreading

During **lipreading**, a person relies only on the visual cues provided by the speaker's mouth and face for recognizing speech. For most people, this is a difficult task. Researchers have studied eye movement patterns during lipreading using instruments that track the center of the pupil. During **speechreading**, a person uses residual hearing and attends carefully to the speaker's visual messages (nonverbal communication, such as facial expressions and body language), clues from the setting of the conversation, and the likely conversational topics in the setting. Good lip-readers are likely good speech-readers. Normal-hearing people rely on speechreading in probably most conversations each day. Because people often are not tuned into every word that is said in a conversation, they use speechreading to fill in the "blanks" that they do not fill from an auditory message (Hull, 2009; Tye-Murray, 2009). The **oralism** philosophical approach in the education of the deaf maintains that language should be oral, that is, from the mouth, and sign language and teachers who are deaf should be excluded from the classroom.

lipreading

The process of recognizing speech using only the visual cues from the speaker's mouth and face.

speechreading

The process of recognizing speech by attending to the speaker's auditory and visual messages (nonverbal communication, such as facial expressions and body language), clues from the setting of the conversation, and the likely conversational topics in those settings.

oralism

A philosophy in the education of the deaf that maintains language should be oral, that is, from the mouth, and sign language and teachers who are deaf should be excluded from the classroom.

Application Question

Have you ever tried to read someone's lips while the person was talking? How difficult was it? How do you use speechreading in conversation?

Speech Skills

The speech skills of children with hearing impairments need to be determined. In Chapter 5, the section on Assessment of Articulation and Phonology provides general information for assessing speech intelligibility of children with hearing impairments. Standardized articulation and phonology tests are appropriate; however, it is particularly important to assess spontaneous, continuous speech to determine conversational intelligibility.

Goals for a comprehensive speech development program may include the following (Carney & Moeller, 1998; Hull, 2009; Tye-Murray, 2009):

- Increase vocalizations that have appropriate timing characteristics and that require numerous vocal tract movements
- Expand phonetic and phonemic repertoires
- Establish links between audition and speech production
- Improve suprasegmental aspects of speech
- Increase speech intelligibility

Phonetic and phonological process errors are targeted in therapy. Therapy goals, for example, may focus on increasing a child's phonetic repertoire and reducing phonological process errors. Auditory modeling, often combined with visual and tactile input, is used extensively.

Ling (1976) developed a program based on the premise that there is a hierarchy of speech skills. The most effective and efficient way to learn these is to build new skills on existing skills. For example, a child should be able to rapidly say a sequence such as *bee-bee-bee-bee* before being expected to say a sequence such as *bee-boo-bee-boo*. Following a natural sequence of progression in therapy allows hearing impaired children to develop speech skills in a similar sequence as normal-hearing children.

Language Skills

The language skills of children with hearing impairments need to be determined. Analyzing a child's receptive and expressive language using language samples can be informative. Therapy goals in language development may include the following (Carney & Moeller, 1998; Hull, 2009; Tye-Murray, 2009):

- Increase communication between parents and child
- Promote an understanding of complex concepts and discourse units
- Enhance vocabulary growth
- Increase world knowledge
- Enhance self-expression
- Enhance growth in use of language syntax and pragmatics
- Develop narrative skills

Therapy goals are often based on information about the language development of normal-hearing children. For preschool children, the emphasis may initially be on vocabulary development and simple sentences. For school-age children, the focus is on development of syntax and semantics. Throughout therapy, form, content, and pragmatics are developed. *Naturalistic methods* are typically used in which language instruction optimizes everyday events and structuring the environment so that certain events occur to promote the growth of form, content, and pragmatics.

Sign Language and Manual Communication

The use of gestures and hands, as well as facial expressions and body language, are as much a part of natural communication as is speaking. Facial expressions (*microgestures*) and gestures of the hands, arms, and body posture (*macrogestures*) are used almost unconsciously in everyday conversation for illustration, emphasis, and emotional content. *Nonverbal communication* or *body language* has been recognized as a form of communication since the beginning of human communication. In a way, it is our first language. Infants communicate with parents through facial expressions and body language long before they can communicate with spoken words. Likewise, infants recognize their parents' nonverbal communications before they clearly recognize the meanings of words and sentences.

Sign language is a natural form of communication for many deaf children and adults when communicating among themselves. Sign language has two main forms of communicating with the fingers and hands: finger spelling and signing. **Finger spelling** is the use of certain finger and hand shapes to represent letters of the alphabet and spell individual words. Sign language is a visual means of communication using hand and arm shapes and gestures to represent words and concepts, along with some finger spelling. Sign language users typically use the force or speed of a sign along with facial expressions to help communicate the emotional content of their messages (e.g., No! or Stop!). Sign language does not depend on spoken language and is used within Deaf communities and learned naturally by interaction with other signers. **Manualism** is a philosophy in the education of the deaf that emphasizes the learning and use of sign language and finger spelling as a natural form of communication among the deaf.

Many countries have their own sign language systems (e.g., **American Sign Language** or **ASL**; British Sign Language, or BSL; Chinese Sign Language, or CSL; French Sign Language, or FSL; German Sign Language, or GSL; Swedish Sign Language, or SSL, etc.), and within countries there are often various systems of sign language used (e.g., in America there is ASL, Signing Exact English, Seeing Exact English, and others). Many normal-hearing people take courses in sign language out

sign language

A visual means of communication using finger, hand, and arm shapes and gestures to represent words and concepts, along with some finger spelling; communication that does not depend on spoken language and is used within Deaf communities and learned naturally by interaction with other signers.

finger spelling

The use of certain finger and hand shapes to represent letters of the alphabet and spell individual words.

manualism

A philosophy in the education of the deaf that emphasizes the learning and use of sign language and finger spelling as a natural form of communication among the deaf.

American Sign Language (ASL)

A manual system of communication commonly used by members of the Deaf culture in the United States; sometimes referred to as *Ameslan*.

of interest or, in some cases, with the intention of becoming sign language interpreters in various settings where deaf individuals may be a part of a larger hearing community, such as in a church service.

ASL is unique to the Deaf community and is its own language that closely follows the French Sign Language system. A person does not use ASL and speak at the same time because ASL has a different grammar than spoken English. One ASL sign might represent a concept that would require several English words to express. Facial expressions and body language can impart a variety of shades of meanings to the signs. In both ASL and manually coded English, finger spelling may be used if there is no sign for a particular word or concept (Tye-Murray, 2009).

Manually coded English (*signed English*) is composed of manual signs corresponding to the words of English, and it has the same syntactic structures. Typically, a person using manually coded English speaks simultaneously while signing, signing each word that she says, including articles such as *the, a,* and *an.* The combined use of sign and speech as an educational philosophy is referred to as *simultaneous communication.*

The Deaf Community Today

(Note: In keeping with Woodward, 1972, *Deaf* with a capital "D" refers to a linguistic and cultural minority of people and *deaf* with a lowercase "d" is related to an audiometric hearing level.)

Normal-hearing people in countries around the world have long tried to determine how deaf individuals should communicate, and there are strong opinions from manualists and oralists. Some teachers of the deaf advocate that all deaf people need to learn and become proficient in speechreading to integrate within the normal-hearing community. On the other hand, manualists recognize that the **Deaf community** is a genuine culture (i.e., **Deaf culture**, and a culture in which they should take pride) and that they should be allowed to communicate in the language of their choosing and not be forced into being marginalized into the hearing world. Whether born into Deaf culture or enculturated later in life, the Deaf have chosen sign language as their primary method of communication and associate primarily with those who have made the same choice (Clark & English, 2004). Another opinion is that deaf individuals should learn sign language to communicate with one another but also learn speechreading and develop speech the best they can to communicate with hearing individuals to some degree (**total communication**).

Most children who are deaf have normal-hearing parents, and most deaf parents have children with normal hearing. Only about 10% of children born deaf have parents who are also deaf (Miles, 2005). Deaf children who have deaf parents are brought up learning the sign language of their parents as their first language. They become a part of the Deaf community from babyhood. Some deaf individuals can trace their deaf ancestors back generations.

In many communities around the world there are Deaf social clubs where sign language is the natural form of communication.

---

manually coded English

A form of communication in which manual signs correspond to English words and syntax.

Deaf community

Those deaf and hard of hearing individuals who share a common language (usually manual communication), common experiences and values, and a common way of interacting with each other and with hearing people.

Deaf culture

Ideology, beliefs, and customs shared by many individuals with prelinguistic deafness that may include communication, social protocol, entertainment, art, recreation, worship, and other aspects of culture.

total communication

A philosophy calling for every possible means of communication to be used by deaf individuals, including hearing aids and assistive devices, speechreading, signing, and spoken English.

Notable scenes in Deaf culture include the standing joke of the club committee trying to push people out at closing time and crowds standing around in the street signing for a good hour afterward, or of people of all ages staying up half the night together telling jokes and stories (a major part of Deaf culture), signing songs or poems or playing sign language games, or of a regional rally, where a town center is taken over by sign language for a weekend and people from all over the country greet old school friends across the street without a word spoken. Overall, although educators of the deaf may try to be multiculturally sensitive to various cultures and ethnic groups, they may still have difficulty accepting the natural communication system of the Deaf culture (Miles, 2005).

EMOTIONAL AND SOCIAL EFFECTS OF HEARING IMPAIRMENTS

The parents and family of newborns with hearing impairments have emotional reactions (challenges) to the news of their baby's loss and must work through the stages of grief (denial, anger, bargaining, depression, and acceptance). The emotional and social effects of hearing loss can be influenced by the different stages of life. Each stage (infancy, preschool, school age, adolescence, young adulthood, late adulthood, old age) has unique problems for both the hearing impaired person and the family (Tye-Murray, 2012).

Infants with hearing impairment do not respond normally to parent-initiated verbal play or attempts to be soothed when crying or distraught, leaving the parents feeling rejected, inadequate, and like failures. Infant–parent bonding can be significantly affected. Children with hearing loss are more likely than other children to have poor self-concepts, feel unlikeable, overly shy, and socially isolated. Hearing impaired adolescents feel covert or overt rejection from peers, and these feelings can continue throughout the rest of their lives (DeLuzio & Girolametto, 2011; Hull, 2009; Tye-Murray, 2009; Tye-Murray, 2012).

Young adults who have acquired hearing losses from listening to very loud music (Shafer, 2006) or being exposed to loud noises (e.g., from being in the military [Chandler, 2006]), or from traumatic brain injuries from motor vehicle accidents typically feel angry and frustrated. Acquired hearing loss during the early years of adulthood causes many people to reevaluate their life expectations and goals. Adults with severe-to-profound hearing losses often feel that they do not fit into any social group: they are not part of the Deaf community because they have a newly acquired hearing loss, and they are no longer comfortably a part of their normal social group because they are out of touch with normal conversation. Compared to normal hearing elderly people, elderly people with hearing losses who choose not to wear hearing aids or are unable to get them report feeling more sad or depressed, anxious, insecure, irritable, fearful, tense, and isolated (National Council on Aging, 1999) (see Figure 14–27).

- DO be facially expressive when communicating.
- DO NOT break eye contact when communicating with Deaf people. Lack of eye contact is considered rude when communicating with a visually oriented person.
- DO get a Deaf person's attention by tapping the shoulder, waving your hand in the person's line of sight, blinking the lights, and so on.
- DO NOT take offense at direct questions regarding qualifications or personal life. Direct questions between one Deaf person and another Deaf person are culturally quite common and can spill over into interactions with hearing people with no attempt to be rude.
- DO be conscious of hearing-loss terminology. Within Deaf culture, the norm is *profound deafness* and a *mild hearing loss* may mean "hard of hearing" to the Deaf person.
- DO NOT touch the Deaf person's hands while that person is signing.
- DO define Deaf individuals by their abilities rather than their disabilities—for example, not by their inability to perform well on a standard speech-reception test, but rather by their abilities in auditory pattern perceptions or environmental sound identification.
- DO NOT talk with another hearing person in the presence of a Deaf person without signing or ensuring a clear line of sight for speechreading. Just as those with acquired hearing loss may be suspicious when they do not understand what others are saying, so may Deaf individuals. Use sign language, use written communication, or ensure the Deaf person can speech-read what is said.
- DO attempt to use sign language with the Deaf. Any attempt is appreciated, but if you are not fluent, the services of an interpreter should be obtained.
- DO NOT use the term *oral* as it implies oral ideologies (*oralists*). Rather, use the term *spoken English* or *spoken communication*. Similarly, *communication training* may be preferred to *aural rehabilitation* because the former implies improvements in aspects of communication, such as written communication, that are not aurally based.

Figure 14-27

Some dos and don'ts when communicating with deaf and hard of hearing people and individuals in the Deaf community.

Adapted from Kaplan, 1996.

Multicultural Considerations

Clark and English (2004) state that audiologists often feel insecure in their counseling interactions with the hearing impaired and even more so when working with multicultural patients. In addition, the Deaf culture is nearly as foreign to audiologists as might be any other cultural group, and few audiologists are fluent in sign language. Clark and English (2004, p. 173) further state:

> Our own [audiology] professional culture and its very trappings are diametrically opposed to the Deaf culture. Audiologists are heavily steeped within a pathology model of health care. We perform diagnostic measures to characterize hearing loss, assess the impact of hearing loss on the individual and family, help those with hearing loss find effective means to overcome the negative impact of the loss with which they suffer, and refer to those we see as "patients."

In contrast, the Deaf culture views deafness as a difference and not as a pathology, disorder, or defect that needs treatment. A person is considered a member of the Deaf culture not on the basis of an audiometric profile but rather on the basis of a chosen identity through adoption of its values, practices, and natural language—signing (Kaplan, 1996). To be a part of the Deaf community does not require deafness. Many normal-hearing individuals are fluent signers and are actively involved in the Deaf culture, including being proponents of its goals and causes.

Just as there are minority groups within the hearing community, there are minority groups in the Deaf community, and these groups can have as much diversity in cultural values and beliefs as any multicultural group. The common denominator among these heterogeneous and international communities is that they all use sign language (Schirmer, 2001; Clark & English, 2004). Just as racial and cultural status among people with normal hearing can affect a person's socioeconomic status, being a minority within a minority in the Deaf community tends to have a far greater effect (MacLeod-Gallinger, 1993; Schirmer, 2001).

Application Question

What are some things you could do to become involved in the Deaf culture?

CHAPTER SUMMARY

The hearing mechanism and auditory system are remarkable in their simplicity and complexity. They take physical energy (i.e., acoustic air pressure waves) and transform it into chemical and electrical activity to allow us to hear the world around us. The physical processing of acoustic information occurs in the outer, middle, and inner ear. Physiological processing begins primarily in the inner ear and continues along the auditory nerve (VIII cranial nerve) to the central auditory nervous system.

Hearing loss is the most common of all physical impairments. A hearing loss can involve a communication handicap with psychosocial disadvantages, including delays in development of speech, language, social skills, and educational achievement. There are two primary types of hearing impairments in children and adults: hearing sensitivity impairments and auditory nervous system impairments. Hearing sensitivity impairments and peripheral hearing loss are the most common type of hearing loss. When the sensory or neural cells or their connections within the cochlea are absent or not functioning normally, a sensorineural hearing loss occurs. When both the conductive mechanism (outer ear, middle ear, or both) and the cochlea are not functioning normally, there is a mixed hearing loss.

The main purpose of a hearing evaluation is to define the nature and extent of the hearing impairment. From this information, decisions can be made about appropriate steps in the rehabilitation of the hearing disorder and handicaps that may result from the impairment. The fundamental purpose of an audiological evaluation is similar for most children and adults, although the specific focus of the evaluation can vary considerably depending on the nature of the individual and the problem. Screening the hearing of newborn infants is now a routine procedure in many hospitals and is both beneficial and justifiable. Detection of hearing loss in newborns may help alert medical professionals to the possibility of other complications.

The fundamental goal of hearing rehabilitation is to limit the extent of any communication disorder that results from a hearing loss. The first step in reaching that goal is to maximize the use of residual hearing.

A hearing aid is a miniature electronic amplifier that has three main components: a microphone, an amplifier, and a speaker. Cochlear implants are the latest and most sophisticated devices to help children and adults with severe or profound bilateral hearing losses. Sign language has two main forms of communicating with the fingers and hands: finger spelling and signing. The Deaf community is a genuine culture and the community has chosen sign language as its primary method of communication.

STUDY QUESTIONS

Knowledge and Comprehension

1. Describe the tympanic membrane and its functions.
2. Explain pure-tone audiometry.
3. Explain the three major types of hearing impairments seen in children and adults.
4. What are the adenoids and how might they contribute to middle ear infections and mouth breathing?
5. Briefly explain aural rehabilitation.

Application

1. How might you explain the hearing mechanism to a client?
2. What are the signs and symptoms of middle ear infections that you might alert a parent to watch for in her child?
3. What can you do to protect your hearing?
4. What are some emotional challenges (reactions) parents may have when an infant is diagnosed with a hearing impairment, and what treatment philosophy may be most helpful when working with parents?
5. What are five dos and don'ts when relating to culturally Deaf people?

Analysis/Synthesis

1. Explain the similarities and differences between air conduction and bone conduction.
2. Compare and contrast a conductive hearing loss and a sensorineural hearing loss.
3. What are the similarities and differences between otitis media with effusion and dormant otitis media?
4. What are the differences between audiologists' professional culture and the Deaf culture?
5. How might hearing impairments affect young adults and older adults emotionally and socially?

REFERENCES

Agrawal, Y., Platz, E. A., & Niparko, J. K. (2008). Prevalence of hearing loss and differences by demographic characteristics among US adults. *Archives of Internal Medicine, 168*(14), 1522–1530.

Allen, T. E. (1986). Patterns of academic achievement among hearing impaired students: 1973–1974. In A. N. Schildroth & M. A. Karchmer (Eds.), *Deaf children in America.* San Diego, CA: College-Hill Press.

Amatuzzi, M. G., Northrop, C., Bento, R. F., & Eavey, R. (2005). Histopathological patterns of hearing loss. *International Archives of Otorhinolaryngology, 9*(3), 213–219.

American Industrial Hygiene Association. (2007). Available at http://www.aiha.org/Content/AccessInfo/consumer/.

American Speech-Language-Hearing Association. (2008a). *Incidence and prevalence of hearing loss and hearing aid use in the United States—2008 edition.* Rockville, MD: ASHA.

American Speech-Language-Hearing Association. (2008b). *Guidelines for audiologists providing adjustment counseling to families of infants and young children with hearing loss birth to 5 years of age.* Available from www.asha.org/policy.

Bamford, J., & Saunders, E. (1985). *Hearing impairment, auditory perception, and language disability.* London: Edward Arnold.

Barton, G., Davis, A., Mair, I., Parving, A., Rosenhall, U., & Sorri, M. (2001). Provision of hearing aid service: A comparison between the Nordic countries and the United Kingdom. *Scandinavian Audiology, 30*(3), 16–20.

Bellis, T. (2003). *Assessment and management of central auditory processing disorders in the educational setting: From science to practice* (2nd ed.). Clifton Park, NY: Delmar Cengage Learning.

Bess, F. H., & Humes, L. E. (2008). *Audiology: The fundamentals* (3rd ed.). Philadelphia, PA: Lippincott Williams & Wilkins.

Campbell, K. C. M. (2007). *Pharmacology and ototoxicity for audiologists.* Clifton Park, NY: Delmar Cengage Learning.

Carney, A., & Moeller, M. P. (1998). Treatment efficacy: Hearing loss in children. *Journal of Speech, Language, and Hearing Research, 41*(Supplement), S61–S84.

Chandler, C. W. (2006, July 11). Blast-related ear injury in current U.S. military operations: Role of audiology on the interdisciplinary team. *The ASHA Leader.*

Chen, W., Campbell, C., Green, G., Van Den Bogaert, K., Komodikis, L., Manolidis, et al. (2002). Linkage of otosclerosis to a third locus (OTSC3) on human chromosome 6p21.3-22.3. *Journal of Medical Genetics, 39,* 473–477.

Chen, W., Lin, C., Hwang, Y., & Ku, C. (2003). Epidemiology of otitis media in Chinese children. *Clinical Otolaryngology and Allied Sciences, 28*(5), 442–445.

Chermak, G. D., & Musiek, F. E. (2007). *Handbook of (central) auditory processing disorders: Comprehensive intervention* (Vol. II). San Diego, CA: Plural Publishing.

Clark, J. G., & English, K. M. (2004). *Counseling in audiologic practice: Helping patients and families adjust to hearing loss.* Boston, MA: Pearson Allyn and Bacon.

Cohen, N., & Waltzman, S. (1996). Cochlear implants in infants and young children. *Seminars in Hearing, 17*(2), 215–222.

Davis, A., & Refaie, A. E. (2000). Epidemiology of tinnitus. In R. Tyler (Ed.), *Tinnitus handbook.* Clifton Park, NY: Delmar Cengage Learning.

DeLuzio, J., & Girolametto, L. (2011). Peer interactions of preschool children with and without hearing loss. *Journal of Speech, Language, and Hearing Research, 54,* 1197–1210.

Diefendorf, A. O. (2005). Early hearing detection and intervention: New ASHA guidelines available on children, ages birth to 5. *The ASHA Leader, 7,* 13.

Ertmer, D. J. (2005). *The source for children with cochlear implants.* East Moline, IL: LinguiSystems.

Forner, L., & Hixon, T. (1977). Respiratory kinematics in profoundly hearing-impaired speakers. *Journal of Speech and Hearing Research, 66,* 383–408.

Geffner, D., & Ross-Swain, D. (2007). *Auditory processing disorders: Assessment, management and treatment.* San Diego, CA: Plural Publishing.

Gold, S. L. (2003). Clinical management of tinnitus and hyperacusis. *ASHA Leader,* Nov. 4–5, 23–25.

Golding-Meadow, S., & Mayberry, R. I. (2001). How do profoundly deaf children learn to read? *Learning Disability Research and Practice, 16,* 222, 229.

Harris, J. D. (1986). Anatomy and physiology of the peripheral auditory system. In *The Pro-Ed studies in communication disorders.* Austin, TX: Pro-Ed.

Hayes, D., & Northern, J. L. (1997). *Infants and hearing.* Clifton Park, NY: Delmar Cengage Learning.

Hixon, T. J., Weismer, G., & Holt, J. D. (2008). *Preclinical speech science: Anatomy, physiology, acoustics, perception.* San Diego, CA: Plural Publishing.

Hoover, A., & Krishnamurti, S. (2010). Survey of college students' MP3 listening: Habits, safety issues, attitudes, and education. *American Journal of Audiology, 19,* 73–83.

Hull, R. H. (2009). *Introduction to aural rehabilitation.* San Diego, CA: Plural Publishing.

Isaacson, J. E., & Vora, N. M. (2003). Diagnosis and treatment of hearing loss. *American Family Physician, 68*(6), 1125–1134.

Jerger, J., & Musiek, F. (2000). Report of the consensus conference on the diagnosis of auditory processing disorders in children. *Journal of the American Academy of Audiology, ii,* 467–474.

Kaplan, H. (1996). The nature of Deaf culture: Implications for speech and hearing professionals. *Journal of the Academy of Rehabilitative Audiology, 25,* 71–84.

Katz, J. (2001). *Handbook of clinical audiology.* Philadelphia, PA: Lippincott Williams & Wilkins.

Katz, J., Medwetsky, L., Burkard, R., & Hood, L. (2009). *Handbook of clinical audiology.* Philadelphia, PA: Lippincott Williams & Wilkins.

Klein, J. O. (2000). The burden of otitis media. *Vaccine, 8*(19), 2–8.

Kraemer, M., Richardson, M., Weiss, N., Furukawa, C., Shapiro, G., Pierson, W., & Bierman, C. (1983). Risk factors for persistent middle ear effusions. *Journal of the American Medical Association, 249,* 1022–1025.

Lee, K. (2012). Language and children with auditory impairment. In V. A. Reed, *An introduction to children with language disorders* (4th ed.). Boston: Pearson Allyn & Bacon.

Ling, D. (1976). *Speech and hearing-impaired child: Theory and practice.* Washington, DC: Alexander Graham Bell Association for the Deaf.

Lutter, S., Currie, M., Mitz, L., & Greenbaum, L. (2005). Antibiotic resistance patterns in children hospitalized for urinary tract infections. *Archives of Pediatric and Adolescent Medicine, 159*(10), 924–928.

MacLeod-Gallinger, J. (1993). *Deaf ethnic minorities: Have they a double liability?* Paper presented at the annual meeting of the American Educational Research Association, Rochester, NY: Office of Postsecondary Career Studies in Deafness, National Technical Institute of the Deaf.

Mahshie, J., Moseley, M. J., Scott, S. M., & Lee, J. (2006). *Enhancing communication skills of deaf and hard of hearing children in the mainstream.* Clifton Park, NY: Delmar Cengage Learning.

Mann, T., Cuttler, K., & Campbell, C. (2001). Newborn hearing screens may give a false sense of security. *Journal of the American Academy of Audiology, 12,* 215–219.

Martin, F. N., & Clark, J. G. (2009). *Introduction to Audiology* (10th ed.). Boston, MA: Pearson Allyn and Bacon.

Miles, D. (2005). *British Sign Language: A beginner's Guide.* London: BBC Books.

Mohr, P. E., Feldman, J. J., Dunbar, J., McConkey-Robbins, A., Niparko, J., Rittenhouse, R., & Skinner, M. (2000). The societal costs of severe to profound hearing loss in the United States. *International Journal of Technology Assessment in Health Care, 16*(4), 1120–1135.

Moore, M. (2010, September 21). Teens at risk: We're on the edge of an epidemic: Research on hearing loss has long-term implications for audiologists. *The ASHA Leader.*

Mosby. (2009). *Mosby's dictionary of medicine, nursing, & health professions* (8th ed.). St. Louis, MO: Mosby Elsevier.

Munos, K., Nelson, L., Goldgewicht, N., & Odell, D. (2011). Early hearing detection and intervention: Diagnostic hearing assessment practices. *American Journal of Audiology, 20,* 123–131.

Musiek, F. E., Baran, J. A., & Pinheiro, M. L. (1994). *Neuroaudiology case studies.* Clifton Park, NY: Delmar Cengage Learning.

Musiek, F. E., & Chermak, G. D. (2007). *Handbook of (central) auditory processing disorders: Auditory neuroscience and diagnosis* (Vol. I). San Diego, CA: Plural Publishing.

Nadler, N. (1997). Noisy toys: Hidden hazards. *Hearing Health,* November/December, 18–21.

National Council on Aging. (1999). *The consequences of untreated hearing loss in older persons.* Washington, DC: National Council on Aging.

National Information Center for Children and Youth with Disabilities. (2004, January). *Deafness and hearing loss* (Pub. No. FS3). Washington, DC: Author.

National Institute of Deafness and Communication Disorders. (2002). Report of the ad hoc committee on epidemiology and statistics in communication. Bethesda, MD: National Institutes of Health.

Nicholas, J. G., & Greers, A. E. (2003). Personal, social, and family adjustment in school-aged children with cochlear implants. *Ear and Hearing, 24,* 69–81.

Northern, J. L., & Downs, M. P. (2012). *Hearing in children* (6th ed.). Baltimore, MD: Lippincott Williams & Wilkins.

O'Neil, J. (2007). Audiologic/Aural rehabilitation is valued and necessary. *The ASHA Leader,* June 19, 5–6.

Pichora-Fuller, M. K. (1997). Language comprehension in older listeners. *Journal of Speech-Language Pathology and Audiology, 21,* 125–142.

Samore, M., Magill, M., Adler, S., Severina, E., Morrison, L., De Boer, L., Lyon, L., & Carroll, K. (2001). High rates of multiple antibiotic resistance in streptococcus pneumonia from healthy children living in isolated rural communities. *Pediatrics, 108*(4), 856–865.

Sandlin, R. E., & Olsson, R. T. (2000). Subjective tinnitus: Its mechanism and treatment. In M. Valente, H. Hossford-Dunn, & R. Roeser (Eds.), *Audiology treatment.* New York, NY: Thieme.

Schirmer, B. (2001). *Psychological, social, and educational dimensions of deafness.* Boston, MA: Allyn and Bacon.

Seikel, J. A., King, D. W., & Drumright, D. G. (2010). *Anatomy and physiology for speech, language, and hearing* (4th ed.). Clifton Park, NY: Delmar Cengage Learning.

Shafer, D. N. (2006, April 11). Noise-induced hearing loss hits teens: ASHA holds national press club event to highlight dangers of MP3 players, media coverage goes worldwide. *The ASHA Leader.*

Shargorodsky, J., Curhan, S. G., Curhan, G. C., & Eavy, R. (2010). Change in prevalence of hearing loss in U.S. adolescents. *Journal of the American Medical Association, 304*(7), 772–778.

Shirin, D. A., & Reed Susanne. (2005). Written language of deaf and hard-of-hearing students in public schools. *Journal of Deaf Studies and Deaf Education, 10*(3), 244–255.

Siegel, R. M., & Bien, J. P. (2004). Acute otitis media in children. *Pediatrics in Review, 25,* 187–193.

Stach, B. A. (2010). *Clinical audiology: An introduction* (2nd ed.). Clifton Park, NY: Delmar Cengage Learning.

Stiles, D. J., McGregor, K. K., & Bentler, R. A. (2012). Vocabulary and working memory in children fit with hearing aids. *Journal of Speech, Language, and Hearing Research, 55,* 154–167.

Strom, K. E. (2004, March). A brightening Future? A review of today's hearing instrument market. *Hearing Review.*

Tomblin, J. B., Barker, B. A., Spencer, L. J., Zhang, X., & Gantz, B. J. (2005). The effect of age at cochlear implant initial stimulation on expressive language growth in infants and toddlers. *Journal of Speech, Language, and Hearing Research, 48,* 853–867.

Tye-Murray, N. (2009). *Foundations of aural rehabilitation: Children, adults, and their family members* (3rd ed.). Clifton Park, NY: Delmar Cengage Learning.

Tye-Murray, N. (2012). Counseling for adults and children who have hearing loss. In L. V. Flasher & P. T. Fogle, *Counseling Skills for Speech-Language Pathologists and Audiologists.* Clifton Park, NY: Delmar Cengage Learning.

Tye-Murray, N., & Folkins, J. (1990). Jaw and lip movements of deaf talkers producing utterances with known stress patterns. *Journal of the Acoustical Society of America, 87,* 2675–2683.

Van Bereijk, W., Pierce, J., & David, E. (1960). Waves and the ear. *Science, 131* (339), 219–220.

Vaughn, L. (2005, February 8). Diagnosis and follow-up of hearing loss in infants. *ASHA Leader, 1,* 4.

Vinson, B. P. (2011). *Preschool and school-aged language disorders.* Clifton Park, NY: Delmar Cengage Learning.

Walker, J. D. (2003). *Universal newborn screening: Saving money, saving lives.* Annual meeting of the Texas Chapter of the American Academy of Pediatrics, Galveston, TX.

Wilson, P. L., & Roeser, R. J. (1997). Cerumen management: Professional issues and techniques. *Journal of the American Academy of Audiology, 8,* 421–430.

Woodward, J. (1972). Implications of sociolinguistic research among the deaf. *Sign Language Studies, 1,* 1–7.

Yoshinaga-Itano, C., & Gravel, J. S. (2001). The evidence for universal newborn hearing screening. *American Journal of Audiology, 10,* 62–64.

Yoshinaga-Itano, C., Sedey, A., Coulter, D., & Mehl, A. (1998). Language of early- and later-identified children with hearing loss. *Pediatrics, 102*(5), 1161–1171.

Epilogue

Congratulations! You have completed your introductory course on speech-language pathology and audiology and have read this textbook on the essentials of these professions—not an easy task. There likely were some surprises in what you learned about the professions. For one, there is much more to these professions than what anyone can imagine who has not studied them. The scope, breadth and depth of information that you will use as your daily base of knowledge includes understanding what is normal and what is abnormal about human communication. Within this understanding, you have knowledge of the anatomy and physiology of each of the speech systems: respiratory, phonatory, resonatory, articulatory, and auditory. You also have a foundational understanding of the neurology that makes the speech systems function independently and together.

Appreciating the complex interactions of these systems adds to the amazement of what it takes to understand the simplest messages we hear and to provide the simplest responses. Fortunately, in our everyday communication we are able to take all of these for granted and hardly give them a second thought. If we had to consciously think of all that takes place every second while we are communicating, we would be continually stumbling over our thoughts, words, and muscle movements that are required to talk.

Another surprise for many students is how much of the study of speech-language pathology and audiology can be applied to their everyday lives. To truly appreciate the knowledge you acquire, it helps to relate it to your personal life. From my perspective, studying speech-language pathology and audiology are the best majors for preparation for adult life and parenthood. You learn about normal and abnormal development of infants and children. You learn how to work with children one-on-one and in small groups of two or three. You learn how to motivate children to work hard to improve their communication and academic skills. You learn how to manage the sometimes delicate task of talking with parents about their concerns regarding their children. You learn how to work with adults and elderly people with a variety of neurological problems and the sensitive issues that accompany impairment or loss of communication abilities. You learn about the problems of hearing impairments at all ages and the effects on not only the person with a loss but the family. And you learn how to be a patient, active listener—a trained listener—which is perhaps the most important interpersonal skill you can develop. On a personal level, it is inevitable that sometime in your life you will be confronted with a few of the disorders discussed within this text. What problems you escape, someone you care about may not.

If you choose not to take further course work in speech-language pathology, consider that you can always draw on the information you have learned and apply it to yourself and people you care about when needed. There is also a possibility that you may be a resource to your family and friends by having some basic education in this area, as well as having a textbook that you can keep for reference. This textbook was written and designed to be "a keeper." The book can be a valuable reference when someone asks you a question that relates to anything you studied in the course. You cannot present yourself as an "armchair" speech-language pathologist or audiologist, but you can speak with some knowledge that could help another person recognize the importance of seeking help from a professional speech-language pathologist or audiologist who is state licensed and nationally certified. For example, over the years, you may refer to this text to refresh your memory on middle ear infections in your own children or problems in speech and language development. Some years down the line, you may be amid the "sandwich generation"—trying to raise your own family at the same time you are taking care of elderly parents or grandparents. Having an understanding of neurological disorders and dementia can help you communicate with medical and rehabilitation staff.

This text also was written to be "a keeper" for SLP and Aud majors. The extensive glossary was carefully developed to provide a resource for terms and definitions for students to have many of the important words used in our professional vocabularies. Another reason for holding on to this text is that it can be helpful when taking graduate courses. For example, when beginning a graduate course on neurological disorders, a quick rereading of Chapter 11, Neurological Disorders in Adults, will be an excellent memory refresher for many of the concepts you will learn in graduate-level textbooks. Likewise, rereading that chapter can get you off to a good start in the clinic with your first client who has had a CVA or TBI if you have not yet completed your coursework in that area. Clinical supervisors are impressed when they hear a student say, "I reread the chapter on neurological disorders in adults in the text we used in the intro course and I think I have a basic understanding of aphasia, but there is still a lot more for me to learn."

Beyond the academic preparation for your profession, so often it seems that when there is a fully qualified SLP or Aud in a family, that person becomes an important resource to other family members. SLPs and Auds know a considerable amount about the human body and various medical problems that can result in disorders and handicaps of various kinds. SLPs and Auds also learn how to negotiate many of the complexities of the medical system, including how to talk with doctors and nurses at a professional level. SLPs and Auds learn about the educational system and how to talk to and interact with teachers and administrators at a professional level—a valuable skill for parents.

Not to sound overly dramatic, but your education and training in speech-language pathology and audiology will change you for the better. Your best character traits will be enhanced. If you consider yourself a patient, understanding, caring, and insightful person, those traits will become stronger. Your character weaknesses may become apparent as well. For example, if you have difficulty tolerating ambiguity—not being able to handle knowing there are few absolutes when working with people who have complex problems—that trait will be magnified and will likely result in considerable frustration. Having disorders neatly contained in boxes with specific therapy approaches and techniques to help empty the boxes is an ideal that is not based on reality.

If communication disorders were mechanical problems where parts could be repaired or replaced, our work would be "cleaner." However, it is the human elements such as emotions, motivation, amount of physical energy, and even the will to want to improve that can make the difference in the success of therapy. The final section of each chapter in this text was always about the emotional and social effects of the disorder. No matter how much we know about a disorder, the variables that determine success in therapy often depend on the emotional makeup and social support of the people who need our help.

Finally, you the student and future clinician are an essential variable in a child's or an adult's success in therapy. If, while taking this course, you continually found it difficult to devote time to studying the material because it did not grab your interest, there is a reasonably good chance that this is not the kind of information you want to spend the next few years delving deeper into, much less spending decades working with. If, on the other hand, you found most chapters of study interesting and even fascinating and could hardly wait to reach the next chapter to see what lies in store, this could be the kind of information you could find endlessly intriguing and captivating. There is an added joy to life when your chosen profession never becomes boring or "old," where you are always interested in the new discoveries, want to learn new ways of viewing familiar problems, and can hardly wait to try new therapy procedures and materials on your clients and patients.

SLPs or Auds whom you happen to meet while on vacation or holiday any place in the country or the world are never strangers; you always have common bonds and things to talk about. It seems that SLPs and Auds never tire of talking about their favorite subject. I have seen people marvel at watching SLPs and Auds who have just met talk animatedly and with a sense of camaraderie about the subject that binds them together. The bottom line for SLPs and Auds is always the children and adults we are trying to help. The treatment approaches, techniques, and materials we use are merely tools for helping people communicate and improve their quality of life. It is hoped that your study of speech-language pathology and audiology further enhances *your* quality of life.

Best wishes to you all,
Paul T. Fogle, Ph.D., CCC-SLP

Glossary

A

abduct/abduction—The opening of the vocal folds away from the midline; (L. *abducto,* to take away).

accent—Usually considered the speech pronunciation and inflections used by nonnative American English speakers (foreign accent); (L. *ac-* [variation of *ad-*], to, + *cantus,* song; i.e., to sing).

acoustic trauma—Damage to hearing from a transient, high-intensity sound; (Gk. *akoustikos,* hearing, + *trauma,* wound).

acquired disorder—A disorder that begins after an individual has developed normal communication abilities, such as a hearing loss from loud noise exposure or a speech, language, or cognitive disorder caused by a traumatic brain injury; (L. *acquirere,* to seek in addition to; *dis,* apart or impaired, + *ordo,* rank).

activities of daily living (ADLs)—The normal activities and tasks people perform in the course of a day, such as ablutions (washing, bathing, brushing the teeth, toileting), dressing, and eating.

acute—Intense and of short duration, usually referring to a disease or injury; (L. *acutus,* sharp).

acute care hospital—A hospital where patients are treated for brief but severe episodes of illness, injury, trauma, or during recovery from surgery; (L. *acutus,* sharp; Old Ger. *chara,* lament; L. *hospitium,* guesthouse).

acute laryngitis/traumatic laryngitis—An abrupt, intense, and usually relatively brief inflammation of the mucous membrane lining in the larynx, accompanied by edema of the vocal folds with hoarseness and loss of voice that is often caused by severe vocal abuse.

adaptive behavior—The ability to act as independently and responsibly as other people of the same age and cultural background in everyday social and practical skills; includes conceptual skills (e.g., language and money concepts), social skills (e.g., following rules and pragmatics), and practical skills (e.g., dressing appropriately and work skills); (L. *adaptare,* to fit).

addition—The insertion of a sound or sounds not part of a word itself, such as *animamal* for *animal;* (L. *ad-,* before, + *dere,* to put).

adduct/adduction—The closing of the vocal folds toward the midline; (L. *adducto,* to bring to).

adenoids (pharyngeal tonsils)—Lymphoid tissue (tissue that produces lymphocytes, which are helpful in fighting infection) found on the pharyngeal wall in the nasal–pharyngeal region; begin to develop about 6 months of age and may continue to grow and possibly interfere with or occlude the openings of the Eustachian tubes; when enlarged, they may block the passage of air from the nasal cavity into the pharynx, preventing normal nasal breathing and requiring mouth breathing; sometimes removed to allow nasal breathing and help prevent middle ear infections; (Gk. *aden,* gland, + *eidos,* form; Gk. *pharynx,* throat, L. *tonsillae,* tonsil).

admittance—The ease and flow of energy transmission through a system; the reciprocal of impedance; (L. *admittere,* to allow in).

affect/affective—Relating to, arising from, or influencing feelings or emotions; *affect* is revealed by facial expressions, body posture and gestures, tone of voice, and choice of words; (L. *afficio,* to have influence on).

agrammatic/agrammatism—Impairment of the ability to produce words in their correct sequence and with all necessary morphemes; (Gk. *agrammatos,* unlearned; from *a-,* without, + *grammatikos,* letters).

agraphia—A disorder of writing resulting in difficulty writing letters, words, and sentences; (Gk. *a-,* without or loss of, + *graphos,* write).

air conduction—The transmission of sound to the inner ear through the external auditory canal and the structures of the middle ear; (L. *con* [variation of *com*], together, + *ducere,* to lead).

alexia (acquired dyslexia)—Impaired ability to read as the result of neurological damage; (Gk. *a-,* without or loss of, *dys,* impairment or disorder, + *lexis,* word; L. *acquirere,* to seek or obtain).

allophone—Slight variation in the way different people produce individual phonemes that can be affected by the initial, middle, or final position of a word, or what sounds precede or follow an individual phoneme; (Gk. *allos,* other or different, + *phonema,* sound).

alphabetic principle—Letters and combinations of letters represent speech sounds; speech can be turned into print; and print can be turned into speech; (L. *alpha,* letter *a,* + *beta,* letter *b;* L. *princep,* first or chief).

alveolar ridge—The upper portion of the mandible and the lower portion of the maxilla that contain sockets for the roots of the teeth; (L. *alveolus,* little hollow—in reference to the sockets for the teeth).

Alzheimer's disease (AD)—A disease that causes progressive dementia that usually begins after age 65 and in many cases is related to genetic factors that cause neuronal degeneration, cerebral atrophy, neurofibrillary tangles, neuritic plaques, white matter changes, and diminished neurotransmitters; characterized by decline in memory, intellect, disorientation, delusions, personality changes, and communication impairments (named after Alois Alzheimer, German neuropsychiatrist, 1864–1915).

American Sign Language (ASL)—A manual system of communication commonly used by members of the

Deaf culture in the United States; sometimes referred to as *Ameslan*.

American Speech-Language-Hearing Association (ASHA)—The professional organization that represents speech-language pathologists and audiologists and sets standards for their education, training, and certification. The organization was formerly called the American Speech and Hearing Association, and retained the ASHA abbreviation.

amyotrophic lateral sclerosis (ALS, Lou Gehrig's disease)—A rare, rapidly progressive degenerative disease of motor neurons that control movement of all muscle systems, including the speech systems; (Gk. *a-*, without, + *myo*, muscle, + *trophe*, nourishment; *latus*, side; *sklerosis*, hardening).

anarthria/anarthric—The complete inability to articulate or speak that is usually caused by brain lesions or damage to peripheral nerves that innervate the articulatory muscles; (L. *an-*, without, + Gk. *arthron*, joined; i.e., [speech] that is not joined).

anesthesia—The administration of a topical, local, regional, or general drug or agent capable of producing a partial or complete loss of sensation or consciousness; (Gk. *an-*, without or loss of, + *aisthesis*, feeling, sensation, or perception).

aneurysm—A localized dilation of a blood vessel wall, resulting in the thinning of the wall at that site (much like a balloon being blown up) and increasing the likelihood of hemorrhaging, especially with high blood pressure; (Gk. *aneurysma*, to dilate).

anomia—Impaired ability to retrieve (remember) names of people, places, or things, as well as to retrieve other parts of speech (e.g., verbs and adjectives) while speaking; (Gk., *a-*, without, + *noma*, name).

anomic aphasia—A syndrome whose primary feature is persistent and severe difficulty retrieving names of people, places, and objects, as well as all classes of words (e.g., verbs and adjectives); (Gk. *a-*, without or loss of, + L. *nomen*, name; *a-*, without or loss of, + *phasos*, to speak).

anosognosia—Decreased awareness of deficits or disabilities often seen in right-hemisphere damage; impairment of an individual's ability to relate to parts of the body; (Gk., *a*, without, + *nosos*, disease, + *gnosis*, knowledge).

anoxia—A complete lack of oxygen to the brain that is relatively rare and is usually caused by asphyxiation (e.g., near-drowning or loss of airway from choking) or inadequate blood circulation (e.g., heart attack) that results in unconsciousness and death of brain tissue; (Gk. *a*, without, + *oxys*, sharp).

aphasia (dysphasia)—A deficit in language processing that may affect all input modalities (auditory, visual, and tactile) and all output modalities (speaking, writing, and gesturing); (Gk. *a-*, without or loss of, + *phasos*, to speak; *dys*, impairment or disorder, + *phasos*).

aphonia—A complete loss of voice followed by whispering for oral communication that typically has psychological causes such as emotional stress; (Gk. *a-* without or loss of, + *phone*, voice).

apraxia of speech (speech apraxia, verbal apraxia, acquired apraxia)—A deficit in the neural motor planning and programming of the articulatory muscles for voluntary movements for speech in the absence of muscular weakness; primarily interferes with articulation and prosody; (Gk. *a-* loss, + L. *praxis*, movement or action).

arteriosclerosis—A common disorder characterized by thickening, hardening, and loss of elasticity of arterial walls as a result of build-up of atherosclerotic plaque, leading to decreased blood supply; (Gk. *arteria*, artery, + *sclerosis*, hardening).

articulation/articulator—In speech, the mandible, lips, tongue, and soft palate are the articulators; *articulation* refers to the movements of the articulators for speech sound production that involves accuracy in placement, timing, direction of movement, and pressure of the articulators on one another; the totality of motor processes involved in the planning and execution of speech; (L. *articulatus*, joined).

articulation disorder—The incorrect production of speech sounds due to faulty placement, timing, direction, pressure, speed, or integration of the movements of the mandible, lips, tongue, or velum; (L. *articulatus*, joined; L. *dis-* apart or impaired, + *ordo*, arrangement or group; i.e., arrangement apart from what is [normally] joined—misarticulated).

arytenoid cartilages—A pair of pyramid-shaped cartilages that sit on top of the posterior edge of the cricoid cartilage and rotate to open and close the vocal folds and pivot back and forth to help change the pitch of the voice; (Gk. *arytaina*, ladle, + *eidos*, form; L. *cartilago*, cartilage).

aspiration—A term in reference to material (food, liquid, saliva, etc.) penetrating the larynx and entering the airway below the true vocal folds; food or liquid entering the lungs rather than the stomach after the swallow; (L. *aspirare*, to breathe upon).

aspiration pneumonia—An acute inflammation of the lungs caused by foreign material (e.g., food or liquid) entering the lung tissue and resulting in infection; alveolar and bronchiole congestion with substances discharged from the alveolar walls as a protection against foreign material; (L. *aspirare*, to breathe upon; (Gk. *pneumon*, lung, + *-ia*, suffix meaning disease).

assessment—See *evaluation*.

assistive listening device—Amplification systems, other than conventional hearing aids, that are designed for specific listening situations (e.g., personal amplifiers, telephone amplifiers, personal text telephones, and personal FM systems); (L. *ad-*, to or toward, + *sistere*, take a stand or cause to stand).

atherosclerosis—A common disorder characterized by yellowish plaques of cholesterol and other lipids (fats) in the inner layers of the walls of arteries; often associated with tobacco use, obesity, hypertension, diabetes mellitus, and aging; (Gk. *athere*, meal, + *sklerosis*, hardening).

atrophy—A shrinking in size or wasting away that is usually caused by injury, disease, lack of use (e.g., muscles), or natural reduction in size over time (e.g., adenoids and tonsils); (Gk. *atrophia*, wasting away [*a-*, not, + *trophe*, nourishment]).

attainable treatment—The expectation that an individual can achieve a specific target within a reasonably specified time; (L. *at-*, before, + *tangere*, to touch, + *abilis*, capable; L. *tractare*, to handle or deal with, + *mentum*, result).

attention deficit/hyperactive disorder (AD/HD, ADD)—A broad syndrome relating to children who demonstrate three primary problems: inattention, impulsivity, and hyperactivity; (L. *addendere*, to stretch; *deficere*, to want; Gk. *hyper-*, excess, + L. *activus*, active).

attention impairments—Difficulty staying focused on a task, difficulty appropriately shifting attention from one task to another, and dividing attention between auditory and visual stimuli; (L. *prejorare*, make worse).

audiogram—A standard graph used to record pure-tone hearing thresholds with air- and bone-conduction thresholds graphed by frequency in hertz (Hz) and hearing level (HL) in decibels (dB); (L. *audire*, to hear, + Gk. *gramma*, record).

audiologist—A professional who is specifically educated and trained to identify, evaluate, treat, and prevent hearing disorders, plus select and evaluate hearing aids, and habilitate or rehabilitate individuals with hearing impairments; (L. *audire*, to hear, + *logia*, study of).

audiometer—An electronic device designed to measure the sensitivity of hearing of pure-tone frequencies (*hertz*) and *intensities* (decibels); sounds are delivered to the ears either through earphones or *free field* (i.e., through loudspeakers in a testing environment with no reverberating surfaces) in an audiometry booth; (L. *audio-*, to hear, + Gk. *metron*, measure).

auditory brainstem response (ABR)—An *electrophysiological response* (the relationship between electrical activity and biologic function, in this case, brain activity) to sound that consists of five to seven identifiable peaks that represent neural function of auditory pathways.

auditory comprehension—The ability to understand spoken language at the single word, phrase, simple sentence, complex sentence, paragraph, and conversational speech levels; (L. *com*, with, + *prehendere*, to grasp).

auditory discrimination training (ear training)—The ability to distinguish sounds from one another; involves a comparison of heard sounds with other sounds; a technique used in articulation therapy that stresses careful listening to differentiate among speech sounds; (L. *dis-*, apart, + *crimin*, distinction).

auditory nervous system impairment—The result of reduced ability to clearly hear sounds above the hearing threshold; occurs less often than hearing sensitivity impairments, which may occur concurrently, causing a dual hearing problem.

auditory processing disorder (APD)/central auditory processing disorder (CAPD)—A disorder in children and adults who have difficulty using auditory information to communicate and learn; may affect their abilities to listen, understand speech, develop language, and have academic success; (L. *auditorius*, hearing; *pro-*, forward, + *cedere*, to go; *centrum*, center).

auditory training—Aural rehabilitation methods designed to optimize use of residual hearing by structured practice in listening, altering the environment, use of hearing aids, etc.

augmentative and alternative communication (AAC) or assistive technology (AT)—Any approach designed to support, enhance, or supplement the communication of individuals who are not independent verbal communicators in all situations; (L. *augmentum*, increase, + *ativus*, tending to; *alter*, other or another; *assistere*, cause to stand; Gk. *techne*, art or skill, + *logos*, study of).

aural habilitation—Sometimes used synonymously with *aural rehabilitation*; intervention for people who have not developed listening, speech, and language skills; may include diagnosis of communication and hearing-related difficulties, speech perception training, speech and language therapy, manual communication, and educational management.

aural rehabilitation—A broad term that involves intervention aimed at minimizing and alleviating the communication difficulties associated with hearing loss; includes identification and diagnosis, patient and family counseling and education, selection and fitting amplification devices, communication training strategies, speech perception training, speech-language therapy, promotion of literacy, and educational management; (L. *auris*, ear, *-alis*, related to; L. *re-* again, + *habitare*, make fit).

autism—A highly variable neurodevelopmental disorder in the broad *autism spectrum disorders (ASD)*, which is in the still broader group of *pervasive developmental disorders*. Autism is a lifelong complex behavioral syndrome that appears by 3 years of age, with children having a markedly absent interest in social interactions and relationships; severely impaired communication skills; and repetitive, stereotyped movements; and restricted interests that are often obsessive or fixated; (Gk. *autos*, self).

autism spectrum disorder (ASD)—A range of developmental disorders from mild to severe, with autism being the most severe form; (Gk. *autos*, self; L. *specere*, to look at or appearance).

automatic speech—Over-learned sequences of words that can be recited without much conscious thought, such as counting to 10; saying the days of the week, months of the year, and the alphabet; and singing some songs (e.g., the birthday song); (Gk. *auto-*, self, + *matos*, thinking).

autonomy—Respect for the patient's right to determine his or her own choices in making health care decisions; (Gk. *auto-*, self, + *nomos*, custom or law).

autopsy (postmortem)—A medical examination performed to determine or confirm the cause of death; (Gk. *auto*, self, + *opsis*, view; L. *post*, after, + *mors*, death).

axon—The cellular extension of a neuron that carries impulses away from the cell body; (Gk. *axon*, axis or axle).

B

babbling—The production of a consonant and vowel in the same syllable, either reduplicated (*ba-ba, gaa-gaa*) or nonreduplicated (*baa-da-gi*), that tends to appear about 6 or 7 months of age; (L. *babulus*, prattle).

behavioral theory (behaviorism)—In reference to speech and language, a perspective of development that asserts that speech and language are behaviors learned through operant conditioning.

Bernoulli's law—A law in physics that states when air flowing through a tube (e.g., trachea) reaches a constriction (e.g., vocal folds) there is an increase in speed of the flow of air that causes decreased pressure on the walls of the constriction that results in a slight negative pressure (i.e., slight vacuum) at the constriction; in voice, this slight negative pressure contributes to the vocal folds closing during vibration; (Daniel Bernoulli, Swiss scientist, 1700–1782).

bilabial—Referring to the two lips; (L. *bi-* two, + *labia*, lips).

bilingual—Children who often speak the parents' native language in the home environment and speak American English in school or other environments; (L. *bi-*, two, + *lingua*, tongue).

bioethics—The attempt to understand and resolve ethical issues and problems in the health care setting; (*bio-*, life, + Gk. *ethos*, moral character).

biofeedback—The process of becoming aware of various physiological functions of the body using instruments that provide information on the activity of muscles or systems being monitored, with the goal of being able to control or manipulate those muscles or systems voluntarily.

blend (consonant cluster)—A blend or consonant cluster occurs when two or more sounds appear together with no vowel separation (e.g., /tr, sp, bl, str, spl, str, skw/).

board and care home—A homelike environment where there may be a few to several elderly or physically impaired individuals residing and meals, laundry, and other services are provided.

bone conduction—Transmission of sound to the inner ear through vibration applied to the bones of the skull; allows determination of the cochlea's hearing sensitivity while bypassing any outer or middle ear abnormalities.

brainstem—The structure (pons and medulla oblongata) that connects the brain to the spinal cord; it is important in sensory and motor functions and contains neurons for the cranial nerves that exit the pons and medulla.

breathiness—Incomplete closure of the vocal folds during phonation that results in excessive unvibrated air escaping.

Broca's aphasia—A nonfluent expressive aphasia characterized by agrammatic language with omissions of articles, conjunctions, prepositions, plurals, possessives, and verb morphemes and auxiliary verbs; speech is often limited to high-frequency content words, making it sound telegraphic; apraxia of speech, dysarthria, or both often coexist; (named after Paul Broca, French neurosurgeon, 1824–1880).

Broca's area—The center for motor speech control (planning, sequencing, coordinating, and initiating) of the articulators located in the lower posterior portion of the left hemisphere's frontal lobe.

bruxing—A compulsive, unconscious clenching and grinding of the teeth, especially during sleep or as a mechanism for releasing tension during periods of extreme stress in waking hours; (Gk. *brychein*, to gnash the teeth)

C

cancer (carcinoma)—A malignant *neoplasm* (new growth) characterized by uncontrolled growth of cells that tend to invade surrounding tissue and *metastasize* (spread) to distant body sites; (L. *cancer*, crab; Gk. *karkinos*, crab, + *oma*, tumor).

cartilage—Firm, fibrous, and strong connective tissue that does not contain blood vessels; (L. *cartilage*, gristle).

central nervous system (CNS)—The brain, cerebellum, brainstem, and spinal cord; (Gk. *kentron*, center; *neuron*, nerve; *systema*, system).

cerebellum—The CNS structure largely concerned with the coordination of muscles and the maintenance of balance and body equilibrium; (L. *cerebellum*, little cerebrum; i.e., little brain).

cerebral embolism (embolus)—An abnormal condition in which a blood clot, piece of tumor, or other material (embolus) circulates in the bloodstream until it becomes lodged in a cerebral blood vessel, causing an occlusion; at the location of the occlusion, the embolus begins to function as a thrombus; (Gk. *embolus*, wedge-shaped object used as a stopper).

cerebral hemisphere—Either of the two halves of the brain that contains a frontal lobe, parietal lobe, occipital lobe, and temporal lobe; (L. *cerebrum*, brain; Gk. *hemi*, half, + *sphaira*, ball).

cerebral hemorrhage (hemorrhagic stroke)—The result of a blood vessel under pressure rupturing and sending blood into the brain tissue; hemorrhages may be arterial, venous, or capillary; (Gk. *haimo*, blood, + *rrhagia*, to break or burst).

cerebral palsy (CP)—A developmental neuromotor disorder that is caused by damage to the central nervous system *prenatally* (before birth), *natally/ perinatally* (during birth), or *postnatally* (during childhood) and results in a nonprogressive, permanent neuromuscular disorder; dysarthria affecting all speech systems is the most common speech problem; (L. *cerebrum*, brain; Gk. *para*, beyond, + *lysis*, loosening; *palsy* is a modification of the word *paralysis*).

cerebral thrombosis (thrombus)—An abnormal condition in which a clot (thrombus) develops within a blood vessel; (Gk. *thrombos*, clot).

cerumen—A yellowish or brownish waxy secretion produced by ceruminous glands in the ear canal that protects the ear canal from intrusion by insects; (L. *cera*, wax).

childhood apraxia of speech (CAS)—A childhood motor speech disorder in the absence of muscle weakness that affects the planning, programming, sequencing, coordinating, and initiating motor movements of the articulators that interferes with articulation and prosody; (Gk. *a-*, loss, + *praxis*, movement or action).

chronic—Of long duration with slow progress, usually in reference to a disease or disorder; (Gk. *chronos*, time).

chronic laryngitis—A persistent laryngitis lasting more than 10 days with inflammation of the mucous membrane lining in the larynx, accompanied by edema of the vocal folds with hoarseness and loss of voice that is often caused by heavy smoking, coughing, allergies and chemical irritants, and ongoing vocal abuse and misuse; (Gk. *chronos*, time, *larynx*, larynx, + *itis*, inflammation).

chronic traumatic encephalopathy (CTE)—A degenerative brain disease caused by repeated brain traumas (particularly concussions) that results in behaviors similar to Alzheimer's disease; (Gk. *chromos*, time; *trauma*, wound; *enkephalos*, brain, + *pathos*, disease).

chronological age—The actual age of a person that is derived from date of birth and expressed in days, months, and years; (Gk. *khronos*, time, + *logia*, study of).

circumlocution—The use of a description or "talking around" a word when the specific word cannot be recalled; (L. *circum*, around, + *locutio*, speech).

client-specific measurements (clinician devised assessments)—Assessments that are not standardized tests that a clinician constructs to make decisions about a specific client's communication abilities; (L. *clientem*, follower; *species*, sort; *mensurare*, to measure).

Clinical Fellowship—A 36-week full-time (35 hours per week) or the equivalent part-time mentored clinical experience totaling a minimum of 1,260 hours begun after all academic coursework and university clinic training are completed; required by ASHA to be eligible for the Certificate of Clinical Competence (CCC).

clinical intuition—A decision-making process that is used unconsciously by experienced clinicians that is rapid, subtle, and based on the entire context of the situation, but does not follow simple, cause-and-effect logic; (L. *intuititus*, look at or consider).

clinicians—Health care professionals, such as physicians, nurses, physical therapists, occupational therapists, speech-language pathologists, audiologists, psychiatrists, or psychologists involved in clinical practice who base their practice on direct observation and treatment of a patient or client; (Gk. *kline*, bed).

closed head injury (CHI) (nonpenetrating brain injury)—Severe impact to the skull that damages the brain, often with a blunt object such as the windshield of a vehicle or a bat, or the head striking the ground after a fall; the skull may be fractured but is not penetrated (e.g., by a bullet).

cluttering—A fluency disorder with speech that is abnormally fast with omission of sounds and syllables of words, abnormal patterns of pausing and phrasing, and often spoken in bursts that may be unintelligible; frequently includes abnormalities in syntax, semantics, and pragmatics; (ME, *clotteren,* to clot).

cochlea—The part of the inner ear containing the sensory mechanism of hearing; a spiral tunnel with 2¾ turns about 30 mm (about 1¼ inches) long, resembling a tiny snail shell; (L. *cochlea*, snail shell).

code switching—An occurrence for bilingual individuals in which sounds, words, semantics, syntactic, or pragmatic elements from one language are included when speaking another language, either automatically or intentionally; also can be expanded to include nonstandard and standard dialects; (L. *caudex*, book).

cognate—Two sounds that differ only in voicing (e.g., /p/ - /b/); (L. *cognatus*, of common descent; from *co-*, with, + *gnatus* [*natus*], to be born).

cognition—The act or process of thinking or learning that involves perceiving, memory, abstraction, generalization, reasoning, judgment, and problem solving; closely related to intelligence; (L. *cognitio*, knowledge; *co-*, with or together, + *gnoscere*, to know).

cognitive behavioral therapy—A model of counseling designed to help individuals recognize and examine problematic beliefs and replace them with more adaptive and flexible ways of thinking.

cognitive development—The progressive and continuous growth of perception, memory, imagination, conception, judgment, and reasoning; it is the intellectual counterpart of a person's biological adaptation to the environment; (L. *cognitio*, knowledge; Fr. *desvoluper*, to unwrap or expose).

cognitive disorder—An impairment of attention, perception, memory, reasoning, judgment, and/or problem solving (i.e., thinking) to allow adequate functioning in activities of daily living (L. *cognitio*, knowledge; *dis*, apart or impaired, + *ordo*, rank).

coma—A prolonged period of unconsciousness in which a patient has minimal, if any, purposeful responses to stimuli; (Gk. *koma*, deep sleep).

communicate/communication—Any means by which individuals relate their wants, needs, thoughts, knowledge, and feelings to another person; (L. *communicare*, to share).

communication (communicative) disorder—Speech, language, voice, resonance, cognitive, or hearing that noticeably deviates from that of other people, calls attention to itself, interferes with communication, or causes distress in both the speaker and the listener; any speech, language, voice, resonance, cognitive, or hearing impairment, disability, or handicap that interferes with a person conveying his wants, needs, thoughts, knowledge, and feelings to another person; (L. *communicare*, to share; *dis-*, apart or impaired, + *ordinare*, to order; i.e., communication that is not in order).

communication (conversation) board—An apparatus or simple board upon which common communication symbols and messages (e.g., alphabet, numbers, pictures, symbols, and common words and expressions) are represented, allowing expressive communication by pointing or gazing; communication boards may be no-tech, low-tech, or sophisticated high-tech electronic devices.

communicative competence—A child's grammatical knowledge of phonology, morphology, syntax, semantics, and pragmatics; (L. *com* [variation of *cum*] with or together, + *petitio*, request or seek).

compliance—The ease with which the tympanic membrane and middle ear mechanism function; (L. *complere*, to complete).

computerized tomography (CT) scan—A radiographic technique to visualize body tissue not able to be seen on standard X-ray images; formerly called computerized axial tomography (CAT) scan; (L. *com-*, with or together, + *putare*, to consider; Gk. *tomos*, section, + L. *graphos*, write).

concussion—Mild traumatic brain injury caused by a violent jarring or shaking that often occurs during a closed head injury and results in at least a brief loss of consciousness; (L. *concutere*, to shake violently).

conductive hearing loss—A reduction in hearing sensitivity because of a disorder of the outer or middle ear; (L. *conducere*, to conduct).

congenital disorder—A disorder that is present at birth; (L. *congenitus*, born with; *dis*, apart or impaired, + *ordo*, rank).

congruent/congruence—The agreement among a person's thoughts, feelings, words, tone of voice, and body language; communication in which a person sends the same message on both verbal and nonverbal levels; (L. *con*, with, + *gruere*, to suit; i.e., to suit with—to be in agreement).

consonant—Speech sounds articulated by either stopping of the outgoing air stream or creating a narrow opening of resistance using the articulators; (L. *con* [variation of *cum*], with or together, + *sonare*, to sound; literally, sound together).

contact ulcer—A benign vocal fold ulceration at the juncture of the middle one-third and posterior one-third of a fold that is caused by persistent and excessive vocal hyperfunction that is most commonly seen in adults males; (L. *contactus*, contact; *ulcus*, sore).

context—The circumstances or events that form the environment within which something exists or takes place; also, the words, phrases, or narrative that come before and after a particular word or phrase in speech or a piece of writing that helps to explain its full meaning; (L. *contextus*, join together).

continuing education units (CEUs)—Additional education or training required by ASHA and most states throughout a professional's career to help the professional remain current in the field.

contracture—An abnormal, usually permanent condition of a muscle group (e.g., bicep and muscle of the forearm) characterized by flexion and fixation of the limb that may be caused by shortening of muscle fibers; in severe cases, the bone (e.g., humerus [upper arm]) may develop an abnormal curvature; (L. *contractura*, pulling together).

contrecoup injury—In closed head injuries damage to the brain occurring on the opposite side of the trauma site; for example, when an impact to the left frontal side of the skull results in brain damage on the right posterior side; (L. *contra*, in opposition, + F. *coup*, impact or blow).

convalescent hospital—A medical facility, such as a skilled nursing facility, extended care facility, or nursing home, that provides extended medical, nursing, or custodial care for individuals over a prolonged period, e.g., during the course of a chronic illness or the rehabilitation phase after an acute illness or injury; (L. *convalescere*, to grow strong; *hospitium*, guesthouse).

conventional literacy—Reading and writing according to the rule-governed system of the alphabetic principle and being able to read to learn; (L. *con-*, with or together, + *venire*, to come; *litterae*, letters).

conversion reaction (disorder)—An ego defense mechanism in which *intrapsychic conflict* (mental struggle of opposing impulses or wishes within oneself) is expressed symbolically through physical symptoms that may manifest as actual illness or delusions of illness or incapacity (including voice disorders); causal factors may include a conscious or unconscious desire to escape from or avoid some unpleasant situation or responsibility, or to obtain sympathy or some other secondary gain; (L. *convertere*, to turn around; *re*, again, + *agrere*, to act).

cooing—The production of vowel-like sounds (usually /u/ and /oo/ with occasional brief consonant-like sounds similar to /k/ and /g/; usually produced by infants when feeling comfort or pleasure and interacting with a caregiver; (the term is in reference to the low, soft sounds of doves).

cortex (gray matter)—The outer layer (approximately one-fourth to one-half inch) of brain tissue containing nerve cell bodies (neurons); (L. *cortex*, bark).

cortical atrophy—Shrinkage and wasting away of cortical (brain) tissue that is common in dementia; (Gk. *a*, without, + *trophe*, nourishment).

cricoid cartilage—A solid circle of *cartilage* (nonvascular dense supporting connective tissue) shaped like a signet (class) ring located below and behind the thyroid cartilage and on top of the first tracheal ring; (Gr. *krikos*, ring, + *edios*, form).

cul-de-sac resonance—A variation of hyponasality that differs in the place of obstruction (anterior, compared to posterior in hyponasality or denasality), resulting in distortion (a muffled quality) of the nasal consonants /m/, /n/, and /ng/; (Fr. *cul-de-sac*, bottom of the sack).

cultural—linguistic diverse (CLD) theory—A perspective of language development that emphasizes the similarities and differences of the people and the languages spoken around the world, and that stresses how one language or dialect is no better than another.

culture—The philosophies, values, attitudes, perceptions, religious and spiritual beliefs, educational values, language, customs, child-rearing practices, lifestyles, and arts shared by a group of people and passed from one generation to the next; (L. *cultura*, culture).

custodial care—Services and care of a nonmedical nature (e.g., bathing and feeding) provided long term, usually for convalescent and chronically ill patients; (L. *custodia*, guarding).

D

Deaf community—Those deaf and hard of hearing individuals who share a common language (usually manual communication), common experiences and values, and a common way of interacting with each other and with hearing people.

Deaf culture—Ideology, beliefs, and customs shared by many individuals with prelinguistic deafness that may include communication, social protocol, entertainment, art, recreation, worship, and other aspects of culture.

decibel (dB)—A basic unit of measure of the intensity of sound; it is one-tenth of 1 bel (B); an increase in 1 bel is perceived as a 10-fold increase in loudness; (L. *decimus*, one-tenth, + *bel*, named after Alexander Graham Bell, American inventor, 1847–1922).

deciduous teeth—The set of 20 teeth that appear during infancy and early childhood (10 uppers, 10 lowers), with the front teeth appearing (erupting) through the gums about 6 months of age; all 20 teeth normally have erupted by 18–24 months. Shedding (losing) the deciduous teeth occurs between 6 and 13 years of age; (L. *decidere*, to fall off).

degenerative disease—Any condition that causes gradual deterioration of normal body functions; (L. *de-*, down from, + *generare*, to produce [i.e., decreased production]; *dis-*, opposite of; Fr. aise, ease).

deglutition—The act of swallowing; (L. *de-*, down, + *gluttire*, swallow).

dementia—A medical term for a syndrome caused by a progressive neurological disease that involves intellectual, cognitive, communicative, behavioral, and personality deterioration that is more severe than what would occur through normal aging; (L. *de-*, loss of, + *mens*, mind).

dendrite—A branching extension of a neuron that carries impulses to the cell body; (Gk. *dentron*, tree).

dentition—The type, number, and arrangement of teeth in the maxilla and mandible, including the incisors, cuspids (canines), bicuspids (premolars), and molars; (L. *dens*, tooth).

developmental coordination disorder—Impairment of groups of gross and fine muscles that prevents smooth and integrated movements, which results in clumsiness during walking, jumping, and athletic movements, and during more refined movements such as using eating utensils and writing; often associated with learning disabilities and complicated by low self-esteem, repeated injuries from accidents, and weight gain as a result of avoiding participating in physical activities.

developmental (intellectual) disability (DD or ID)—A disability that originates before 18 years of age and is characterized by significant limitations in intellectual functioning (intelligence) and adaptive behavior as expressed in conceptual, social, and practical skills.

diadochokinetic (diadochokinesis, diadochols)—In speech, the ability to execute rapid repetitive or alternating movements of the articulators; *diadochokinetic rate* is the speed at which the movements can be performed; (Gk. *diadochos*, successive, + *kinesis*, motion or movement).

diagnosis—The determination of the type and cause of a speech, language, cognitive, swallowing, or hearing disorder based on the signs and symptoms of the client or patient obtained through case history, observations, interviews, formal and informal evaluations, and other methods; (Gk. *dia*, through, + *gnosis*, knowledge).

dialect—A specific form of speech and language used in a geographical region or among a large group of people (social or ethnic dialects) that differs significantly from the standard of the larger language community in pronunciation, vocabulary, grammar, and idiomatic use of words; (Gk. *di-*, two, + *logos*, word or speech, becoming *dialecktos*, conversation).

diaphragm—A large, dome-shaped muscle that separates the thoracic and abdominal cavities and is the main muscle of respiration; during inspiration it moves down to increase the volume in the thoracic cavity, and during expiration it moves up to decrease the volume; (Gk. *diaphragma*, partition).

differential diagnosis—The process of narrowing possibilities and reaching conclusions about the nature of a deficit.

differential threshold—The smallest difference that can be detected between two auditory signals.

diphthong—A combination of two vowels in which one vowel glides continuously into the second vowel;

in American English: /eɪ/, /aɪ/ /oʊ/, /ɔɪ/ and /aʊ/; (Gk. *di-*, two, + *phthongos*, voice or sound).

diplophonia—Two distinct pitches perceived simultaneously during phonation that is caused by the two vocal folds vibrating under different degrees of tension (as in unilateral vocal fold paralysis) or vibration of the ventricular folds concurrently with the true vocal folds; (Gk. *diplos*, double, + *phone*, voice).

direct laryngoscopy—Examination by an ENT physician of the interior of the larynx by direct vision with the aid of a laryngoscope, usually while the patient is anesthetized; (L. *directus*, straight, + Gk. *larynx*, larynx, + *skopein*, to look).

disability—Any restriction or lack (resulting from an impairment) of ability to perform an activity in the manner or within the range considered normal for a human being (World Health Organization [WHO]); the impairment, loss, or absence of a physical or intellectual function; *physical disability* is any impairment that limits the physical functions of limbs or gross or fine motor abilities; *sensory disability* is impairment of one of the senses (e.g., hearing or vision); *intellectual disability* encompasses intellectual deficits that may appear at any age; (L. *dis*, apart, + *ablen*, to make fit, + *-itas*, suffix for condition or state).

discourse—An extended verbal exchange on a topic (i.e., a conversation or long narrative); (L. *dis-*, apart, + *currere*, to run).

disorder—A disruption of or interference with normal functions; (L. *dis*, apart, + *ordo*, rank).

distinctive feature—The smallest individual differences required to differentiate one phoneme from another in a language; (L. *distinctus*, separate [*dis-*, apart, + *tinct*, colored or tinged]; L. *facere*, to make).

distortion—A sound that does not have a phonetic symbol to represent the sound that is produced in place of the intended sound (e.g., a lateral lisp that is not a clear "sh" sound, or a distorted /r/ sound that cannot be clearly represented by a phonetic symbol); (*dis-*, apart, + *torquere*, to twist).

Down syndrome—A common chromosome disorder due to an extra chromosome number 21 (trisomy 21) that results in intellectual disability, small head, small ears, flat face with upward slant of the eyes, and abnormal physical development; (named after the English physician John Down, 1828-1896).

dysarthria—A group of motor speech disorders caused by *paresis* (weakness), *paralysis* (complete loss of movement), or incoordination of speech muscles as a result of central and/or peripheral nervous system damage that may affect respiration, phonation, resonation, articulation, and prosody; dysarthric speech sounds "mushy" because of distorted consonants and vowels; (Gk. *dys-*, difficult, impaired, + *arthroo*, articulate).

dysgraphia—A developmental motor disorder that affects a child's or adult's ability to write, characterized by messy or illegible handwriting, misspellings, and difficulty with grammar and organizing sentences; note: *agraphia* is a loss of ability to write resulting from injury to the brain; (Gk. *dys*, impaired or difficult, + *graphein*, write).

dysphagia (swallowing disorders)—Difficulty swallowing that occurs when impairments affect any of the four phases of swallowing (oral preparatory, oral, pharyngeal, or esophageal); puts a person at risk for aspiration of food and/or liquid and potential aspiration pneumonia; (Gk. *dys*, difficult or impaired, + *phagein*, to eat).

dysphonia—A general term that means a voice disorder, with the person's voice typically sounding rough, raspy, or hoarse; (Gk. *dys-*, impaired, + *phonia*, voice).

dystonia—A general neurological term for a variety of problems characterized by excessive contraction of muscles with associated abnormal movements and postures; (Gk. *dys-*, impaired, + L. *tonus*, sound).

E

echolalia—The automatic and involuntary repetition of another person's utterance that is normal for 18–24-month-old children, but which also can occur at later ages (including adulthood) in individuals who are autistic or have neurological damage; (Gk. *ekhe*, sound + *lalia*, talk).

edema—Accumulation of excessive fluid in tissue that is associated with inflammatory conditions and results in swelling of the tissue; (Gk. *oidema*, swelling).

effective treatment—Treatment with a particular method or approach that has been shown by research to be better than no treatment; (L. *effectus*, to bring about; L. *tractare*, to handle or deal with, + *mentum*, result).

electrolarynx/artificial larynx—An electronic (battery powered) device used by laryngectomees that produces a vibrated mechanical sound that is held against the neck, with the sound entering the pharynx and oral cavity where it is articulated for speech.

elicit—Behavior that is drawn out of a person by presenting certain stimuli, e.g., asking a child to name or describe objects to observe his speech and language; (L. *elicitus*, draw forth).

emergent literacy (preliteracy) skills—Early skills developed in the preschool years that precede or are presumed prerequisites for later-developing reading and writing skills; (L. *e-* out, + *mergere*, to plunge).

endoscopy (videoendoscopy, videostroboscopy)—Methods of viewing the velopharyngeal mechanism, vocal tract, or both that use a rigid endoscope introduced *intraorally* (through the mouth) or flexible fiberoptic endoscope *transnasally* (through the nose) with a camera lens and fiberoptic light source at the tip of the scope that can illuminate the nasopharynx, oropharynx, and larynx; the structures may be videotaped (*videoendoscopy*), and the light source can be put in *strobe mode* (rapid flashing) so that the vibrating vocal folds appear to move in slow motion for more detailed viewing (*videostroboscopy*); (note: SLPs may be trained to perform endoscopic evaluations and in most states are allowed to perform them); (Gk. *endon*, within, + *skopein*, to look).

English as a second language (ESL)—Learning English after a child's native (home) language has been established.

enteral feeding—The delivery of hydration and nutrition into the gastrointestinal (GI) tract by way of tube feedings through the nose or stomach; (Gk. *enteron*, bowel).

epiglottis—A large cartilage that is wide at the top and narrow at the bottom that is attached to the anterior edge of the cricoid cartilage and drops over the vocal folds like a lid to prevent food and liquid from entering the trachea and lungs when swallowing; (Gk. *epi*, on or upon, + *glossa*, tongue).

esophageal speech—The compression of air within the oropharynx and injection of it into the esophagus, followed by the rapid expelling of the air out of the esophagus that causes it to vibrate the upper esophageal valve, which produces a low-pitched, monotone "voice" that is shaped by the articulators to produce "burp" speech; (Gk. *oisophagos*, gullet).

etiology—The cause of an occurrence (e.g., a medical problem that results in a disorder or disability); (Gk. *aitia*, cause, + *logos*, science; i.e., the science of causes).

Eustachian (auditory) tube—A tube lined with mucous membrane that joins the nasopharynx and the middle ear cavity; normally closed but opens during yawning, chewing, and swallowing to allow equalization of air pressure in the middle ear with atmospheric pressure (named after Bartolomeo Eustachio, an Italian anatomist, 1524–1574).

evaluation/assessment—The overall clinical activities designed to understand an individual's communication abilities and disabilities before a treatment program is determined and established; (L. *e-* [variation of *ex-*], missing or absent, + *valuer*, value, i.e., missing value; *assidere*, to sit beside).

evidence-based practice—The quality of treatment that is measurable in terms of some form of functional outcomes and maintained in the face of cost-containment efforts (L. *evidentia*, proof; *practicare*, to do or perform).

evidence-based treatment (best practices)—The integration of (a) clinical expertise, (b) the current best evidence based on controlled and replicated research, and (c) the client's values, needs, and choices to provide high-quality service; (L. *evidentia*, proof; *tractare*, manage or handle).

executive functions—A composite of the following activities related to goal completion: anticipation, goal selection, planning, initiation of activity, self-regulation or self-monitoring, and use of feedback to adjust for future responses; (L. *executio*, accomplish; *functio*, performance).

expiration (exhalation)—The process of breathing air out of the lungs; (L. *ex*, out, + *spirare*, to breathe).

expressive aphasia—Difficulty formulating verbal, written, and/or gestural language; (L. *expressus*, clearly presented; Gk. *a-*, without or loss of, + *phasos*, to speak).

expressive language—The words, grammatical structures, and meanings that a person uses verbally; (L. *ex-*, out of or from, + *pressare*, to press; *pro-*, before, + *-ducere*, leading to; *in-*, in, + *codex*, trunk of a tree [originally, document carved from wooden tablets]).

external motivation—Motivation that is provided by the encouragement of someone else, often family or an employer; (L. *externus*, beyond or outside; *motus*, move).

F

facilitating techniques—The selected therapy exercises that help to achieve a "target" or a more optimal vocal response by the patient; (L. *facilis*, easy to do; Gk. *tekhne*, art, skill, or method).

failure to thrive—The abnormal retardation of growth and development of an infant resulting from conditions that interfere with normal metabolism, appetite, and activity.

false vocal folds (ventricular folds)—Paired, thick folds of mucous membranes with few muscle fibers that lie just above the true vocal folds in the larynx at the level of the Adam's apple; they do not vibrate during speech but close tightly during swallowing to prevent material from entering the trachea; (L. *ventriculus*, little belly).

family systems therapy—A model of counseling in which each family member is part of a system (the family), each member affects the others, and the system is interdependent; within the system there are sub-systems: e.g., mother–father, mother–son, father–son, grandparent–grandchild; (L. *familia*, household; Gk. *syn-* with or together, + *histanai*, to stand; L. *consilium*, consult; *modulus*, small measure).

family therapy—The counseling theory that emphasizes that a person's emotional reactions and problems must be viewed in the context of the family's roles and communication and interaction patterns; the focus is on family relationships and interdependent family systems (e.g., husband-wife, parent-child) rather than individuals within the family.

fiberoptic endoscopic evaluation of swallowing (FEES)—A procedure used to provide visual information about the pharyngeal phase of swallowing; a flexible endoscope is passed through the nasal passageway into the nasopharynx to view the laryngopharynx and the patient is asked to swallow food or liquid that has been dyed green for contrast; (L. *fibra*, fiber, + Gk. *optikos*, sight, Gk. *endon*, inward, within, + *skopia*, to look).

fine motor skills—Movements that require a high degree of dexterity, control, and precision of the small muscles of the body that enable such functions as grasping small objects, drawing shapes, cutting with scissors, fastening clothing, and writing.

finger spelling—The use of certain finger and hand shapes to represent letters of the alphabet and spell individual words.

fluency shaping (modification)—A therapy approach for children and adult stutterers that attempts to directly train individuals to speak with relaxed respiration, relaxed vocal folds, and relaxed articulation muscles; the approach attempts to teach stutterers how to talk fluently; (L. *fluens*, relaxed; *modificare*, to limit or restrain).

fluent aphasia—Aphasia that results from damage to posterior regions of the cortex (i.e., temporal or temporal-parietal lesions) characterized by language with normal pauses and articulation but with frequent syntactic errors, paraphasias, and circumlocutions (L. *fluens*, relaxed; Gk. *a-*, without or loss of, + *phasos*, to speak).

formulate—In language, the choice of words and grammatical structures in the construction of a meaningful verbal expression; (L. *formula*, form or rule).

frenum/frenulum—A fold of mucous tissue connecting the floor of the mouth to the midline underside of the tongue; (L. *frenum*, bridle, reins, and bit used to control a horse; *frenulum* is the diminutive for *frenum*).

frequency—In speech, the number of complete cycles (opening, closing) per second that the vocal folds vibrate; *pitch* is the psychological perception of frequency; (L. *frequens*, repeated).

fricative—A sound formed by forcing the air stream through a narrow opening between articulators (tongue-teeth - /θ/, /ð/ [th]; lips - /f/, /v/; tongue-alveolar ridge /s/, /z/, and tongue-hard palate /ʃ/).

functional—An incorrect production of standard speech sounds for which there is no known anatomical, physiological, or neurological basis; (L. *functico*, to perform).

functional aphonia—A hyperfunctional voice disorder in which a person speaks mostly with a whisper although is able to use a normal voice when laughing, coughing, clearing the throat, and humming; often associated with psychological stressors or conflicts; (Gk. *a-*, without or loss of, + *phone*, sound or voice).

functional disorder—A problem or impairment with no known anatomical, physiological, or neurological basis that may have behavioral or emotional causes or components; (L. *functico*, to perform; *dis*, apart or impaired, + *ordo*, rank).

functional dysphonia—A voice disorder that may be either hyperfunctional or hypofunctional and has no organic, physical, or neurological cause but is heard in patients with extreme tension in both the laryngeal and the supralaryngeal regions; the voice may have hypofunctional qualities such as low-pitch and breathy or hyperfunctional qualities such as high-pitch, strident, or hoarse; (L. *functio*, performance; Gk. *dys-*, disturbance or impaired, + *phonia*, voice).

functional outcomes—The results of treatment intended to clearly show a person's improved ability to communicate in the hospital setting with medical and rehabilitation staff; at home, performing activities of daily living (ADLs); in the community; and on the job (if the person returns to work).

functional treatment—Treatment results that improve communication abilities useful in a person's natural environments (e.g., home, school, and community); (L. *functio*, performance; L. *tractare*, to handle or deal with, + *mentum*, result).

functor (function) words—Words whose grammatical functions are more obvious than their semantic content and that serve primarily to give order to a sentence, such as articles, conjunctions, determiners, prepositions, and modal and auxiliary verbs.

G

gastroenterologist—A physician who specializes in diseases of the gastrointestinal tract; (Gk. *gaster*, stomach, + *enteron*, intestine, + *logos*, science).

gavage feeding—The use of a *nasogastric (NG) tube* (see definition) to provide sufficient nutrition and hydration for newborns who have a failure-to-thrive condition, with infant milk or specialized formulas (e.g., PediaSure®) inserted into the tube; (Fr. *gaver*, to gorge).

General American English (GAE)—The speech of native speakers of American English that is typical of the United States and that excludes phonological forms easily recognized as regional dialects (e.g., Northeastern or Southeastern) or limited to particular ethnic or social groups, and that is not identified as a nonnative American accent; the norm of pronunciation by national radio and television broadcasters.

generalization—The transfer of learning from one environment to other environments; usually considered the therapy or classroom to a natural environment, such as the home and community); (L. *generalis*, relating to all).

glide/semivowel—A type of consonant that has a gradual (gliding) change in an articulator (lips or tongue) position and a relative long production of sound; /w/, /j/.

global aphasia—A severe-to-profound aphasia resulting from a diffuse lesion involving portions of the left temporal, frontal, and parietal lobes that is characterized by severely impaired receptive and expressive language in all input and all output modalities, with motor speech disorders of apraxia of speech, dysarthria, or both; (L. *globus*, globe; Gk. *a-*, without or loss of, + *phasos*, to speak).

glottal stops—Compensatory articulation productions primarily for plosive sounds (e.g., /p/, /b/, /t/, /d/) used by individuals with velopharyngeal inadequacy; characterized by the forceful adduction of the vocal folds and the buildup and release of air pressure under the glottis, resulting in a grunt-type sound.

goal (target behavior)—Any verbal or nonverbal skill a clinician tries to teach a child; (OF *targe'*, shield, i.e., a warrior would try to hit what a shield was trying to protect).

grammar—The rules of the use of morphology and syntax in a language; (Gk. *grammatikos,* letter, + L. *ars,* art; literally, the art of letters).

gross motor skills—Involvement of the large muscles of the body (e.g., trunk, legs, arms) that require tone, strength, and coordination that enable such functions as standing, lifting, walking, and throwing a ball; (L. *grossus,* thick or course).

H

habilitation/habilitate—The process of developing a skill in order to function within the environment; the initial learning and development of a new skill; (L. *habilitatus,* ability, to make able).

handicap—Loss or limitation of opportunities to take part in the life of the community on an equal level with others (World Health Organization [WHO]); a congenital or acquired physical or intellectual limitation that hinders a person from performing specific tasks; (*hand in cap,* 17th-century game of betting).

hard glottal attack—Forceful approximation (closing) of the vocal folds during the initiation of phonation.

hard palate—The bony anterior two-thirds of the roof of the mouth that separate the oral cavity from the nasal cavity; (L. *palatum,* palate).

harshness—A "rough" sounding vocal quality resulting from a combination of hard glottal attacks, low pitch, and high intensity caused by *overadduction* (hyperfunction) of the vocal folds.

hearing aid—Any electronic device (usually battery operated) designed to amplify and deliver sound to the ear and consists of a microphone, amplifier, and receiver.

hearing impairment—Abnormal or reduced function in hearing resulting from an auditory disorder; (L. *im-* [variation of *in-*], in or into, + *pejorare,* make worse).

hearing sensitivity impairment—The most common type of hearing loss; a reduction in the sensitivity of the auditory mechanism that results in sounds needing to be a higher intensity than normal before they can be heard by the listener; (L. *sentire,* feel or perceive).

hearing threshold—In audiometry, the level at which a stimulus sound, such as a pure tone, is barely perceptible; usual clinical criteria demand that the level be just high enough for the subject to be aware of the sound at least 50% of the time it is presented.

hertz (Hz)—The unit of vibration adopted internationally to replace *cycles per second* (CPS); 1 hertz = 1 cycle per second = fundamental frequency (1 Hz = 1 CPS = f_0); (Heinrich R. Hertz, German physicist, 1857–1894; first person to broadcast and receive radio waves).

heterogeneous—Consisting of dissimilar or diverse individuals or constituents; (Gk. *heteros,* other or different, + *genos,* kind).

high blood pressure (hypertension)—A common disorder in middle age and later (although now often being seen in obese children and young adults) in which blood pressure is persistently above 140 over 90 mm Hg (120/80 is considered normal).

hoarseness—A common dysphonia that is a combination of breathiness and harshness that may affect loudness (usually decreased loudness or a monoloudness), pitch (usually a low pitch with reduced pitch range), and quality (usually decreased "pleasantness" of the sound of the voice).

holistic—A philosophic concept in which an entity (e.g., person) is seen as more than the sum of its parts; a prominent approach to psychology, biology, nursing, medicine, and other scientific, sociologic, and educational fields of study and practice; (Gk. *holos,* whole).

holophrastic language—The use of a single word to express a complete thought; (Gk. *holos,* whole, + *phrazein,* to declare; i.e., to declare the whole [meaning]).

hyperadduction—Difficulty with the vocal folds closing too tightly or for too long that results in a voice that sounds tense and strained and tends to fatigue with use as a result of hypertonicity; (Gk. *hyper-,* excess, + *adducere,* to bring to).

hyperfunction—A pervasive pattern of excessive effort and tension that affects many different structures and muscles in the phonatory system and, in some cases, the respiratory, resonatory, and articulatory systems; signs of hyperfunction include a tense sounding voice and hard glottal attacks; (Gk. *hyper,* over or beyond; + L. *functio,* performance or execution).

hypernasal/hypernasality—A resonance disorder that occurs when oral consonants and vowels enter the nasal cavity because of clefts of the hard and soft palates or weakness of the soft palate, causing a person to sound like he is "talking through his nose"; (Gk. *hyper-,* excess, + L. *nasus,* nose).

hypertonicity—Excessive tone or tension in a muscle or muscle group (e.g., chest muscles, articulatory muscles); (Gk. *hyper,* over or above [normal], + *tonos,* tone).

hypoadduction—Difficulty making the vocal folds close strongly enough or long enough for normal phonation that results in a weak, breathy voice that often deteriorates with increasing amounts of vocal use throughout the day; (Gk. *hypo-,* under, + L. *adducere,* to bring to).

hypofunction—Inadequate muscle tone in the laryngeal mechanism and associated structures, including the muscles of respiration; signs of hypofunction include breathiness because of inadequate closure of the vocal folds, weak vocal power that can affect speech intelligibility, and reduced vocal endurance; (*hypo,* under; + L. *functio,* performance).

hyponasal/hyponasality (denasal/denasality)—Lack of normal resonance caused by partial or complete obstruction in the nasal tract resulting in the three English phonemes /m/, /n/, and /(ŋg)/ being perceived as /b/, /d/, or /g/ respectively; (Gk. *hypo-* under, [L. *de-,* down], + L. *nasus,* nose).

hypotonicity—Weak or absent tone or tension in a muscle or muscle group (e.g., laryngeal muscles or abdominal muscles); (Gk. *hypo,* under or below [normal], + *tonos,* tone).

I

idiom—An expression in the usage of a language that is peculiar to itself either grammatically (e.g., "Zip your lip.") or in having a meaning that cannot be derived from the normal combination of words (e.g., "Keep your eyes on the ball, your shoulder to the wheel, and your nose to the grindstone."); (Gk. *idioma,* to appropriate or acquire).

idiopathic—A disease or disorder of unknown etiology; (Gk. *idio,* own or personal, + *pathos,* suffering).

idiosyncratic language—An individual's choice of words and use of words in sentences that have their own unique meaning, which may or may not be interpretable to a listener; (Gk. *idios,* one's own, + *syn,* together, + *krasis,* to blend or mix; i.e., blending together one's own [language]).

immittance audiometry—A routinely used objective assessment of the functioning of the middle ear; a general term to describe measurements made of tympanic membrane impedance, compliance, or admittance; (a combination of *impedance* and *admittance*; L. *audio-,* to hear, + Gk. *metron,* measure).

impairment—Any loss or abnormality of psychological, physiological, or anatomical structure or function that interferes with normal activities (World Health Organization [WHO]); (L. *impejorare,* to make worse).

impedance—The opposition of sound-wave transmission, which includes frictional resistance, mass, and stiffness and is influenced by frequency; (L. *impedire,* to entangle).

incidence—The rate at which a disorder appears in the normal population over a period, typically 1 year; (L. *incidere,* to fall into).

incisors—The four front upper and lower teeth (central and lateral incisors); (L. *incidere,* to cut into, as in *incision*).

incontinence—The inability to control or retain urination or defecation; (L. *incontinentia,* inability to retain).

indirect laryngoscopy—A method of examining the larynx and vocal folds by placing a *laryngeal mirror* (a small round mirror attached to a long handle) into the back of the mouth and directing a reflected light source onto the mirror to shine on the vocal folds; (L. *in-,* not, + *directus,* straight; Gk. *laryngos,* upper windpipe, + *skopein,* to look).

infantile hypoxia—In newborns and infants, inadequate oxygenation of the blood leading to *tachycardia* (rapid heart rate) and rapid, shallow breathing that quickly affects the brain and other organs and systems; severe hypoxia can result in cardiac failure; (L. *infans,* unable to speak; Gk. *hypo,* below or deficient, + *oxys,* sharp or quick).

infantile (primitive) reflex—Any reflex normal in infants that is an automatic, uncontrolled movement; normally disappears (becomes "integrated") by about 6 months of age; (L. *infans,* unable to speak; *primivus,* primitive; *reflectere,* to bend back).

infarction (necrosis)—A localized area of necrotic (dead) tissue resulting from lack of blood supply and oxygen to the tissue; (L. *in* + *farctus,* to fill; Gk. *nekros,* dead).

inner speech (internal discourse, stream of consciousness)—The nearly constant internal monologue a person has with himself at a conscious or semi-conscious level that involves thinking in words; a conversation with oneself.

inpatient—A patient who has been admitted to a hospital or other health care facility for at least an overnight stay.

inspiration (inhalation)—The process of drawing air into the lungs; (L. *in,* in, + *spirare,* to breathe).

integrate—In neurology, the process of combining information from various input modalities, attaching meaning and interpreting the information, storing (remembering), and making decisions about responding; (L. *integrare,* to make whole).

intelligence—A global construct involved in the collective capacity to act purposely, think rationally, and deal effectively with the environment; (L. *intelligentia,* intelligent).

intelligence quotient (IQ)—An estimate of intellectual status based on an index determined by dividing the *mental age* (MA) in months by the *chronological age* (CA) in months and reducing the result to a percentage; 100 is considered the mathematical average; (L. *intellentia,* intelligent; *quot,* how many).

intelligible—The degree to which a person's utterances are understood by the average listener; influenced by articulation, rate of speech, fluency, vocal quality, and intensity of voice.

intensity—In reference to voice, the force with which the vocal folds open and close and the amount of air that escapes between the open vocal folds; *loudness* is the psychological perception of intensity; (L. *intensus,* strained or tight).

interdisciplinary team—A group of professionals from various disciplines who work together to coordinate the care of a patient through collaboration, interaction, communication, and cooperation; (L. *inter,* between, + *disciplina,* teaching).

internal motivation—Motivation that is self-generated or intrinsic in which a person decides what is important and needed; (L. *internus,* between; *motus,* move).

International Phonetic Alphabet (IPA)—Specially devised signs and symbols designed to represent the individual speech sounds of all languages.

intonation—Variations in pitch on syllables, words, and phrases that produce *stress* to give emphasis and meaning to utterances; (L. *in-,* in or into, + Gk. *tonus,* tone).

intraoral breath pressure—A buildup of air pressure in the oral cavity that provides the force for the production of oral consonants, particularly plosives, fricatives, and affricates; (L. *intra,* within, + *os,* mouth).

intubation—The passage of a breathing tube through the mouth, through the nose, or directly into the trachea through a *tracheotomy* (endotracheal intubation) to ensure a *patent* (open; pronounced "pAtent") airway for delivery of oxygen; (L. *in,* in or within, + *tubus,* tube, + *atio,* process).

J

jargon aphasia—Continuous but unintelligible speech with various combinations of literal and verbal paraphasias and neologisms, with little or no conveying of information; often with the speaker having little awareness of the problem and occurring in both speech and writing; (O.Fr. *gargon*, gibberish).

L

labia—Pertaining to the lips; (L. *labia*, lips).

labiodental—The /f/ and /v/ sounds, where the upper front teeth are in contact with the lower lip; (L. *labia*, lips, + *dentes*, teeth).

language—A socially shared code or conventional system for representing concepts through the use of arbitrary symbols [sounds and letters] and rule-governed combinations of those symbols [grammar]; (L. *lingua*, tongue or language).

language arts—Academic activities such as listening, speaking, reading, handwriting, spelling, and written composition.

language comprehension—An active process in which, from instant to instant, a listener infers the meaning of an auditory message based on the context of the information and long-term stored memory of words and general knowledge; (L. *com-*, with, + *prehendere*, to grasp or seize).

language delay—An abnormal slowness in developing language skills that may result in incomplete language development; (L. *de-*, down or from, + Fr. *laier*, leave).

language development—The progressive growth of a receptive and expressive communication system for representing concepts using arbitrary symbols (sounds and words) and rule-governed combinations of those symbols (grammar); (L. *lingua*, tongue or language; Fr. *desvoluper*, to unwrap or expose).

language differences—Variations in speech and language production that are the result of a person's cultural, linguistic, and social environments; (L, *differentia*, diversity).

language disorder—An impairment of receptive and/ or expressive linguistic symbols (morphemes, words, semantics, syntax, or pragmatics) that affects comprehending what is said or verbally expressing wants, needs, thoughts, information, and feelings; (L. *dis*, apart or impaired, + *ordo*, rank).

language-learning disability—An impairment of receptive and/or expressive linguistic symbols that affects learning and educational achievement and, consequentially, possible occupational and professional choices, in addition to emotional and social development.

language sample—An audio recording of a child's spontaneous conversation or naturalistic verbal interaction with the clinician, family member, or both.

laryngectomy—Surgical removal of the larynx because of cancer and includes the trachea being brought forward and sutured to the skin in the lower midline of the neck to create a permanent stoma; the pharynx is closed as a separate tract for swallowing; (Gk. *larynx*, larynx, + *ektome*, excision).

laryngitis—An acute or chronic inflammation of the mucous membranes of the larynx that often results in hoarseness or loss of voice; (Gk. *larynx*, larynx, + *-itis*, disease or inflammation).

laryngopharyngeal reflux (LPR)—Gastric reflux (stomach acids causing "heart burn") that flows through the esophagus, past the upper esophageal valve, and into the larynx or pharynx; reflux may spill over onto the vocal folds and irritate them, causing coughing and inflammation; (L. *refluere*, to flow back).

larynx (pl. larynges)—Located just above the trachea, the structure that contains cartilages, muscles, and membranes that produce voice by air passing between the vocal folds; (Gk. *larynx*, larynx).

learning disability (LD)—A disorder in one or more of the basic psychological processes involved in understanding or using language, spoken or written, that may manifest itself as difficulty listening, speaking, reading, writing, spelling, mathematical calculations, reasoning, and problem solving; (L. *dis-*, apart or impaired, + *habilitas*, aptitude or easy to manage).

lesion—A wound, injury, or area of pathological change in tissue; (L. *laesus*, injury).

letter—An arbitrary written or printed symbol or character representing a speech sound (L. *littera*, letter of the alphabet).

lexicon—Refers to all morphemes, including words and parts of words, that a person knows; (Gk. *lexikos*, of words).

linguadental (interdental)—Voiced and unvoiced /th/ sounds with the tongue tip placed lightly between the top and the bottom front teeth; (L. *lingua*, tongue, + *dens*, tooth).

linguapalatal—The /ʃ/ [sh] and /ʒ/ [zh] sounds, where the top center of the tongue is near the hard palate; (L. *lingua*, tongue, + *palatum*, palate).

linguavelar—The /k/ and /g/ consonants, where the back of the tongue moves near the soft palate; (L. *lingua*, tongue, + *velum*, curtain or veil).

linguistics—The scientific study of the structure and function of language and the rules that govern language; includes the study of phonemes, morphemes, syntax, semantics, and pragmatics; (L. *lingua*, tongue).

lipreading—The process of recognizing speech using only the visual cues from the speaker's mouth and face.

literacy (reading, writing)—The ability to communicate through written language, both reading and writing; (L. *litterae*, letters; Old English [OE] *raedan*, to advise; OE *writan*, to scratch).

literacy disorder (disability)—Reading and writing impairments in a heterogeneous population of children; (L. *litterae*, letters).

literal or phonemic paraphasia—Sounds and syllables that are correctly articulated but may be extraneous, transposed, or substituted, usually with the preservation of the vowels and intended number of syllables in a word (e.g., *tar* for *car*); often occurring in both speech and writing; (L. *littera*, of a letter;

Gk. *phonema,* sound or voice; *para,* near or alongside, + *phasos,* speech).

loss of consciousness (LOC)—Impaired responsiveness, usually caused by diffuse brain dysfunction or damage to the brainstem and the reticular activating system; duration is often used as a measure of traumatic brain injury severity; (L. *conscius,* to know).

low birth weight—An infant whose weight at birth is less than 5.5 pounds (2,500 grams), regardless of gestational age.

M

magnetic resonance imaging (MRI)—An imaging study that does not expose the patient to radiation and often provides images with sharper detail than those from computerized tomography (CT) scans; medical imaging based on the resonance of atomic nuclei in a strong magnetic field; (Gk. *magnesia,* lodestone [a type of iron that attracts other iron]; *resonare,* to sound again; *imago,* image).

malignant—A neoplasm with uncontrollable growth and dissemination that invades and destroys neighboring tissue; (L. *mal-,* bad, poor, or abnormal + *ignari,* disposition).

malocclusion—Misalignment of the maxillary teeth with the mandibular teeth; (L. *malus,* bad, poor, or abnormal, + *occludere,* to shut).

mandible—The lower jaw that is hinged to the temporal bone for opening and closing and contains sockets for the lower teeth; (L. *mandibula,* jaw).

manner—The way in which the air stream is modified as a result of the interaction of the articulators; direction of airflow (e.g., oral or nasal sounds), or the degree of narrowing of the vocal tract by the articulators in the various places; (L. *manus,* hand, in reference to how a sound is made; [*manufactured,* made by hand]).

manualism—A philosophy in the education of the deaf that emphasizes the learning and use of sign language and finger spelling as a natural form of communication among the deaf; (L. *manus,* hand, + *-isma,* feature).

manually coded English—A form of communication in which manual signs correspond to English words and syntax.

masking—In audiology, the process that occurs when two sounds occur simultaneously and one sound is sufficiently loud to cause the other to be inaudible; (L. *maschera,* mask).

mastication—The act of chewing food in preparation for swallowing and digestion; (L. *masticare,* to chew).

mastoiditis—An infection of one of the mastoid bones (just behind the ear) that is usually an extension of a middle ear infection, characterized by earache, fever, headache, and malaise; medical treatment may require intravenous antibiotics for several days, and residual hearing loss may follow the infection; (Gk. *mastos,* breast [e.g., mastectomy], + *edios,* form, + *itis,* inflammation).

maxilla—The upper jaw that includes the hard palate and contains sockets for the upper teeth; forms much of the midfacial structure; (L. *maxilla,* upper jaw).

mean length of utterance (MLU)—The average length of oral expressions as measured by representative sampling of oral language (e.g., 50–100 spontaneous utterances); usually calculated by counting the number of morphemes per utterance and dividing by the number of utterances; e.g.,

$$\frac{150 \text{ morphemes}}{50 \text{ utterances}} = 3.0 \text{ MLU.}$$

measurement—Procedures that quantify observed behaviors and can be calculated as mathematical results, such as percentages and percentiles; (L. *mensurare,* to measure).

Meniere's disease—A chronic disease of the inner ear characterized by recurrent episodes of vertigo, tinnitus, and sensorineural hearing loss, which may be bilateral; (named after Prosper Meniere, French physician, 1799-1862).

mental status examination—A structured interview and observations conducted by a psychologist or neuropsychologist of a patient's orientation, attention, concentration, memory, language comprehension and expression, visual–spatial skills, abstraction abilities, general cognitive functioning, and insight into problems, with impairments typically treated by an SLP.

metalinguistics—The ability to think about and talk about language; (Gk. *meta-,* changed or beyond, + L. *lingua,* tongue).

metastasis—The process by which tumor cells travel or spread to distant parts of the body; (Gk. *methistanai,* to change; from *meta,* beyond, + *stasis,* standing).

middle ear—An air-filled chamber located within the temporal bone of the skull; beginning at the inner side of the tympanic membrane and attaching the ossicular chain to the oval window of the cochlea.

mixed hearing loss—A reduction in hearing because of a combination of a disordered outer or middle ear and inner ear.

modality—Any sensory avenue through which information may be received, i.e., auditory, visual, tactile, taste, and olfactory (smell); (L. *modus,* measure or quantity).

modified barium swallow study (MBSS)—A dynamic (moving) imaging radiographic (x-ray) procedure focusing on the mouth, pharynx, larynx, and cervical esophagus used to examine the process of swallowing; a video recording of real-time movement of a bolus from entering the mouth to entering the stomach.

morpheme—The smallest unit of language having a distinct meaning, for example, a prefix, root word, or suffix; (Gk. *morphe,* form, + *pheme,* sound).

morphology—The study of the structure (form) of words; (Gk. *morphe,* form, + *logia,* study of).

motor—Pertaining to motion or movement; nerve cells that initiate and regulate contracting and relaxing of muscle fibers; (L. *movere,* to move).

motor speech disorders—Neurological impairments that affect the motor planning, programming, neuromuscular control, and/or execution of speech and include the dysarthrias and apraxia of speech; they typically have a sensory component and should be thought of as sensorimotor disorders.

multicultural—A society characterized by a diversity of cultures, languages, traditions, religions, and values, as well as socioeconomic classes, sexual orientations, and ability levels; ideally, where individuals are respected and valued for their contributions to the whole of that society; (L. *multus,* many, + *cultura,* culture).

multifactorial—Referring to the likelihood of two or more causes contributing to the etiology or development of an impairment or disorder; (L. *multi,* many, + *factus,* made by hand; i.e., many hands [causes] make the disorder).

muscle tension dysphonia (MTD)—A hyperfunctional voice disorder in which the voice is adversely affected by excessive muscle tension that ranges from mild to severe; characteristics include a weak voice that lacks intensity, range and variation, a rough, hoarse, or thin vocal quality that lacks resonance, and a voice that fatigues easily; (L. *musculus,* little mouse; *tension,* stretch; *dys,* impaired or difficult, + Gk. *phone,* sound or voice).

mutational falsetto (puberphonia)—A high-pitched, breathy voice produced by the vibration of the anterior one-third of the vocal folds, with the posterior two-thirds being held tightly in a slightly open position or else so tightly adducted that little or no posterior vibration occurs; (L. *falsus,* false, + *ete,* small; L. *puberatus,* age of maturity, + Gk. *phonia,* voice).

mutism—The inability or unwillingness to speak; usually used in reference to voice disorders where an individual may use selective or elective mutism, that is, unconsciously or consciously not be able to use voice or speak; (L. *mutus,* mute).

myasthenia gravis—A neuromuscular disorder more commonly seen in women than men; characterized by chronic fatigue and muscle weakness, especially in the facial and articulatory muscles, resulting in dysarthria.

myofunctional therapy—Treatment designed to correct a tongue thrust or habitual forward-resting position of the tongue against the front teeth; (Gk. *myos,* muscle, + L. *functio,* performance).

N

narrative—The orderly, sequenced relating of accounts or events; (L. *narratus,* to know).

nasal—Sound resulting from the closing of the oral cavity, preventing air from escaping through the mouth, with a lowered position of the soft palate and a free passage of air through the nose (/m/, /n/, and /ŋ/ [ng]); (L. *nasus,* nose).

nasal air emission/nasal escape—The inappropriate release of air pressure through the nose during speech, causing distortion of the speech; (L. *e-,* out, + *mittere,* to send).

nasogastric (NG) tube—A medical device consisting of a long flexible tube that is passed through the nose, down the esophagus, and into the stomach for the delivery of liquids, nutrition, and medications; (L. *nasus,* nose, + Gk. *gastros,* stomach).

nasometer—A computer-based instrument that measures the relative amount of nasal acoustic energy in a person's speech; (L. *nasus,* nose, + Gk. *metron,* measure).

nasopharyngoscopy—A minimally invasive procedure commonly used by SLPs for evaluation of velopharyngeal dysfunction that allows visual observation and analysis of the velopharyngeal mechanism during speech; equipment includes a flexible fiberoptic endoscope, the same that is used in laryngoscopy; (L. *nasus,* nose, + Gk. *pharynx,* throat, + *skopein,* to look).

National Student Speech-Language-Hearing Association (NSSLHA)—The preprofessional association for students interested in the study of communication sciences and disorders.

nativistic theory—A perspective of language development that emphasizes the acquisition of language as an innate, physiologically determined, and genetically transmitted phenomenon; (L. *nativus,* innate, produced by birth).

natural processes—The processes that are common in the speech development of children across languages.

neologism—A form of paraphasia in which a person combines consonants and vowels that sound like they could be words and uses inflection to give them emotional meaning; for example, *bingtema* and *hitican*; (Gk. *neos,* new, + L. *logos,* word).

neonate—A child within the first 28 days after birth; (Gk. *neos,* new, + L. *natus,* born).

neural plasticity—The brain's ability to reorganize itself throughout life by forming new neural connections. Neural plasticity allows neurons to compensate for injury and disease and to adjust their activities in response to new situations or to changes in their environment; (Gk. *neuro,* nerve; *plastikos,* to mold).

neuritic (senile) plaques— Neuronal abnormalities and degeneration seen in cortical and subcortical brain regions of people with Alzheimer's disease.

neurofibrillary tangles—Neuronal abnormalities seen in Alzheimer's disease where there are filamentous bodies (fine, threadlike fibers) in nerve cells, axons, and dendrites.

neuron—The basic nerve cell of the nervous system, containing a nucleus within a cell body and extending an axon and multiple dendrites (Gk. *neuron,* nerve).

neuropsychologist—A Ph.D. psychologist specialized in the area of practice in clinical psychology and neurogenic disorders who assesses cognitive functioning, discriminates between psychiatric and neurological conditions, distinguishes among different neurological conditions, and predicts the course of a patient's recovery; however, most of the cognitive-linguistic therapy is provided by SLPs (Gk. *neuron,* nerve, + *psyche,* breath, life, or soul).

noise-induced hearing loss—A permanent sensorineural hearing loss caused by exposure to excessive loud noise, often over long periods of time.

nonfluent aphasia—Aphasia that results from damage to anterior cortical regions (i.e., frontal lobe lesions) characterized by sparse, perseverative language with disturbed prosody, misarticulations, errors in syntax, and a reduction in phrase length (L. *non*, not, + *fluens*, relaxed; Gk. *a-*, without or loss of, + *phasos*, to speak).

normal disfluency—The repeating, pausing, incomplete phrasing, revising, interjecting, and prolonging of sounds that are typical in the speech of young children; (L. *normalis*, according to pattern).

normative data (norms)—Data that characterize what is usual in a defined population and that describe rather than explain a particular occurrence; an average of performance of a sample drawn randomly from a population; (L. *norma*, rule or pattern; *datum*, thing given).

NPO (nothing by mouth)—A patient care instruction advising that a patient is prohibited from orally ingesting food, beverage, or medicine; patients must receive nutrition through enteral feeding; (L. *nil per os*, nothing by mouth).

O

occlusion—The process of bringing the upper and lower teeth into contact; (L. *occludere*, to shut).

occlusive (ischemic) stroke—A partial or complete blockage (occlusion) of a cerebral artery, causing decreased blood supply to brain tissue; (L. *occludere*, to close up; Gk. *ischein*, to hold back, + *haima*, blood).

occupational therapist (OT)—A rehabilitation specialist who is licensed to evaluate and treat developmental, physical, and cognitive impairments that interfere with functional independence for daily living and work skills by facilitating the development of sensory–motor (sensorimotor) integration, perceptual functioning, and neuromuscular functioning; (L. *occupare*, work; Gk. *therapia*, treatment).

omission—The absence of a speech sound where one should occur in a word, e.g., *k-on* for *crayon*; (L. *omittere*, to let go).

open bite—An abnormal vertical space between the anterior maxillary and mandibular teeth that often allows the tongue tip to be seen when a person smiles.

open head injury (OHI)—Head injury in which the skull and brain are penetrated by a severe impact or a projectile (bullet, fragment of glass, or shrapnel from an explosion).

operant (instrumental) conditioning—A learning model for changing behavior in which a desired behavior is reinforced immediately after it spontaneously occurs; (L. *opera*, work; *instruere*, to arrange; *condicio*, agreement or stipulation).

operationally defined goal—A specific behavior that is observable (can be heard or seen) and measurable; (L. *opera*, work, + *-atio*, action or process).

oral apraxia (nonverbal apraxia, facial apraxia, buccofacial apraxia)—Difficulty with volitional nonspeech movements of the articulators (e.g., puffing the cheeks, clicking the tongue, protruding the tongue, whistling, or smiling; (L. *buccus*, cheeks, + *facies*, make or form).

oralism—A philosophy in the education of the deaf that maintains language should be oral, that is, from the mouth, and sign language and teachers who are deaf should be excluded from the classroom; (L. *os*, mouth, + *isma*, feature).

oral reflex—Infantile primitive reflexes that are present at birth or soon after that are specifically designed to assist the infant in finding and obtaining oral nutrition; for example, the *rooting reflex*, *sucking reflex*, and *swallowing reflex*; (L. *os*, mouth; *reflexus*, bending back).

orbicularis oris—The muscle surrounding the opening of the mouth; the muscular structure of the lips; (L. *orbis*, circle, + *biculus*, little; *or*, mouth; i.e., the little circle of the mouth).

organic—Inability to correctly produce standard speech sounds because of anatomical, physiological, or neurological causes; (L. *organum*, to work).

organic disorder—A problem or impairment with a known anatomical, physiological, or neurological basis; (L. *organum*, to work; *dis*, apart or impaired, + *ordo*, rank).

orthography—The part of language study concerned with letters and spelling; the representation of the sounds of a language by written or printed symbols; (Gk. *orthos*, correct or straight, + *graphe*, to write).

orthopedic—A branch of health care concerned with the prevention and correction of disorders of the musculoskeletal systems of the body; an *orthopedist* is a physician who specializes in orthopedics; (Gk. *orthos*, straight, + *pais*, child).

ossicular chain—The three small bones (ossicles) of the middle ear named after their basic shapes: *malleus*, for the mallet or hammer; *incus*, for the anvil; and *stapes*, for the stirrup; (L. *os*, bone; *ossiculum*, small bone).

otitis media with effusion—Any inflammation or infection of the middle ear; particularly common in childhood and often associated with a common cold, allergies, sinus infections, and sore throats; Eustachian tube malfunction typically is the physiological cause; effusion—the escape of fluid from tissue as a result of seepage (Gk. *ous*, ear, + *itis*, inflammation, L. *medius*, middle; *effundere*, to pour out).

otolaryngologist/otorhinolaryngologist—A medical doctor who specializes in diseases of the ears, nose, and throat; often referred to as an "ear, nose, and throat" (ENT) doctor; (Gk. *ot-*, ear, + *rhin-*, nose, + *larynx*, larynx, + *logos*, study of).

otosclerosis—A hereditary condition of unknown cause in which irregular ossification occurs in the ossicles of the middle ear, especially of the stapes, causing hearing loss; typically first observed between 11 and 30 years of age; women are affected twice as often as men and may begin during pregnancy; (Gk. *ous,* ear, + *skelos,* hard, + *osis,* condition).

ototoxic—Drugs that have harmful effects on the central auditory nervous system, including aspirin, aminoglycoside antibiotics, furosemide, and quinine; (Gk. *ous,* ear, + *toxikon,* poison).

outer (external) ear—The concave, somewhat funnel-like structure that collects, resonates, and directs sound waves to the tympanic membrane, assists in localizing the direction from which sound is coming, and helps protect the middle ear; composed of the auricle (pinna), ear canal, and outer layer of the tympanic membrane.

outpatient—A patient who is not hospitalized but is being treated in an office, clinic, or medical facility.

P

palatal fistula—Usually a small opening or passage between the oral cavity and the nasal cavity that allows air or sound to escape from the oral cavity into the nasal cavity, causing some hypernasality; (L. *palatum,* palate; *fistula,* pipe).

palatal lift—A prosthetic appliance that can be used to raise the velum for speech if the velum is long enough to achieve velopharyngeal closure but does not move well, often because of central or peripheral neurological impairment.

palatal obturator—A prosthetic appliance that can be used to cover an open palatal defect, such as an unrepaired cleft palate or a palatal fistula; it can be used to improve an infant's ability to achieve compression of the nipple for suction or can be used to close a cleft palate for speech; (L. *palatum,* palate; obturare, to close).

palatine tonsils—Two almond-shaped masses of lymphoid tissue between the anterior and the posterior faucial pillars; (L. *palatum,* plate, *tonsillae,* tonsil).

palatoplasty—The surgical repair of a cleft palate; (L. *palatum,* palate, + Gk. *plastikos,* to mold or form).

papilloma—Soft, wart-like, benign growths on the vocal folds of children that have a viral origin and may grow to a size that can obstruct the airway; (L. *papilla,* nipple, + Gk. *oma,* tumor).

parallel speech—Naming, describing, and explaining what the child is experiencing and probably feeling, almost as if the caregiver is the child; a technique used by some parents, as well as clinicians, to help children develop receptive and expressive language; (Gk. *para,* beside, + *allos,* one another).

parentese (motherese, baby talk, child-directed speech)—The often automatic speech pattern of parents and caregivers with infants in which the person uses a high pitched voice with an unusual amount of inflection, one- and two-syllable words in short, simple sentences, and a slower than normal rate of speech with clear articulation that sometimes emphasizes every syllable.

perception—The process of detecting, discriminating, and recognition of a stimulus; (L. *per,* through, + *capere,* to grasp or take).

perinatal—Pertaining to the time and process of giving birth or being born; (Gk. *peri,* around, + L. *natus,* birth).

peripheral nervous system (PNS)—The cranial nerves that exit the brainstem and the spinal nerves that exit the spinal cord that allow the body to communicate sensory information to the brain and the brain to communicate motor information to the body; (Gk. *peripheria,* circumference).

perseverate/perseveration—An automatic and involuntary repetition or continuation of a thought or behavior after it is no longer appropriate, including repetition of a sound, syllable, word, or phrase when speaking; (L. *perseverare,* to persist; *per,* through, + *severus,* severe).

persistent vegetative state (PVS)—A medical diagnosis made only after numerous neurological and other tests that, due to extensive and irrevocable brain damage, a patient is highly unlikely ever to achieve higher functioning above a vegetative state; (L. *persistere,* continue steadfastly; *vegere,* to be alive; *status,* condition).

pervasive developmental disorder (PDD)—Serious multiple developmental impairments typically diagnosed in children before the age of 3 and in males approximately four times as often as in females; autism spectrum disorders are the more severe extreme; (L. *per-,* through, + *vadere,* to go).

pharyngeal fricatives—Compensatory articulation productions primarily for fricatives and affricates (e.g., /f/, /v/, /s/, /z/, /ʃ/ [sh], and /tʃ/ [ch]) used by individuals with velopharyngeal inadequacy; characterized by tongue retraction so that the base of the tongue approximates, but does not touch, the pharyngeal wall, which causes a friction sound as air pressure passes through the narrow opening.

pharyngoplasty—A surgical procedure of the pharynx that is designed to correct velopharyngeal dysfunction; (Gk. *pharynx,* throat, + *plastikos,* to mold or form).

phonation—The vibration of air passing between the two vocal folds that produces sound that is used for speech; (Gk. *phone,* voice; L. *vox,* voice).

phoneme—The shortest arbitrary unit of sound in a language that can be recognized as being distinct from other sounds in the language; (Gk. *phone/phonema,* voice or sound).

phonetics—The study of speech-sound production and the special symbols that represent speech sounds.

phonics method—The method of teaching reading and pronunciation by learning the sounds of letters and groups of letters ("sounding out words"); the association of the sounds (phonemes) of a language with the equivalent written forms (graphemes).

phonological awareness—Recognition and understanding of sound–letter associations; that individual sounds can be combined to form words; that a single-syllable word is heard as one word but can be segmented into its beginning, middle, and ending sounds; and that longer words have more "middle" sounds.

phonological disorder—Errors of phonemes that form patterns in which a child simplifies individual sounds or sound combinations; (Gk. *phonos*, sound + *logia*, study of).

phonological processes—The simplification of sounds that are difficult for children to produce in an adult manner; phonological processes help explain errors of substitution, omission, and addition that children may use to simplify the production of difficult sounds.

phonology—The study of speech sounds and the system of rules underlying sound production and sound combinations in the formation of words; (Gk. *phone/phonema*, voice or sound, + *logia*, study of).

phonotrauma—Deleterious acute or chronic vocal behaviors, such as excessive yelling, screaming, cheering, coughing, throat clearing, inappropriate pitch or loudness, singing beyond the range of the vocal mechanism, hard glottal attacks, inadequate respiratory support, talking loudly over noise, poor hydration, and smoking that are damaging to the vocal folds and the laryngeal and pharyngeal muscles and tissues; (Gk. *phone*, sound or voice, + *trauma*, wound).

physical therapist (PT)—A rehabilitation specialist who is licensed to evaluate and treat developmental and physical impairments through the use of special exercises or other modalities to assist individuals to maximize independence and mobility, self-care, and functional skills necessary for daily living; (Gk. *physikos*, body; *therapia*, treatment).

place—The location in the mouth where two articulators come together (constrict) to produce specific sounds; places may include the lips, teeth, alveolar ridge, tongue, and hard and soft palates.

plateau—A patient's general leveling off of improvement in rehabilitation, after which gains are slower and less easily documented; often the reason for discharging from rehabilitation; (Fr. *plateau*, platter).

polypoid thickening (degeneration)—A condition in which a vocal fold becomes edematous, flabby, and almost jelly-like as the result of vocal hyperfunction, making the voice chronically low pitched and hoarse; (L. *poly*, many, + Gk. *oeides*, form).

positive emission tomography (PET)—A computerized radiographic scanning technique that examines metabolic activity, blood flow, and biochemical activity of the brain and other body parts; (L. *positivus*, positive; *emissio*, send out; Gk. *tomos*, slice or section, + *graphia*, describe).

positive reinforcement (positive feedback, reward)—A technique used to encourage a desired behavior by presenting something the person wants soon after the desired behavior is made; (L. *positivus*, positive; L. *re-*, again, *en*, in, + *fortis*, strong).

postconcussion syndrome (PCS)—A constellation of symptoms seen in some patients with mild traumatic brain injury, including headache, poor concentration, short-term memory deficits, and affective disturbances (e.g., anxiety, depression, and irritability); (L. *post*, after, + *concussio*, shaking; Gk. *syn-* with, + *dromos*, running or course).

post-traumatic stress disorder (PTSD)—A set of symptoms after exposure to a psychologically extreme traumatic stressor that involves intense fear, horror, or helplessness; symptoms include persistent reexperiencing of the traumatic event or events, avoidance of stimuli associated with the trauma, and symptoms of increased arousal (*hypervigilance*); (L. *post*, after; *trauma*, wound).

pragmatics—The rules governing the use of language in social situations; includes the speaker–listener relationship and intentions and all elements in the environment surrounding the interaction— the context; (L. *pragmaticus*, skilled in law or business).

prelinguistic (preverbal) vocalizations—The sounds produced by an infant before the production of true words (e.g., crying, cooing, babbling, and echolalia); vocal behaviors that precede the acquisition of true language; (L. *prae*, before, + *lingua*, tongue; L. *vocalis*, sound).

premature (infant)—Any infant born before the gestational age of 37 weeks; often associated with low birth weight that results in high risk for incomplete organ system development, causing poor temperature regulation, respiratory disorders, and poor sucking and swallowing reflexes; (L. *prae*, before, + *maturare*, to ripen; i.e., before ripe).

premorbid—In medicine, the wellness or functioning of a patient before a significant illness or injury; (L. *prae-*, before, + *morbus*, disease).

presbycusis—Hearing loss associated with old age, usually involving both a loss of hearing sensitivity and a reduction in clarity of speech; (Gk. *presbys*, old man, + *akousis*, hearing).

pressure-airflow technique—A procedure using *aerodynamic instrumentation* to evaluate the dynamics of the velopharyngeal mechanism during speech; also used to evaluate nasal respiration and to quantify upper airway obstruction through measurements of nasal airway resistance; (L. *pressus*, to press).

pressure-equalizing (PE) tube—A small silicone tube inserted into the tympanic membrane following a myringotomy to equalize air pressure between the middle ear cavity and the atmosphere as a substitute for a nonfunctional Eustachian tube; (L. *pressus*, to press; *aequalis*, uniform or equal).

prevalence—The estimated total number of individuals diagnosed with a particular disorder at a given time in a population, or the percent of people in a population with the disorder; (L. *praevalere*, to be powerful).

process—In reference to neurological functioning, the activation of neurons (hundreds to millions at any instant) with their impulses sent through axons and dendrites to other neurons to bring about general and specific cognitive, linguistic, and motor activity; (L. *processus*, process).

produce—In speech, to create an utterance (sound, syllable, word, sentence, or longer) that is spontaneous or imitated; (L. *productus,* lead forth).

prognosis—A prediction of the probable course, duration, recovery, or termination of a disease or disorder; a prediction of the outcome of a proposed course of treatment, its effectiveness and duration, and the individual's progress; (Gk. *pro,* first or before, + *gnosis,* knowledge).

prosody (prosodic)/melody (melodic)—The qualities of stress and intonation in the voice that are influenced by the pitch, loudness, and duration of individual speech sounds; (Gk. *prosoidia,* song sung to music).

prosopagnosia—Difficulty recognizing familiar faces (including those of family members) and famous people; (Gk. *prosopon,* mask; + *gnosis,* knowledge).

prosthetic device (prosthesis)—An artificial device to replace or augment a missing or impaired part of the body; (Gk. *pros-,* in addition to, + *tithenai,* to put).

protrude—In speech, the puckering of the lips forward or the movement of the tongue forward past the lips; (L. *pro-,* in front of or forward, + *trudere,* to thrust).

psychophysiological (psychosomatic) disorder—A disorder with physical signs and symptoms that have a psychological origin, often with common ailments such as tension headaches, gastrointestinal disorders, or both that are attributed to psychological stress; (Gk. *psyche,* breath, life, or soul, + *physikos,* of nature; *somatikos* [soma], body).

pure-tone audiometry—Audiometry using tones of various frequencies and intensities as auditory stimuli to measure hearing using both air conduction and bone conduction.

Q

quality of life—A global concept that is difficult to measure but often is considered to involve a person's standard of living, personal freedom, and the opportunity to pursue happiness; a measure of a person's ability to cope successfully with the full range of challenges encountered in daily living; the characterization of health concerns or disease effects on a person's lifestyle and daily functioning; (L. *qualis,* of what sort).

R

range of motion (ROM)—For speech, the limits the mandible can open and close, the lips can protrude and retract, and the tongue can protrude and retract, elevate and lower, and move side to side (lateralize).

reading disability (dyslexia, developmental dyslexia)—An inability or difficulty reading that is of neurological origin; (OE *raedan,* to advise or interpret; Gk. *dys,* impaired or difficult, + *lexis,* word).

receptive aphasia—Difficulty comprehending verbal, written, and/or gestural language; (L. *recipere,* to receive; Gk. *a-,* without or loss of, + *phasos,* to speak).

receptive language—What a person understands of what is said; (L. *recipere,* to receive; *lingua,* tongue or language).

referred pain—Pain felt at a site different from that of an injured or diseased organ or part of the body, e.g., *angina,* the pain of coronary artery insufficiency, may be felt in the left shoulder, arm, or mandible; (L. *referre,* to bring back; *poena,* punishment).

reflex—An involuntary response to a sensory input, such as the corneal reflex in which both eyes blink in response to something irritating an eye; the gag reflex, caused by something touching the posterior wall of the pharynx; and the knee jerk (deep tendon) reflex, caused by a sharp tap just below the knee; (L. *reflectere,* to bend back).

rehabilitation—Restoration of impaired functions and abilities to normal or to as satisfactory a status as possible; (L. *re-,* back or return, + *habilitatus,* ability, to make able).

reliable/reliability—The dependability of a test or treatment procedure as reflected in the consistency of its scores on repeated measurements of the same group; (L. *re-,* again, + *ligare,* to bind).

replicate—Evaluation or treatment procedures that can be repeated by either the same investigator or other investigators to determine reliability of the data; (L. *re-,* again, + *plicare,* to make parallel).

residential care facility—Often a fairly large complex of small "apartments" where individuals or couples live; there is communal dining, and various services (e.g., security, trips to the mall, and outings) are provided to residents; (L. *residere,* to rest).

resonance—The quality of the voice that results from the vibration of sound in the vocal tract (i.e., spaces and tissues of the pharynx, oral cavity, and nasal cavity); (L. *resonantia,* echo; *re-,* again, + *sonare,* to sound).

resonance disorder—Abnormal modification of the voice by passing through the nasal cavities during production of oral sounds (*hypernasality*) or not passing through the nasal cavities during production of nasal sounds (*hyponasality*).

respiration (ventilation, pulmonary ventilation, breathing)—The movement of air into and out of the lungs that allows for the exchange of oxygen and carbon dioxide; (L. *respirare,* to breathe).

retract—In speech, the pulling back of the lips past their neutral or resting position, or the movement of the tongue back into the oral cavity after protrusion or past the neutral, resting position; (L. *re-,* back or again + *trudere,* to thrust).

retrocochlear hearing loss—A hearing disorder resulting from a *neoplasm* (tumor) or other lesion located on cranial nerve VIII or beyond in the auditory brainstem or cortex; (L. *retro-,* back or behind, + *cochlea,* snail shell).

right-hemisphere syndrome—Damage to the right hemisphere of the brain that can result in impairments of attention, visual–spatial abilities, orientation to person, place, time, and purpose, emotions, cognition, subtle to overt communication problems, and left-side neglect.

rule of 10s—A guideline for the appropriate time for a cleft lip repair, which says that the infant must be at least 10 weeks of age, weigh 10 pounds, and have a hemoglobin count of 10 grams before the lip repair; the purpose of the rule is to help insure the infant will survive the anesthesia during surgery.

S

savant syndrome—The co-occurrence with autism of unexpected or unusual high-level skills with generally limited intelligence (e.g., mathematical calculations, days and dates in history or the future, or remarkable memory for unrelated information); (Fr. *savoir*, to know).

scaffolding—Support that adults provide to children for them to achieve competence in an activity (e.g., reading and writing), with the support gradually removed until the child is able to perform independently.

scope of practice—ASHA's delineation of the general and specific areas in which speech-language pathologists and audiologists may engage with the appropriate and necessary education, training, and experience.

screening—In speech, any gross measure used to identify individuals who may require further assessment in a specific area (e.g., articulation, language, hearing, fluency, or voice).

secondary/overt/concomitant stuttering behaviors—Extraneous sounds and facial and body movements a person who stutters uses during moments of stuttering; e.g., repetitions of "uh" or "um," eye blinks, and unusual head, hand, or other body part movements.

seizure (epilepsy, convulsion)—A hyperexcitation of neurons in the brain that causes a sudden, sometimes violent, involuntary series of contractions of groups of muscles; (Fr. *saisir*, to seize; Gk. *epilepsia*, seizure; L. *convulsion*, to cramp).

semantic-cognitive theory—A perspective of language development that emphasizes the interrelationship between language learning and cognition, that is, the meanings conveyed by a child's productions; (Gk. *semantikos*, meaning; L. *co-*, with, + *gnosticus*, knowledge).

semantics—The study of meaning in language conveyed by words, phrases, and sentences; (Gk. *semantikos*, to mean or signify).

senility—A medical term that refers to the normal loss of cognitive functioning with advanced age; (L. *senilis*, old or aged).

sensorimotor—The combination of input of sensations and output of motor activity; motor activity reflects what is happening to the sensory systems; (L. *sentire*, to perceive or feel, + *movere*, to move).

sensorineural hearing loss—A reduction of hearing sensitivity produced by disorders of the cochlea and/or the auditory nerve fibers of the vestibulocochlear (VIII cranial) nerve; (L. *sentire*, to perceive or feel, + Gk. *neuron*, nerve).

sensory—Pertaining to sensation or awareness of stimuli that are received in the central nervous system; (L. *sentire*, to feel).

sensory–motor (sensorimotor) integration—The ability to take information (*stimuli*) in through the senses of vision, hearing, touch, taste, and smell, and to combine the information with previously stored memories to develop a coherent concept or appropriate motor response; (L. *sentire*, to perceive or feel; *movere*, to move; *integrare*, make whole).

sibilant—A fricative sound whose production is accompanied by a "hissing" sound (/s/, /z/, /ʃ/ [sh], and /ʒ/ [dj]); (L. *sibilare*, to hiss).

sign—An objective finding of a disease or change in condition as perceived by an examiner, such as a physician; (L. *signum*, mark).

significant—A term often used to specify the impairment level a child must exhibit before he is considered to have a speech or language disorder; no "gold standard" is available to use to define this term as it applies to speech and language disorders. In statistics, the probability that a given finding (e.g., an individual test score) may have occurred by chance; usually a finding that occurs fewer than 5 times in 100 by chance alone ($p < .05$).

sign language—A visual means of communication using hand and arm shapes and gestures to represent words and concepts, along with some finger spelling; communication that does not depend on spoken language and is used within Deaf communities and learned naturally by interaction with other signers.

silent aspiration—Penetration of food or liquid (including saliva) into the larynx and passing below the vocal folds without a protective cough or choking occurring; (L. *aspirare*, to breathe upon).

social-pragmatic theory—A perspective of language development that considers communication as the basic function of language.

social reinforcer—A word, phrase, or short statement said with warmth and enthusiasm as a reward and encouragement for an accurate response or good attempt at a specific task or target; (L. *socius*, companion, associate; *re-*, again, + *en-*, in, + *fortis*, strong).

social worker—A professional who helps families coordinate appointments, deal with insurance and other funding sources, and manage their stress and emotional reactions to the many problems associated with the child's treatment.

soft palate (velum)—The muscular tissue in the posterior one-third of the roof of the mouth that separates the oral cavity from the nasal cavity when raised and in contact with the posterior pharyngeal wall; (L. *palatum*, palate; *velum*, curtain or veil).

spasmodic dysphonia (SD)—A relatively rare voice disorder that may have either or both neurological and psychological etiologies; characterized by a strained, strangled, harsh voice quality, or an absence of voice because of tight abduction of the vocal folds; clients typically do not respond well to voice therapy; (Gk. *spasmodes,* spasm or convulsion; *dys-,* disturbance or impaired, + *phonia,* voice).

specific language impairment (SLI)—Significant receptive and/or expressive language impairments that cannot be attributed to any general or specific cause or condition.

speech—The production of oral language using phonemes for communication through the process of respiration, phonation, resonation, and articulation.

speech audiometry—A key component of audiological assessment that uses auditory signals present in everyday communication; assessment involves, in part, the presentation of single-syllable words at a fixed intensity level above the threshold with the client aurally discriminating the sounds in the words to correctly say words aloud for the examiner to score.

speech bulb obturator—A prosthetic device that may be considered when the velum is too short to close completely against the posterior pharyngeal wall; it consists of a retaining appliance and a bulb (usually made of acrylic) that fills in the pharyngeal space for speech; (L. *obturare,* to close).

speech development—The progressive evolving and shaping of individual sounds and syllables that are used as arbitrary symbols and applied in rule-governed combinations to produce words to communicate a person's wants, needs, thoughts, knowledge, and feelings; (Fr. *desvoluper,* to unwrap or expose).

speech disorder—Any deviation of speech outside the range of acceptable variation in a given environment; (L. *dis,* apart or impaired, + *ordo,* rank).

speech-language pathologist/speech pathologist/ speech therapist—A professional who is specifically educated and trained to identify, evaluate, treat, and prevent speech, language, cognitive, and swallowing disorders; (Anglo Saxon *speche,* to speak; [Gk. *spharageisthai,* to crackle]; Anglo Saxon *langue,* tongue; [Gk. *lingua,* tongue]; Gk. *pathos,* suffering or disease; Gk. *logia,* study of).

speech-language pathology assistant (SLPA)— A support person who performs tasks as prescribed, directed, and supervised by ASHA certified SLPs.

speechreading—The process of recognizing speech by attending to the speaker's auditory and visual messages (nonverbal communication, such as facial expressions and body language), clues from the setting of the conversation, and the likely conversational topics in those settings.

spinal cord—A thick "cord" of nerve fibers that passes through the vertebral column that conducts sensory and motor impulses to and from the brain and controls many body reflexes; (L. *spina,* backbone).

spontaneous (connected, running) speech sample— A sample of a child's oral discourse in conversation or while describing a picture, usually 50 to 100 consecutive utterances; (L. *sponte,* voluntary).

spontaneous recovery—The physiological healing of the brain's damaged tissue, including reduction of cerebral edema, development of collateral blood vessels, and rerouting of neural pathways.

Standard American English (SAE)—See *General American English* (GAE).

standard dialect—The dialect of a language that is commonly spoken or established by individuals with considerable formal education; (Gk. *dia-,* two or apart, + *lektos,* discourse, way of speaking).

standardized test (norm-referenced test)—A test that has been administered to a large group of individuals to determine uniform or standard procedures and methods of administration, scoring, and interpretation, and has adequate normative data on validity and reliability; tests that are administered to compare one child's performance to others the same age.

stereotyped movements—Persistent and inappropriate mechanical repetition of actions, body postures, or speech patterns, often seen in autism (Gk. *stereos,* solid, + *typos,* mark).

stimulability—The evaluation of a child's ability to produce a correct (or an improved) sound in imitation after the clinician models the sound for the child or after the child is given specific instructions on the articulatory placement or manner of production; (L. *stimulare,* to goad).

stoma—An opening about the diameter of a finger or thumb made surgically into the neck that allows a person to breathe directly through the trachea; (Gk. *stoma,* mouth).

stop—Sound made by building up air pressure in the mouth and then suddenly releasing it; the airflow can be blocked momentarily by pressing the lips together (bilabial—/p, b/) or by pressing the tongue against either the gums (lingua [tongue]-alveolar—/t, d/) or the soft palate (linguavelar—/k, g/).

stress—Variations in intensity, frequency, and duration on one syllable more than another in a word, which usually results in the syllable sounding both louder and longer than other syllables in the same word.

stroke (cerebrovascular accident, CVA)—A disruption of blood supply to the brain caused by an occluded (blocked) artery or an artery that has hemorrhaged; (from the concept that a person has been *stricken*).

stuttering (disfluency)—A disturbance in the normal flow and time patterning of speech characterized by one of more of the following: repetitions of sounds, syllables, or words; prolongations of sounds; abnormal stoppages or "silent blocks" within or between words; interjections of unnecessary sounds or words; circumlocutions (talking around an intended word); or sounds and words produced with excessive tension; (Teutonic, *steut,* stop; L. *dis-,* apart or impaired + *fluere,* to flow [i.e., impaired flow]).

stuttering modification—A therapy approach for children and adult stutterers that requires the speaker to recognize and confront his fears, avoidances, and struggles to escape his stuttering, and the speaker reducing and managing those fears, avoidances, and struggles.

subacute hospital—A level of care needed by patients who do not require acute care but who are medically fragile and require special services, e.g., respiratory therapy, intravenous tube feeding, and complex wound management care; (L. *sub,* under or beneath; *hospitium,* guesthouse).

submucous cleft—A defect in the hard palate in the absence of an actual opening into the nasal cavity or a defect in the muscles of the soft palate that cannot be seen through the mucosal tissue but may cause disunity of the velar muscles, resulting in velopharyngeal inadequacy and hypernasality; (L. *sub,* under or beneath, + *mucus,* slime).

substitution—The replacement of one standard speech sound by another, e.g., /th/ for /s/; (L. *substituere,* to put in place of).

suprasegmentals/paralinguistics/prosody (prosodic) features—Voice inflections used in a language such as stress, intensity, changes in pitch, duration of a sound, and rhythm that help listeners understand the true intent of a message and that convey the emotional aspects of a message, such as happiness, sadness, fear, or surprise; (L. *supra,* above or beyond, + *segmentum,* cut or divide).

swallow/swallowing—The process of moving food from the mouth to the stomach via the esophagus that involves smooth coordination of muscles in the mouth, pharynx, and esophagus.

syllable—Either a single vowel (V) or a vowel and one or more consonants (C); e.g., V+ consonant (VC), VCC, CV, CCV, CVC, etc.; (Gk. *syn-* together, + *lambanein,* to take).

symmetry (symmetrical)—Both sides (e.g., the lips) in balanced proportions for size, shape, and relative position; (Gk. *syn,* with or together, + *metron,* measure).

symptom—A subjective indication of a disease or change in condition as perceived by the patient or other nonmedical or rehabilitation specialist, such as a family member; (Gk. *symptoma,* that which happened).

synapse—The junction at which two neurons communicate with each other; (Gk. *syn,* with or together, + *haptein,* to fasten).

syndrome—A complex of signs and symptoms resulting from a common etiology or appearing together that presents a clinical picture of a disease or inherited anomaly; (Gk. *syn,* together, + *dromos,* course).

syntax—Rules that dictate the acceptable sequence and combination of words in a sentence to convey meaning; the study of sentence structure; (Gk. *syntaktos,* order or arrange together).

T

telecommunication devices for the deaf (TDD)—Telephone systems used by those with significant hearing impairments in which a typewritten message is transmitted over telephone lines and is received as a printed message; (Gk. *tele-,* afar, + L. *commicare,* to share).

telegraphic speech (language)—Condensed language in which only the essential words are used, such as nouns, verbs, and adjectives; often used by 3-year-old children and college students taking lecture notes (Gk. *tele,* afar, + *graphos,* written).

teratogen—Any substance, agent, or process that interferes with prenatal development, causing the formation of one or more developmental abnormalities in a fetus; (Gk. *teras,* monster, + *genein,* to produce).

therapy/treatment—The care of any significant condition to prevent, alleviate, or cure it; (Gk. *therapeia,* medical treatment; L. *tractare,* manage, handle, or deal with, + *mentum,* result.

thoracic cavity—The upper part of the trunk that contains the organs of respiration (lungs) and circulation (heart); (Gk. *thorax,* chest; *cavus,* hollow).

thyroid cartilage—The largest of the *laryngeal cartilages* that is the main structure of the larynx and encloses and protects the vocal folds; its *anterior* (front) point is popularly referred to as the "Adam's apple"; (Gk. *thyreos,* shield; L. *cartilago,* cartilage).

tinnitus—A subjective noise sensation, often described as a ringing, roaring, or swishing in the ear that may be heard in one or both ears; associated with a variety of hearing disorders in both adults and children; can affect concentration, sleep, education, employment, personal relationships, and social functioning and sometimes is debilitating; treatment success varies; (L. *tinnire,* to tinkle).

tongue (lingua, glossus)—The primary articulator, whose movement creates consonants and vowels as well as performs biological functions; (L. *lingua,* tongue; Gk. *glossa,* tongue).

tongue thrust—The habitual pushing of the tongue against the inner surface of the front teeth (incisors), or the protrusion of the tongue between the upper and the lower teeth.

total communication—A philosophy calling for every possible means of communication to be used by deaf individuals, including hearing aids and assistive devices, speechreading, signing, and spoken English.

toxin—A substance that poisons or causes inflammation of tissue, including in the central nervous system; (Gk. *toxikon,* poison).

trachea (windpipe)—The tube that begins just below the larynx and continues down to where it divides into the lungs; (Gk. *tracheia,* rough [from the appearance of the numerous tracheal rings]).

tracheoesophageal prosthesis (TEP)—A surgical procedure (*tracheoesophageal puncture*) in which an incision through the trachea and esophageal walls is created to fit a one-way plastic valve (*prosthesis*) that directs air from the trachea into the esophagus where it can reach the oral cavity and be articulated for speech; (Gk. *tracheia*, rough, + *oisophagos*, gullet; Gk. *prostithenai*, add to).

transient ischemic attack (TIA)—An episode of cerebral vascular insufficiency with partial occlusion of a cerebral artery by atherosclerotic plaque or an embolus; disturbances of vision in one or both eyes, dizziness, weakness, numbness, dysphasia, or unconsciousness may occur; TIA (sometimes called "ministroke") usually lasts a few minutes, and in rare cases symptoms may continue for several hours; (L. *transire*, to go through; Gk. *ischein*, to hold back; L. *attacco*, attack).

traumatic brain injury (TBI) (head trauma, acquired brain injury [ABI])—An acquired injury to the brain caused by an external force and resulting in partial or total functional disability; applies to both closed and open head injuries, affecting speech, language, cognition, psychosocial behavior, and physical functioning; (Gk. *trauma*, wound; L. *injurus*, injury).

treatment effectiveness—The extent to which services are shown to be beneficial under typical (or real-world) conditions.

treatment efficacy—The extent to which an intervention can be shown to be beneficial under optimal (or ideal) conditions; (L. *tractare*, manage, handle, or deal with; *efficacere*, accomplish or efficiency).

tremors at rest—Tremors that occur when the head, limbs, hands, or fingers are not intentionally being moved; when movement is initiated, the tremors subside until the body part is again no longer moving; (L. *tremere*, to shake).

true vocal folds—Paired muscles (thyroarytenoid and vocalis) covered with mucous membranes with a pearly white appearance inside the thyroid cartilage at the level of the Adam's apple that open and close extremely rapidly to produce voice; closure during swallowing protects the trachea and lungs from penetration of food and liquid.

tumor (neoplasm)—Any abnormal growth of new tissue, either benign or malignant, caused by aberrant increases in the rate of cell reproduction; (L. *tumor*, swelling; Gk. *neos*, new, + *plasma*, something formed).

tympanic membrane (eardrum)—A thin, semitransparent membrane that separates the ear canal from the middle ear and transmits sound vibrations into the middle ear; (Gk. *tympanon*, drum; L. *membrana*, thin skin or covering).

tympanometry—A measurement of middle ear pressure that is determined by the mobility of the tympanic membrane as a function of various amounts of positive and negative air pressure in the external ear canal (the more positive or negative the air pressure in the external ear canal, the more the normal middle ear system becomes immobilized); (Gk. *tympanon*, drum, + *metron*, measure).

U

utterance—A unit of vocal expression preceded and followed by a pause or silence; may be a single sound, word or words, phrase, clauses, or sentence; (ME. *utter*, outward, + L. *ans*, relating to).

uvula—The cone- or teardrop-shaped structure that hangs from the back of the soft palate but does not have any known function; (L. diminutive or *uva*, cluster of grapes; i.e., one grape).

V

valid/validity—The extent to which a test measures what it is intended to measure; (L. *validus*, strong).

Valsalva maneuver—The procedure of closing the mouth and pinching the nostrils closed with the fingers and forcefully exhaling air, usually causing the Eustachian tubes to open and air to flow into the middle ear to equalize middle ear cavity air pressure with atmospheric air pressure, for example, when going up or down in an elevator or ascending or descending in an airplane, causing the ears to "pop"; any exhaling of air against tightly closed vocal folds, as when lifting heavy objects; (named after Antonio Valsalva, Italian surgeon, 1666–1723).

vegetative state—A condition in which a person may have some minimal level of wakefulness but has not regained awareness (i.e., they lack cognitive function).

velopharyngeal closure—The upward and backward movement of the soft palate to make contact with the posterior pharyngeal wall to close off the coupling of the oral and nasal cavities; (L. *velum*, curtain or veil, + Gk. *pharyngos*, throat; L. *clausura*, closing).

velopharyngeal incompetence—A term generally used to describe abnormal velopharyngeal function, regardless of the cause (i.e., an anatomical or structural defect [e.g., a cleft] or a neuromotor or physiological disorder [e.g., weakness of the soft palate caused by a CVA or TBI]) that typically results in hypernasality and/or nasal emission; various authors use different terms, such as *incompetence*, *inadequacy*, *insufficiency*, and *dysfunction*; (L. *velum*, curtain, + Gk. *pharyngos*, throat; L. *in*, variation of *im*, not, + *competere*, able).

ventricular folds—See *false vocal folds*.

verbal or semantic paraphasia—Unintended substitution of one word for another word that is often semantically related to the intended word (e.g., *sister* for *brother* and *horse* for *dog*); often occur in both speech and writing; (Gk. *semantikos*, significant; *para*, near or alongside, + *phasos*, speech).

vestibular system—The inner ear structures associated with balance and position sense, including the vestibule and semicircular canals of the vestibular mechanism, with interactions of the visual and proprioceptive systems and connection to the cerebellum; (L. *vestibulum*, courtyard).

visual–spatial impairments—Difficulty associating seen objects with their spatial relationships, that is, what is around the objects and the environment; often results in disorientation.

vocal abuse—Deleterious acute or chronic vocal behaviors that are damaging to the vocal folds and laryngeal and pharyngeal muscles and tissue, such as yelling, screaming, cheering, coughing, frequently clearing the throat, and talking loudly over loud noise; (L. *vocalis*, sound; *abusus*, to use or consume).

vocal fold paralysis—Unilateral (one side) or bilateral (two sides) loss of laryngeal movements (including vocal fold opening or closing) that may be caused by damage to the brainstem, vagus (X cranial) nerves, recurrent laryngeal nerves, or the neuromuscular junctions (where the nerve fibers connect with the muscle tissue), resulting in a weak, breathy voice, or possible difficulty breathing if the vocal folds are paralyzed in the closed position; (L. *vocalis*, sound; Gk. *paralyein*, disable or feeble).

vocal hygiene—Behaviors that are helpful to achieve and maintain a healthy vocal mechanism and prevent or decrease vocal pathologies, such as eliminating phonotrauma, speaking in an appropriate pitch, turning the television or radio down while talking, using amplification when speaking to an audience in a large room, and singing within the optimal pitch range; (L. *vocalis*, sound; Gk. *hygieinos*, healthful).

vocal misuse—Deleterious chronic vocal behaviors that may have a cumulative effects on the structure and functioning of the laryngeal mechanism, such as chronic inappropriate loudness or pitch, singing beyond the range of the vocal mechanism, frequent hard glottal attacks, and speaking with inadequate respiratory support (L. *vocalis*, sound).

vocal nodule—A *benign* (nonmalignant or not cancerous) vocal fold growth that tends to be *bilateral* (both sides, i.e., both vocal folds) and occur at the same location as vocal polyps (i.e., juncture of the anterior 1/3 and middle 1/3 of the vocal folds), caused by continuous vocal fold hyperfunction (abuse and misuse); (L. *nodus*, knot).

vocal play—The longer strings of syllables that extend babbling (e.g., *baa-da-gi-daa-um-ma*).

vocal polyp—A benign vocal fold growth that may take various forms and is caused by vocal abuse and misuse and results in vocal hoarseness; (Gk. *polys*, many, + *pous*, foot).

voice—The distinctive feature that refers to a sound produced either with the vocal folds vibrating (*voiced*) or not vibrating (*unvoiced*); (L. *vox* and *vocalis*, voice).

voice box—See *larynx*.

voice disorder (dysphonia)—Any deviation of loudness, pitch, or quality of voice that is outside the normal range of a person's age, gender, or geographic cultural background that interferes with communication, draws unfavorable attention to itself, or adversely affects the speaker or listener; (L. *vox*, voice or sound; *dis-* apart or impaired, + *ordinare*, to order).

voice quality—The auditory aspects of the function of the vocal folds that is affected by adequate closure, efficient timing of closure, and the amount of muscle tone of the vocal folds; normal voice quality is a described as nontense, no extraneous noise, nonbreathy, and easily produced and sustained throughout phonation.

vowel—Voiced speech sounds from the unrestricted passage of the air stream through the mouth without audible stoppage or friction; (L. *vocalis*, voice).

W

Wernicke's aphasia—A fluent aphasia characterized by impaired comprehension, integration, and formulation of language caused by damage to the perisylvian regions in or around Wernicke's area in the posterior superior left temporal lobe (auditory association cortex); characteristics include impaired auditory comprehension, integration of information, and formulation of language; (named after Karl Wernicke, German neurologist, 1848–1905).

working memory—Temporary information storage that is limited in capacity and requires rehearsal; often thought of as "what is on your mind" at any given moment.

World Health Organization (WHO)—An agency of the United Nations established in 1948 to further international cooperation in improving health conditions throughout the world.

Index

Page numbers in italics indicate figures, tables, and boxes.

A

Abduction, 53
Academic achievement, 188–189
Accents, 80
Accessory nerve, 70
Acoustic correlates, of voice, 259
Acoustic trauma, 457–458
Acquired apraxia. *See* Apraxia of speech
Acquired brain injury. *See* Traumatic brain injury (TBI)
Acquired disorders
    effects of, 27
    explanation of, 15, 16
Acquired dyslexia, 328
Acute care hospitals, 38
Acute laryngitis, 241, 242, *242*
Adaptive behavior, 400
Addition, of sound, 120
Adduction, 53
Adenoids, 454
Adolescents. *See also* Children
    with expressive language problems, 155–156
    with hearing loss, 458, 493
    with language-learning disabilities, 154–156
    with receptive language problems, 155
    with repaired clefts, 303–304
    stuttering in, 224–229
    voice disorders in, 269 (*See also* Voice disorders)
Adults
    acquired communication disorders in, 27
    acquired resonance disorders in, 18–19
    attention deficit disorder in, 409
    language disorders in, 17
    neurological disorders in, 314–352 (*See also* Neurological disorders in adults)
    repaired clefts in, 304
    stuttering in, 224–229
    voice disorders in, 269–270 (*See also* Voice disorders)
Affective mode, 225
African American English (AAE), 81–82
African Americans
    incidence for high blood pressure and strokes in, 319

language development in, 81–82
Agrammatic expressive language, 332–333
Agraphia, 331
AIDS. *See* HIV/AIDS
Air conduction, 472
Air paddle, 296
Alexia, 328
Allophones, 105
Alphabetic principle, 181
Alphabet knowledge, 8–9, 182
Alphabet symbols, 105, *106*
Alstrom syndrome, 130
Alveolar consonants, 107
Alveolar ridge, 56, 280
Alveolar sacs, 50–51
Alzheimer, Alois, 344
Alzheimer's disease (AD). *See also* Dementia
    assessment of, 347, 350
    care for individuals with, 350
    explanation of, 19, 344–345
    stages of, 345–348, 350
Alzheimer's units, 350
American Academy of Audiology (AAA), 40, 43
American Academy of Speech Correction (AASC), 28
American Audiological Association (AAA), 30
American Cleft Palate-Craniofacial Association, 291–292
American Heart Association, 315
American Indians. *See* Native Americans
American Sign Language (ASL), 491–492
American Speech and Hearing Association (ASHA), 28
American Speech-Language-Hearing Association (ASHA)
    on bilingual assessment and remediation, 163
    on childhood apraxia of speech, 131, 133
    code of ethics of, 31
    on dialects of speech-language pathologists, 80
    establishment of, 28
    function of, 30
    on language disorders, 142
    on literacy development, 185

    membership in, 30
    position paper on social dialects, 17
    on prevention strategies, 216
    professional credentials offered by, 30, 31, 36, 40, 42, 43
Americans with Disabilities Act (ADA) (Public Law 101-336) (1990), 29
Amplification, real-time, 262
Amplification devices
    assistive listening, 383–486, *483–485*
    cochlear implants as, 486–487, *487*
    hearing aids as, *481*, 481–482, *482*
Amyotrophic lateral sclerosis (ALS), 366
Anarthria, 366
Anesthesia, 292
Ankyloglossia, 113, *113*
Anomia, 329
Anomic aphasia, 331, 332
Anosognosia, 342
Anoxia, 65, 116
Anterior spillage, 378
Anticipatory struggle behavior theories, 209
Anxiety
    attention deficit disorder and, 409
    dysphagia and, 388
    stuttering and, 230
Aperiodicity, 243
Apgar scores, *114*
Aphasias
    anomic, 331, 332
    assessment of, 334–335
    Broca's, 331–333
    classifications and terminology associated with, 326–327
    cognitive impairments associated with, 333
    explanation of, 17, 18, 326
    expressive, 326–327
    fluent and nonfluent, 327, *328*
    global, 333
    jargon, 331
    multicultural considerations related to, 319, 335–336
    receptive, 326–327
    study of, 135
    therapy for, 336–337
    Wernicke's, 328–331
Aphonia
    explanation of, 18, 19
    functional, 247–249